Sports Medicine for the Emergency Physician

Written by sports-trained emergency physicians, *Sports Medicine for the Emergency Physician: A Practical Handbook* is the only resource of its kind. Created specifically for the emergency medicine provider, it is designed to be used as a reference tool, and includes high-yield musculoskeletal physical exam skills and key management of sport injuries in the emergency department.

Each chapter is dedicated to a specific joint(s) and includes the basics of a high-yield musculoskeletal physical examination, including inspection, palpation, range of motion, special tests, and neurovascular and skin exams. Corresponding figures of essential anatomy, pictures of physical exam maneuvers, and clinical correlations are also featured.

Emergent and common musculoskeletal conditions for each joint(s) are discussed, as well as the appropriate emergency department management for each condition. Additional chapter topics include sports-related concussions, sports cardiology, heat illness, and common splints used in the emergency department.

Anna L. Waterbrook, MD, FACEP, CAQSM, graduated from the University of Arizona Medical School in 2004, completed her residency in Emergency Medicine at Maine Medical Center in 2007, and completed her Sports Medicine fellowship at the University of Arizona in 2008. She is board-certified in both emergency and sports medicine. She is currently practicing both specialties at the University of Arizona, where she is Associate Professor of Emergency Medicine, Assistant Team Physician for Intercollegiate Athletics, Associate Fellowship Director for the Sports Medicine Fellowship and Associate Residency Program Director for the South Campus Emergency Medicine Residency. She has authored several book chapters and manuscripts in scholarly journals, contributed to the AMSSM Sports Medicine CAQ Study Guide, and given numerous lectures both locally and nationally.

Sports Medicine for the Emergency Physician

A Practical Handbook

Anna L. Waterbrook

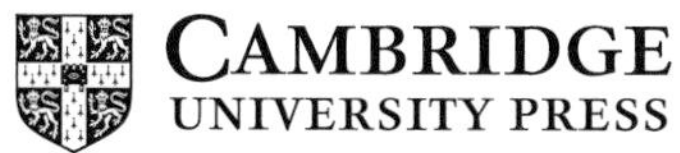

CAMBRIDGE
UNIVERSITY PRESS

Cambridge, New York, Melbourne, Madrid, Cape Town, Singapore, São Paulo, Delhi, Mexico City

Cambridge University Press

32 Avenue of the Americas, New York, NY 10013-2473, USA

www.cambridge.org
Information on this title: www.cambridge.org/9781107449886

First published 2016

Printed in the United States of America by Sheridan Books, Inc.

A catalog record for this publication is available from the British Library.

Library of Congress Cataloging in Publication Data
Sports medicine for the emergency physician :
a practical handbook / [edited by] Anna Waterbrook,
Includes bibliographical references and index.
ISBN 978-1-107-44988-6 (Paperback)
1. Sports emergencies–Handbooks, manuals, etc.
2. Sports medicine–Handbooks, manuals, etc.
3. Emergency medicine–Handbooks, manuals, etc.
4. Physicians–Handbooks, manuals, etc.
I. Waterbrook, Anna.
RC1210.S6753 2015
617.1′027–dc23 2015018952

Contents

Contributors

Amanda Akin, DO
Emergency Medicine Resident
John Peter Smith Health Network
Fort Worth, Texas
Emergency Medicine
Albany Medical College
Albany, New York

Matthew Baird, MD
Emergency and Sports Medicine Physician
Greenville Health System
Steadman Hawkins Clinic of the Carolinas
Assistant Program Director of Primary Care
Sports Medicine Fellowship Program
Assistant Professor of Emergency and Sports
Medicine – USC-Greenville SOM

Brenden J. Balcik, MD
Assistant Professor
Department of Emergency Medicine
West Virginia University

Yvonne C. Chow, MD, CAQSM, FACEP
Assistant Professor of Emergency Medicine and
Internal Medicine
Associate Residency Program Director
Department of Emergency Medicine
Albany Medical College
Albany, New York

Moira Davenport, MD, CAQSM
Associate Residency Director
Allegheny General Hospital Emergency Medicine
Residency
Associate Professor, Temple University School of
Medicine
Pittsburgh, PA

Jeffrey P. Feden , M.D., FACEP
Assistant Professor of Emergency Medicine
(Clinical)
Alpert Medical School of Brown University
Providence, RI

Christopher A. Gee, MD, MPH
Assistant Professor
Division of Emergency Medicine
University of Utah

Christopher Guyer, MD, FACEP, CAQ-SM
Senior Staff Physician,
Henry Ford Health System
Division of Orthopaedics and Division of
Emergency Medicine
Assistant Director, Physical Diagnosis Program,
Wayne State University School of Medicine
Clinical Assistant Professor,
Wayne State University
Adjunct Physician Instructor, University of
Michigan

Christopher Hogrefe, MD
Assistant Professor
Department of Emergency Medicine
Department of Medicine – Sports Medicine
Department of Orthopaedic Surgery – Sports
Medicine
Northwestern Medicine
Northwestern University Feinberg School of
Medicine

William Krantz, MD
Assistant Professor
Department of Radiology
West Virginia University

Allison Lane, MD
Assistant Professor
Emergency Medicine
Sports Medicine
University of Arizona
Banner- University Medical Center

Melissa D. Leber, MD
Assistant Professor of Orthopedics
Assistant Professor of Emergency Medicine

Director of Emergency Department Sports Medicine
Icahn School of Medicine at Mount Sinai Hospital

Ross Mathiasen, MD
Assistant Professor
Department of Emergency Medicine
Department of Orthopaedic Surgery
University of Nebraska Medical Center

Aaron J. Monseau, MD FACEP
CAQ, Primary Care Sports Medicine
Assistant Professor
Department of Emergency Medicine
West Virginia University

Christopher R. Pruitt, MD
Attending Emergency Medicine Physician
Dept. of Emergency Medicine
Maine Medical Center
Portland, Maine

Brian L. Springer, MD, FACEP
Associate Professor,
Wright State University Department of Emergency Medicine
Dayton, OH

Timothy W. Thomsen, MD
Primary Care Sports Medicine Fellow
Department of Emergency Medicine
Department of Family Medicine
University of Iowa Hospitals and Clinics

Anna L. Waterbrook, M.D., FACEP, CAQ-SM
Associate Professor
Department of Emergency Medicine
Associate Program Director, South Campus Residency Program
Associate Program Director, Sports Medicine Fellowship
Assistant Team Physician, Intercollegiate Athletics
The University of Arizona
Tucson, Arizona

Acknowledgments

This book is the result of a vision I had many years ago, and the opportunity to create and edit this book is a dream come true for me.

This project is dedicated to my family: my parents, for teaching me that the sky is the limit; my children, who inspire me every day to be the best that I can be; and my husband, who has always unconditionally supported me.

I want to thank all of the contributors to this project, who put in endless hours writing and revising their chapters. None of this would be possible without all of them.

They say that it takes a village to raise a family. Well, it also takes a village to complete a great project. I could have never completed this book without support from my family, mentors, colleagues, and students. I am truly blessed to work with exceptional colleagues in both sports and emergency medicine, and to be a part of a growing community of dual-boarded sports and emergency physicians.

Introduction

Anna L. Waterbrook

Musculoskeletal training is generally underrepresented in medical training and residency curriculums. There is a general deficit in musculoskeletal knowledge amongst current medical students, residents and practicing medical providers despite the fact that musculoskeletal complaints are among the most common complaints seen in the emergency department (ED). Currently, most educational resources on this subject are geared towards orthopedists and nonoperative sports medicine physicians however they are often too detailed for the average practicing emergency medicine (EM) provider. EM providers need a few, high-yield musculoskeletal physical exam skills to help them diagnose and rule out life-threatening conditions, while also recognizing common conditions.

This is a handbook written by trained sports EM physicians for EM providers as a guide to high-yield physical exam skills and management of sports injuries appropriate for the EM provider practicing in the ED. This book may also be useful for the sports-fellowship-bound EM resident, or the EM provider with a special interest in sports medicine. Each chapter is dedicated to a specific joint or joints and includes the basics of a high-yield musculoskeletal physical examination, including inspection, palpation, range of motion, special tests, as well as neurovascular and skin exam. Corresponding figures of essential anatomy, pictures of physical exam maneuvers, and clinical correlations are included. Emergent and common musculoskeletal conditions for each joint are discussed, as is the appropriate ED management for each condition. Additional chapter topics include sports-related concussions, sports cardiology, heat illness, and common splints used in the ED.

This book is not meant to be a comprehensive sports medicine book. Thus, each chapter does not include every possible diagnosis or physical exam skill for each joint, but rather focuses on the emergent and common conditions seen in the ED. While every effort has been made to ensure the accuracy of the information presented, neither the author nor the publishing company assumes any responsibility for injury to persons or property.

Shoulder

Christopher Guyer

Background/Epidemiology

- Shoulder pain is a common chief complaint in the emergency department (ED). Prevalence estimates of shoulder pain vary widely across different populations.[1]
- Limited data on the epidemiology of upper extremity injuries presenting to the ED currently exist.
- Recent data show the incidence of shoulder injury is 190 injuries per 100,000 persons per year.[2]
- Traumatic shoulder injuries account for 17 percent of upper extremity injuries presenting to EDs. The most common type of injuries seen are fractures (29 percent), strains/sprains (16 percent), and dislocations (5 percent).[2]
- Shoulder injuries are sustained as a result of many scenarios such as participation in sports, accidental trauma sustained in the home and at work, overuse injuries, and motor vehicle accidents.
- Shoulder injuries can be categorized as acute and nonacute.
  - Acute shoulder injuries include traumatic instability, acromioclavicular (AC) and sternoclavicular (SC) joint injury, proximal humerus fractures, scapular fractures, and clavicle fractures.
  - Anterior and anteroinferior instability account for more than 90 percent of shoulder dislocations.
  - Nonacute shoulder injuries include impingement, rotator cuff tendinopathy and tear, biceps tendinopathy and tear, multidirectional instability, and labrum tears.

Anatomical Considerations/Pathophysiology

- The shoulder is the most mobile joint in the body.
- It is comprised of three bones and four articulations (Figure 1.1).
  - Three bones:
    - Clavicle, scapula, and humerus.
    - The acromion is an extension from the spine of the scapula and forms a roof over the shoulder joint.
      - A type I acromion has a flat undersurface.
      - A type II acromion has a downward curve and decreased angle of inclination.
      - A type III acromion has a hooked appearance with further decreased angle of inclination.
    - The proximal humerus has four main parts:
      - Humeral head
      - Greater tuberosity
      - Lesser tuberosity
      - Metaphyseal portion of the shaft
  - Four articulations:
    - SC, AC, glenohumeral, and scapulothoracic.
    - The SC joint is the only true articulation between the upper extremity and the axial skeleton.
    - The scapulothoracic articulation is the interface between the scapula and the thorax and does not represent a true joint.
- The glenoid labrum is composed of dense fibrocartilage and increases the surface area of the glenohumeral joint to deepen the socket and provide stability for the joint.
- The muscles of the shoulder attach to the scapula, clavicle, and humerus (Figures 1.2 and 1.3).

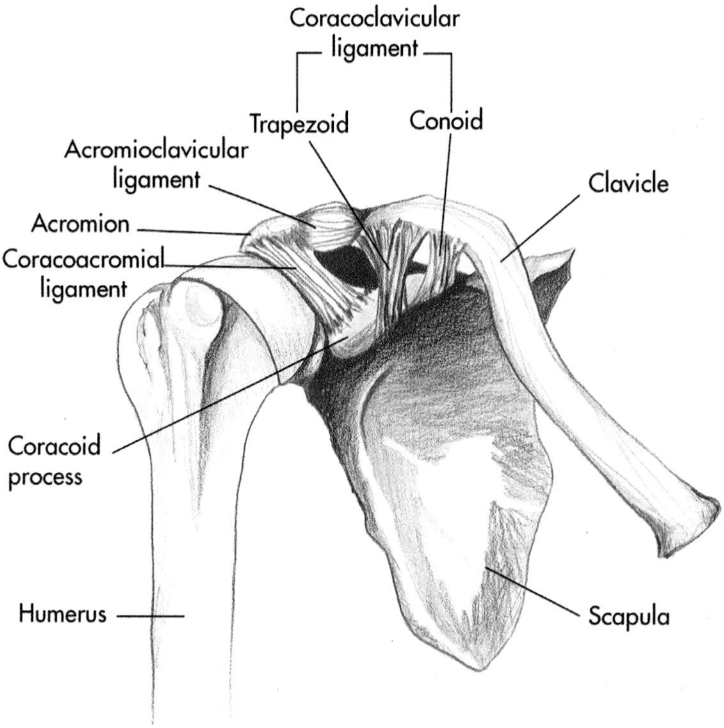

Coracoclavicular ligament
Trapezoid
Conoid
Acromioclavicular ligament
Acromion
Coracoacromial ligament
Clavicle
Coracoid process
Humerus
Scapula

Figure 1.1. Bony anatomy of the shoulder.

Trapezius
Sternocleidomastoid
Subscapularis
Deltoid
Pectoralis Minor
Pectoralis Major
Serratus Anterior
Biceps Brachii

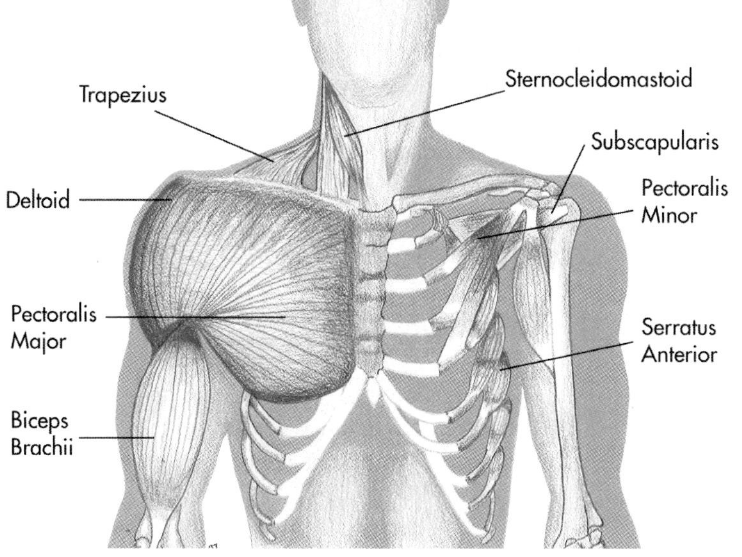

Figure 1.2. Anterior shoulder muscular anatomy.

- The deltoid muscle provides primary motor power at the glenohumeral joint.
  - It functions in elevation, forward flexion, abduction, and extension of the shoulder.
  - It is innervated by the axillary nerve.
- The rotator cuff comprises four muscles and provides dynamic stability to the glenohumeral joint:
  - Supraspinatus
  - Infraspinatus
  - Teres Minor
  - Subscapularis

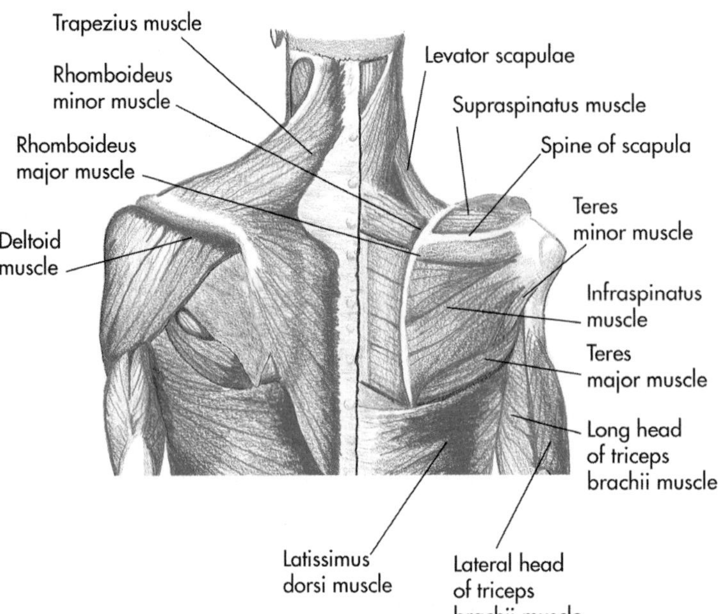

Figure 1.3. Posterior shoulder muscular anatomy.

- The supraspinatus functions in shoulder elevation and is innervated by the suprascapular nerve.
- The infraspinatus functions in external rotation of the shoulder and is innervated by the suprascapular nerve.
- The teres minor functions in external rotation of the shoulder and is innervated by the axillary nerve.
- The subscapularis functions in internal rotation of the shoulder and is innervated by the subscapular nerve.
- Other muscles involved with motion at the shoulder include the following:
  - Pectoralis major
  - Latissimus dorsi
  - Biceps brachii
  - Trapezius
  - Rhomboids
  - Levator scapulae
  - Serratus anterior

Focused History and Physical Exam

- Assessment of shoulder complaints requires taking a focused history.
- Important historical features regarding the onset of pain or dysfunction include eliciting a traumatic mechanism of injury, degenerative or inflammatory conditions, or causative factors from other regions in the body.
  - In adolescents and young adults traumatic injury and poor postural habits are common causes of shoulder complaints.
  - In older patients shoulder complaints can be attributed to overuse in sports or occupational activities, and to wear of articular and periarticular structures.
- The history should include the site and type of pain, duration, and time of occurrence.
  - Referred pain occurs in the subacromial bursa.
  - Pain from a rotator cuff tear is commonly referred to the proximal upper arm or felt diffusely in the deltoid.
  - AC symptoms are usually located directly over the joint.
  - Night pain is common in rotator cuff injury and in advanced impingement syndromes like calcific tendinitis.
- Some patients cannot precisely describe the location of pain and radiation into the arm, trunk, and head can occur.
  - It's important to distinguish shoulder disorders from neurovascular disorders such as distal compression neuropathies, thoracic outlet syndrome, cervical rib

  - syndrome, cervical spine disorders or injury, and other disorders such as splenic rupture and cardiopulmonary disease.
- Additional historical features include:
  - Right or left handedness
  - Occupation, hobby, or sports participation
  - Chronic or recurrent symptoms
  - Previous diagnosis
  - Past surgical interventions
  - Treatments the patient has tried, including the use of oral and topical medications, heat and cold therapy, and a sling or brace
  - Restrictions with range of motion
  - Difficulty with activities of daily living
    - Males will commonly note difficulty reaching a wallet in their back pants pocket, putting on a shirt, or fastening a seatbelt.
    - Women will commonly note difficulty hooking a bra or doing their hair.[3]
- Physical examination of the shoulder should be systematic and include inspection, palpation, range of motion, special maneuvers, and neurovascular evaluation.
- Inspection begins with looking for joint symmetry, alignment, bony deformities, swelling, scars, ecchymosis, atrophy, and hypertrophy.
  - Note any abnormalities on observation of the shoulder, shoulder girdle, and related musculature anteriorly and posteriorly.
  - Identify any swelling, deformity, muscle atrophy, hypertrophy, fasciculations, or abnormal positioning.
  - Observe for swelling of the joint capsule anteriorly or a bulge in the subacromial bursa.
  - Examine the entire upper extremity for color change, skin alteration, and abnormal bony contours.
- Palpate bony structures of the shoulder first, then palpate any areas of pain.
  - While palpating, watch for any areas of tenderness or swelling.
  - First palpate the SC joint medially and follow the clavicle laterally with your fingers.
  - Posteriorly palpate the spine of the scapula and follow it laterally and upward until you reach the anterior tip of the acromion.
  - With your index finger on top of the acromion, posterior to the tip, press your thumb medially and find the slightly elevated ridge that marks the distal edge of the clavicle at the AC joint.
  - Medially and a short step down, palpate the coracoid process of the scapula.
  - On the lateral aspect of the humerus, palpate the greater tubercle, where the rotator cuff muscles insert.
  - Move your fingers just medial to the greater tubercle to palpate the biceps tendon within the intertubercular groove.
  - To palpate the subacromial bursa, subdeltoid bursa, and the rotator cuff muscles, extend the humerus to bring these structures anterior to the acromion.
    - Supraspinatus lies directly under the acromion.
    - Infraspinatus sits posterior to the supraspinatus.
    - Teres minor is found posterior and inferior to the supraspinatus.
    - Subscapularis inserts anteriorly and is not palpable.
    - Looking down on the shoulder from above, assess for swelling in the fibrous articular capsule and synovial membrane.
    - Palpate the capsule and synovial membrane under the anterior and posterior acromion.
- Range of motion should be assessed starting with active range of motion, then with passive range of motion if any active restrictions are noted.
  - All range of motion assumes a neutral-zero method, where 0° is represented by the patient's arm hanging down at his or her side.
  - The shoulder girdle is capable of moving in six directions: flexion, extension, abduction, adduction, and internal and external rotation.
  - Stand in front of the patient and observe for smooth movement.
  - Note muscle strength for each direction.

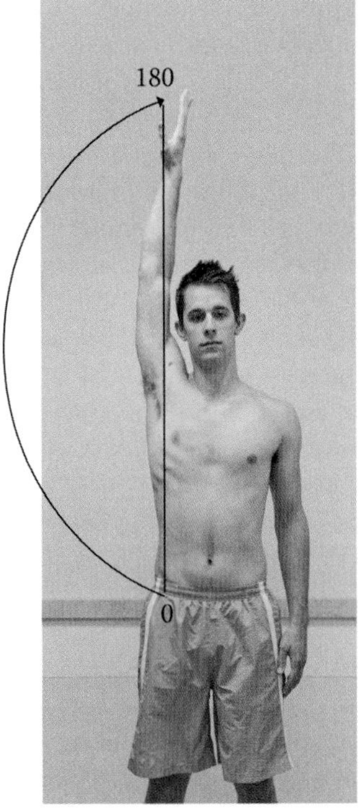

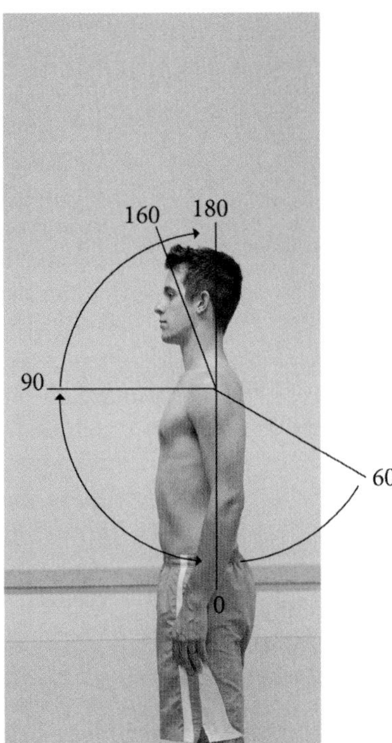

Figure 1.4. Forward elevation, extension and abduction.

- For flexion or forward elevation (Figure 1.4), ask the patient to raise the arms in front and overhead.
  - Normal range of motion is from 0° to 160–180°.
- For extension (Figure 1.4), ask the patient to raise the arms behind the body.
  - Normal range of motion is 0–60°.
- To test abduction (Figure 1.4), ask the patient to raise the arms above the head.
  - Normal range of motion is 0–180°.
  - Glenohumeral range of motion is 0–90°.
  - Scapulothoracic motion is 90–150° of abduction.
  - Both glenohumeral and scapulothoracic motion account for the last 30° of motion.
  - Painful arc is present when the patient experiences pain between 60° and 120° of active abduction.
- For adduction, ask the patient to cross the arm in front of the body.
  - Normally, a patient should be able to touch the opposite shoulder.
- To test internal rotation, ask the patient to place one hand behind the back and touch the shoulder blade.
  - Identify the highest spinous process the patient can touch.
  - Normally patients will be able to reach T7–T10. T9 is near the lower border of the scapula and serves as a good landmark.
  - Often patients will be able to reach higher with the nondominant hand.
- For external rotation, ask the patient to raise the arm to shoulder level, bend the elbow, and raise the forearm to the ceiling.
  - Normal range of motion is up to 90°.

- There are more than twenty special maneuvers for testing shoulder function but not all are well studied. Commonly performed maneuvers are described later.
  - The *crossover test* (Figure 1.5) is used to assess for injury to the AC joint.
    - While palpating the AC joint, adduct the patient's arm across the chest.

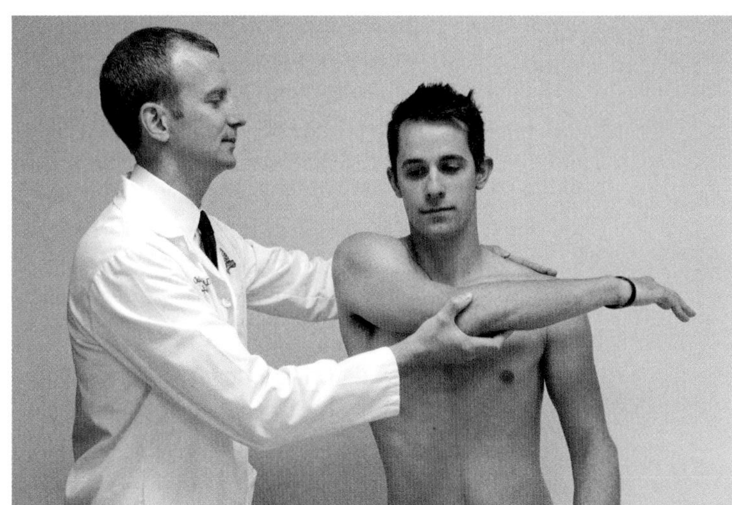

Figure 1.5. Crossover test for AC joint disorders.

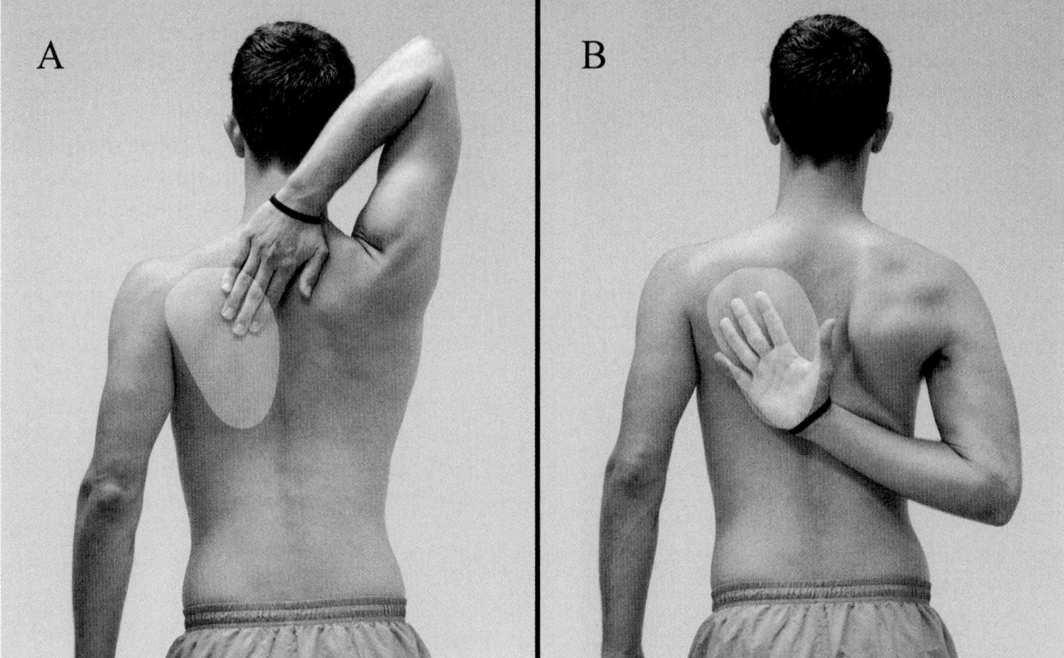

Figure 1.6 A and B. Apley scratch test.

- A positive test will elicit pain at the AC joint.

- *Apley scratch test* (Figures 1.6 A and B) assesses overall shoulder rotation.
  - Ask the patient to reach behind the head and touch the top of the scapula (Figure 1.6A). This tests abduction and external rotation.
  - Next, ask the patient to reach behind the back and touch the bottom of the scapula (Figure 1.6B). This tests adduction and internal rotation.
  - Difficulty with either of these motions is suggestive of a rotator cuff disorder, adhesive capsulitis, or glenohumeral osteoarthritis.

- *Neer's impingement sign* (Figure 1.7) evaluates for dynamic subacromial impingement, including constriction, inflammation, or injury to the rotator cuff.
  - Stabilize the scapula with one hand and with the other hand internally rotate the shoulder and then move the patient's arm into forward flexion.
  - A positive test will elicit pain as the shoulder is placed into forward flexion as the greater tuberosity of the humerus rotates below the acromion.

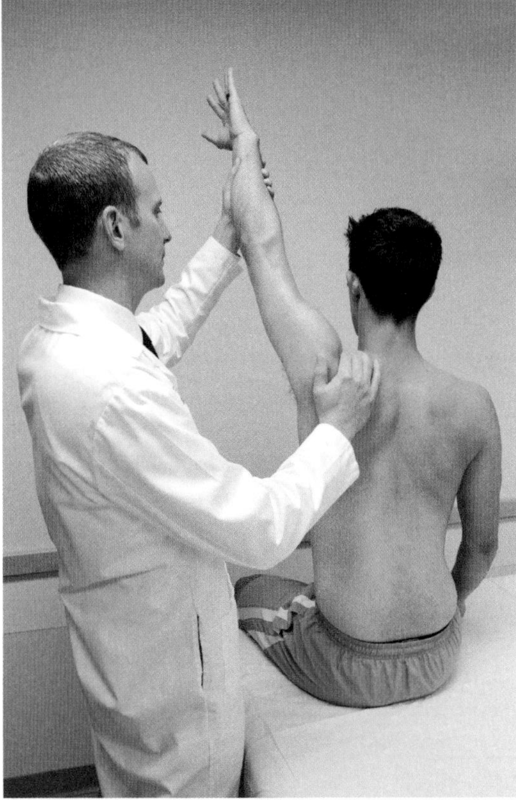

Figure 1.7. Neer's impingement sign.

- *Hawkins–Kennedy impingement sign* (Figure 1.8) is similar to Neer's impingement sign and also evaluates for subacromial impingement.
  - Flex the patient's shoulder and elbow to 90° with the palm facing down. Place one hand on the patient's forearm and another on the arm and rotate the arm internally.
  - A positive test will elicit pain as the greater tuberosity is compressed against the coracoacromial ligament.
- The *empty can test* (Figure 1.9) evaluates supraspinatus strength.
  - Elevate the arms to 90° in the scapular plane and internally rotate them at the shoulder so the thumbs are facing down. Ask the patient to resist as you press down on the arms.
  - A positive test is indicated by weakness.
- The *infraspinatus test* (Figure 1.10) can help you evaluate for an infraspinatus disorder or tear.
  - With the arms at his or her side, ask the patient to bend the elbows to 90° and

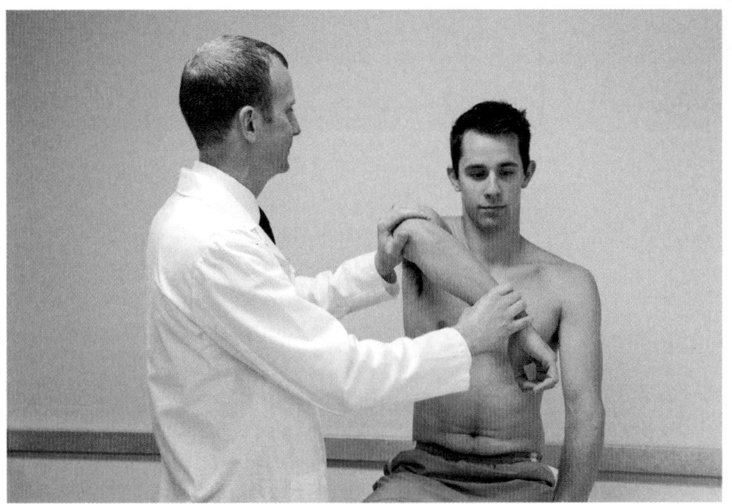

Figure 1.8. Hawkins–Kennedy impingement sign.

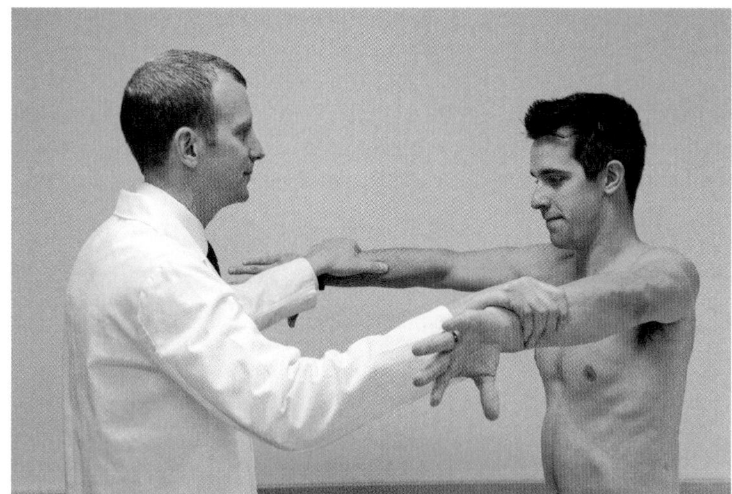

Figure 1.9. Empty can test.

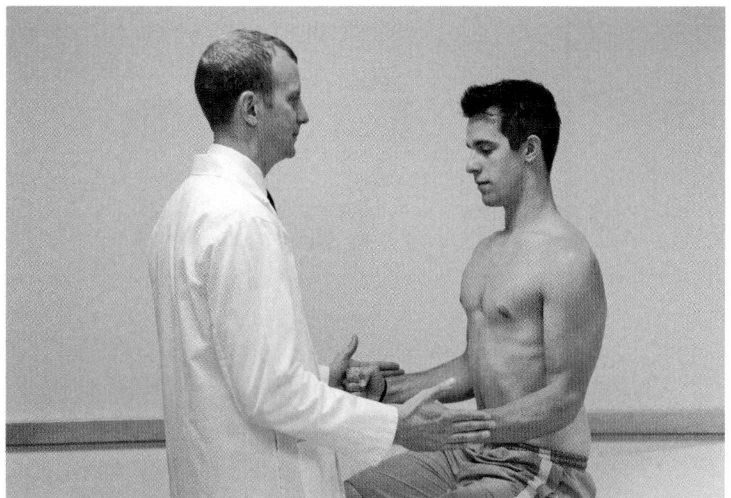

Figure 1.10. Infraspinatus test.

provide resistance as he or she presses the forearms outward.
- A positive test is indicated by weakness.

- The *lift-off test* (Figure 1.11) tests for subscapularis strength.
  - Ask the patient to place the arm in internal rotation with the dorsum of the hand on the back as you provide resistance.
  - A patient with a subscapularis tear will be unable to perform this maneuver.

- The *drop arm test* (Figures 1.12A and B) is a good test in evaluating for a supraspinatus tear.
  - With the patient seated, passively abduct the arm to 120° (Figure 1.12A). Ask the patient to hold the arm in that position without support and then slowly bring it to his or her side (Figure 1.12B).
  - A positive test is indicated by failure to maintain an abducted position or a sudden drop of the arm as the patient brings the arms back down towards the side.

- *Speed's test* (Figure 1.13) is an indicator for biceps injury.
  - Ask the patient to elevate the arm in supination and 60° of forward flexion, and to maintain this position as you

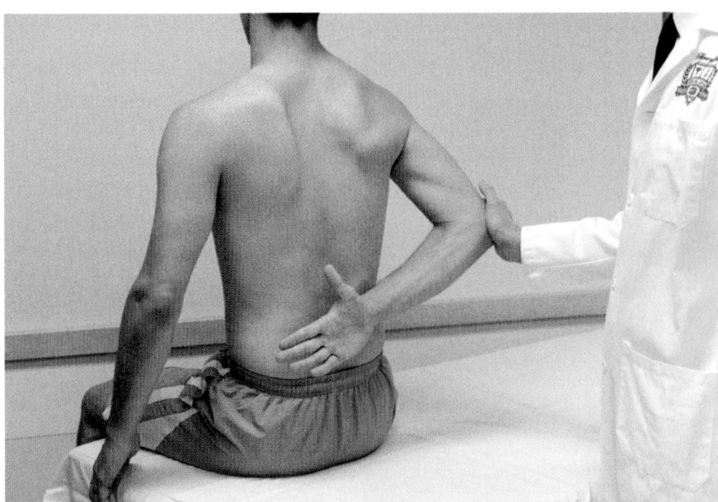

Figure 1.11. Lift-off test.

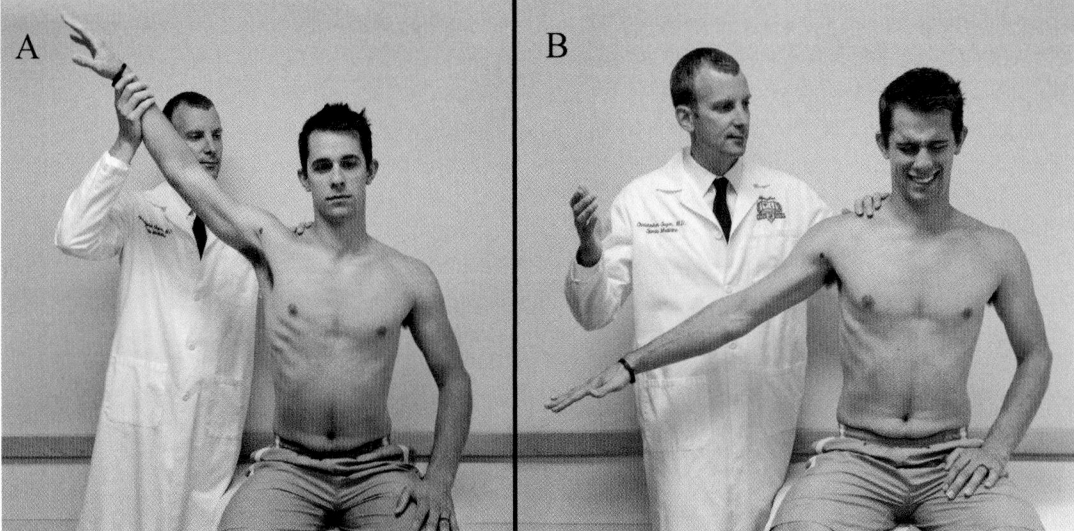

Figure 1.12A and B. Drop arm test.

provide downward pressure on the arm.
- Asymmetrical strength and pain in the region of the bicipital groove suggests a disorder of the long head of the biceps tendon.

- *Popeye sign* (Figure 1.14) indicates a proximal long head of the biceps tendon rupture.
  - Ask the patient to abduct the arm to 90° and flex at the elbow (i.e., ask them to flex the muscles).
  - This sign is present when there is a large bump in the area of the biceps muscle belly.
  - It may only be obvious when compared to the contralateral side.
- *O'Brien's active compression test* (Figures 1.15a and b) is used to detect labral pathology.
  - Stand behind the patient and ask him or her to flex the affected arm to 90°, adduct 15° medially, and internally rotate the arm.

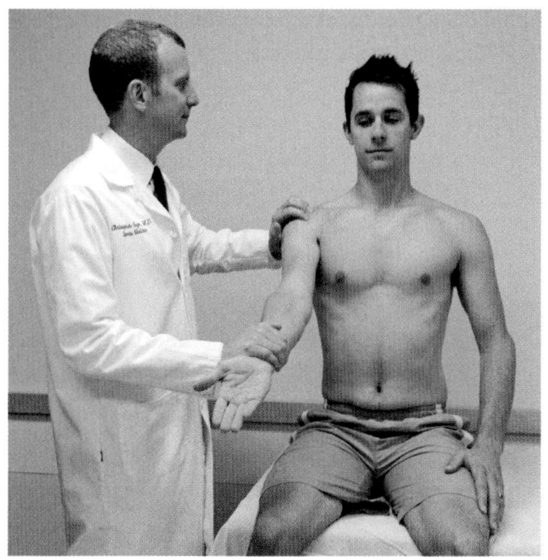

Figure 1.13. Speed's test.

Figure 1.14. Popeye sign.

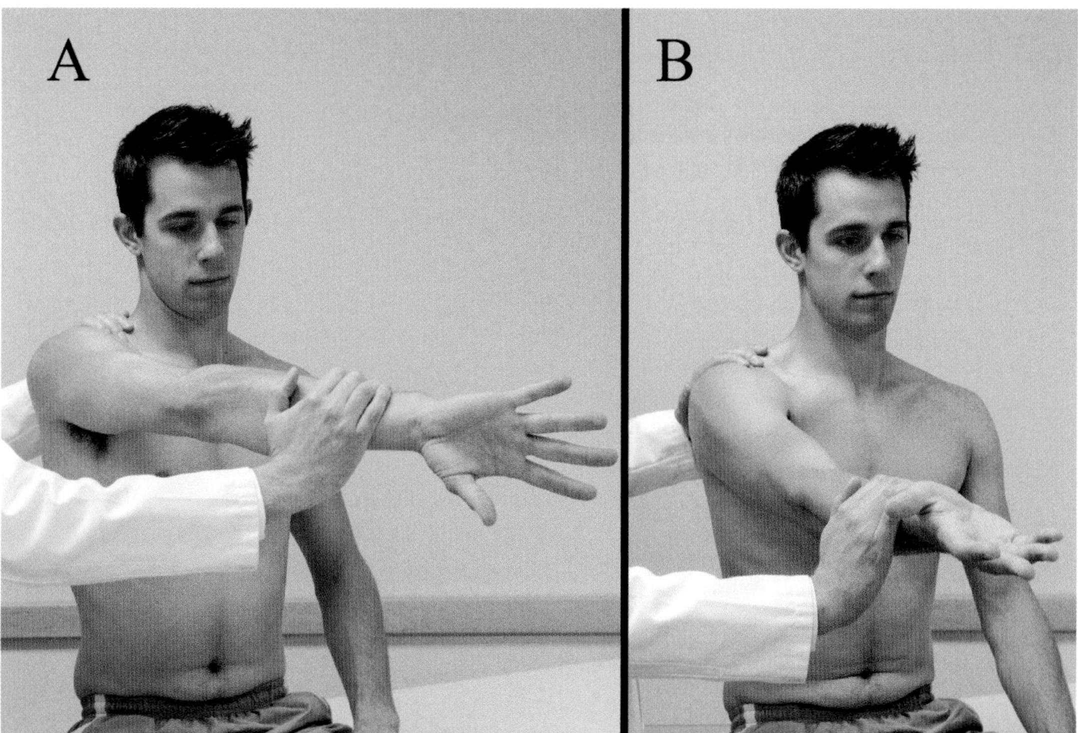

Figure 1.15 A and B. O'Brien's active compression test.

- Place a downward force to the patient's arm (Figure 1.15A).
- Observe for pain that localizes to the AC joint or the shoulder joint.
- Repeat the test with the arm maximally supinated (thumb up) (Figure 1.15B).
- A positive test is indicated if pain is decreased with the second maneuver.
  - Superficial pain is associated with AC joint pathology, while deep pain or a click is associated with labral abnormalities.

- A thorough neurovascular exam of the upper extremity is important in evaluation of patients with shoulder complaints.
  - Long thoracic nerve (C5–7) and spinal accessory nerve (CN XI) function is indicated by scapular winging.
    - While standing, have the patient forward flex the arm to 90° and push against a wall.
    - Medial scapular winging is indicative of serratus anterior weakness or long thoracic nerve dysfunction.
    - Lateral scapular winging is an indicator for trapezius weakness or spinal accessory nerve (CNXI) dysfunction.
  - The supraclavicular nerve (C4) provides sensory innervation to the skin over the superior shoulder and clavicular area.
  - The suprascapular nerve (C5–6) provides motor innervation to the supraspinatus and infraspinatus.
    - Its function is tested by resisted abduction and external rotation.
  - The axillary nerve (C5) functions in sensation of the shoulder joint and the skin covering the inferior area over the deltoid. It supplies motor innervation to the deltoid and teres minor muscles.
    - Motor function is tested by resisted abduction and external rotation.
  - The dorsal scapular nerve (C5) innervates the levator scapula and rhomboid muscles.
    - Motor function is tested by having the patient shrug the shoulders.
  - The lateral pectoral nerve (C5–7) innervates the pectoralis major.
    - Motor function is tested via resisted adduction.
  - The thoracodorsal nerve (C7–8) innervates the latissimus dorsi.
    - Motor function is tested with resisted shoulder adduction.
  - The upper and lower subscapular nerve (C5–6) innervates the teres minor and subscapularis.
    - Motor function is tested by resisted internal rotation.
  - The T2 segmental nerve provides sensory innervation to the axilla.
  - Vascular examination of the shoulder includes checking brachial, radial, and ulnar artery pulses, as well as capillary refill.
- Neck examination should also be included when evaluating certain shoulder conditions, as radicular pain from C5–6 can mimic rotator cuff disorders.

Differential Diagnosis – Emergent and Common Diagnoses

Anterior Shoulder Dislocation

General Description

- Glenohumeral dislocations make up more than half of all dislocations seen by emergency medicine physicians.
- The glenohumeral joint can dislocate anteriorly, inferiorly, posteriorly, or superiorly.

Table 1.1. Emergent and Common Diagnoses in the Emergency Department

Emergent Diagnoses	Common Diagnoses
Shoulder dislocation	Acromioclavicular separation, types I-III
Acromioclavicular separation, types IV-VI	Proximal humerus fracture (elderly)
Posterior sternoclavicular dislocation	Clavicle fracture
Certain proximal humerus fracures	Rotator cuff impingement
Certain scapula fractures	Subacromial bursitis
Certain clavicle fractures	Rotator cuff tendinopathy
Septic arthritis	Adhesive capsulitis
Any open fracture	
Any injury associated with neurovascular compromise	

Mechanism

- In anterior or anteroinferior dislocations, the humeral head becomes dissociated from the glenoid fossa and can rest under the inferior rim of the glenoid, beneath the coracoid process and less commonly in an intrathoracic or subclavicular position (Figure 1.16).[4]
  - Anterior or anteroinferior shoulder dislocation is the most common type of traumatic instability, representing more than 90 percent of dislocations.
  - A Bankart lesion (Figure 1.17) and avulsion of the inferior glenohumeral ligament and labrum complex from the glenoid is the most common structural injury with shoulder dislocation occurring in greater than 90 percent of injuries.
    - A Bankart lesion occurs when the labrum detaches with or without a bony fragment.
  - Humeral avulsion of the glenohumeral ligament occurs less than 10 percent of the time.
  - A Hill–Sachs lesion (Figure 1.18) is an impression fracture on the posterior humeral head that results from abutment against the anterior glenoid rim as it dislocates.
  - A Hill–Sachs lesion, glenohumeral ligament avulsion and Bankart lesion can all contribute to instability.
  - Anterior and anteroinferior dislocation occurs after a force is applied to an abducted and externally rotated arm.
  - The risk of dislocation is higher in individuals with a prior dislocation and they may dislocate during general daily activities.
  - The younger a patient is at the initial injury, the higher the likelihood of recurrence: age less than 20, 80 percent or greater; age 20–40, 26–48 percent; age greater than 40, 0–10 percent.

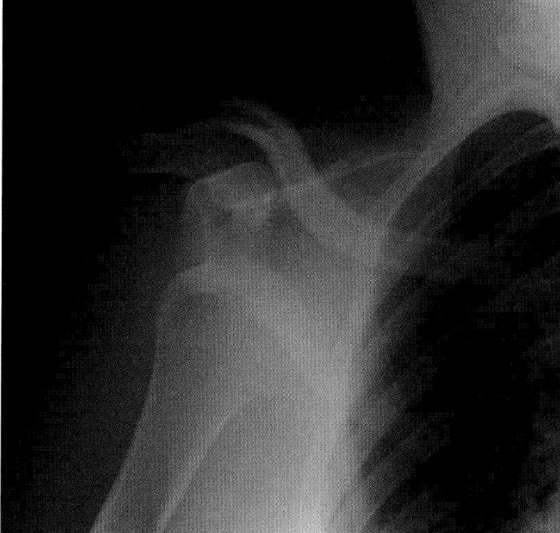

Figure 1.16. Anterior-posterior shoulder x-ray demonstrating characteristic appearance of an anterior shoulder dislocation.

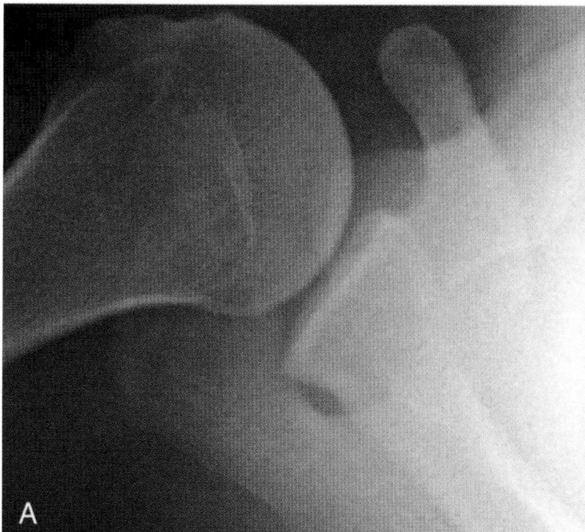

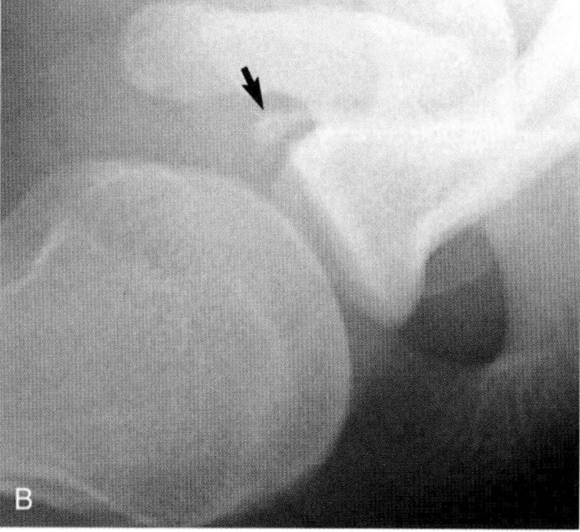

Figure 1.17. Bankart lesion. A West Point view shows a fracture of the inferior aspect of the glenoid fossa (*arrow*). *From* Eiff, MP. *Fracture Management for Primary Care.* Elsevier 2012; 8:170, with permission.

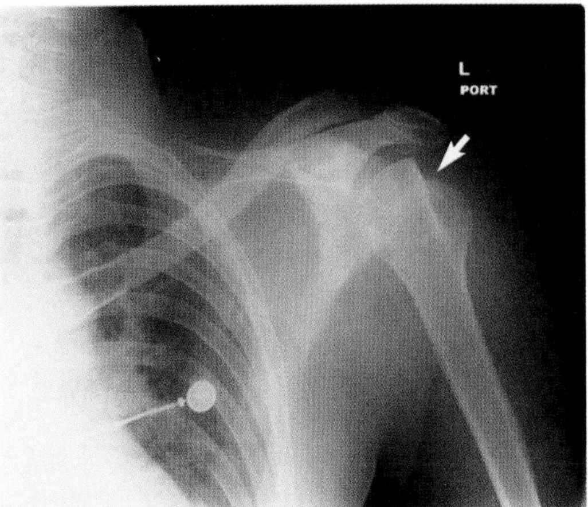

Figure 1.18. Hill–Sachs lesion. Note the cortical depression of the posterosuperior humeral head caused by impaction with the glenoid rim (*arrow*). *From* Eiff, MP. *Fracture Management for Primary Care.* Elsevier 2012; 8:170, with permission.

Presentation

- Dislocations commonly happen following a traumatic injury.
  - This can occur in contact sports like football and hockey, or from activities like throwing or reaching for an overhead object where the shoulder is flexed greater than 90° with slight external rotation.
  - Other scenarios where dislocation may occur include falls, motor vehicle accidents, lightning strikes, and seizures.
- Patients usually complain of severe shoulder pain.
- Additionally, patients may note deformity and inability to use the arm.

Physical Exam

- Typically, "squaring" of the shoulder is present with a loss of normal deltoid contour when compared to the uninjured shoulder.
- Decreased active and passive range of motion will be present.
- Patients will often refuse to move the shoulder.
- The humeral head may be prominent anteriorly.
- It is essential to document neurovascular findings pre and post reduction.
  - The axillary nerve is the most commonly injured nerve as the neurovascular bundle passes anterior to the glenohumeral joint.

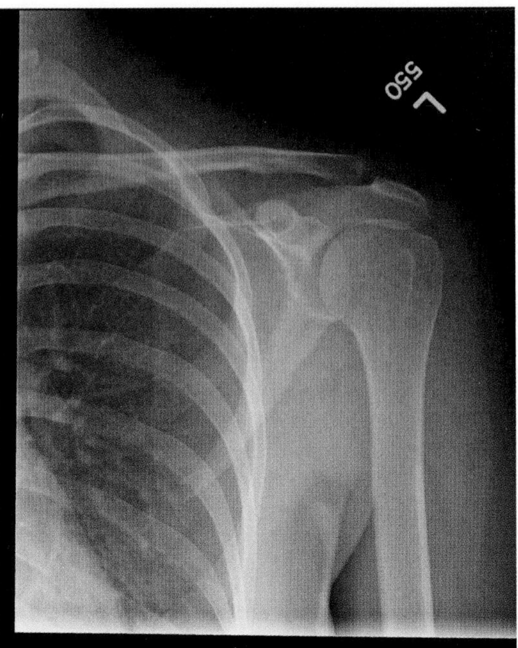

Figure 1.19. Normal anterior-posterior (AP) x-ray of the shoulder. Note the normal alignment of the humeral head and glenoid contours.

Essential Diagnostics

- X-rays are always indicated when a dislocation is suspected.
  - A shoulder trauma series should include an anterior-posterior (AP) view with the beam at right angle to the scapula (Figure 1.19), a "Y" view (true lateral) with the scapular wing seen "edge on," (Figure 1.20) and an axillary view (Figure 1.21).
- At a minimum, post-reduction radiographic views include an AP view and an axillary view.
- It has been suggested that point-of-care ultrasound can also be an imaging modality used to diagnose glenohumeral dislocation and confirm reduction.[5]
- Generally, CT scan and MRI are not indicated in the ED setting.

ED Treatment

- ED treatment includes prompt pain control and reduction of the dislocation.
- Reduction is easiest before the onset of muscle spasm and pain; however, this is not common in the ED setting.
- Recurrent dislocations are often more easily reduced.

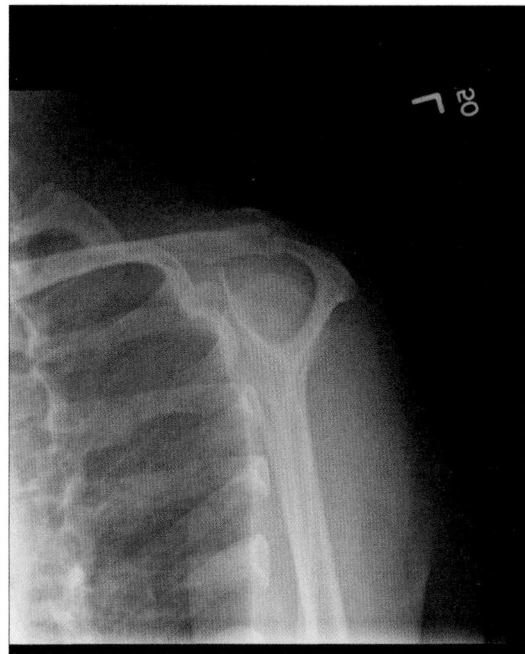

Figure 1.20. Normal scapular Y-view showing the humeral head overlying the glenoid positioned posterior to the coracoid. The Y-view gets its name from the Y shape of the scapula seen when looking at it laterally.

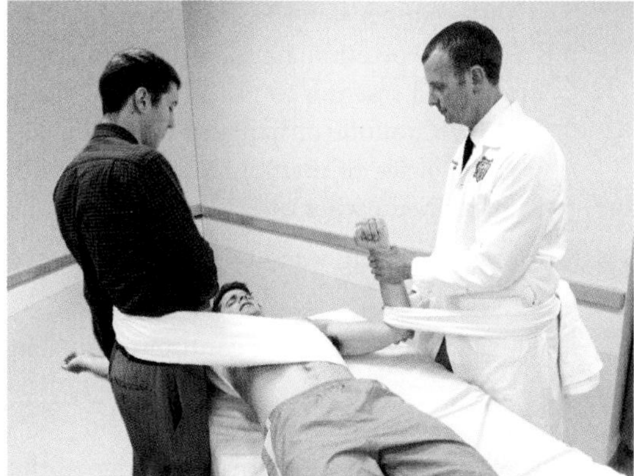

Figure 1.22. Traction–countertraction shoulder reduction technique.

- Procedural sedation can be utilized to allow for reduction maneuvers.
- Recent systematic review has suggested that reduction can be obtained using intra-articular lidocaine injection as an alternative to procedural sedation.
  - This study demonstrated decreased emergency department time and complications for intra-articular lidocaine compared with IV sedation.

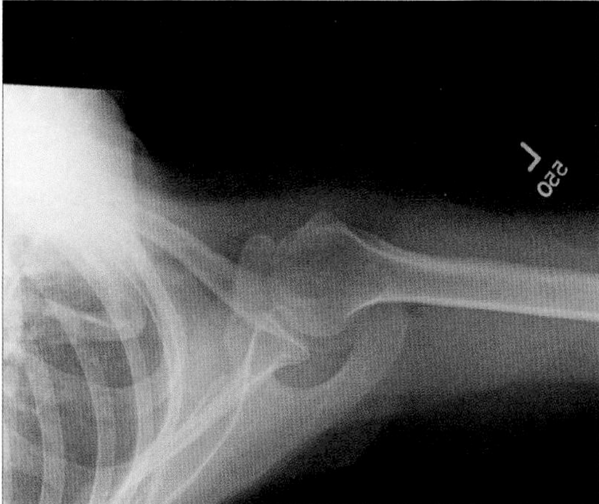

Figure 1.21. Axillary x-ray view of the shoulder shows normal alignment at the glenohumeral joint and the acromioclavicular joint.

  - This method may be considered as the first option for reducing shoulder dislocations.[6]
- Ultrasound-guided brachial plexus and interscalene nerve blocks are additional alternatives to procedural sedation and intra-articular lidocaine injection.
- Many reduction maneuvers exist. The most common are described here.
- Traction/countertraction technique (Figure 1.22)
  - With the patient in a supine position, have an assistant wrap a sheet around the waist, through the patient's axilla, and across the patient's chest to provide counter traction. Alternatively, the patient can be secured to a stationary object if no assistant is available.
  - The operator then applies axial traction to the patient's arm with a sheet wrapped around his or her own waist and the patient's forearm with the elbow bent to 90°.
  - Successful reduction is usually indicated by a soft, palpable clunk and return of mobility.
- Scapular manipulation technique (Figure 1.23)
  - This is most easily accomplished with the patient prone but can also be performed with the patient seated.
  - In the seated position, brace the uninjured shoulder firmly against a rigid support like

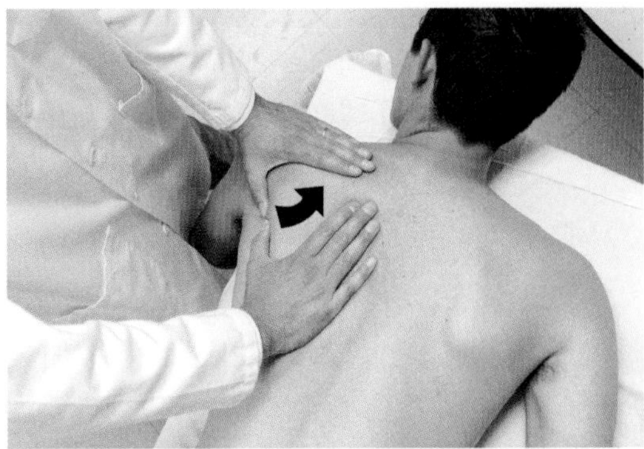

Figure 1.23. Scapular manipulation technique for shoulder reduction.

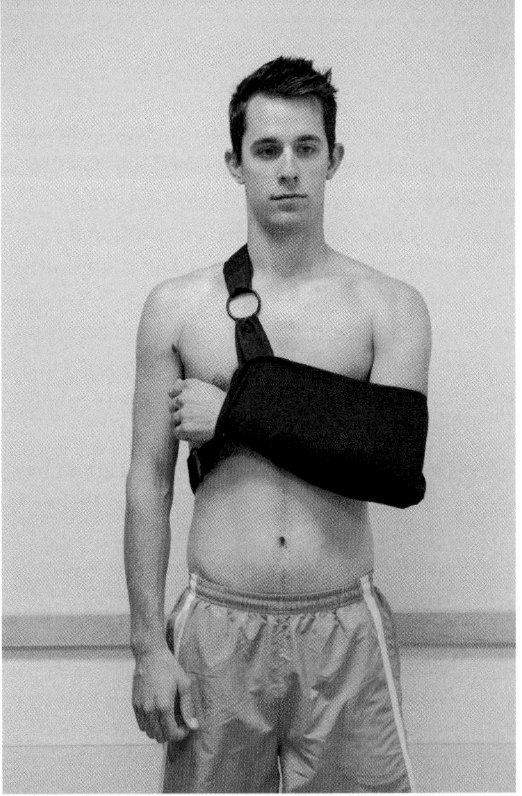

Figure 1.25. Shoulder sling.

a wall or the raised head of a hospital stretcher.

- Have an assistant face the patient and gently raise the wrist of the affected arm until the shoulder is flexed to 90°.
- The assistant then places the palm of his or her free hand against the midclavicular area of the injured shoulder for stabilization and gently puts anterior traction on the patient's arm.

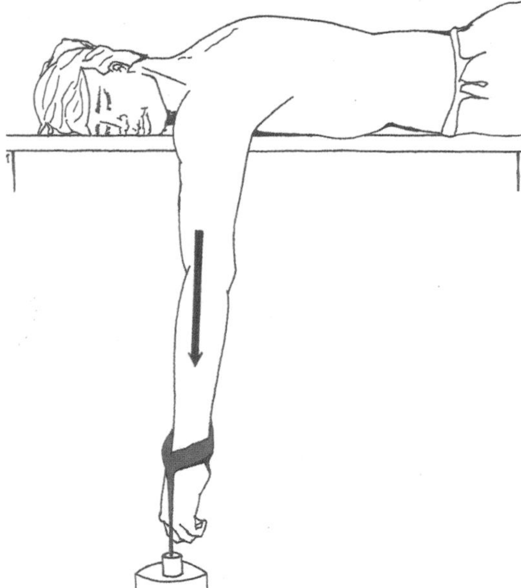

Figure 1.24. Stimson hanging weight technique for shoulder reduction.

- While forward traction is applied, the operator manipulates the scapula by adducting the inferior tip using thumb pressure and stabilizing the superior aspect with the upper hand.
- In a prone position, have an assistant apply downward traction to the affected arm or use 5–10 pounds of hanging weight for traction prior to manipulating the scapula as described earlier.

- Stimson or hanging weight technique (Figure 1.24)
  - This technique requires continuous patient observation.
  - Place the patient in a prone position.
  - Hang the affected arm over the edge of the bed with 10 pounds of weight for traction.
  - Spontaneous reduction usually occurs within 10–20 minutes.
  - If reduction is not accomplished, use the prone scapular manipulation technique.
- After successful reduction the patient will require immobilization with a sling, sling and swathe, or shoulder immobilizer (Figure 1.25).
- Significant controversy exists regarding the type and position of immobilization and duration of immobilization.
- Studies have suggested that immobilization in external rotation (Figure 1.26) increases

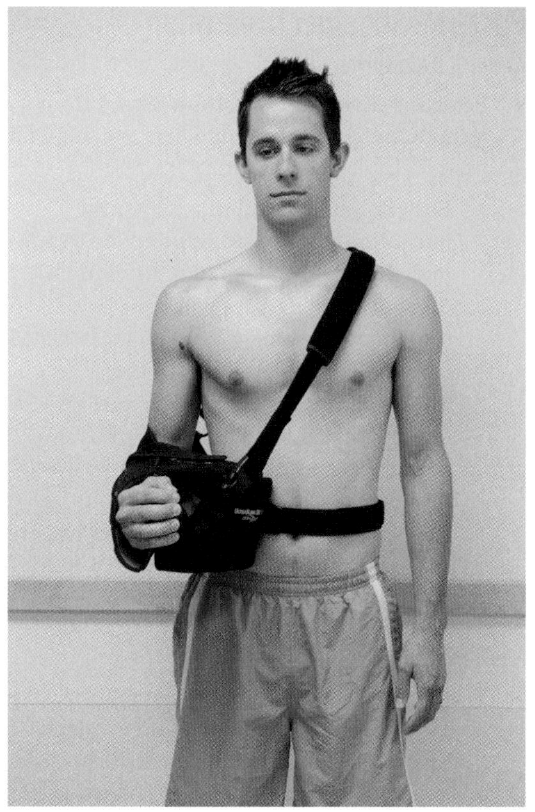

Figure 1.26. Shoulder external rotation brace.

contact force between a Bankart lesion and the anterior glenoid rim, possibly influencing healing. In another study, decreased rate of recurrence (26 vs. 42 percent) was found following immobilization in external rotation compared with internal rotation; however, both remained high and noncompliance complicates treatment (53 vs. 72 percent).[4]

- Patients should be counseled on non-weight bearing of the arm during the initial immobilization treatment phase.
- For pain control, NSAIDs are the first line of treatment for pain and inflammation.
- Providers might also consider adjunctive treatment with acetaminophen and narcotic pain relievers in certain cases.
- Cold treatment modalities might also provide pain relief for patients.
- Patients may be discharged safely after successful reduction of their shoulder dislocation.
- Definitive treatment will most likely require rehabilitation and may include surgical stabilization.

Disposition

- Patients may be discharged safely after successful reduction of their shoulder dislocation.
- An orthopedic surgery consult is indicated when ED providers are unable to perform a successful reduction, a fracture is present, or there is neurologic or vascular compromise.
- Some patients may require admission if one of these complications is present.
- Uncomplicated shoulder dislocation patients should follow-up with an orthopedic or sports medicine specialist within 3–5 days after discharge.
    - It is important to encourage close outpatient follow-up to ensure reassessment and avoid prolonged immobilization, which can lead to frozen shoulder (adhesive capsulitis), especially in older patients.
- Return to work or sports occurs when the patient has full range of motion and near symmetric strength.

Complications

- Several complications from shoulder dislocation are possible.
    - If attempts at closed reduction fail or signs of neurovascular injury develop, patients may require closed or open reduction in the operating room under general anesthesia.
    - Reduction injuries can occur, and it is important to use the least amount of force during reduction to avoid creating or exacerbating existing fractures, nerve and vascular injuries.
    - In patients greater than 40 years old, the risk of rotator cuff tear occurring with shoulder dislocation is significant increased, up to 40 percent in those older than 60.
    - Failure to recognize neurologic or vascular injury can lead to significant morbidity.
    - Patient noncompliance can lead to increased risk of recurrent dislocation.
    - Recurrent dislocations can lead to development of osteoarthritis.

  - Younger patients are more susceptible to recurrent dislocation.
  - While it is important to immobilize the affected shoulder initially, the patient should also be warned about complications of prolonged immobilization.

Pediatric Considerations

- Shoulder dislocations in general are rare in children.
- Most often they occur near the time of skeletal maturity in adolescents participating in contact sports.
- Children have weaker epiphyseal growth plates that are more likely to fracture before dislocation occurs.
- Chronic instability can occur in pediatric patients and is often due to an underlying connective tissue disorder (e.g., Marfan and Ehler–Danlos syndromes) or multidirectional instability.
- On examination the shoulder may be unstable in several planes and these patients may demonstrate multiple lax joints.

Pearls and Pitfalls

- Ensure patient's pain is controlled and muscles are relaxed prior to attempting reduction.
- In patients with recurrent dislocation, ask what reduction method has been successful in the past.
- When choosing a reduction method, consider patient volume, staffing, and available equipment.
- Consider intra-articular lidocaine injection as a first line option for reduction.
- Use the minimum amount of force necessary during reduction to avoid causing new injury or exacerbating an existing one.
- In elderly and pediatric patients, use extra caution during reduction and avoid causing friction injury to skin if sheets or straps are utilized.
- Always consider alternative diagnoses, like coexisting cervical spine injury.
- Other disorders such as myocardial infarction and splenic rupture can present with shoulder pain.[7]

Posterior Shoulder Dislocation

General Description

- Posterior shoulder dislocation results from glenohumeral dissociation where the humeral head is displaced posteriorly.
  - Posterior shoulder dislocation is an uncommon injury, accounting for less than 4 percent of shoulder dislocations.
  - Most of these injuries will reduce spontaneously unless there is an associated fracture.[8]
  - These injuries are commonly missed initially (up to 80 percent) by treating physicians and diagnosis within six weeks of injury is considered acute.
  - Reverse Hill–Sachs and Bankart lesions are common injuries associated with posterior shoulder dislocations.

Mechanism

- The mechanism of injury is traumatic, usually occurring after a direct force to the anterior shoulder or a force directed posteriorly on an adducted, flexed, and internally rotated upper extremity.

Presentation

- Common historical features include direct blow to the anterior shoulder, seizure, electrocution, high-speed motor vehicle accident, and fall on an outstretched arm.

Physical Exam

- On physical exam, findings are less obvious than in anterior dislocation.
  - Patients generally hold their arm internally rotated and tight at their side.
  - Patients will be unable to actively or passively externally rotate or abduct their arm.
  - Fullness may be palpated posteriorly.

Essential Diagnostics

- Essential imaging includes a shoulder trauma series.
  - The shoulder may appear normal on the AP view.
  - An axillary or Y view is required for diagnosis.

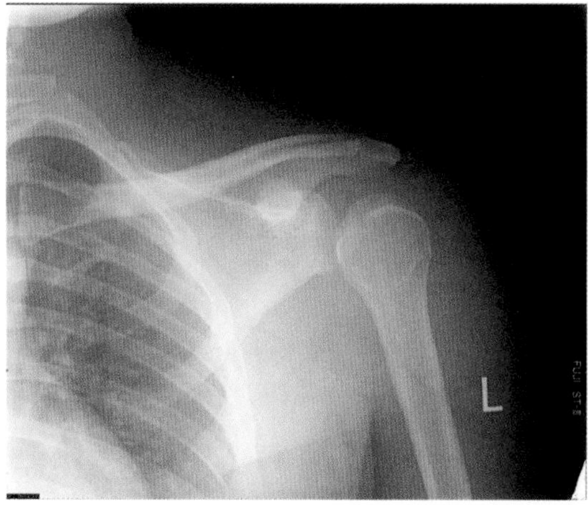

Figure 1.27. AP radiograph of a patient with posterior shoulder dislocation.

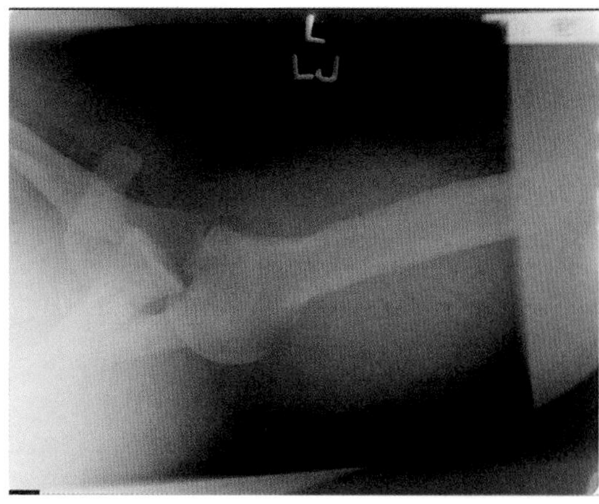

Figure 1.28. Axillary x-ray view in a patient with posterior shoulder dislocation and associated reverse Hill–Sachs lesion.

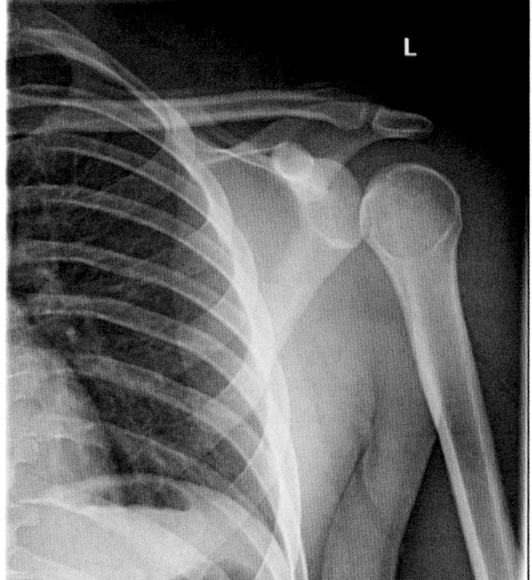

Figure 1.29. Abnormal AP x-ray view demonstrating a "lightbulb sign" in a patient with posterior shoulder dislocation. Courtesy of Lorna Breen, MD, New York.

- Abnormalities include loss of the normal elliptical overlap between the glenoid rim and humeral head on the AP view, and loss of normal alignment at the glenohumeral joint on the axillary view (Figures 1.27 and 1.28).
- A "lightbulb sign" may be present on the AP view.
  - This occurs when the humerus dislocates and internally rotates in posterior shoulder dislocation, causing the head contour to resemble a lightbulb when viewed from the front.[9] (Figure 1.29)
  - If x-ray is not diagnostic, consider CT for definitive diagnosis.

ED Treatment

- ED treatment is similar to anterior shoulder dislocation. A traction/countertraction technique should be used to achieve reduction.
  - The patient is placed in a supine position and a sheet is fixed around an assistant's waist or a stationary object and wrapped around the patient's chest through the axilla.
  - The operator then will loop a sheet around his or her waist and provide traction on the patient's forearm with the elbow flexed to 90°.
  - Traction is applied smoothly and firmly with the shoulder held in adduction and internal rotation.
  - The assistant can provide gentle pressure on the humeral head in a posterior and lateral direction to disengage it from the glenoid.
  - After the humeral head is disengaged, the arm can be externally rotated with caution as humeral fracture can occur if the humerus is not completely disengaged from the glenoid.

Disposition

- Post-reduction treatment and disposition is identical to anterior shoulder dislocation and should include radiographic imaging, repeat exam with careful attention to neurovascular exam, immobilization, and follow-up instructions.

Complications

- Complications from posterior shoulder dislocation include the following:
  - Humerus fracture
  - Acute redislocation
  - Avascular necrosis
  - Posttraumatic osteoarthritis
  - Joint stiffness and functional limitation

Pediatric Considerations

- Posterior shoulder dislocation in pediatric patients is extremely rare and has not been well studied.

Pearls and Pitfalls

- Making the correct diagnosis is critical in posterior shoulder dislocation.
- A complete shoulder trauma x-ray series is essential for diagnosis and includes AP, axillary, and Y views.
  - An axillary view is essential to rule out a posterior shoulder dislocation, and if needed, help the x-ray technician to achieve appropriate patient positioning.
- Chronic posterior dislocation and complex fracture dislocation will likely require open reduction and internal fixation or humeral head replacement.
- Intra-articular lidocaine injection is more difficult to perform in posterior shoulder dislocation, but can be used by experienced providers.
- Smooth, firm traction is required for successful reduction. Providers should not become impatient and use excessive force or impatient maneuvers.
- Impatience or excessive force can lead to increased likelihood of complications.
- Aftercare must include complete neurovascular examination and postreduction radiographs.
- Seek input from orthopedic surgery consultant, as this injury is rare.

Inferior Shoulder Dislocation (Luxatio Erecta)

General Description

- Inferior shoulder dislocation is a rare but serious type of shoulder dislocation.

Mechanism

- The mechanism of injury is hyperabduction of the arm where the neck of the humerus is leveraged against the acromion and the humeral head is forced out inferiorly.
- This requires significant force, such as during a motor vehicle accident.

Presentation

- Patients will present with an obvious visual dislocation with the arm stuck overhead, and will complain of severe pain and inability to move the shoulder.

Physical Exam

- On exam the patient's shoulder will be locked in abduction with their arm held against or behind their head.
  - The dislocated humeral head may be palpable along the lateral border of the chest wall.

Essential Diagnostics

- A complete shoulder trauma x-ray series including AP, axillary, and Y views is essential due to the high incidence of associated fractures.
  - The humeral shaft will be seen parallel to the spine of the scapula with the humeral head sitting inferior to the glenoid (Figure 1.30).

ED Treatment

- ED treatment is similar to anterior and posterior shoulder dislocation. An axial (in-line) traction or two-step method should be utilized for reduction.
- To perform the axial traction method, place the patient in a supine position. The operator should be at the patient's head on the affected side.
  - An assistant can provide countertraction using a sheet wrapped around the waist and across the patient's chest and above the affected shoulder.
  - The operator then applies axial traction in line with the abducted arm.
  - Increase the degree of abduction and apply cephalad pressure to the humeral head to assist in reduction.

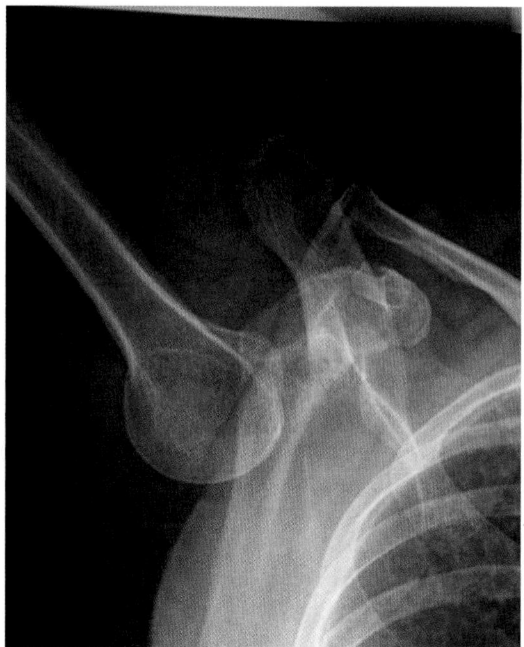

Figure 1.30. X-ray image demonstrating luxatio erecta. Note the abducted arm with the humeral head dislocated inferiorly. Courtesy of Trevor Lundstrom, MD, Birmingham, Alabama.

  - After the reduction the arm should be immobilized in full adduction and supination.
- The two-step reduction method requires converting the inferior dislocation to an anterior dislocation (step one) then reducing the anterior dislocation (step two).
  - With the patient supine, the operator stands at the patient's head on the affected side.
  - The hand closest to the patient is placed on the lateral aspect of the patient's mid-humerus with the other on the medial condyle.
  - The operator pushes anteriorly with the hand on the mid-humerus and pulls posteriorly with the hand on the medial condyle. This will bring the humeral head into an anterior position.
  - Next, adduct the patient's arm and move the hand on the medial condyle to grasp the wrist.
  - With the arm in adduction, externally rotate the shoulder by pulling on the wrist.
  - After reduction is accomplished, immobilize the arm in adduction and supination.[10]

Disposition

- Post-reduction treatment and disposition is identical to anterior and posterior shoulder dislocation and should include radiographic imaging, repeat exam with careful attention to neurovascular exam, immobilization, and follow-up instructions.

Complications

- Complications of inferior shoulder dislocation include:
  - Avulsed capsule
  - Rotator cuff tear
  - Fracture of the acromion, clavicle, inferior glenoid fossa, or greater tuberosity
  - Neurovascular injury including brachial plexus injury
  - Vascular injury including axillary vein thrombosis[11]

Pediatric Considerations

- There is limited literature regarding inferior shoulder dislocation in pediatric patients. Evaluation and treatment should follow that for adult patients.

Pearls and Pitfalls

- 80 percent of patients with inferior shoulder dislocation will have associated fracture of the greater tuberosity or rotator cuff tear.
- 60 percent will have neurologic compromise and 3 percent will have vascular injury.

Acromioclavicular Joint Injuries

General Description

- AC joint sprain and separation occurs from trauma to the joint and the surrounding AC ligaments and coracoclavicular (CC) ligament. It is commonly referred to as a separated shoulder.
- In adults, the normal width of the AC joint is 1–3 mm.
  - May be wider in children or adolescents and narrower in older adults.
- There are six types of injuries classified by the Rockwood classification system:
  - Type I: Ligament sprain without tearing or rupture of ligaments

    - Type II: AC ligaments are torn and the CC ligaments are sprained.
    - Types III–VI: AC and CC ligaments are torn and further classification is based upon direction of displacement of the distal clavicle.

Mechanism

- The mechanism of injury is typically impact from a collision or from a fall onto the shoulder with the arm in the adducted position.
- This type of injury will cause a sprain or disruption of the AC ligaments first, followed by the CC ligament.
- Indirect injury to the AC joint can occur, for example, from a fall on an outstretched hand.
    - These injuries will usually only affect the AC ligaments and spare the CC ligament.

Presentation

- The patient with AC joint injury will typically present complaining of shoulder pain that localizes to the AC joint.
    - They will often splint the arm in an adducted position and will be hesitant to range the shoulder when asked.
    - There may be an obvious deformity of the shoulder, depending on the severity of injury.
        - This injury may be confused with a shoulder dislocation.

Physical Examination

- On physical examination, an abnormal contour of the shoulder may be present when compared to the contralateral side.
    - On inspection, bruising, swelling, and tenting can all be noted near the AC joint.
    - Patients will have significant tenderness at the AC joint.
    - To assess for stability of the AC ligaments, attempt to translate the clavicle in an anterior-posterior direction.
    - Vertical stability confirms the integrity of the CC ligament and is tested by moving the clavicle in the cephalad and caudal directions.
    - The *crossover test* will be positive in these patients.
    - Neurovascular injury is possible, and one should perform a complete neurovascular examination of the affected extremity.

Essential Diagnostics

- Essential diagnostics include a shoulder trauma x-ray series.
    - An AP view is necessary and should include both clavicles and shoulders.
    - An axillary view will help to assess the anterior posterior displacement of the clavicle (important for diagnosing type IV injuries).
    - Stress views are generally not required in the ED setting.
- There are six types of ligamentous injuries to the AC joint (Figure 1.31):
    - Type I: X-rays will be normal.
    - Type II: X-rays will demonstrate slight widening of the AC joint and the distal clavicle may be slightly elevated compared to the contralateral side.
    - Type III: X-rays will show significant increased displacement of the distal clavicle as well as widening of the CC space.
    - Type IV: Axially x-ray will show posterior displacement of the clavicle.
    - Type V: X-rays will show significant increased displacement of the distal clavicle as well as of the CC space.
    - Type VI: These types of injuries are extremely uncommon. On x-ray the distal clavicle will be visualized in a subcoracoid or subacromial position.

ED Treatment

- The type of injury sustained drives treatment in the ED.
- Type I: X-rays will be normal. Advise patients on rest, ice, and use of a sling for 7–10 days.
- Type II: X-rays will demonstrate slight widening of the AC joint. Advise patients to use a sling for up to two weeks. They will often require rehabilitation in physical therapy.

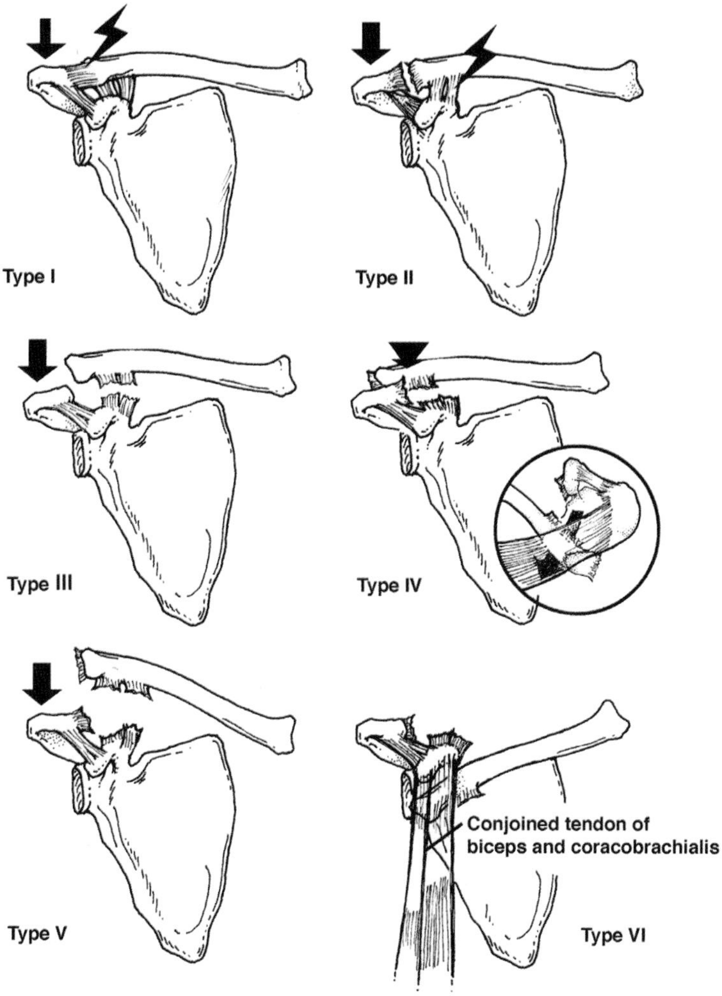

Figure 1.31. Classification of ligamentous injuries to the acromioclavicular joint.

- Type III: X-rays will show significant increased displacement with stress views. Definitive treatment is usually nonsurgical but surgical repair may be advised by some surgeons, especially for athletes or laborers.
- Type IV: Axillary x-ray will show posterior displacement of the clavicle. If closed reduction is possible, treat like a type III injury, otherwise these patients will require emergency orthopedics consult for surgical reduction and repair.
- Type V: Gross displacement is noted on x-ray. Patients will require emergency orthopedic surgery consult. Definitive treatment is generally with open reduction and internal fixation.
- Type VI: These types of injuries are extremely uncommon. On x-ray the distal clavicle will be visualized in a subcoracoid or subacromial position. If closed reduction is possible, treat like a Type III injury, otherwise these patients will require ORIF.
- Fracture of distal clavicle associated with rupture of the CC ligament often will require surgical intervention.

Disposition

- Patients with Type I, Type II, and Type III injuries can be safely discharged from the ED. They will require routine follow-up with their primary care provider or in the orthopedic or sports medicine clinic.
- Patients with Type IV, Type V, and Type VI injuries and injuries associated with fractures will require orthopedic consultation and disposition.

- NSAIDs are first line of treatment for pain control. More significant injuries may require opiates for analgesia.
- Patients may return to work or sports once they have normal strength, and full pain-free range of motion.

Complications

- Complications may occur with both nonsurgical and surgical treatment of AC joint injury.
  - Complications of nonoperative treatment include skin breakdown as well as osteolysis at the distal clavicle and degenerative changes at the AC joint.

Pediatric Considerations

- In pediatric patients, consider performing a Zanca (AC joint) view (Figure 1.32) to exclude associated fractures.
  - A Zanca view is an AP view with the beam directed toward the AC joint with 10° cephalic tilt, with the voltage idealized for soft tissue to avoid over penetration.
- Pediatric injuries are classified using the Dameron and Rockwood classification system, which is very similar to the Rockwood adult classification system.
- Treatment for pediatric injuries essentially follows that for adult injury.

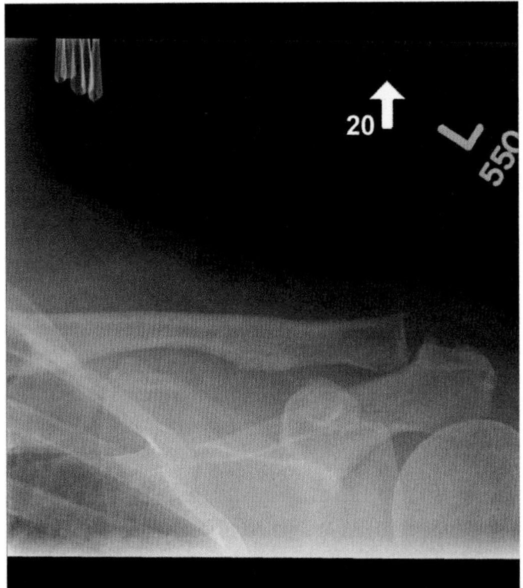

Figure 1.32. A normal Zanca view in an adult patient.

Pearls and Pitfalls

- Concomitant injuries do occur and can be masked by the more painful AC joint injury.
- Stress views are generally not obtained in the ED.[12, 13]

Sternoclavicular Joint Injury

General Description

- Sternoclavicular (SC) joint dislocation occurs when the medial end of the clavicle becomes displaced anteriorly or posteriorly relative to the sternum.

Mechanism

- The most common mechanism of injury is a direct blow to the anterior chest, such as a steering wheel injury that occurs during a motor vehicle accident.
  - This typically results in posterior SC joint dislocation.
  - Posterior SC joint dislocation can be associated with occlusion of the superior vena cava or esophagus.
- A lateral or posterior force to the shoulder girdle will result in an anterior SC joint dislocation.
  - This type of dislocation is generally benign.
- Scapulothoracic dissociation occurs as a result of severe high-energy trauma and can cause complete disruption of the SC joint.
  - These injuries can be associated with axillary artery and brachial plexus injury.

Presentation

- On presentation, patients will localize pain with possible deformity at the SC joint after traumatic injury.
  - Patients may complain of dysphonia, dysphagia, or dyspnea.

Physical Exam

- Physical exam will demonstrate soft tissue swelling and tenderness at the medial clavicle.
  - Patients may laterally flex their neck toward the affected side to relieve pressure on the SC joint.

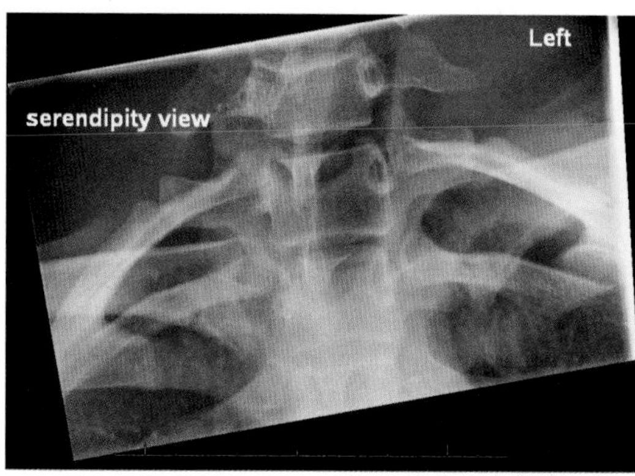

Figure 1.33. A normal serendipity x-ray view.

- In posterior dislocation, there will be a palpable step-off at the lateral manubrium.
- Swelling and a prominent medial head of the clavicle may be palpable in anterior SC joint dislocation.
- SC joint sprain will present with mild to moderate pain at the SC joint without instability on physical exam.

Essential Diagnostics

- Essential radiographic views include AP, and serendipity or tilt views.
  - In a serendipity view the beam is aimed at the manubrium with a 40°cephalic tilt (Figure 1.33).
  - CT is the most reliable imaging modality to determine dislocation.
  - CTA and MRA are useful in assisting with determining the direction of dislocation and in evaluation for vascular injury.

ED Treatment

- Treatment for SC joint sprain is conservative with a sling for comfort, analgesia as needed, and cold therapy. These injuries will generally resolve in one week.
- A SC joint subluxation can occur and treatment follows that for SC joint sprain. Sling immobilization will be required for a longer duration.
- Reduction is not typically needed for anterior dislocation.
  - Closed reduction may be needed for patients who engage in strenuous activity involving the upper extremities.
  - These patients may be safely discharged from the ED.
- Closed reduction can be attempted in the ED for patients with posterior dislocation without evidence of airway, vascular, or esophageal injury.
  - Procedural sedation is recommended to accomplish these maneuvers.
  - General anesthesia is usually required for patients with severe pain and muscle spasms.
  - If reduction is unsuccessful, orthopedic surgery and thoracic surgery consults will be required for open or closed reduction in the operating room.
- Classic method (abduction-traction technique) (Figure 1.34)
  - To perform this reduction maneuver, place a rolled-up towel or sandbag posteriorly between the shoulder blades with the patient positioned supine.
  - Traction is applied to the abducted arm against countertraction in an abducted and slightly extended position.
  - Direct pressure over the medial clavicle may reduce the joint in anterior dislocations.
  - Successful reduction is indicated by an audible snap or pop.
  - For posterior dislocations, manual manipulation of the medial clavicle may be necessary to dislodge it from behind the manubrium.
  - For difficult posterior dislocations, the medial clavicle may need to be prepared sterilely, followed by use of a towel clip to grasp the medial clavicle and lift it into a normal position.
- Buckerfield and Castle technique (adduction-traction technique)
  - In this method, place a rolled towel between the supine patient's shoulder blades.
  - The operator applies traction to the adducted arm while an assistant applies a posteriorly directed pressure to the shoulder.
  - This will lever the clavicle over the first rib into its normal position.[14]
- In both of these techniques, the medial end of the clavicle may need to be manipulated using a towel clip or fingers.

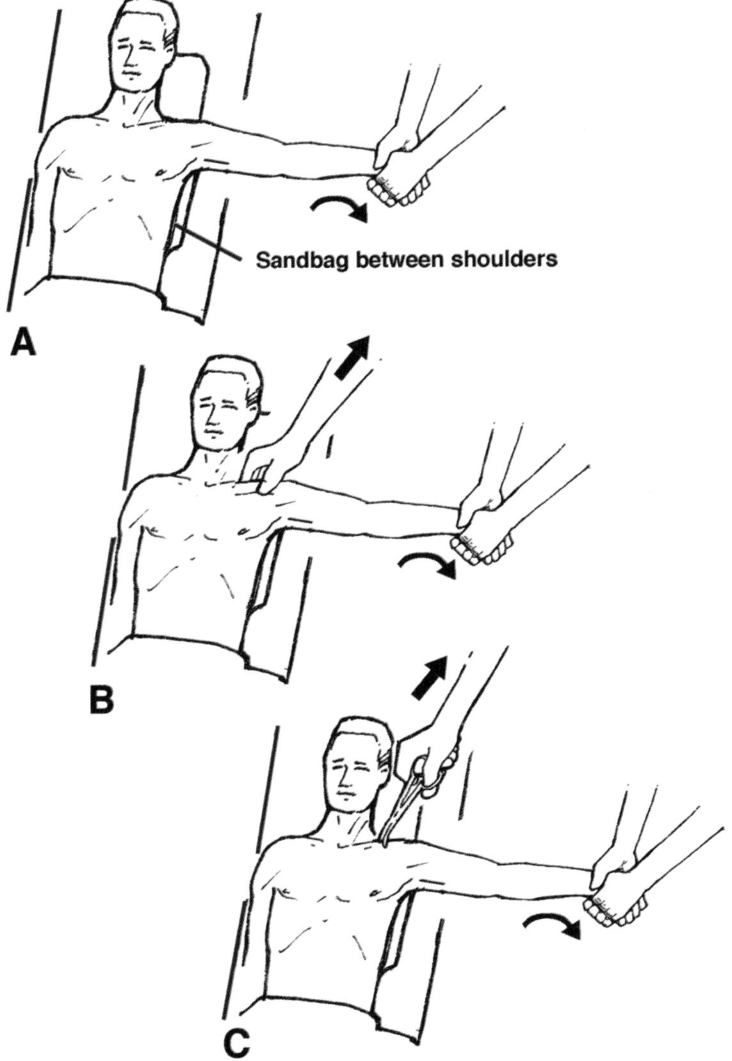

Figure 1.34. Technique for closed reduction of the sternoclavicular joint. **A.** Patient position with sandbag and traction in abduction and slight extension. **B.** Manual manipulation of the medial end of the clavicle in posterior dislocation. **C.** Use of a towel clip for difficult posterior dislocations.

- Following reduction, the arm should be placed in a figure-of-eight brace (Figure 1.35) for immobilization.
  - Alternatively a Velpeau bandage or sling may be utilized.[15]
- NSAIDs and cold therapy are first-line treatment for pain. More severe injuries may require opioid analgesics.

Disposition

- Generally, patients with anterior SC joint dislocation and uncomplicated posterior SC joint dislocation can be discharged from the ED.
- If attempts at posterior SC joint dislocation reduction fail or if complicated SC joint dislocation is present, orthopedic surgery and/or thoracic surgery consult is warranted in the ED.
- Routine sports medicine or orthopedic surgery follow-up is necessary after anterior SC joint dislocation.
- After reduction, patients with posterior SC joint dislocation require close orthopedic surgery and/or thoracic surgery follow-up.
- Patient may recover quickly from SC joint sprain, subluxation, and anterior dislocation. Return to work or sports can occur when patients regain full pain-free range of motion and near symmetric strength.
  - Patients with posterior SC joint dislocation will take longer to heal.

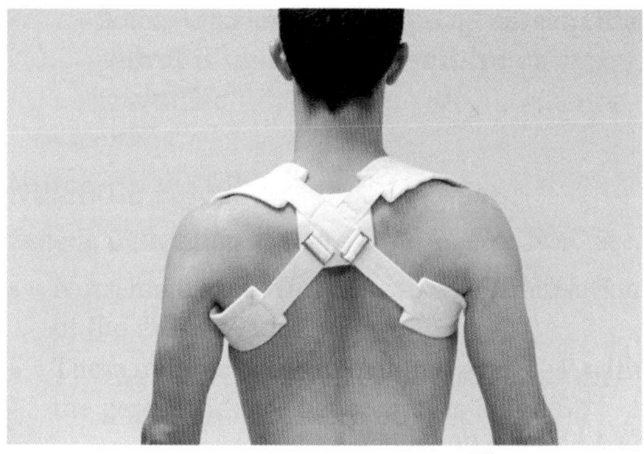

Figure 1.35. Figure-of-eight brace, also called a clavicle strap.

- Recurrent instability may delay or preclude return to pre-injury levels of activity.

Complications

- Cosmetic deformity
- Superior vena cava syndrome occurs rarely and will require emergent reduction.
- In posterior dislocation, potential SC joint instability, airway, vascular, and esophageal complications can occur.
- The reduction can be unstable and repeat dislocation can occur.
- Late SC joint instability and persistent pain can occur.
- Significant posterior instability and associated injury may preclude a patient from returning to work or sports activity.[16]

Pediatric Considerations

- In pediatric patients with an anterior SC joint dislocation, reduction can be accomplished by applying gentle pressure over the area.
- Posterior SC joint dislocation in pediatric patients can be reduced with an abduction-traction technique.
  - In this technique the patient should be placed supine with the affected arm abducted and axial traction applied.
  - The medial clavicle is then pulled forward to reduce the dislocation.
  - A towel clip can be utilized to assist with manipulation of the medial clavicle.[17]

Pearls and Pitfalls

- SC joint dislocation is rare.
- Posterior dislocation can be associated with airway or vascular injury and should be treated emergently with closed or open reduction by an orthopedist with a vascular surgeon standing by.
- An orthopedic and thoracic surgeon must closely follow all patients with posterior dislocation.

Proximal Humerus Fractures

General Description

- Proximal humerus fractures occur in four anatomic areas: the greater tuberosity, lesser tuberosity, anatomic neck, and surgical neck.
  - Proximal humerus fractures account for 4–5 percent of all fractures.
    - 75 percent occur in patients older than 60 years.
    - Women are three times as likely to sustain this type of fracture due to their risk of decreased bone density.

Mechanism

- In older adults, these injuries usually occur as a result of a fall on an abducted arm or onto an outstretched hand.
- In younger patients proximal humerus fractures are more likely to occur from high-energy trauma.
- Other mechanisms of injury include violent muscle contractions from seizure, electrical shock, sports injuries, and a direct blow to the proximal humerus.

Presentation

- Patients with proximal humerus fractures will generally present with complaints of diffuse pain at the shoulder following traumatic injury.
  - They may also note loss of shoulder function and swelling of the involved extremity.

Physical Exam

- Physical exam will demonstrate swelling and ecchymosis over the upper arm and shoulder.
  - Patients will generally hold the arm in adduction and will resist movement.
  - Extensive ecchymosis can be present 2–3 days following injury and may spread to involve the chest, back, flank, and entire upper extremity.

- The examiner should palpate the entire upper extremity, neck, and chest wall to evaluate for additional injuries.
- The fracture can be difficult to pinpoint on palpation because of diffuse swelling and overlying structures.
- Gross deformity at the shoulder and drooping of the arm are not usually caused by an isolated fracture and can suggest the presence of a dislocation.
- Careful neurovascular examination must be performed.
  - Pseudoparalysis (where the patient will not move the arm due to pain from the fracture) can limit your examination of motor function.
  - Close attention should be paid to the axillary nerve, looking for deltoid muscle weakness and decreased sensation over the mid-deltoid region, and the suprascapular nerve, looking for weakness with internal rotation.

Essential Diagnostics

- Radiographic evaluation should include AP, axillary, and trans-scapular Y views, in addition to a minimum of two views of the humerus (AP and lateral).
  - Supporting the patient's arm during the axillary view can allow for adequate abduction.
  - CT scan is useful if plan radiographs are difficult to interpret.

ED Treatment

- Neer developed the most commonly used classification scheme for proximal humerus fracture (Figure 1.36).
  - In this method, fractures are grouped based on the number of parts and displacement.
  - Criteria of displacement is 45° of angulation or greater than 1cm of displacement between fracture parts, otherwise they are termed "minimally displaced."
- Nondisplaced or two part fractures can usually be treated conservatively with immobilization in a sling, shoulder immobilizer, sling and swath, or collar and cuff sling. Gentle range of motion can start at 7–10 days for patients with stable fractures.

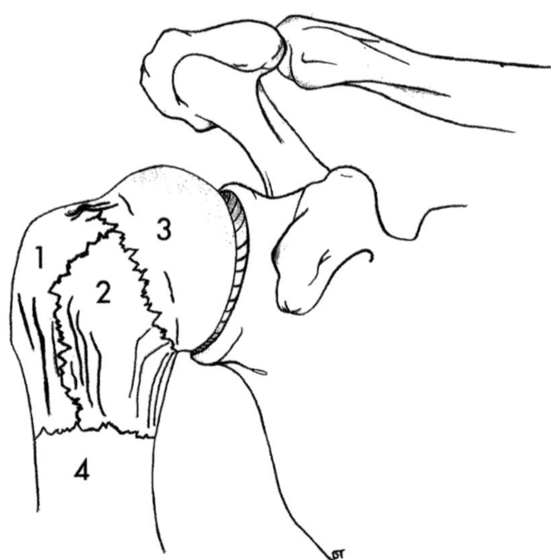

Figure 1.36. The four parts of the proximal humerus referred to in the Neer classification: 1. greater tuberosity, 2. lesser tuberosity, 3. head, and 4. shaft.

  - A sling is recommended for fractures with minimal angulation and minimal displacement.
  - A collar and cuff sling is used for fractures with significant angulation as the weight of the unsupported elbow can improve the degree angulation by downward traction.
  - A shoulder immobilizer sling and swath may be required for unstable fractures and should only be used for short time.
- Greater tuberosity fractures – if less than 5mm of displacement is present after closed reduction these can be observed carefully.
  - Displacement can indicate a rotator cuff tear is present and these may need surgical treatment.
  - In fractures associated with anterior shoulder dislocation, reduce the dislocation and treat as mentioned earlier.
- Lesser tuberosity fractures are often associated with posterior shoulder dislocation.
  - Operative repair is considered if there is more than 5mm of displacement after reduction. Otherwise these can be treated by observation.
- Anatomic neck fractures without displacement can be treated conservatively;

those with displacement will likely require open reduction and internal fixation.

- Surgical neck fractures that are isolated, displaced less than 1 cm, or impacted can be treated conservatively.
  - Displaced fractures will usually require open reduction and internal fixation.
- Fractures associated with shoulder dislocation require urgent orthopedic surgery consult for consideration of closed reduction under general anesthesia.
  - Following reduction, fractures can usually be treated as those not associated with dislocation.
- Young patients with three- and four-part fractures will likely require ORIF, while older patients may require hemiarthroplasty.

Disposition

- The majority of these injuries can be treated initially in the ED and discharged with early orthopedic surgery or sports medicine follow-up (3–7 days).
- Patients should be counseled to avoid weight-bearing on the affected extremity and the importance of wrist and finger range of motion exercises.
- These fractures are quite painful and ice and narcotic analgesics will be required for pain control.
  - Patients are usually more comfortable sleeping in a semi-recumbent position with sufficient support under the arm.
- Orthopedic surgery consult is indicated in the ED for patients with open fractures, unstable fractures, fracture-dislocations, or signs of neurological or vascular injury.
- Return to work can usually occur within a week following the injury.
  - The patient will be able to use the hand for many tasks and this may actually help with range of motion of the wrist, hand and fingers.
  - Patients with strenuous jobs that require use of both arms or heavy lifting will not be able to return to work until bony callus is present, and they have sufficient range of motion and strength to perform duties safely.

Complications

- Neurovascular injury
- Avascular necrosis of the humeral head
- Adhesive capsulitis

Pediatric Considerations

- Proximal humerus fractures are uncommon in children.
- In adolescents, the most common type seen is Salter–Harris type II fractures.
- Mechanisms of injury are similar to those in adults.
  - Stress from repetitive throwing can lead to widening of the physis and is known as Little League shoulder.
  - Child abuse should be suspected in otherwise healthy children with a reported mechanism and consistent with the fracture pattern.
  - Metaphyseal corner fractures of the proximal humeral physis can occur when the arm is twisted or pulled.
- In children with nondisplaced fractures physical findings may be minimal.
  - In those with displaced fractures the arm is usually shortened and held in extension. Anterior swelling and irregular shoulder appearance is usually present.
- Comparison views of the contralateral shoulder may be useful to determine if physeal widening is present.
- Orthopedic surgery consultation is indicated for patients with associated shoulder dislocation, neurovascular injury, and injury involving the physis.
  - Consider consultation if you are unsure about the acceptability of the fracture position.
- Treatment for pediatric nondisplaced or minimally displaced proximal humerus fractures includes immobilization in a sling and swath or shoulder mobilizer appropriately sized for the patient.
- Follow-up should usually occur 3–5 days after the injury.
- Complications of physeal injury include abnormal growth and limb length discrepancy.

Pearls and Pitfalls

- Proximal humerus fractures are most common in patients over 60 years old and are three times more likely to occur in women.
- Pseudoparalysis can limit motor function exam.
- Careful examination of axillary and suprascapular nerve function should be performed to exclude neurological injury.
- These fractures are described using the Neer classification scheme.
- Proximal humerus fractures are quite painful and will require narcotic analgesics.
- In pediatric patients, physeal injuries are the most likely injury one will encounter.[18]

Scapula Fractures

General Description

- Scapula fractures (Figure 1.37) occur as a result of significant force.
  - The most common cause of these injuries is motor vehicle accidents.
  - Fractures may occur to the body, coracoid process, acromion, glenoid fossa, spine, and glenoid neck.
  - Body and spine fractures occur as a result of direct trauma from a blow or a fall.
  - Neck fractures may happen from indirect injury like a fall on an outstretched hand or impact on the point of the shoulder.

Mechanism

- The mechanism for glenoid fractures is a fall on the lateral shoulder or on a flexed elbow.
  - Glenoid fractures may be associated with shoulder dislocation, clavicle fracture, and AC joint separation.
- Acromion fractures occur from direct downward force on the shoulder.

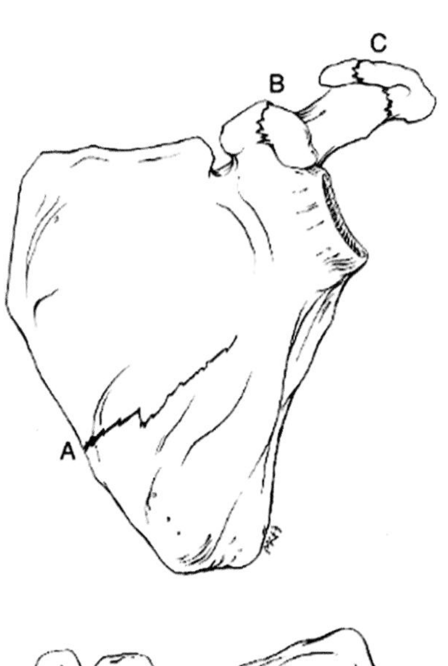

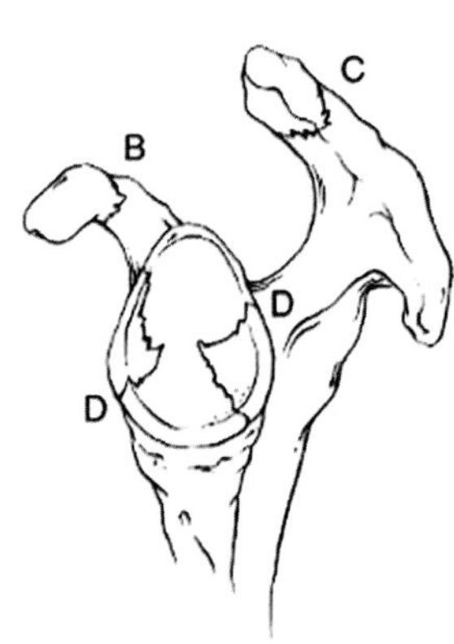

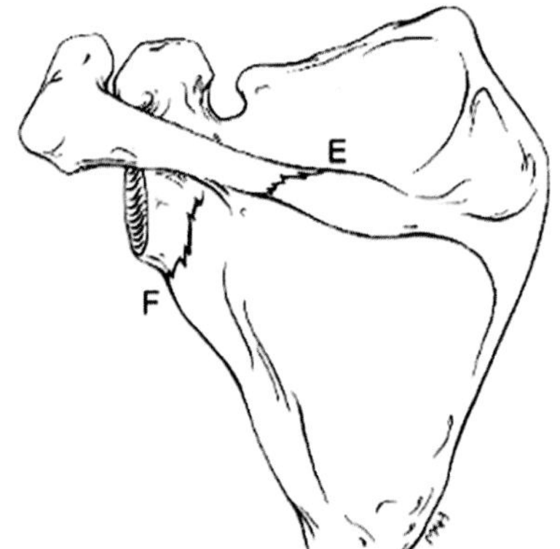

Figure 1.37. Fractures of the scapula: body (A), coracoid process (B), acromion (C), glenoid fossa (D), spine (E), and glenoid neck (F). *From* Eiff, MP. *Fracture Management for Primary Care.* Elsevier 2012; 9:183, with permission.

- Direct trauma to the point of the shoulder or violent muscle contraction may cause coracoid process fracture.

Presentation

- Patients with scapula fractures will often present with complaints of pain over the shoulder blade following traumatic injury.

Physical Exam

- On physical exam the patient may hold the arm in abduction and resist any motion at the shoulder, particularly abduction.
  - Localized tenderness and soft tissue swelling may be present.
  - Displaced glenoid neck or acromion fracture may be present with a flattened appearance at the shoulder.
  - Deep swelling from a body fracture may mimic a rotator cuff tear.

Essential Diagnostics

- A shoulder trauma x-ray series should be obtained and includes AP, axillary, and Y views.
- A cephalic tilt view can be helpful when assessing for coracoid fractures.
- CT scan is recommended for evaluation of glenoid fractures.
- An os acromiale is a normal variant that results from failed fusion of the ossification center of the acromion and can be confused with an acute fracture.

ED Treatment

- Patients may be placed in a sling or a sling and swath for comfort.
- Patients should be non-weight bearing on the affected extremity.
- Pain control with ice and narcotic analgesics is appropriate.

Disposition

- Patients with an isolated scapula fracture can be discharged from the ED.
- Indications for orthopedic surgery consult include:
  - Displaced glenoid neck fractures with clavicle fracture, more than 1 cm displacement or > 20° inferior angulation
  - Glenoid fractures with more than 25 percent articular involvement, greater than 5 mm step-off or displaced humeral head
  - Displaced coracoid and acromion fractures
- Patients should follow-up with orthopedic surgery or sports medicine within 1–2 weeks following the injury.
- Patients can return to less strenuous occupations once pain is controlled. They should be counseled that it may take several months before they regain normal function following a scapula fracture.

Complications

- Pneumothorax.
- Rib fracture.
- Pulmonary contusion.
- Clavicle fracture.
- Brachial plexus injury.

Pediatric Considerations

- Scapula fractures are rare in children.
- Most of these injuries will be nondisplaced and require only symptomatic treatment.[19]

Pearls and Pitfalls

- Neck and body fractures are most common (10–15 percent and 50–80 percent, respectively).
- These injuries occur as the result of significant force.
- Scapula body fractures can mimic rotator cuff tears.
- CT scan is useful in evaluation of glenoid fractures.
- An os acromiale is a normal variant and can be confused with an acute fracture.
- Thoracic and neurologic injuries are complications of scapula fractures.[18]

Clavicle Fractures

General Description

- Clavicle fractures account for 2 percent of all fractures.
  - The majority occur in the middle third (69 percent) (Figure 1.38) followed by distal third (28 percent), with only 3 percent in the proximal third.

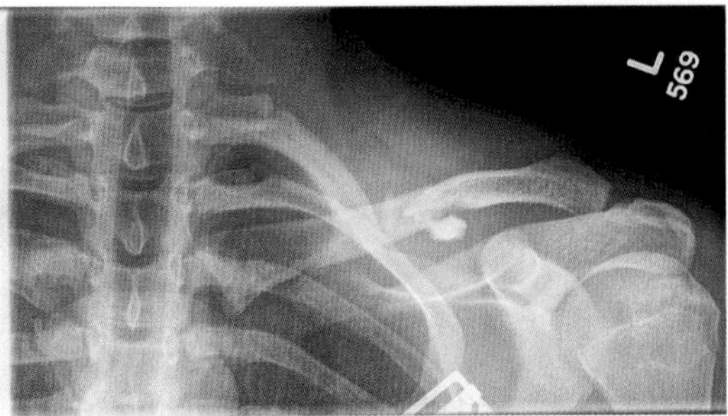

Figure 1.38. Anterior-posterior clavicle x-ray demonstrating a midshaft clavicle fracture.

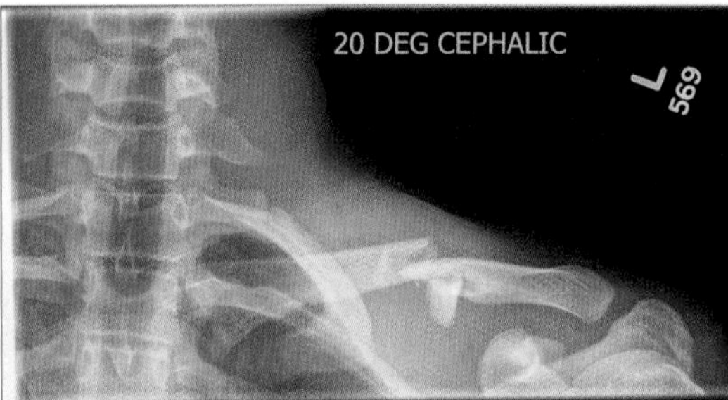

Figure 1.39. Cephalic tilt x-ray view demonstrating a midshaft clavicle fracture with a large inferior osseous fragment.

Mechanism

- Middle and distal third clavicle fractures usually occur as a result of a fall onto the shoulder.
  - A direct injury to the shoulder and indirect trauma from a fall on an outstretched hand can also cause fracture to the clavicle.
  - No correlation exists between the fracture location and mechanism of injury.
- Proximal clavicle fractures are usually the result of motor vehicle accidents or other severe trauma.

Presentation

- Patients will present with complaints of shoulder pain with any shoulder movement.
  - They will often hold the shoulder adducted against their chest to minimize motion.
  - Fractures involving the distal third of the clavicle can mimic AC joint injury.
  - Patients with proximal third clavicle fractures will complain of pain, tenderness, and swelling in the SC region. They are often more comfortable in a sitting position.

Physical Exam

- Physical exam can demonstrate a bulge at the fracture site.
  - This is a result of fracture hematoma or bone displacement.
  - In displaced and shortened fractures, the shoulder will be displaced downward and inward.
  - Patients will have point tenderness over the fracture site.
  - Patients with fractures of the distal third will have tenderness over the AC joint and pain will increase when the arm is adducted across the chest.
  - Crepitus or palpable motion at the fracture site may be present.
  - Ecchymosis and tenting of the skin can occur if fracture fragments are displaced or with significant ligamentous injury.
  - Lung and neurovascular injuries can be associated with clavicle fractures, and patients should be examined for these coexisting injuries.

Essential Diagnostics

- An AP clavicle radiograph is usually all that is necessary to diagnose middle and distal third clavicle fractures. However, additional x-rays may be necessary if you are considering other injuries.
  - If the diagnosis is unclear, a 45°cephalic tilt view can aid in diagnosis.
  - Comminution is typically seen with middle third fractures.
  - Stress views can be beneficial in fractures of the distal third to assist with determination of the degree of separation of the fracture fragments.
  - Proximal clavicle fractures can be difficult to visualize on AP radiographs because of bony overlap.
    - A cephalic tilt view (Figure 1.39) can be useful to diagnose these fractures.
    - Approximately 20 percent of these fractures will be missed on x-ray.
    - CT scan is useful to evaluate for these fractures and associated injuries.

ED Treatment

- Treatment is aimed at limiting motion at the fracture site.
- Middle third fractures
    - Patients should be placed in a sling, or a figure-of-eight brace may be considered to immobilize the injury.[20]
    - Both treatments will limit range of motion to less than 30° of abduction, forward flexion, and extension.
    - A sling is preferred for treatment of nondisplaced fractures.
    - Figure-of-eight bracing can minimize displacement and should be considered for treatment of significantly displaced fractures.
        - Treatment with this brace allows the elbow and hand to remain free for use for activities of daily living.
        - The brace requires regular tightening to maintain tension and may not be a good option for patients who won't have someone to assist them at home.
        - This brace is less comfortable than a sling.
    - Treatment outcomes are the same for both devices.[21]
- Distal third fractures
    - Distal third clavicle fractures are classified into three types (Figure 1.40).
        - Type I fractures are nondisplaced and AC and CC ligaments remain intact.
        - Type II fractures are displaced and the CC ligament is torn.
        - Type III fractures are nondisplaced with the fracture extending intra-articularly through the AC joint. Ac and CC ligaments remain intact.
    - Patients with type I and type III distal clavicle fractures should be placed in a sling for comfort.
    - Patients with a type II fracture should be placed in a sling and swath or shoulder immobilizer until follow-up.
- Proximal third fractures
    - Treatment is with sling immobilization.
- Patients should be counseled on activity modification.
- Analgesics and cold therapy will be required for pain control. Narcotic analgesics may be required.

Disposition

- The majority of patients with clavicle fractures can be discharged from the ED after treatment.
- Indications for orthopedic surgery consult in the ED include neurovascular compromise, intrathoracic injury, open fracture, and tenting of the skin.
- For middle third fractures, initial follow-up with orthopedic surgery or sports medicine should occur within one week following the injury.

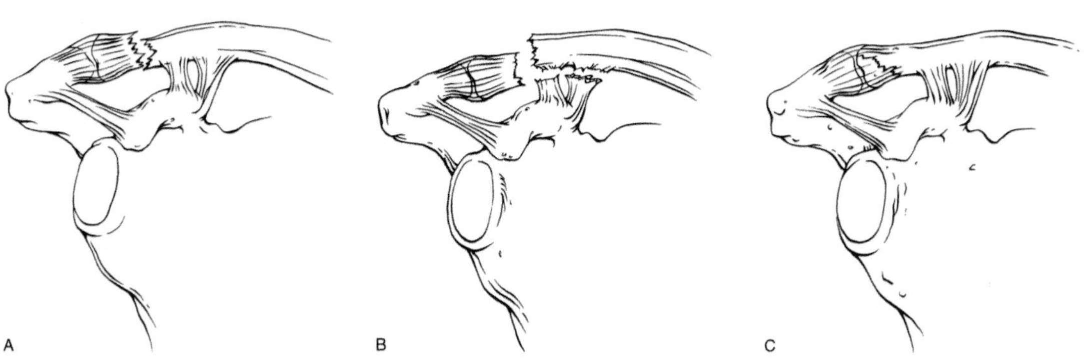

Figure 1.40. Classification of fractures of the distal clavicle. A, Type I: Nondisplaced, intact ligaments. B, Type II: Displaced coracoclavicular ligament tear. C, Type III: Nondisplaced, intra-articular through the acromioclavicular joint. *From* Eiff, MP. *Fracture Management for Primary Care.* Elsevier 2012; 9:10, with permission.

- Patients can gradually return to work and sports activities as pain allows.
  - Return to strenuous activities and contact sports can generally occur 8–12 weeks following middle third clavicle fractures.
- For distal third fractures, follow-up should occur within three days after injury.
  - Patients with type II injuries may require open reduction and internal fixation.
  - Return to work and sports may occur sooner for patients with distal third clavicle fractures (4–6 weeks).
- Most proximal third fractures can be referred for follow-up in one week.
  - Patients who have proximal third fractures that are significantly displaced or associated with SC dislocation should be seen within three days for follow-up.

Complications

- Malunion can result in angulation, shortening, poor cosmetic outcome, ongoing tenderness, and reduced shoulder function.
- Nonunion
- Delayed union
- Symptomatic degeneration of the AC joint
- Brachial plexus compression neuropathy can occur as a result of hypertrophic callus formation.

Pediatric Considerations

- Middle third fractures in pediatric patients can be treated the same as in adult patients.
- Bowing injuries of the clavicle can occur in younger children and should be treated with a sling for protection.
- Distal clavicle fractures in children are classified similar to those in adults.
  - Type II fractures are much more stable than similar fractures in adults.
  - Type I, II, and III fractures can all be treated with a sling for comfort and are expected to heal well within 4–6 weeks.
- Proximal clavicle fractures in children are very uncommon.
  - Late presentation is common because of the lack of deformity and symptoms.
  - Children can present later with concerns about a mass that represents callus formation at the fracture site.
  - Uncomplicated fractures can be treated with a sling for comfort.

Pearls and Pitfalls

- The majority of clavicle fractures occur in the middle third.
- Proximal fractures are less common and are often the result of severe trauma.
- Lung and neurovascular injury are associated with clavicle fractures.
- X-ray is the test of choice for diagnosis and a 45°cephalic tilt view can be used if the diagnosis is not clear.
- Proximal fractures can be particularly difficult to diagnose and CT scan may be required.
- Treatment outcomes are the same for both sling and figure-of-eight bracing.[18]

Rotator Cuff Impingement

General Description

- Prevalence and incidence of these injuries are not well described in the literature.
- Rotator cuff impingement (Figure 1.41) occurs as a result of many diagnoses.
  - It is caused by irritation or inflammation of the subacromial space and may include the subacromial bursa, rotator cuff tendons, and/or biceps tendon.
  - Neer described 3 stages of rotator cuff impingement:
    - Stage 1 occurs generally in patients younger than 25 years. This stage is characterized by inflammation, edema, and hemorrhage in the rotator cuff.
    - Stage 2 occurs in patients 25–40 years old. In this stage there is progression to rotator cuff tendonitis and fibrosis.
    - Stage 3 will typically affect those older than 40 years. In this stage, mechanical disruption of the rotator cuff and osteophytosis of the acromion can occur.

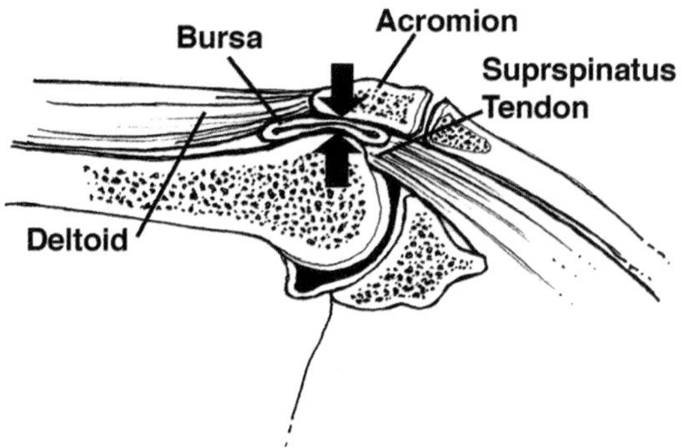

Figure 1.41. When the arm is abducted past 90° the greater tuberosity of the humerus compresses the rotator cuff against the acromion.

Mechanism

- Primary rotator cuff impingement (Figure 1.41) results from mechanical impingement on the rotator cuff tendon.
  - Commonly impingement occurs as a result of mechanical compression of the rotator cuff by the acromion, coracoacromial ligament, or AC joint.
- Secondary impingement occurs as the result of a functional decrease in the supraspinatus outlet space.
  - This can be caused by underlying glenohumeral instability and is the most common cause in athletes with rotator cuff impingement.
- Additional causes for both primary and secondary impingement exist.
- Risk factors for developing rotator cuff impingement include a hooked acromion; shoulder instability from glenohumeral instability, labral lesions, and muscle imbalance; and repetitive overhead activities.

Presentation

- Symptoms of rotator cuff impingement include pain over the lateral, anterior, or superior part of the shoulder.
  - Pain can be referred to the deltoid region.
  - Pain is gradual in onset and made worse with overhead activities.
  - Patients may work in an occupation or participate in sports where repetitive overhead activity is required.

Physical Exam

- A thorough shoulder exam is necessary to determine the cause of the patient's pain and to evaluate shoulder function.
- Useful special tests for impingement include the *Hawkins–Kennedy sign*, *Neer's sign*, *empty can test*, and *painful arc*.
- Strength of the rotator cuff muscles is normal, or may be slightly decreased due to pain.
- A subacromial injection of lidocaine can assist in diagnosis.
  - Inject 5ml of 1 percent lidocaine into the subacromial space.
  - Following the injection, repeat impingement testing.
  - Patients who have impingement or tendinopathy will have temporary relief of their symptoms following the injection.[22]
- C5–C6 radiculopathy can cause referred pain to the shoulder and the neck should be examined in addition to the shoulder.
  - Spurling's test can be useful in eliciting radicular pain.

Essential Diagnostics

- Plain radiographs should be obtained to exclude fracture and arthritis.
  - X-ray series should include a true AP (Grashey), lateral, and axillary views.
    - A true AP (Grashey) view is performed with the patient's arm in neutral rotation compared with a standard AP view where the patient's arm is positioned in external rotation.
    - This view allows for better evaluation of glenohumeral joint space narrowing, rotator cuff calcifications and acromial spurring compared to a standard AP view.
- Ultrasound allows for dynamic assessment of rotator cuff impingement and tearing.
  - Shoulder ultrasound is not used frequently in the ED.
  - Ultrasound is less expensive than MRI.
  - The test is user dependent.
  - Musculoskeletal ultrasound is gaining in popularity.

- MRI is the diagnostic study of choice for evaluating shoulder pathology.
  - Like ultrasound, MRI is generally not required for diagnosing shoulder disorders in the ED.

ED Treatment

- Treatment in the ED is generally directed at symptom control.
  - Patients should be counseled on activity modification and avoiding repetitive overhead activities.
  - Patients may require analgesics and NSAIDs as the first line of treatment.
  - Cold therapy can also provide analgesia.
  - Subacromial injection with lidocaine and corticosteroid can be both diagnostic and therapeutic.
  - Patients may require outpatient physical therapy.
  - Additional treatments that may benefit patients in the outpatient setting include transcutaneous electrical nerve stimulation, iontophoresis, and surgical intervention.
  - Work restrictions might include lifting restrictions, no pushing or pulling, and no over the shoulder work.
  - No immobilization is necessary. Immobilization may lead to frozen shoulder.[23]

Disposition

- Patients diagnosed with rotator cuff impingement will not require admission and may be discharged from the ED.
- There are no indications for orthopedic surgery consult in the ED for rotator cuff impingement.
- Patients can be advised on routine outpatient follow-up with their primary care physician for further treatment. Patients may require evaluation by an orthopedic or sports medicine specialist if they have significant rotator cuff weakness or are failing conservative treatment.
- Return to work or sports can typically occur within 6–12 weeks when the patient demonstrates pain-free range of motion, no impingement signs, and near symmetric strength.

Complications

- Rotator cuff degeneration and tear
- Progression to adhesive capsulitis
- Cuff tear arthropathy
- Reflex sympathetic dystrophy[24]

Pediatric Considerations

- In the pediatric population, sports participation (swimmers, tennis players, gymnasts, and most overhead throwing sports) is a common cause of shoulder impingement syndrome.
- Historical features and physical exam findings are similar to those found in adults.
- Diagnostic imaging is not routinely indicated in pediatric patients unless rotator cuff tear or glenoid labral tear is suspected and surgical intervention is a consideration.
- Treatment strategies for shoulder impingement follow that for adults. Surgical intervention is rarely indicated.

Pearls and Pitfalls

- Care must be taken to differentiate subacromial impingement syndrome from a rotator cuff tear.
- History of significant trauma and decreased strength is more likely to be a rotator cuff tear than rotator cuff impingement syndrome.
- Rotator cuff impingement syndrome is treatable.
- Proper evaluation includes a good history, physical exam, and diagnostic testing.
- Imaging is not usually required for pediatric patients.
- Treatment is focused on activity modification, modalities for pain control, and rehabilitation.
- Sling immobilization can lead to complications.[25]

Rotator Cuff Tendinopathy and Tear

General Description

- Rotator cuff tendinopathy and tear encompasses a broad range of disease involving the rotator cuff tendons.
- Current understanding of tendon disorders is limited.

- Tendinitis became a common term to describe painful tendon injuries before the pathology was well understood.
- Inflammation might play a role initially; however, current research supports that tendinopathy is more of a degenerative process.
- Tendinopathy and tendinosis are the preferred terminology because they better describe chronic tendon disorders.
- Tendinopathy refers to the clinical presentation of a symptomatic tendon.

Mechanism

- It is thought that biomechanical and vascular factors both play a role in rotator cuff pathology.
- Two mechanisms have been suggested as causes: intrinsic and extrinsic.
- The intrinsic mechanism suggests that injury within the tendon occurs as a result of tendon overload, degeneration, or other insult.
  - Age can be a factor in degeneration of tendons through microtears, calcification, and fibrovascular proliferation.
  - Comorbid medical conditions like diabetes and connective tissue disorders can also contribute to tendinopathy.
- The extrinsic mechanism proposes that tendinopathy occurs as a result of compressive forces described in the rotator cuff impingement section.
- The mechanism for rotator cuff tears in many patients is multifactorial.
  - Degeneration, impingement, and overload are all thought to contribute to the development of atraumatic rotator cuff tears.
  - Acute trauma, such as a fall or a motor vehicle accident, may also cause a rotator cuff tear.
    - Rotator cuff tears can be associated with shoulder dislocation.
- Rotator cuff tears in older patients may be asymptomatic.

Presentation

- Patients with rotator cuff tendinopathy will complain of pain in the shoulder with overhead activity.
  - Pain can be localized to the lateral deltoid area.
  - They may have pain with activities of daily living such as getting dressed, doing their hair, and reaching backwards (for males, getting their wallet; for females, hooking a bra).
  - Night pain may be present when they lie on the affected shoulder.
- Patients who participate in overhead sports or whose occupation requires overhead work may note decreases in their performance.
- History may reveal risk factors for developing rotator cuff tendinopathy or tear:
  - Repetitive overhead activities in work or sports
  - Anatomic variants
  - Scapular instability and dyskinesia
  - Older age
  - Increased body mass index
  - Glenohumeral joint instability and hypermobility

Physical Exam

- On inspection, observe for atrophy of the supraspinatus and infraspinatus.
  - Scapular motion may be asymmetric.
- Neck examination is essential to exclude referred pain and cervical radiculopathy.
  - Spurling's test is useful in eliciting radicular pain.
- The role of palpation is limited given the deep location of the rotator cuff.
  - Tenderness over the supraspinatus, infraspinatus, greater and lesser tuberosity, lateral and posterior-lateral border of the acromion may be present.
- Pain elicited with range of motion above 90° of abduction or with internal rotation is suggestive of rotator cuff tendinopathy.
  - When testing range of motion, the painful arc test is useful, especially when combined with *Neer's impingement* and *Hawkins-Kennedy signs.*
  - Passive range of motion is generally greater than active range of motion in patients with rotator cuff pathology.
- Strength testing can assist with making a diagnosis.

  - The *empty can* test evaluates supraspinatus strength.
  - The *infraspinatus test* assesses strength of the infraspinatus.
  - The *lift-off test* evaluates subscapularis strength.
- Special tests include the *Neer's* and *Hawkins–Kennedy signs.*
  - Both evaluate for impingement, but can also be positive in patients with rotator cuff tendinopathy.
- Three tests are particularly useful when evaluating for rotator cuff tears.
  - Patients with rotator cuff tear will often demonstrate painful arc.
  - *Drop arm test* may be positive.
  - Patients may demonstrate weakness with external rotation.
- Subacromial lidocaine injection can be useful in distinguishing rotator cuff tendinopathy from rotator cuff tear.
  - Following adequate analgesia, patients with rotator cuff tendinopathy will have pain relief and normal strength.
  - Patients with a rotator cuff tear will still have weakness following the injection.

Essential Diagnostics

- A shoulder radiograph series is not directly indicated for diagnosis of rotator cuff tendinopathy or tear.
  - X-ray cannot make a definitive diagnosis but can help exclude other pathology.
  - Radiographic views include a true AP (Grashey), Y, and axillary.
  - Findings on plain radiographs which may be associated with rotator cuff tendinopathy or tear include:
    - Greater tuberosity sclerosis
    - Greater tuberosity osteophyte
    - Greater tuberosity cyst
    - Subacromial osteophyte
    - Humeral head osteophyte
    - Decreased acromiohumeral distance (<7mm)[26]
    - Calcific tendonitis
- Musculoskeletal ultrasound is a useful modality for evaluation of rotator cuff disorders including rotator cuff tendinopathy and rotator cuff tears.
  - Ultrasound allows for dynamic evaluation of tendons.
  - Contralateral comparison views are easy to obtain.
  - Ultrasound is operator dependent.
  - Partial rotator cuff tears can be difficult to visualize on ultrasound.
  - Advantages to use of musculoskeletal ultrasound include the absence of radiation exposure and low cost compared to MRI.
- Magnetic resonance imaging is sensitive for diagnosing full thickness rotator cuff tears but is not indicated in the ED.

ED Treatment

- Patients should be counseled on avoidance of overhead activities.
  - Work restrictions include lifting restrictions and avoidance of any work performed over the level of the shoulder.
- Pain can usually be controlled with NSAIDs and cold therapy.
- Patients with tendinopathy will generally require a home rehabilitation program and may need referral to physical therapy.
  - For cases refractory to conservative treatment, surgical intervention may be necessary.
- The use of a sling should be avoided to reduce the risk of developing frozen shoulder.
- Subacromial corticosteroid injection can be considered for pain control.
- Patients with chronic rotator cuff tears will generally do well with conservative treatment.
- Active patients and those with traumatic rotator cuff tears may be candidates for surgical repair.
  - Surgical repair should also be considered in patients with impaired function after a trial of conservative treatment.

Disposition

- Patients with rotator cuff disorders can be discharged from the ED.
- Orthopedic surgery consultation is not indicated in the acute setting.

- Routine follow-up with the patient's primary care physician or sports medicine physician is advised after discharge.
  - Orthopedic surgery follow-up should be considered in certain cases:
    - Patients younger than 60 years
    - Acute full thickness tear
    - Failure to improve after a trial of conservative treatment
    - Patients whose sport or occupation requires shoulder use
- Return to work and sports can occur once the patient has full pain free range of motion of the shoulder and near symmetric strength.

Complications

- Development of adhesive capsulitis
- Missed work or sports activity

Pediatric Considerations

- Rotator cuff tears are rare in children, when they do occur, they are usually small and partial thickness.
- Mechanism of injury is usually a sudden forceful elevation of the arm against resistance.
  - Examples include heavy lifting or a direct fall on the shoulder.
  - Injuries are often associated with shoulder instability or impingement.
- Pediatric patients will typically present with sudden onset of anterolateral shoulder pain that worsens with continued activity or sports.
- Physical exam findings are similar to those in adults.
- Ultrasound and magnetic resonance imaging are both useful if advanced imaging is required to evaluate for rotator cuff tear and magnetic resonance arthrogram can be utilized for imaging a suspected labral tear.
- Treatment should follow that for adults.
  - Surgical intervention is the last treatment option and most patients respond well to conservative treatment.

Pearls and Pitfalls

- Rotator cuff tendinopathy encompasses a broad range of diseases.
- Tendinopathy refers to the clinical presentation of a symptomatic tendon and is thought to represent more of a degenerative process than an inflammatory one.
- Cervical pathology should be considered in the differential diagnosis.
- Patients with rotator cuff tear will often demonstrate painful arc and may have positive *drop arm test* and weakness with external rotation.
- Certain abnormal X-ray findings can be associated with rotator cuff tendinopathy or tear.
- Ultrasound and MRI are useful tests in making a diagnosis and are commonly used outside of the ED.
- Sling use should be avoided to reduce the risk of developing frozen shoulder.
- Conservative treatment is generally indicated but most patients with acute full thickness rotator cuff tears will require early orthopedic surgery evaluation.[27]

Frozen shoulder

General Description

- Adhesive capsulitis is a disease of variable severity signified by shoulder pain and gradual limitation of active and passive range of motion in the absence of significant radiographic findings.
- Frozen shoulder is also commonly called adhesive capsulitis, painful stiff shoulder, and periarthritis.
- The condition is thought to affect 2–5 percent of the population and occurs most commonly in patients in their 50s and 60s.
- Frozen shoulder usually occurs unilaterally and the disease process is typically self-limited lasting 2–3 years.[28]

Mechanism

- Frozen shoulder can be primary (idiopathic) or associated with other diseases including diabetes, thyroid disorders, prolonged immobilization, stroke, autoimmune disease, Parkinson disease, and antiretroviral therapy.
- More often, frozen shoulder develops secondary to shoulder injury including rotator cuff tear, proximal humerus fractures, shoulder surgery, cardiac surgery, and neurosurgery.
- The pathophysiology of frozen shoulder is poorly understood.

- It is thought that inflammation occurs initially with subsequent development of adhesions and fibrosis of the synovial lining.
- Thickening and contraction of the glenohumeral joint capsule and surrounding collagenous tissue reduces the joint volume.
- In stroke patients, stiffness can result from muscle spasticity and glenohumeral subluxation.

Presentation

- Patients can present with complaints of atraumatic severe or nagging shoulder pain, night pain, progressive stiffness, and restriction in range of motion.
- Patients will often note limitation with reaching and rotation of the shoulder and will have difficulty with work activities, activities of daily living, and sports and recreational activity.
- Frozen shoulder progresses through three clinical phases.
- This freezing, or first phase, usually lasts 2–9 months and is characterized by generalized severe shoulder pain that is usually worse at night and increasing stiffness.
- The second, frozen, phase typically lasts 4–12 months and patients will note less pain but will have stiffness and severe loss of range of motion.
- The third, recovery or thawing phase, is signified by gradual return of range of motion and usually takes 5–24 months to conclude.

Physical Exam

- A complete shoulder examination in patients with frozen shoulder is difficult due to pain and stiffness.
- Significantly reduced active and passive range of motion will be present.
- There is usually a clear endpoint with range of motion and this is typically painful.
- External rotation and abduction are the most commonly restricted motions but patients will often also have difficulty with internal rotation.
- A diagnostic lidocaine injection in the subacromial bursa can help to differentiate frozen shoulder from other conditions like bursitis or tendinopathy.
  - Patients with frozen shoulder will still have painful restricted range of motion following the injection while patients with other conditions will usually have decreased pain and improved range of motion.

Essential Diagnostics

- Radiographs are necessary to exclude other pathology such as glenohumeral osteoarthritis.
- AP, true AP (Grashey), Y, and axillary views should be obtained.
- Shoulder x-rays are usually normal in patients with frozen shoulder.
- Osteopenia may be present in some cases.
- Advanced imaging is not usually indicated in the ED.
- Ultrasound can be a useful test to exclude rotator cuff and bursal pathology.
- MRI and MR arthrogram can be useful in the outpatient setting.

ED Treatment

- Treatment strategies in the ED should be focused on pain control and patient education.
- Patients should be counseled on an early range of motion program and the importance of follow-up.
- Patients with frozen shoulder should not be immobilized.
- Outpatient treatments include physical therapy, intra-articular glenohumeral glucocorticoid injection, capsular hydrodilatation, and manipulation under anesthesia, as well as other surgical options.

Disposition

- Patients with frozen shoulder can be discharged from the ED.
- NSAIDS, acetaminophen, and ice can be effective for outpatient pain control. Opiate analgesics may be necessary, particularly in the freezing stage.
- Patients diagnosed with frozen shoulder do not require orthopedic surgery consultation in the ED.
- Routine outpatient follow-up with an orthopedic or sports medicine provider is recommended.
- Patients may need work and lifting restrictions depending on their occupation or recreational activities.

Complications

- Prolonged pain and stiffness

Pediatric Considerations

- Frozen shoulder does not affect the pediatric population and to our knowledge, no cases have been reported.[29]

Pearls and Pitfalls

- The hallmark of frozen shoulder is painful restricted active and passive range of motion in the absence of other pathology.
- Frozen shoulder is associated with many diseases including diabetes and thyroid disorders.
- Prolonged shoulder immobilization is a risk factor for developing frozen shoulder.
- Physical exam is often limited due to pain and stiffness.
- Diagnostic subacromial lidocaine injection can be a useful test.
- X-ray imaging is useful to exclude other pathology.
- Advanced imaging is not indicated in the ED.
- ED treatment strategies should be focused on pain control, initiating early range of motion and patient education.

Proximal Biceps Tendinopathy and Tear

General Description

- Biceps tendinopathy and tear can be a source of anterior shoulder pain and is generally attributed to injury to the proximal long head of the biceps tendon.
- The musculotendinous junction is subject to overuse injury.
- Biceps tendinopathy is commonly associated with rotator cuff pathology.
- Distal biceps tendon tear is discussed separately in the elbow chapter.

Mechanism

- Biceps tendinopathy can result from both acute and chronic injury.
    - Overload of the tendon can cause microtearing and acute inflammatory changes seen in tendinitis.
    - Chronic degenerative changes can occur in the biceps tendon without evidence of inflammation.
    - Tenosynovitis can occur from direct injury to the tendon as it rubs over a bony prominence causing inflammation of the paratendon or tendon sheath.
    - Tendon subluxation or dislocation from the bicipital groove can also occur.
- Partial and complete tendon tear can occur from acute trauma and chronic degeneration.

Presentation

- Patients will note pain in the bicipital groove at the anterior shoulder. Pain may radiate toward the elbow.
- Patients will note worsening of the pain with initiation of activity, and particularly with shoulder and elbow flexion and forearm supination.
- Night pain can be present.
- Patients with biceps tendon rupture may note a tearing sensation that occurs with lifting.
    - They may also complain of biceps muscle deformity and bruising.

Physical Exam

- Inspection can reveal significant ecchymosis in patients with biceps tendon tear. This can be seen over the proximal arm and can extend to the elbow.
    - Patient with biceps tendon tear can have a *Popeye sign* where there is obvious deformity of the biceps muscle and balling up of the biceps muscle in the arm as a result of the tendon tear.
- In patients with biceps tendinopathy, palpation can elicit tenderness in the bicipital groove.
- *Speed's test* can be positive in patients with biceps tendinopathy.

Essential Diagnostics

- A shoulder radiograph series is not directly indicated for diagnosis of biceps tendinopathy or tear.
    - X-ray can be useful to exclude other shoulder pathology.
    - Calcification of the biceps tendon can be noted on plain radiography.
- Ultrasound can be used to evaluate dynamic biceps tendon function and to assess for tears; however, this is not commonly employed in the ED.

- MRI is not indicated in the ED but can be useful in the outpatient setting for visualizing biceps tendon pathology.

ED Treatment

- Patients diagnosed with biceps tendinopathy can be treated conservatively.
  - NSAIDs are first line treatment for pain control.
  - Cold therapy can be an effective adjunct for analgesia.
  - Patients should be counseled on avoidance of heavy lifting and overhead activities. Work and sports restrictions may be needed.
  - Immobilization is not necessary.
  - Physical therapy may be prescribed as an outpatient.
- Patients with proximal long head biceps tendon tears can be treated with a sling for comfort if needed for a few days. They should be counseled on early range of motion.
  - Strategies for pain control can follow those for tendinopathy.
  - Like those patient with biceps tendinopathy, those with tears will also require rehabilitation.
  - Surgical treatment is not usually indicated, but may be needed for athletes and manual laborers to return to their pre-injury level of function.

Disposition

- Patients with biceps tendinopathy and proximal long head tendon tears can be safely discharged from the ED.
- Orthopedic surgery consultation in the ED is not required.
- Outpatient follow-up with the patient's primary care provider or sports medicine physician can be arranged for patients with biceps tendinopathy.
- Patient with proximal biceps tendon tear should be referred for outpatient orthopedic or sports medicine evaluation within 1–2 weeks following injury.
- Return to work and sports can occur following successful rehabilitation or surgery, once the patient has no pain with lifting and normal range of motion of the elbow and shoulder.

Complications

- Recurrent shoulder pain
- Biceps rupture
- Weakness
- Maladaptive compensation strategies adopted by the patient causing other shoulder pathology

Pediatric Considerations

- These disorders are rare in the pediatric population but can occur in patients with acute trauma and in those who perform repetitive overhead activities.
- Typically no imaging is indicated. Ultrasound and MRI can be performed if needed as an outpatient.
- Treatment strategies follow those for adults.

Pearls and Pitfalls

- Biceps tendinopathy is commonly associated with rotator cuff pathology.
- The mechanism of injury includes tendinitis, chronic degeneration, tenosynovitis, tendon subluxation, dislocation, and tearing.
- *Speed's test* is a useful physical exam maneuver used when evaluating for biceps tendinopathy.
- X-ray is not indicated for diagnosis of biceps tendinopathy.
- Most patients with proximal long head biceps tendon tears can be treated conservatively without surgical intervention.[30]

Multidirectional Instability

General Description

- Multidirectional instability (MDI) is a common atraumatic shoulder condition and often occurs bilaterally.

Mechanism

- MDI is caused by general capsular laxity, altered biomechanics, and muscle activations.

Presentation

- Typical historical features include generalized shoulder pain or soreness that is exacerbated by activity and certain arm positions.
- Patients will deny dislocation but may describe episodes of subluxation or looseness.
- Symptoms are commonly present bilaterally.

- Patients with occupations or who participate in sports requiring repetitive stressful shoulder movements are at increased risk.
- Impingement symptoms may be present and may be secondary to MDI.

Physical Exam

- Hyperlaxity can be demonstrated on range of motion.
- A *load and shift test* may be positive.
    - In the load and shift test, the patient is seated with arms at their side, palms on the hips, with thumbs posterior. The examiner uses one hand to stabilize the shoulder and the other to gently translate the humeral head anteriorly. Increased movement is associated with anterior instability.
- A *sulcus sign* (Figure 1.42) may be present.
    - In this test, the patient's arm should be relaxed at their side. The examiner grasps the patient's arm at the elbow and applies traction inferiorly. A positive test is indicated by the appearance of a depression just below the patient's acromion.

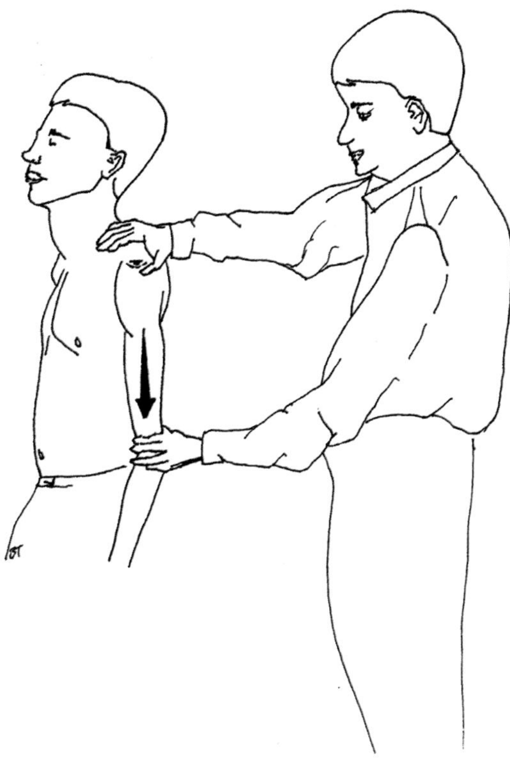

Figure 1.42. Sulcus sign.

- AP laxity may also be demonstrated by the *shoulder drawer sign*.
    - To perform this maneuver, grasp the humeral head with one hand and stabilize the clavicle and scapula with the other.
    - Push the humeral head anterior and posterior and compare the degree of translation with the contralateral shoulder.
    - Increased laxity is a positive test, up to 50 percent posterior translation can be a normal finding.
- Labral tests can also be positive (see section on labral tears) with or without true labral pathology being present.
- Additionally, apprehension testing can be positive.
    - Anterior apprehension can be demonstrated by placing the shoulder in an abducted and externally rotated position. A positive test is indicated by the patient feeling a sense of instability.
    - A similar test called the *Jobe relocation test* can be performed in the same manner as the *apprehension test* with the patient in a supine position. If anterior instability is present the patient will feel pain or a sense of instability during external rotation. The examiner will then apply a posteriorly directed force to the proximal arm, which gives the patient a sense of relief of pain or apprehension.

Essential Diagnostics

- Plain radiographs offer limited utility in the ED when evaluating for MDI.
    - X-ray can be useful to exclude other pathology.
- MRI is also generally not useful in evaluating these patients and is not needed in the ED setting.
- MR arthrography can be a useful test in the outpatient setting in evaluating these patients.
    - Typical findings include a blunted labrum, diffuse capsular laxity, and increased capsular volume.

ED Treatment

- Conservative treatment is indicated initially.
    - Patients can modify work and sports activities as needed.

- NSAIDs are first line treatment if pain is present.
- No immobilization is necessary.
- Patients will require rehabilitation and can be counseled on a shoulder strengthening and stability program.
- Surgical intervention might be considered in cases of conservative treatment failure.

Disposition

- Patients with MDI can be discharged from the ED.
- Orthopedic surgery consultation is not required in the ED.
- Patients should be referred for routine follow-up with an orthopedic or sports medicine specialist for further outpatient management.
- Return to work and sports can occur when the patient can demonstrate normal pain free range of motion.

Complications

- Complications of MDI are generally related to surgical interventions.
- Failure to recognize coexisting pathology is also a consideration.

Pediatric Considerations

- In pediatric patients, shoulder joint laxity can be part of genetic syndromes like Marfan's and Ehler–Danlos as well as systemic disorders.
- MDI is common in young female athletes.
- Patients will generally present with shoulder pain that occurs with overhead movements and weakness.
- Athletes may note decreased performance.
- Family history may be positive for shoulder laxity.
- Physical exam will reveal instability in multiple planes.
- Useful tests include the *load and shift test*, *sulcus sign*, and *relocation test.*
- Treatment follows that for adults and usually requires a prolonged course of rehabilitation.
- Pediatric patients with labral tearing or significant capsular laxity may require surgical reconstruction; however, this is uncommon.[31]

Pearls and Pitfalls

- MDI can occur from congenital laxity, repetitive trauma, or major shoulder injury.
- Symptoms of MDI can be vague and can include looseness, crepitation, and anterolateral shoulder pain.
  - Special tests include *sulcus sign* and *apprehension test.*
- Diagnosis is generally made clinically. X-ray can be useful to exclude other pathology.
- Treatment is focused on rehabilitation.
- Surgical intervention is considered for conservative treatment failure or recurrent dislocation.[32]

Superior Labrum Tears

General Description

- Superior labrum anterior posterior (SLAP) lesions are defined as labral detachment occurring posterior to the long head of the biceps tendon (LHBT) insertion and extending anteriorly.

Mechanism

- SLAP lesions are classified into four injury types.
  - Type I: Degenerative changes and fraying at the edges of the labrum
  - Type II: Degenerative changes and fraying at the edges of the labrum are present in addition to complete detachment of the labrum from the anterosuperior to the posterosuperior glenoid rim.
  - Type III: The free edge of the superior labrum is displaced into the joint (bucket-handle), while the attachment of the labrum and the biceps tendon to the glenoid rim remains intact.

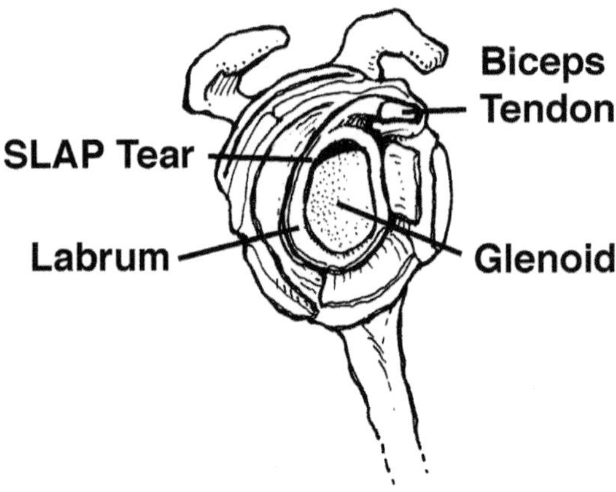

Figure 1.43. Superior labrum anterior posterior (SLAP) lesion.

- Type IV: The free edge of the superior labrum is displaced into the joint as in type III, additionally the long biceps tendon is torn in the direction of the fibers.

Presentation

- SLAP lesions can be difficult to diagnose and can occur with other shoulder conditions.
- Historical features can include traction injury, direct trauma to the shoulder and a fall on an outstretched hand.
- Athletes participating in overhead throwing sports can also develop SLAP lesions from repetitive traction forces.
- Pain can be described as deep and vague, sometimes associated with stiffness or weakness.
- Patients will often complain of nonspecific shoulder pain that occurs with overhead or cross-body activity.
- Patients may note popping, clicking or catching at the shoulder joint.
- Instability symptoms may also be present.

Physical Exam

- A thorough cervical spine and shoulder exam should be performed.
- Commonly performed maneuvers can be positive in patients with SLAP tears.
- *Speed's test* can be positive due to injury at the LHBT attachment site.
- *O'Brien's active compression test* can be used to evaluate for labral injury.
- Patients may also demonstrate a positive *Neer's* or *Hawkins–Kennedy impingement sign.*

Essential Diagnostics

- Plain radiographs offer limited utility in the ED when evaluating for MDI.
  - X-ray can be useful to exclude other pathology.
- MRI and MR arthrography can both be useful in the outpatient setting but are not indicated in the ED evaluation of suspected SLAP tears.

ED Treatment

- Acute treatment in the ED is focused on reducing pain and inflammation, restoring range of motion, and initiating an appropriate rehabilitation program.
- NSAIDs are the mainstay of treatment for pain control.
- Cold modalities can be an effective adjunct for pain control.
- Immobilization is not advised for treatment of SLAP tears.
- Rehabilitation programs should focus on normalizing range of motion, and strengthening scapulothoracic and glenohumeral muscle groups.
- Conservative treatment is not usually successful and many patients will require operative intervention for definitive treatment.

Disposition

- Patients diagnosed with SLAP tears will not require admission and can be discharged from the ED.
- Orthopedic surgery consultation in the emergency department is not indicated for SLAP lesions.
- Routine outpatient orthopedic surgery or sports medicine follow-up in 1–2 weeks is recommended.
- Return to pre-injury level of activity can take 4–6 months following surgery.

Complications

- Failure to recognize coexisting pathology
- Postoperative complications include:
  - Stiffness.
  - Persistent rotator cuff tears adjacent to surgical portal sites.
  - Articular cartilage damage.

Pediatric Considerations

- Most pediatric SLAP tears occur as a result of injury sustained during overhead sports activity.
- The mechanism, presentation, and physical exam for pediatric SLAP tears is similar to that in adults where repeated overhead movements tear or avulse the superior labrum and LHBT attachment.
- Initial treatment with NSAIDs, cold therapy, rest, and sling use is indicated.

- Surgical repair may be indicated if persistent pain and functional limitations are present.[31]

Pearls and Pitfalls

- SLAP tears can be difficult to diagnose.
- Many commonly performed physical exam maneuvers can be positive in patients with SLAP tears.
- MR arthrography can be used in the outpatient setting to confirm the diagnosis of SLAP tear.
- ED treatment is focused on limiting and managing symptoms, initiating a rehab program, and referral to an orthopedic or sports medicine specialist.[33]

Shoulder Arthritis

General Description

- When the smooth, fluid function of the glenohumeral joint is compromised, arthritis is often the result.

Mechanism

- Many types of shoulder arthritis exist.
- In osteoarthritis, progressive narrowing of the glenohumeral joint occurs.
  - Articular cartilage damage is followed by subchondral sclerosis, osteophyte formation, complete loss of cartilage, and finally bony destruction.
- AC joint osteoarthritis can also be a source of pain in patients.
- Secondary arthritis occurs as a result of trauma and is also termed "posttraumatic arthritis."
  - Trauma, fracture, and instability can all be causes.
  - Secondary arthritis is characterized by bony deformities and asymmetrical soft tissue contractures.
- Inflammatory arthritis can occur with many diseases – rheumatoid arthritis, systemic lupus erythematosus, gout, pseudogout, ankylosing spondylitis, and psoriatic arthritis.
  - All of these diseases have similar pathology. This generally starts with synovitis. Inflammatory mediators released can directly cause joint destruction. Painful joint capsule distention occurs and the patient splints the shoulder restricting motion.
  - This restricted motion leads to cartilage erosion in the center of the glenoid.
  - Additionally, marginal erosions and rotator cuff tears can occur as a result of the disease process.
- Cuff tear arthropathy occurs in elderly patients who have long standing massive rotator cuff tears.
  - This is thought to result from loss of superior stability, loss of synovial fluid and hydroxyapatite crystal deposition disease.
- Osteonecrosis, or avascular necrosis, can occur from traumatic and atraumatic causes.
  - Traumatic osteonecrosis results after the vascular supply is interrupted in patients who have 3- or 4-part fractures of the humeral head.
  - Atraumatic osteonecrosis can result from alcohol use, smoking, steroid use, metabolic conditions like Gaucher disease and gout, and hematologic diseases such as sickle cell anemia and thalassemia.
- Septic arthritis is not common in the shoulder but can occur in patients who are immunocompromised (diabetes, sickle cell anemia, human immunodeficiency virus, active chemotherapy, etc.).
  - Bacteria can be introduced following aspiration or injection of the joint.
  - Overlying cellulitis and recent surgical intervention are also known risk factors for septic arthritis.
  - Septic arthritis can result from any organism (bacterial, viral, mycobacterial, or fungal).
- Neuropathic or Charcot arthropathy can result secondarily following nerve injury from conditions such as syringomyelia, diabetes, and cervical spine pathology.

Presentation

- Osteoarthritis
  - Patients describe slowly progressive pain that is poorly localized.
  - Pain can be present at rest and becomes worse with movement and activity.

- Inflammatory arthritis.
  - Patients will note painful restriction of motion.
  - Cervical spine pain and myelopathy may be present and can complicate the picture.
  - Pain can be localized to the AC joint, subacromial bursa, and glenohumeral joint.
- Osteonecrosis.
  - Steroid use is a major risk factor for development of avascular necrosis.
- Septic arthritis.
  - Historical features include a history of intravenous drug use, recent arthrocentesis, immunocompromise, or debilitation.
- Neuropathic.
  - Patients will describe functional limitation and pain.

Physical Exam

- A thorough cervical spine and shoulder exam are required.
- Inspect for muscle wasting and asymmetry.
- Range of motion testing should assess flexion, extension, and internal and external rotation.
- Passive range of motion may be restricted.
  - Limited, painful passive range of motion should increase suspicion for septic arthritis in the right clinical context (this can also be positive in patients with adhesive capsulitis).
- Patients with osteoarthritis may have crepitus with range of motion.
- Patients with inflammatory arthritis can have a warm, swollen joint and demonstrate painful crepitus in addition to tenderness at the AC joint.

Essential Diagnostics

- Radiographic evaluation should include a true AP (Grashey), lateral and axillary views.
  - These views allow for evaluation of joint space narrowing, humeral head position, bone quality, and presence of bony defects, deformity, and osteophytes.
  - Computed tomography can be useful to evaluate the degree of osseous loss but is not necessary in the ED.

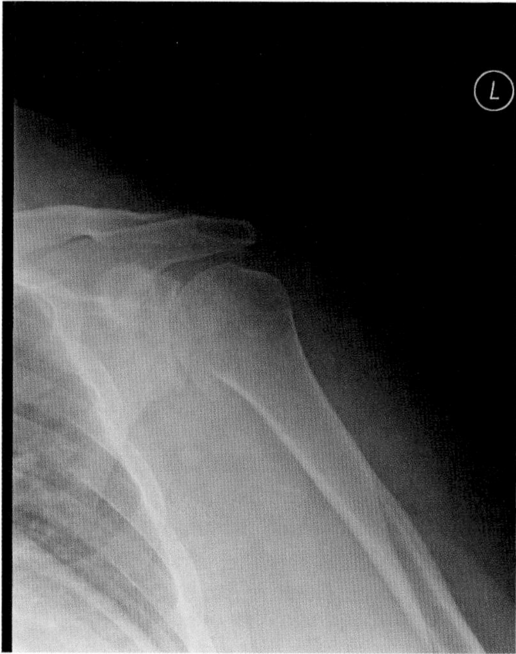

Figure 1.44. AP shoulder x-ray demonstrating degenerative changes at the AC and glenohumeral joints and humeral head osteophyte formation.

Radiographic Findings

- Osteoarthritis.
  - Joint space narrowing, osteophyte and cyst formation, and subchondral sclerosis can all be seen on x-ray (Figure 1.44).
- Inflammatory arthritis.
  - X-ray findings include osteopenia, juxta-articular erosions, symmetric joint space loss, cystic change and in severe cases central glenoid erosion, and humeral head elevation.
- Osteonecrosis.
  - Radiographs will demonstrate bony resorption, and in late stages collapse of the humeral head.
  - MRI is a sensitive test to evaluate for avascular necrosis but is not necessary to perform in the ED.
- Septic arthritis.
  - In late stages bone destruction can be seen.
  - Ultrasound can demonstrate a joint effusion and ultrasound guided diagnostic arthrocentesis can be performed.
- Neuropathic arthritis.
  - Bone destruction, soft tissue calcification, and joint subluxation can all be seen on x-ray.

Table 1.2 Radiographic findings in shoulder arthritis

Arthritis Type	Radiographic Findings
Osteoarthritis	Joint space narrowing, osteophyte and cyst formation, subchondral sclerosis
Inflammatory arthritis	Osteopenia, juxta-articular erosions, symmetric joint space loss, cystic change, central glenoid erosion and humeral head elevation in severe cases
Osteonecrosis	Bony resorption, collapse of the humeral head in late stages.
Septic arthritis	Bone destruction
Neuropathic arthritis	Bone destruction, soft tissue calcification, joint subluxation

Laboratory Evaluation

- Laboratory evaluation can be useful in diagnosing inflammatory arthritis and septic arthritis.
- Inflammatory arthritis.
  - Laboratory testing should be performed based on the suggested diagnosis.
    - Most testing not required in the ED.
  - Gout.
    - Synovial fluid analysis is the gold standard for diagnosis.
      - Demonstrates negatively birefringent needle-shaped crystals under polarized light.
      - WBC 5,000–50,000/mm^3
      - Coexisting septic arthritis should always be considered.
  - Pseudogout.
    - Synovial fluid analysis will reveal rhomboid calcium pyrophosphate crystals that are weakly birefringent.
    - As with gout, coexisting septic arthritis should be excluded.
- Septic arthritis.
  - Joint aspiration is essential for suspected septic arthritis and synovial fluid should be sent for cell count with differential, glucose, protein, crystals, gram stain, and culture.
    - Positive test indicated by
      - Positive synovial fluid culture.
      - WBC >50,000–100,000 (50–100 × 10^9/L), 75 percent PMNs.
      - Low glucose: 25–50mg/dL (1.4–2.8 mmol/L) < serum glucose.
      - Additional biomarkers such as synovial fluid lactate are being studied for use in diagnosing septic arthritis.[34]
  - Presence of crystals does not exclude septic arthritis.
  - Complete blood count can demonstrate leukocytosis, but this is not a sensitive or specific finding.
  - ESR and C-reactive protein can both be elevated in septic arthritis.
  - Blood cultures should be considered.
  - Consider Neisseria gonorrhea cultures of skin lesions, the pharynx, urethra, and cervix in suspected cases of gonococcal arthritis.
  - Additional laboratory testing may be indicated for underlying conditions (Lyme disease, tuberculosis, HIV, etc.).

ED Treatment

- ED treatment for shoulder arthritis is focused on pain control, modification and restriction of activity to avoid triggering symptoms, and initiation of gentle range of motion exercises.
- Immobilization of the shoulder is not recommended due to risk of development of adhesive capsulitis, especially in the older population.
- NSAIDs are first line of treatment for pain control.
- In shoulder osteoarthritis, intra-articular corticosteroid injection can be considered for pain control.
- Additional treatment for inflammatory arthritis is aimed at managing the underlying disease.
  - Additional medications used for treatment include salicylates, gold salts, chloroquine, corticosteroids, and methotrexate.

- Septic arthritis
  - Underlying conditions and sepsis should be treated as appropriate.
  - Orthopedic surgery consultation is required for consideration for irrigation and debridement.
    - Options include serial aspiration, arthroscopic, and open arthrotomy.
  - Intravenous antibiotic treatment for suspected septic arthritis should not be delayed.
    - Treatment should be started based on the suspected organism and local susceptibilities.

Disposition

- Patients with septic arthritis will require admission.
  - Management in the intensive care unit is required if the patient is unstable or if there is evidence of systemic spread of the infection.
- Patients with other types of shoulder arthritis can be discharged from the ED with appropriate outpatient treatment and follow-up.
- Orthopedic surgery consultation is necessary in the ED in patients with suspected septic arthritis.
  - Consultation is not required if septic arthritis is not suspected.
- For patients discharged, appropriate follow-up should be arranged.
  - Osteoarthritis, cuff tear arthropathy, osteonecrosis, and neuropathic arthritis
    - Patients can generally follow-up with their primary care provider or sports medicine physician for further management.
    - In patients where conservative treatment seems to be failing, surgical treatment options may be considered and patients can be referred to an orthopedic specialist.
      - Surgical treatment options include joint arthroplasty, debridement and synovectomy, glenoid or humeral osteotomy, arthrodesis, and resection arthroplasty.
  - Inflammatory arthritis.
    - A multidisciplinary treatment approach may be needed for patients with inflammatory arthritis.
    - Urgency of follow-up will depend on the underlying condition.
    - Patients can be referred to a Rheumatologist for outpatient evaluation ED and for coordination of care.
- Return to work and sports can occur after appropriate treatment of the underlying condition, and when the patient's pain is controlled with appropriate restrictions in place.
  - Patients may need lifting restrictions, restricted range of motion (e.g., no or limited overhead activities) and restrictions for pushing, pulling and carrying.
  - Patients undergoing shoulder arthroplasty can expect to return to light activities of daily living around 6–8 weeks following surgery, and return to less strenuous work and noncontact sports after three months.

Complications

- Worsening function with work and activities of daily living leading to permanent disability
- Failure to recognize septic arthritis can lead to sepsis and joint destruction.
- Numerous complications can occur following shoulder arthroplasty.
  - Infection
  - Glenoid loosening
  - Rotator cuff deficiency
  - Fracture
  - Thromboembolism
  - Heterotopic bone formation

Pediatric Considerations

- Juvenile idiopathic arthritis (JIA) (formerly juvenile rheumatoid arthritis) should be considered in the differential diagnosis of pediatric patients presenting with shoulder arthritis.
  - JIA is not a single disease and is classified into three main types: systemic, oligoarticular, and polyarticular.

  - A specific etiology for JIA is not known. Pathology shows chronic inflammation of the synovium with B lymphocyte invasion.
    - Macrophages and T-cells release cytokines that leads to synovial proliferation and pannus formation.
    - The thickened pannus leads to joint destruction.

General Historical Features

- Morning stiffness and daytime arthralgias
- Weight loss without diarrhea and anorexia
- Fever and chills
- Photophobia
- Preceding illness
- Absence of severe GI symptoms and very severe joint pain and fever
- Systemic onset JIA historical features
  - Short-lived linear rash on the trunk and extremities
  - Arthralgia
  - Myalgia
- Oligoarticular JIA historical features
  - Affects four or fewer joints
  - Usually larger joints
- Polyarticular JIA historical features
  - Affects five or more joints
  - Both large and small joints involved
  - Usually bilateral and symmetric
  - Severe limitations in motion

Physical Exam Findings

- General exam findings
  - Joint swelling, decreased range of motion, and pain with range of motion
  - Photophobia or synechiae
- Systemic onset JIA
  - Salmon-pink linear rash on the trunk and extremities that lasts less than 24 hours
  - Hepatomegaly
  - Splenomegaly
  - Lymphadenopathy
  - Muscle tenderness
- Oligoarticular JIA
  - Usually large weight-bearing joints like the knee and ankle are affected
  - Joint swelling, decreased range of motion, and pain with range of motion
  - Muscle atrophy
- Polyarticular JIA
  - Joint swelling, decreased range of motion, and pain with range of motion affecting both large and small joints

Diagnostic Testing

- Lab evaluation includes ESR, CBC, liver function tests, urinalysis with microscopy, antinuclear antibody, rheumatoid factor, total protein and albumin, fibrinogen, and D-dimer.
- Imaging includes x-ray, bone scan, MRI, and CT.
  - X-ray findings include cartilage loss, erosion, joint space loss, periarticular osteopenia, subluxation, sclerosis, and epiphyseal derangement.
  - Advanced imaging modalities are not routinely used in the ED.
- Echocardiography evaluates for cardiac manifestations such as pericarditis.

Diagnostic Criteria

- General criteria
  - Arthritis in one or more joints for six weeks or greater
  - Exclusion of other types of arthritis or rheumatic disease
- Systemic JIA
  - Arthritis, continuing recurrent fever of 103°F or more with or without rash or other organ involvement
- Oligoarticular JIA
  - Arthritis that involves four or fewer joints in the first six months of disease
- Polyarticular JIA
  - Arthritis that involves five or more joints in the first six months of disease
- Differential diagnosis is extensive and includes rheumatologic, infectious, hematologic, GI and orthopedic etiologies.

Treatment

- Acute treatment in the ED includes treatment for pericarditis if present, excluding infectious causes of fever and joint pain, and initiating treatment with NSAIDs for pain control.

- Chronic treatment in the outpatient setting includes physical therapy, NSAIDs, immunosuppressive agents, and TNF inhibitors.

Disposition

- Indications for admission include persistent fevers of unknown origin, severe exacerbation of disease, inability to ambulate, and pericarditis.

Follow-up

- Patients will need to follow-up with pediatric rheumatology and may require additional specialty care from pediatric orthopedic surgery, ophthalmology, hematology, and physical and occupational therapy.[35]

Pearls and Pitfalls

- Shoulder arthritis can occur at the glenohumeral or AC joint.
- Multiple etiologies for shoulder arthritis exist and include primary, secondary, inflammatory, septic and neuropathic causes, cuff tear, capsulorrhaphy arthropathy, and osteonecrosis.
- Septic arthritis is associated with significant morbidity and mortality and should be considered in the differential diagnosis for patients with atraumatic shoulder pain.
- X-ray, arthrocentesis, and laboratory evaluation can all be useful diagnostic tests to make an accurate diagnosis in the ED.
- Treatment with IV antibiotics for septic arthritis should not be delayed.
- Patients with septic arthritis will require orthopedic surgery consultation and hospital admission.

Table 1.3. Key Diagnoses, History and Physical Exam Findings, and Treatment

Diagnosis	History	Physical Exam Findings	Treatment
Anterior shoulder dislocation	Traumatic injury (sports, MVA, lightning strike, seizure), severe shoulder pain, deformity, and inability to use the arm	Loss of normal deltoid contour, decreased active and passive ROM, refusal to move the shoulder, prominent humeral head anteriorly, axillary neuropathy possible	Prompt pain control, reduction of dislocation, immobilization
Posterior shoulder dislocation	Direct trauma to the anterior shoulder, seizure, electrocution, MVA, fall on outstretched hand	Arm held adducted in internal rotation, inability to actively or passively externally rotate or abduct arm, palpable posterior fullness, prominent coracoid process	Prompt pain control, reduction of dislocation, immobilization
Inferior shoulder dislocation	Obvious visual dislocation (arm overhead), severe pain, inability to move the shoulder	Shoulder locked in abduction with arm held against or behind head, humeral head may be palpable along the lateral chest wall	Prompt pain control, reduction of dislocation, immobilization
AC joint injury	Traumatic injury, possible deformity, pain localized to the AC joint, arm splinted in adduction, hesitant to move shoulder	Abnormal contour, instability, bruising, swelling and tenting near the AC joint, AC joint tenderness, + crossover test	Pain management as necessary. Type I: Sling for comfort; Type II: Sling up to 2 weeks; Type III: Sling until follow-up; Type IV: Reducible – treat as type III

Table 1.3. *(cont.)*

Diagnosis	History	Physical Exam Findings	Treatment
			or consult orthopedic surgery for reduction and repair; Type V: consult orthopedic surgery for ORIF; Type VI: Reducible – treat as Type III otherwise consult orthopedic surgery for ORIF
SC joint injury	Traumatic injury, pain localized to the SC joint, possible deformity, dysphonia, dysphagia, dyspnea	Soft tissue swelling and tenderness at the medial clavicle, neck laterally flexed to the affected side, step-off in posterior dislocation, prominent medial head of the clavicle in anterior dislocation	Pain management as necessary. Sprain and subluxation: sling for comfort; Anterior dislocation: closed reduction if needed and sling immobilization; Posterior dislocation: closed reduction if no airway, vascular, or esophageal injury present, followed by immobilization in a figure-of-eight brace, Velpeau bandage, or sling, if co-existing injury present consult orthopedic/ thoracic surgery
Proximal humerus fracture	Traumatic injury, diffuse shoulder pain, loss of shoulder function, extremity swelling	Upper arm and shoulder swelling and ecchymosis (possibly extending to the chest, back, flank and entire extremity), arm held in adduction, patient resists movement, pseudoparalysis and axillary neuropathy possible	Pain management as necessary. Immobilization with a collar and cuff sling
Scapula fracture	Traumatic injury, pain localized to the shoulder blade	Arm held in adduction, patient resists motion (especially abduction), localized tenderness, soft tissue swelling, possible flattened appearance of the shoulder with displaced glenoid neck or acromion fracture, body fracture may mimic rotator cuff tear	Pain control as needed. Sling or sling and swath for comfort
Clavicle fracture	Shoulder pain with any movement, arm held in adduction, distal third fracture can mimic AC joint injury, proximal third fracture will have pain in SC region	Bulge at fracture site, shoulder displaced downward and inward, point tenderness at fracture site, distal third fractures will have AC joint tenderness and increased pain with cross-	Pain control as necessary. Middle third: sling, consider figure-of-eight brace for significantly displaced fractures; Distal third: Types I & III – sling for comfort, Type II – sling and swath or

Table 1.3. *(cont.)*

Diagnosis	History	Physical Exam Findings	Treatment
		body adduction, crepitus or palpable motion at the fracture site, ecchymosis and skin tenting	shoulder immobilizer; Proximal third: sling
Rotator cuff impingement	Pain over the lateral, anterior, or superior shoulder, may refer to deltoid region, gradual onset, worse with overhead activity, repetitive overhead activity	Positive Hawkins–Kennedy sign, Neer's sign, empty can test, painful arc, normal or slightly decreased strength, relief of pain following diagnostic subacromial injection	Counsel on activity modification, pain control as needed, consider starting home rehab program and subacromial injection, do not immobilize
Rotator cuff tendinopathy and tear	Shoulder pain with overhead activity, pain localized to the lateral deltoid, difficulty with activities of daily living, night pain, risk factors include: repetitive overhead activities at work or sports; anatomic variant; scapular instability and dyskinesia; older age; increased body mass index; glenoid humeral joint instability and hypermobility	Neck exam to exclude referred pain, painful arc, positive Neer's impingement and Hawkins–Kennedy signs, passive range of motion greater than active range of motion, decreased strength with rotator cuff tear, positive drop arm test, subacromial injection to differentiate tendinopathy from tear	Activity modification and avoidance of overhead activity, pain control as needed, consider initiating home rehab program, subacromial corticosteroid injection can be considered for pain control, do not immobilize
Frozen shoulder (AKA adhesive capsulitis)	Atraumatic shoulder pain, night pain, progressive stiffness and restriction in range of motion, three phases: freezing, frozen, and recovery or thawing	Exam limited by pain and stiffness, reduced active and passive range of motion with clear painful endpoint; patients will still have painful restricted range of motion following diagnostic subacromial injection	Pain control as necessary, patient education, early range of motion program, do not immobilize
Proximal biceps tendinopathy and tear	Pain over the anterior shoulder possibly radiating toward the elbow, pain worse with initiation of activity, shoulder and elbow flexion, and forearm supination, night pain; tearing sensation, muscle deformity and bruising with tear	Ecchymosis, Popeye sign, tenderness in bicipital groove, positive Speed's test	Pain control as necessary, lifting restrictions and avoidance of overhead activity, consider sling for comfort for patients with tear, sling not necessary for tendinopathy
Multidirectional instability	Generalized shoulder pain worse with activity, episodes of subluxation or loose feeling, typically bilateral, repetitive shoulder stress is a risk factor, impingement symptoms may be present	Hyperlaxity, positive load and shift test, sulcus sign, positive drawer sign, labral tests may be positive, positive anterior apprehension and Jobe relocation test	Activity modification, pain control as necessary, initiation of a home rehabilitation program, no immobilization is necessary

Table 1.3. *(cont.)*

Diagnosis	History	Physical Exam Findings	Treatment
Superior labrum tear	Traction injury, direct trauma, fall on an outstretched hand, participation in overhead throwing sports, deep vague pain, stiffness, weakness, pain reproduced with overhead and cross-body activity; popping, clicking, catching, and instability symptoms may be present	Positive Speed's test and O'Brien's active compression test, may have positive Neer's or Hawkins–Kennedy impingement sign	Pain control as necessary, immobilization is not recommended, initiation of a home rehabilitation program
Shoulder arthritis	Osteoarthritis: poorly localized, slowly progressive pain worse with movement and activity; inflammatory arthritis: pain localized to the AC joint, subacromial bursa or glenohumeral joint, painful restricted motion, possible cervical spine pain and myelopathy; osteonecrosis: history of steroid use; septic arthritis: history of intravenous drug use, recent arthrocentesis, immunocompromise. or debilitation; neuropathic: functional limitation and pain	Muscle wasting and asymmetry may be present, limitations in active and passive range of motion, crepitus in patients with osteoarthritis, warm, swollen joint, painful crepitus and tenderness at the AC joint can be present in patients with inflammatory or septic arthritis	Pain control as necessary, activity modification to avoid triggering symptoms, initiation of gentle range of motion program, immobilization not recommended, consider intra-articular corticosteroid injection for osteoarthritis; inflammatory arthritis: management of underlying disease; septic arthritis: treat underlying conditions and sepsis, irrigation and debridement, intravenous antibiotic treatment

Table 1.4. Indications for Orthopedic Surgery Consultation in the Emergency Department

Injury	Indication for Consult
Shoulder dislocation	Failed reduction, fracture-dislocation, neurologic or vascular compromise
Acromioclavicular joint injury	Type IV, V, and VI injuries
Sternoclavicular joint injury	Failed posterior dislocation reduction, neurologic or vascular compromise
Proximal humerus fracture	Open fracture, unstable fracture, fracture-dislocation, neurologic or vascular compromise
Scapula fracture	Displaced glenoid neck fracture with clavicle fracture, more than 1cm displacement or > 20° inferior angulation, glenoid fracture with more than 25% articular involvement, greater than 5 mm step-off or displaced humeral head, displaced coracoid, and acromion fractures
Clavicle fracture	Open fracture, intrathoracic injury, tenting of the skin, neurologic or vascular compromise
Septic arthritis	Suspected or confirmed

Recommended Reading

Eiff MP, Hatch R, Calmbach WL. Humerus fractures, clavicle and scapula fractures. In: *Fracture Management for Primary Care*, 3rd ed. Philadelphia: Saunders; 2011.

Della-Giustina D, Harrison B. Shoulder pain. In: Tintinalli JE, Stapczynski JS, Ma OJ, Cline DM, Cydulka RK, Meckler GD, et al., eds. *Tintinalli's Emergency Medicine: A Comprehensive Study Guide*. New York: McGraw-Hill; 2011.

Fitch RW, Kuhn JE. Intraarticular lidocaine versus intravenous procedural sedation with narcotics and benzodiazepines for reduction of the dislocated shoulder: a systematic review. *Academic Emergency Medicine*. 2008 Aug; 15(8):703–8.

Carpenter CR, Schuur JD, Everett WW, Pines JM. Evidence-based diagnostics: Adult septic arthritis. *Academic Emergency Medicine*. 2011 Aug;18(8):781–96.

References

1. Pribicevic M. The epidemiology of shoulder pain: A narrative review of the literature. In: DSG, ed. *Pain in Perspective*. InTech; 2012.
2. Ootes D, Lambers KT, Ring DC. The epidemiology of upper extremity injuries presenting to the emergency department in the United States. *Hand*. 2012 Mar;7(1):18–22. PMID: 23449400. PMCID: 3280373.
3. Buckup K. *Clinical Tests for the Musculoskeletal System: Examination, Signs, Phenomena*, 2nd ed., p. 326. Stuttgart: Thieme; 2008.
4. Marx JA, Rosen P. *Rosen's Emergency Medicine: Concepts and Clinical Practice*, 8th ed. Philadelphia: Elsevier/Saunders; 2014.
5. Riguzze C, Mantuani D, Nagdev A. How to use point-of-care ultrasound to identify shoulder dislocation, 2014 [accessed 2014 July 1]. Available from: www.acepnow.com/article/use-point-care-ultrasound-identify-shoulder-dislocation/.
6. Fitch RW, Kuhn JE. Intraarticular lidocaine versus intravenous procedural sedation with narcotics and benzodiazepines for reduction of the dislocated shoulder: a systematic review. *Academic Emergency Medicine*. 2008 Aug;15(8):703–8. PMID: 18783486.
7. Aponte E. Joint reduction, shoulder dislocation, anterior, 2013 [accessed 2014 July 1]. Available from: emedicine.medscape.com/article/109130-overview - a01.
8. Kibler WB. *American Orthopaedic Society for Sports Medicine: Orthopaedic Knowledge Update; Sports Medicine 4*, 4th ed., xvii, p. 459. Rosemont, IL: American Academy of Orthopaedic Surgeons; 2009.
9. Mudgal P, Dixon A. Lightbulb sign: shoulder dislocation [accessed 2014 July 1]. Available from: radiopaedia.org/articles/lightbulb-sign-shoulder-dislocation.
10. Mallia A. Joint reduction, shoulder dislocation, inferior, 2012 [accessed 2014 July 1]. Available from: emedicine.medscape.com/article/110422-overview - a16.
11. Petty K, Price J, Kharasch M, Novack J. Bilateral luxatioerecta: A case report. *Journal of Emergency Medicine*. 2014 Feb;46 (2):176-9. PMID: 24238597.
12. Reid D, Polson K, Johnson L. Acromioclavicular joint separations grades I–III: A review of the literature and development of best practice guidelines. *Sports Medicine*. 2012 Aug 1;42(8):681–96. PMID: 22784232.
13. Tauber M. Management of acute acromioclavicular joint dislocations: Current concepts. *Archives of Orthopaedic and Trauma Surgery*. 2013 Jul;133 (7):985–95. PMID: 23632779.
14. Rockwood CA, Green DP, Bucholz RW. *Rockwood and Green's fractures in adults*, 7th ed. Philadelphia: Wolters Kluwer Health/Lippincott Williams & Wilkins; 2010.
15. Weatherford B. Sternoclavicular dislocation, 2014 [accessed 2014 July 1]. Available from: www.orthobullets.com/trauma/1009/sternoclavicular-dislocation.
16. Cadogan M. Sternoclavicular joint dislocation, 2010 [accessed 2014 July 1]. Available from: lifeinthefastlane.com/sternoclavicular-joint-dislocation.
17. Lee JT, Nasreddine AY, Black EM, Bae DS, Kocher MS. Posterior sternoclavicular joint injuries in skeletally immature patients. *Journal of Pediatricorthopedics*. 2014 Jun;34 (4):369–75. PMID: 24172671.
18. Eiff MP, Hatch R, Calmbach WL. *Fracture Management for Primary Care*, 3rd ed., viii, p. 398. Philadelphia: Saunders; 2011.
19. Gross R. Fractures of the scapula. Pediatric Orthopaedic Society of North America, 2009 [accessed 2014 July 1]. Available from: www.posna.org/education/StudyGuide/fracturesOfTheScapula.asp.
20. van der Meijden OA, Gaskill TR, Millett PJ. Treatment of clavicle fractures: Current concepts review. *Journal of Shoulder and Elbow Surgery*. 2012 Mar;21(3):423–9. PMID: 22063756.
21. Andersen K, Jensen PO, Lauritzen J. Treatment of clavicular fractures. *Figure-of-Eight Bandage versus a Simple Sling. Actaorthopaedica*

Scandinavica. 1987 Feb;58 (1):71–4. PMID: 3554886.

22. Tallia AF, Cardone DA. Diagnostic and therapeutic injection of the shoulder region. *American Family Physician*. 2003 Mar 15;67(6):1271–8. PMID: 12674455.
23. DePalma AF. The classic loss of scapulohumeral motion (frozen shoulder). *Ann Surg*. 1952;135:193-204. *Clinical Orthopaedics and Related Research*. 2008 Mar;466 (3):552–60. PMID: 18264843. PMCID: 2505213.
24. Chang WK. Shoulder impingement syndrome. *Physical Medicine and Rehabilitation Clinics of North America*. 2004 May;15(2):493–510. PMID: 15145427.
25. Escamilla RF, Hooks TR, Wilk KE. Optimal management of shoulder impingement syndrome. *Open Access Journal of Sports Medicine*. 2014;5:13–24. PMID: 24648778. PMCID: 3945046.
26. Koh KH, Han KY, Yoon YC, Lee SW, Yoo JC. True anteroposterior (Grashey) view as a screening radiograph for further imaging study in rotator cuff tear. *Journal of Shoulder and Elbow Surgery*. 2013 Jul;22 (7):901–7. PMID: 23312822.
27. Factor D, Dale B. Current concepts of rotator cuff tendinopathy. *International Journal of Sports Physical Therapy*. 2014 Apr;9(2):274–88. PMID: 24790788. PMCID: 4004132.
28. Prestgaard T. *Frozen shoulder (adhesive capsulitis)*. Waltham, MA: UpToDate.
29. Modesto C, Crespo E, Villas C, Aquerreta D. Adhesive capsulitis: Is it possible in childhood? *Scandinavian Journal of Rheumatology*. 1995;24(4):255–6. PMID: 7481593.
30. Gonzalez P, Sigmon C, Sullivan W, Sequeira K, Potter P. Biceps tendinopathy, 2013 [accessed 2014 July 1]. Available from: emedicine.medscape.com/article/327227-overview.
31. Patel DR, Greydanus DE, Baker RJ. *Pediatric Practice: Sports Medicine, xiii, p. 534*. New York: McGraw-Hill Medical; 2009.
32. Wnorowski D. Multidirectional glenohumeral instability treatment and management, 2014 [accessed 2014 July 1]. Available from: emedicine. medscape.com/article/1262368-treatment – a17.
33. Williams R, Petrigliano F. Superior labrum lesions, 2013 [accessed 2014 July 1]. Available from: emedicine.medscape. com/article/92512-overview.
34. Carpenter CR, Schuur JD, Everett WW, Pines JM. Evidence-based diagnostics: Adult septic arthritis. *Academic Emergency Medicine*. 2011 Aug;18 (8):781–96. PMID: 21843213. PMCID: 3229263.
35. Prince FH, Otten MH, van Suijlekom-Smit LW. Diagnosis and management of juvenile idiopathic arthritis. *British Medical Journal*. 2010;341:c6434. PMID: 21131338.
36. Della-Giustina D, Harrison B. Shoulder pain. In: Tintinalli JE, Stapczynski JS, Ma OJ, Cline DM, Cydulka RK, Meckler GD, et al., eds. *Tintinalli's Emergency Medicine: A Comprehensive Study Guide*. New York: McGraw-Hill; 2011.

Elbow

Christopher Hogrefe, Ross Mathiasen, and Timothy W. Thomsen

Background/Epidemiology

- The elbow is a relatively complex hinge joint that permits not only flexion and extension but also supination and pronation (Figure 2.1).
  - It is this combination of movements/articulations that can lead to instability of the elbow.
- An estimated 15% of ED visits for upper extremity musculoskeletal injuries involve the elbow/forearm.[1]
- The underlying mechanisms contributing to elbow injuries are varied, although certain mechanisms are more common.
  - Falls on outstretched hands (FOOSH)
  - Motor vehicle collision
  - Specific sports-related activities
    - Baseball pitching/throwing
    - Football passing
    - Tennis serving
    - Volleyball spiking

Figure 2.1. A human cadaver elbow.

- The incidence of sports-related elbow injuries continues to rise.
  - This is driven by an increase in sport participation, particularly by the pediatric population.
  - Overuse and/or early sport specialization can result in acute injuries.
- Injuries to the elbow include fractures, dislocations, muscular/tendon ruptures, and other soft tissue injuries (bursitis, epicondylitis, etc.).
  - The incidence of each injury varies widely, particularly based on age (i.e., adult vs. pediatric).
- Fractures are the most common significant elbow injury presenting to the ED, regardless of age group.
  - Historically, fractures of the elbow are one of the most commonly missed fractures by ED providers evaluating plain films.
  - The miss rate is as high as the miss rate for phalanx fractures despite the fact that phalanx fractures are three times more prevalent in one study.[2]

Anatomical Considerations/Pathophysiology

Bony Anatomy

- The elbow joint itself features three bony constructs: the humerus, radius, and ulna (Figure 2.2).
- The medial and lateral epicondyles of the elbow arise from the widened distal humerus.
- The capitellum is the cartilaginous component of the distal humerus, which articulates with the radial head.
  - This junction facilitates supination and pronation of the forearm.

- The cartilaginous trochlea resides at the medial condyle articular surface of the humerus.
  - The trochlea articulates with the ulna.
  - It permits flexion and extension of the elbow.
- Of note, the radial head is angulated 15° away from the radial tuberosity by design.
  - This facilitates up to 180° of rotation of the forearm.
- The ulna features the coronoid process to articulate with the humerus and the olecranon posteriorly.
  - Disruption of the coronoid and/or the olecranon process can be problematic for maintaining elbow stability.
  - A fracture of the coronoid process without an intact radial head can result in elbow instability even with intact ligaments.

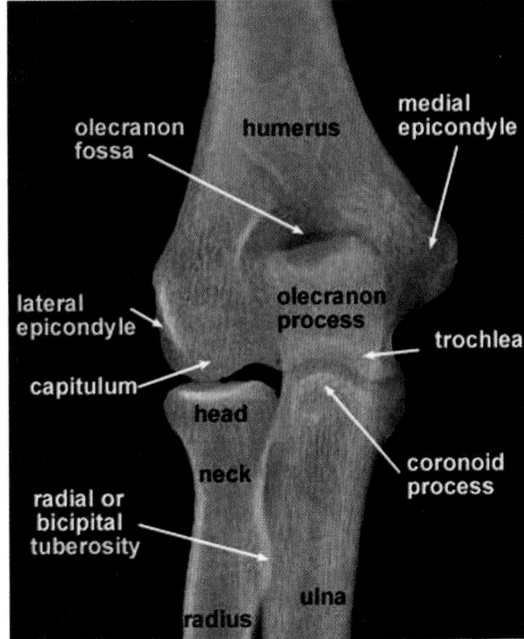

Figure 2.2. The bony anatomy of the elbow.

Muscles

- A significant number of muscles originate, insert, and/or pass through the elbow.
- Flexion of the elbow is produced by the brachialis, brachioradialis, and biceps brachii.
- Extension of the elbow is primarily performed by the triceps.
  - The anconeus, found lateral to the olecranon process, also plays a small role in extension. While trivial, some controversy exists as to whether this muscle is actually part of the triceps brachii or a posterior component of the forearm.
- Forearm pronation is performed by the pronator teres.
  - The medial epicondyle serves as the origin of this muscle.
  - The pronator quadratus also aids in pronation.
- Supination of the forearm is handled by the biceps and supinator muscles.
  - The supinator originates at the lateral epicondyle.
- The muscles that control flexion and extension of the wrist also originate at the elbow. These are listed here for completeness but discussed in more depth elsewhere.
  - The medial wrist/finger flexors, stemming from the medial epicondyle, include:
    - Flexor carpi radialis
    - Palmaris longus
    - Flexor carpi ulnaris
    - Flexor digitorum superficialis
  - Originating from the lateral epicondyle, the muscles responsible for wrist/finger extension are:
    - Extensor carpi radialis longus
    - Extensor carpi radialis brevis
    - Extensor digitorum
    - Extensor digiti minimi
    - Extensor carpi ulnaris

Ligaments

- The ulnar collateral ligament (UCL) stabilizes the elbow in the setting of valgus stress.
  - It is localized along the medial aspect of the elbow, originating at the medial epicondyle and inserting at the coronoid process.
  - This is frequently referred to as the "Tommy John" ligament, often injured due to repetitive stress from overhead throwing activities.

- Some refer to the ligament as the medial collateral ligament of the elbow.
- It is a bundled ligament with an anterior and posterior aspect.
  - The anterior bundle is tight in extension, akin to the ACL of the knee.
  - The posterior bundles are tightest in flexion.
- The UCL is maximally stressed with the elbow flexed between 30° and 120°.[3]

- The radial collateral ligament (RCL) is actually a complex of ligaments.
  - It functions to provide stability against varus stress at the elbow.
  - Primarily composed of the RCL, this complex also includes the annular ligament, accessory collateral ligament, and the lateral ulnar collateral ligament (or LUCL).
  - This ligament complex is rarely injured, particularly in athletes.
- The annular ligament supports the radioulnar joint.
  - Its flexibility permits the radius to rotate freely with forearm rotation.
  - Additionally, it is this ligament that "fails" to keep the radial head articulated in patients with a nursemaid's elbow.

Neurovascular Structures

- The median nerve (Figure 2.3) innervates virtually all of the forearm flexors.
  - It passes along the anterior elbow.
  - Covered by the bicipital aponeurosis, it passes between the pronator teres heads.
  - In the elbow, it provides sensation anteriorly and medially.
- Amongst other muscles, the radial nerve (Figure 2.3) innervates the triceps, brachioradialis, supinator, and extensors of the forearm/hand.
  - It runs between the brachialis and brachioradialis in the anterior elbow.
  - The radial nerve also provides sensation to the posterior medial elbow.
- The ulnar nerve (Figure 2.3) innervates the remaining forearm flexors.

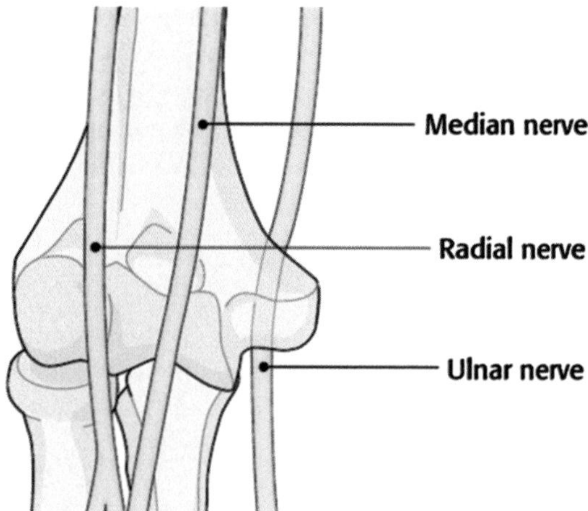

Figure 2.3 The median, radial, and ulnar nerves as they pass through the elbow. Courtesy of the AO Foundation.

  - Specifically, it innervates the flexor carpi ulnaris and the flexor digitorum profundus.
  - The ulnar nerve passes the posterior medial epicondyle and runs through the cubital tunnel.
  - It has no sensory role at/near the elbow.
- The brachial artery courses though the anterior elbow as well, medial to the distal biceps tendon.
  - It runs along the course of the median nerve in the elbow.
  - The brachial artery bifurcates in the cubital fossa to form the radial artery (lateral aspect) and ulnar artery (medial aspect) in the forearm.

Focused Physical Examination

Visual Inspection

- Appreciate any gross visual deformities, such as:
  - Erythema
  - Ecchymosis
  - Swelling (diffuse or focal)
  - Atrophy
- The carrying angle of the arm should be noted.
  - It is the bisection of a line drawn down the humerus and a line that runs along the mid-forearm.
  - The normal carrying angle varies but is generally between 5–15°.[4]

  - This must be assessed with the elbow in extension.
  - An increased angle (cubitus valgus) suggests a lateral epicondyle fracture.
  - A decreased angle (cubitus varus) may indicate a supracondylar fracture.
- Pay attention to the patent's position of comfort (e.g., flexed and abducted).
  - An elbow joint holds the greatest volume at 45° of flexion; holding it in this position may indicate a joint effusion.[5]

Palpation

- The key elbow structures to palpate include:
  - Distal humerus
  - Medial epicondyle
  - Lateral epicondyle
  - Olecranon/olecranon bursa
  - Radial head
  - Distal biceps tendon
  - Distal triceps tendon

Range of Motion

- The flexion/extension arc of motion of the elbow is roughly 0–140° degrees.
  - Some overhead athletes (e.g., baseball pitchers) may have a flexion contracture of up to 10° in the dominant upper extremity.[6]
  - Gymnasts, conversely, may have motion that exceeds these limits.
  - Those with significant muscle mass (football lineman, body builders, etc.) may have generally decreased motion.
- Supination and pronation should allow for 180° of motion at the elbow.
  - This motion should be assessed with the patient's elbow flexed to 90° and held at the waist.
  - Start with the thumb pointed upward.
    - Rotation of the palm to face upward is supination.
    - Rotation of the palm to face downward is pronation.
  - Measure the full distance of the arc, noting which direction of the rotation may be lacking.
  - Utilize the contralateral side if necessary to compare the arc of supination/pronation.

Neurovascular Examination

- Sensation about the elbow is supplied by four different nerves (Figure 2.4).
  - The lateral distal humerus down to the level of the elbow is supplied by C5 (axillary nerve).
  - The lateral forearm is supplied by C6, which is a branch of the musculocutaneous nerve.
  - Sensation of the medial forearm is provided by the medial antebrachial cutaneous nerve (C8).
  - T1 produces the brachial cutaneous nerve, providing sensation to the distal, medial humerus region.
- Injury to the median, radial, and/or ulnar nerves may be assessed via a thorough evaluation of the sensation of the hand, which is discussed elsewhere in this text.
- The brachial artery is the primary artery passing through the elbow.
  - It can be assessed with palpation medial to the distal biceps tendon.
- There are three primary reflexes to evaluate at or near the elbow.
  - For each test, position the patient's arm flexed to roughly 70° and support the arm with your own extremity.
  - Biceps reflex (C5): Place your thumb over the distal biceps tendon and strike the thumb to elicit the biceps reflex.
  - Brachioradialis reflex (C6): Strike the distal radius near the insertion of the brachioradialis muscle and look for a radial jerk.
  - Triceps reflex (C7): Encourage the patient to relax the arm and tap the triceps tendon over the olecranon fossa.

Special Tests

- The *Hook test* evaluates for a ruptured distal biceps tendon. (Figure 2.5)
  - With the forearm supinated, attempt to hook the distal biceps tendon with your index finger from the lateral aspect.

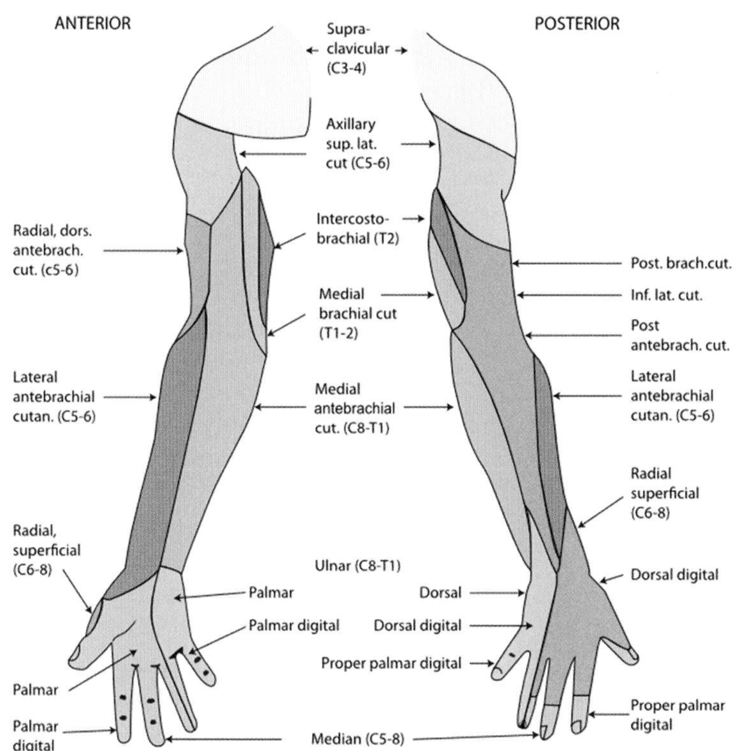

Figure 2.4. The cutaneous innervation of the upper extremity.

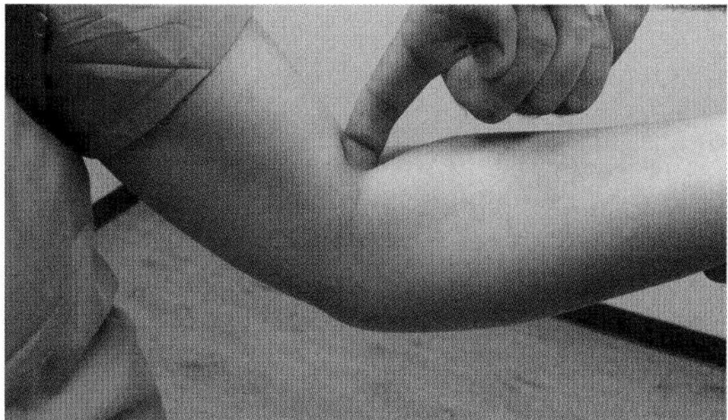

Figure 2.5. A negative hook test.

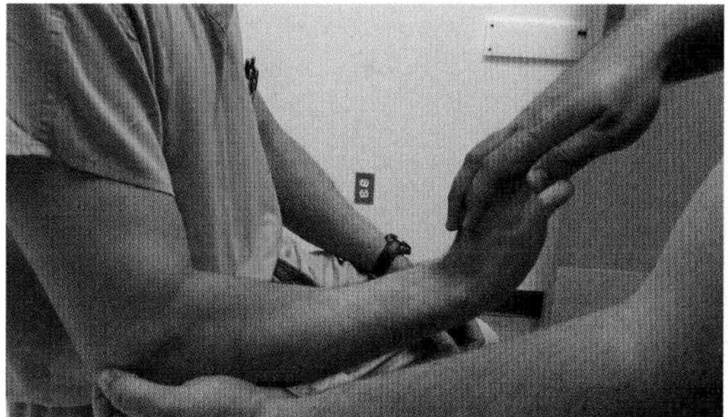

Figure 2.6. Cozen's test.

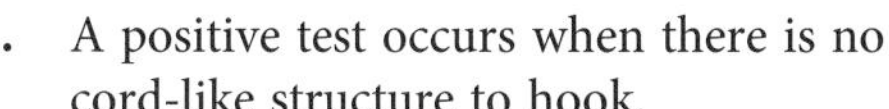

- A positive test occurs when there is no cord-like structure to hook.
- The sensitivity and specificity of this test is 100%; MRI is 92% and 85%, respectively.[7]

- *Tennis elbow test* is utilized to evaluate for lateral epicondylitis.
  - The shoulder is flexed to approximately 60° with the elbow extended, forearm pronated, and wrist extended to 30° while making a fist.
  - The examiner then applies pressure to the dorsum of the hand.
  - A positive test reproduces pain at the extensor carpi radialis brevis tendon.
- *Cozen's test* may also assess for lateral epicondylitis. (Figure 2.6)
  - Place the affected elbow in 90° of flexion with the wrist in flexion, pronation, and radial deviation.
  - The provider should place one thumb over the lateral epicondyle.
  - Ask the patient to extend the wrist against resistance.
  - A positive test reproduces pain at the lateral epicondyle.

- *Golfer's elbow test* may assist in identifying patients with medial epicondylitis.
  - The affected elbow should be slightly flexed with the forearm pronated and the fingers fully flexed.
  - With one hand palpating the medial epicondyle, passively supinate the forearm while extending the elbow and the wrist.
  - Pain at the medial epicondyle signals a positive test.
- The *modified milking maneuver* may be utilized to assess for injuries to the UCL. (Figure 2.7)
  - The forearm of the affected extremity should be supinated and the elbow flexed to 70°, which creates the valgus laxity.
  - The shoulder should be abducted and in maximum external rotation.
  - The examiner then pulls on the patient's thumb to create a valgus stress.
  - Pain, laxity, and/or apprehension about the medial elbow reflect a positive test.
- The *moving valgus stress test* may also be utilized to assess the integrity of the UCL. (Figure 2.7)
  - The shoulder should be held in 90° of both abduction and external rotation.
  - A constant valgus stress is applied to the fully flexed elbow.
  - The elbow is then extended quickly while the force is maintained.
  - A positive test occurs when pain is reproduced at the medial elbow, especially between 120° and 70°.
  - One should also assess for laxity compared to the contralateral elbow.
  - This test has been shown to have a sensitivity of 100% and a specificity of 75%.[8]
- To assess for RCL injuries, a *varus stress test* can be performed. (Figure 2.7)
  - Flex the affected elbow to approximately 20° with the forearm supinated.
  - A varus force is then applied about the elbow by holding the humerus in one

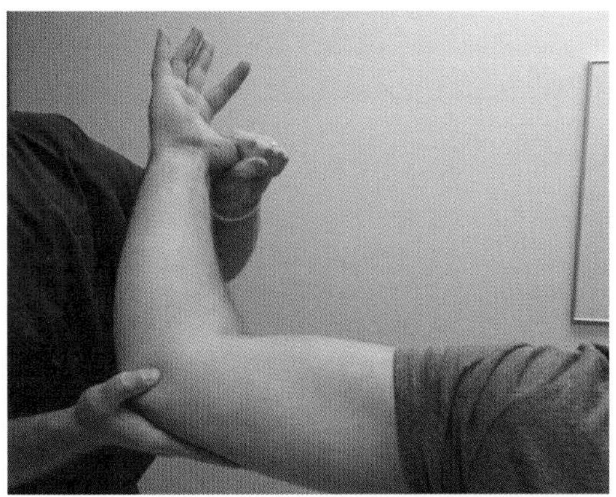

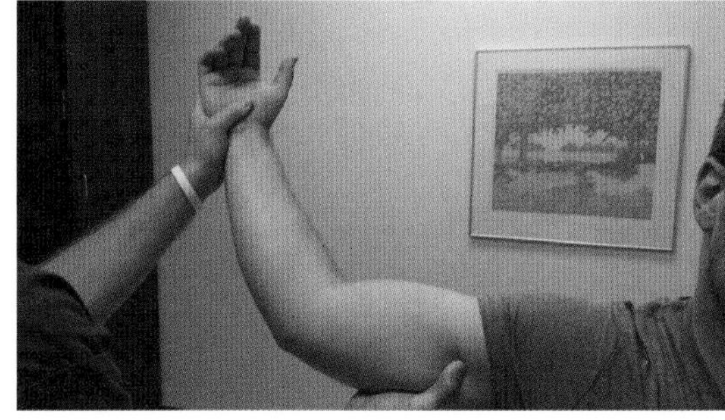

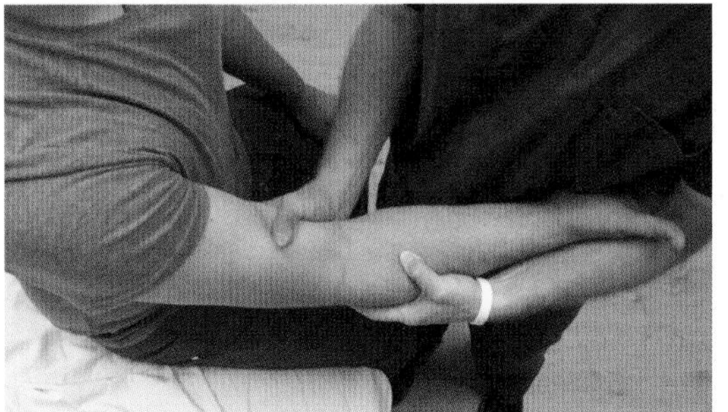

Figure 2.7. Special tests for evaluating the elbow (left to right): modified milking maneuver, moving valgus stress test, and varus stress test.

hand and the ulna in the other to create a fulcrum.
- A positive test results in pain, laxity, and/or apprehension at the lateral elbow.

Differential Diagnosis-Emergent and Common Diagnoses

Elbow Dislocations

General Description

- Elbow dislocations are defined as disruptions of the articulation of the distal humerus, proximal radius, and proximal ulna.
- The elbow is the second-most commonly dislocated major joint (after the shoulder).
  - The rate of elbow dislocation is up to 6.1 cases per 100,000 people.[9]
  - Such injuries represent 10–25% of all elbow injuries.[10]
- These injuries can occur in an anterior fashion, which is rare, or a posterior variation, which accounts for up to 90% of such injuries.[11] (Figure 2.8)

Table 2.1 Emergent and Common Diagnoses in the Emergency Department

Emergent Diagnoses	Common Diagnoses
Elbow Dislocations	Nursemaid's Elbow
Displaced Radial Head Fractures	Elbow Subluxation
Supracondylar Fractures	Occult Radial Head Fractures
Monteggia Fractures	OCD Lesion/Little Leaguer's Elbow
Septic Bursitis	Ligamentous Injuries (UCL/RCL)
Septic Arthritis	Distal Biceps Ruptures
Compartment Syndrome	Distal Triceps Ruptures
	Lateral/Medial Epicondylitis
	Cubital Tunnel Syndrome
	Pronator Syndrome
	Olecranon Bursitis
	Gout/Pseudogout

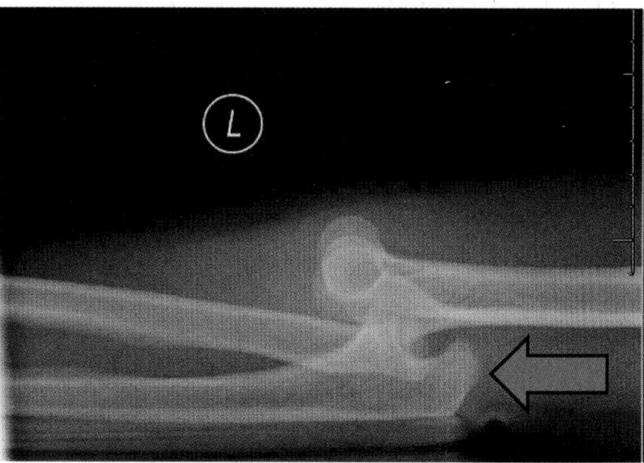

Figure 2.8. Posterior dislocation of the elbow without any associated fractures.

  - Some further divide the dislocations into simple (soft tissue involvement only) vs. complex (associated with a fracture).

Mechanism

- Most commonly, elbow dislocations are the result of a fall on an outstretched hand (FOOSH) injury, which results in a posterior dislocation.
  - Anterior dislocations can be caused by trauma to the flexed posterior elbow.
  - Medial and lateral dislocations can occur, but they are exceedingly rare.
- Inquire about sports participation, as it has been reported that 44.5% of elbow dislocations are sports-related.[12]
  - One study reports a higher incidence in football, rugby, roller skating, ice skating, skateboarding, and wrestling.[12]
- Falls, even from standing, and/or motor vehicle collisions may result in elbow dislocations.
  - Falls have been attributed to greater than 80% of elbow dislocations.[13]
  - The most common location for such a fall is the home (51.5%), vs. the workplace (13.7%).[12]

Presentation

- Males are more affected than females, particularly in the 11-year-old to 20-year-old age demographic.[12,13]
  - The mean age of the presenting patient is 30.[14]

- The nondominant extremity is more commonly affected (60% vs. 40%).[15]
- Elbow dislocations may be acute or chronic (more than seven days old).
- Visual inspection often reveals a gross deformity.
- The position of comfort for the patient may provide insight into the type of dislocation.
  - A flexed elbow is indicative of a posterior elbow dislocation.
  - An extended, supinated elbow/forearm reflects an anterior elbow dislocation.

Physical Exam

- Palpation of the elbow may provide insight into the type of elbow dislocation.
  - Posterior dislocations often result in a prominent olecranon.
  - An extended forearm frequently signals an anterior dislocation.
- An elbow effusion is frequently present.
- Be sure to assess the skin thoroughly to rule out an open dislocation.
- Range of motion (ROM) is often severely limited.
- The neurovascular examination is paramount in these injuries.
  - It is important to clearly document the patient's neurovascular examination before and after reduction.
  - The most commonly injured artery is the brachial artery.
    - This injury is still exceedingly rare, with a reported incidence in one study of 0.47%.[16]
  - The median and ulnar nerves should also be carefully assessed.
    - Ulnar nerve palsies occur in 14% of elbow dislocations.[17]
    - Neuropraxia occurs in 20% of patients.[17]
      - This typically involves the anterior interosseous branch of the median nerve (thumb flexion) or the ulnar nerve.
    - Radial nerve injuries are rare.
  - Most neurologic deficits are transient.
    - Median nerve entrapment after reduction can occur, more commonly in pediatric patients.
- Consider compartment syndrome, particularly with significant antecubital fossa swelling.

Essential Diagnostics

- Anteroposterior (AP) and lateral plain films of the elbow are critical for identifying the type of dislocation and any concomitant fractures. (Figure 2.9)
  - Patients with a shallow olecranon fossa or a prominent olecranon tip are more prone to elbow dislocations.
- Post-reduction plain films (AP and lateral) are equally essential.
  - They ensure adequate alignment and evaluate for a possible iatrogenic fracture.
- In patients with complex elbow dislocations, a CT scan of the elbow is appropriate to facilitate reconstruction.
  - Discuss the necessity of this imaging with the orthopedic consultant.
- Evidence of brachial artery injury on physical examination may necessitate angiography.
  - Given the rarity of this injury, treatment (conservative vs. operative repair) is controversial.[18]

ED Treatment

- Pain control is important, but reduction does not, by definition, require analgesia.
  - These injuries may be reduced on-scene (e.g., the athletic field) without analgesia.
  - Successful reduction may prove sufficient for relieving a patient's pain.
- Procedural sedation may be necessary for complicated reductions or to achieve adequate muscle relaxation.
- Reduction is critical and should be performed as soon as possible.
  - Reduction prior to imaging in the setting of neurovascular compromise is appropriate.
- There are several described methods for reducing a posterior elbow dislocation. (2.10)
  - Supine Traction/Countertraction: Apply traction to the forearm and countertraction to the humerus while flexing and slightly supinating the elbow.
    - One may need to apply downward pressure on the forearm to free

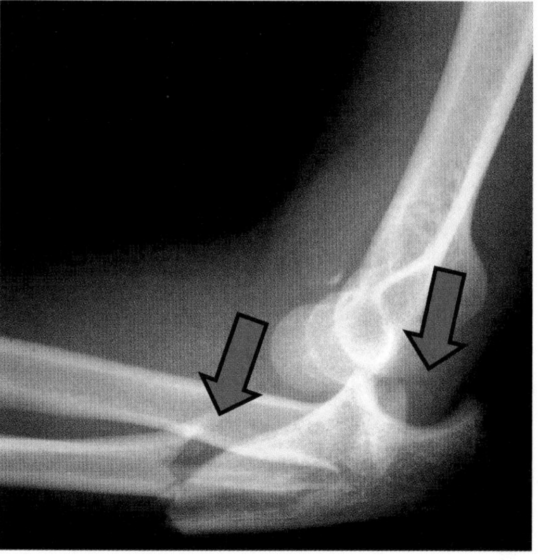

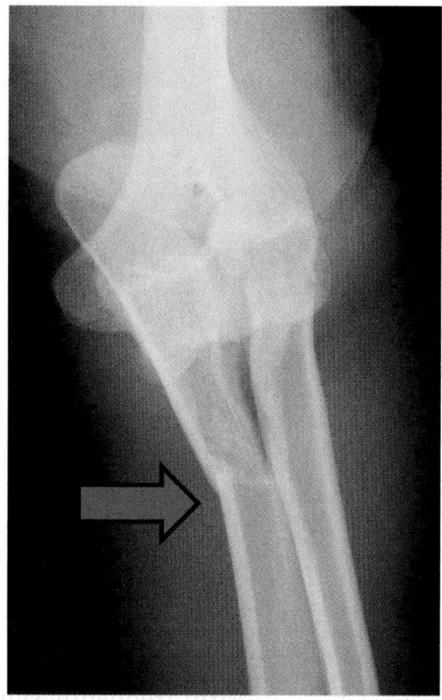

Figure 2.9. Lateral (left) and AP (right) radiographs of a complex posterior elbow dislocation with a proximal ulna fracture.

the coronoid from the olecranon fossa.

- Prone Traction: With the patient's elbow hanging off the bed/table, apply longitudinal traction to the humerus while the elbow is extended.
  - This may take several minutes to be effective.
  - One may have to manipulate the coronoid process to slide it past the trochlea.
  - Weight (5–10 pounds) may be used to apply the aforementioned traction.
- One-Person Technique: Place the patient's arm across the chest while bracing the distal upper extremity; traction is then applied longitudinally at the forearm to allow the coronoid to slide past the trochlea.

- Anterior elbow dislocations are best reduced by applying downward pressure to the forearm with concomitant anterior pressure to the distal humerus.
- Confirmation of a successful reduction should include full passive ROM and post-reduction plain films of the elbow.
  - ROM should be smooth and free of locking.
  - Perform gentle *moving valgus stress* and *varus stress testing* to ensure stability.
- The final ED treatment depends upon the patient's elbow joint stability.
  - If the joint is stable, an upper extremity sling is sufficient.
  - If the elbow feels unstable with pronation, a posterior splint with the elbow at 90° of flexion and the forearm pronated is advised.[14]
    - A hinged elbow brace locked at 90° of flexion is an appropriate alternative.
  - An unstable joint warrants an orthopedic surgery consultation in the ED.
    - A CT scan may be necessary to further evaluate the joint in advance of possible surgical stabilization.

Disposition

- In the absence of neurovascular injury, these patients may be discharged to home.
  - Some advocate a two- to four-hour observation period in the ED.[19]
- Prompt follow-up with an orthopedic surgeon or sports medicine provider is critical.
  - Ideal follow-up should occur in two to three days, at which time the posterior splint is removed and the patient's physical examination repeated.
  - Early ROM exercises and/or physical therapy will likely be recommended to

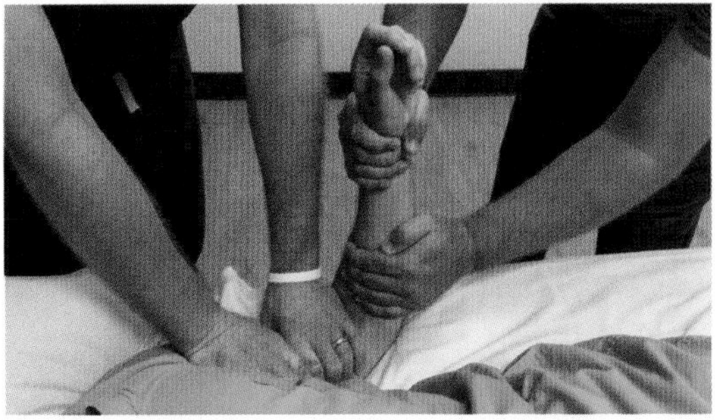

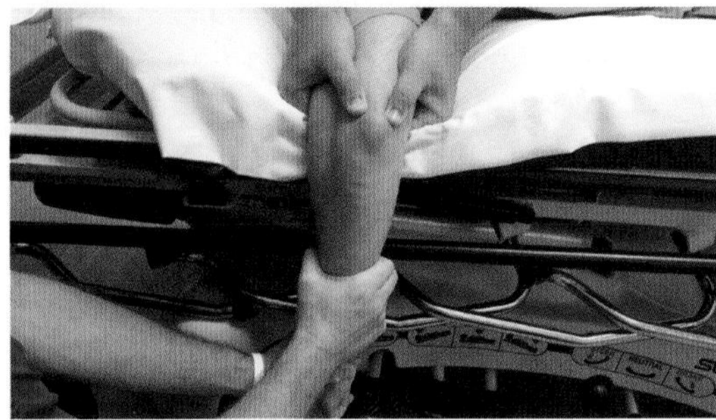

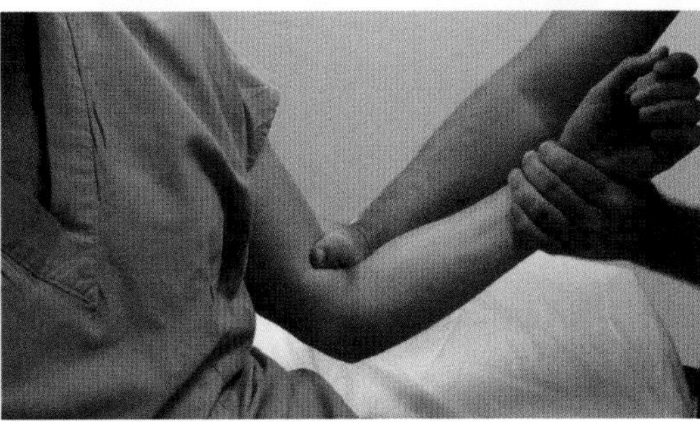

Figure 2.10. Techniques for reducing a posterior elbow dislocation. From left to right: supine traction/countertraction; prone traction; and the one-person technique.

decrease the likelihood of stiffness and/or decreased ROM.

- An inability to reduce the dislocation, neurovascular compromise, and/or concern for compartment syndrome warrant orthopedic consultation and admission.

Return to Work/Sports

- Patients should not return to activities that stress the elbow (e.g., throwing) until a follow-up appointment is completed.
- A full return to activity is typically within four to six weeks.
  - However, it may require up to three months for athletes to return to their pre-injury level of participation.[14]

Complications

- Recurrent dislocations are rare although persistent instability may be more common than previously thought.
  - 15–30% of patients may have instability symptoms (painful clicking, snapping, clunking, etc.), which are often difficult to appreciate on examination.[20]
- Heterotopic ossification has been associated with elbow dislocations.
  - This occurs at a rate of 5–18%.[21]
  - Prescribing NSAIDs at the time of discharge can reduce the possibility of developing heterotopic ossification.[22]
- Compartment syndrome is an associated complication that must be considered.

Pediatric Considerations

- Due to the relative strength of ligaments/ muscles in children compared to bone, this population has a higher prevalence of physeal injuries.
- While still rare (3%), pediatric patients are more prone to median nerve entrapment in the elbow following a dislocation reduction.[23]

Pearls and Pitfalls

- Document a thorough neurovascular examination both before and after reducing the elbow dislocation.
- Prompt reduction is essential; do not wait for an orthopedic surgeon.
- Be sure to obtain post-reduction films.
- Follow-up with an orthopedic surgeon or sports medicine provider within one week, preferably in two to three days, is essential to prevent ROM loss.

- A fixed flexion deformity will develop if a patient is immobilized for three or more weeks.[24]

Nursemaid's Elbow

General Description

- Nursemaid's elbow is defined as a subluxation of the radial head.
- These injuries occur in children ages 1–4, with the peak incidence between ages 2 and 3.[25]
  - This condition is uncommon in those older than 5 due to the development of the orbicular ligament.
  - However, it has been described in adults.
- Other colloquial synonyms for this injury include: temper tantrum elbow and Malgaigne's injury.

Mechanism

- Typically, this injury is the result of a longitudinal force applied to the forearm. (Figure 2.11)
  - This results in subluxation of the radial head and entrapment of the annular ligament in the radiocapitellar joint. (Figure 2.11)
- Subluxing the radial head requires pronation of the forearm, which places the radial head in the narrowest plane.
- Theoretically, it can occur as the result of a fall with the upper extremity trapped between the patient's trunk and the ground.

Presentation

- The left arm is more commonly affected than the right.[25]
- At least 80% of cases involve longitudinal traction of a pronated, extended forearm.[14]
- The patient will often hold the arm in slight flexion with the forearm pronated (known as the "nursemaid's position").
- A tearful child refusing to utilize the affected upper extremity is frequently observed.
- Pain in the wrist may be reported.
- Occasionally, no trauma will be noted; parents may simply report that the patient is not utilizing the upper extremity.

Physical Exam

- Careful observation can be very beneficial.
  - The patient may be playful but simply avoid the use of the affected extremity.
  - One may witness the patient utilize the shoulder, wrist, and hand without difficulty and/or pain.
- No ecchymosis and/or swelling is generally appreciated.
- Flexion and extension of the elbow may be normal; however, supination will be limited or absent.
- Careful palpation of the anterolateral radial head may reveal a subluxation.
- Be sure to evaluate the wrist and shoulder of the patient to rule out concomitant injuries.

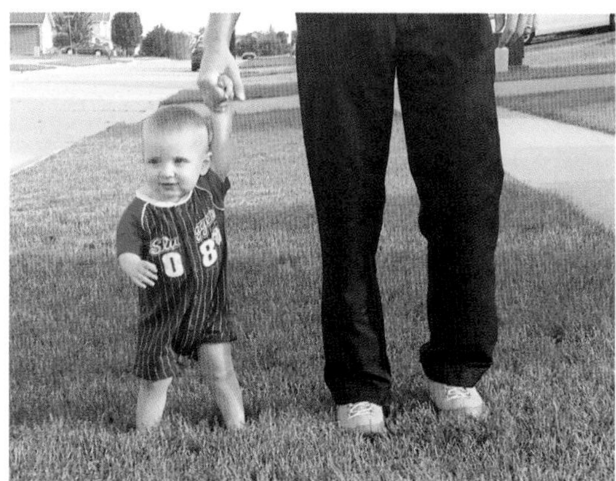

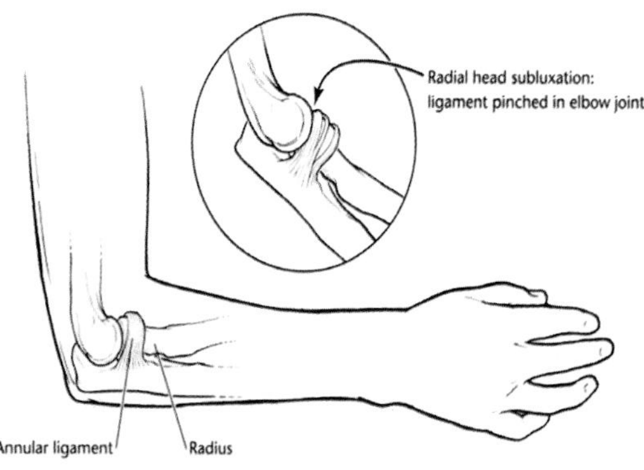

Figure 2.11. The classic mechanism precipitating nursemaid's elbow (left), resulting in subluxation of the radial head and entrapment of the annular ligament (right).

Essential Diagnostics

- Plain films of the elbow are not necessary in the proper age demographic with a classic history, as described earlier.
- In the setting of trauma, AP and lateral plain films of the elbow may be helpful to rule out a concomitant injury.

ED Treatment

- Reduction should be attempted in the ED.
- The hyperpronation technique may be more effective and less painful for reducing nursemaid's elbow.[26] (Figure 2.12)
  - Palpate the radial head.
  - Then, gently rotate the forearm into hyperpronation.
  - Slowly fully extend the elbow until maximum extension is achieved.
  - This is 95% effective, compared to 77% for the supination/flexion method.[26]
- The supination/flexion technique is also an accepted reduction method.
  - Place a thumb on the radial head.
  - With the other hand on the distal forearm, gently yet firmly fully supinate the forearm.
  - Then flex the elbow to 90° or until maximum flexion is achieved.
  - A palpable and/or audible click should be appreciated.
  - This typically results in immediate pain relief and restoration of full range of motion.
- After successful reduction, observe the patient for 15 minutes to ensure full function of the affected extremity.[26]
  - If full function has not returned, a repeated attempt at reduction is recommended.
  - The time to return of normal function may be delayed if the time to treatment is delayed.
- Reconsider the diagnosis if full function does not return after multiple reduction attempts.
  - Plain films of the elbow should be considered at that juncture.
  - If imaging is negative in the setting of failed reduction attempts, the patient should be placed in a posterior splint and follow-up with an orthopedic surgeon in twenty-four to forty-eight hours.[27]
- Post-reduction plain films are not necessary.
- Immobilization is not generally recommended following a successful reduction.

Disposition

- Formal follow-up is not generally recommended/necessary.
- Prevention is essential; counsel parents to avoid longitudinal traction in the future.
- If the patient has a history of recurrent radial head subluxations, a referral to an orthopedist (or pediatric orthopedist) is appropriate.
  - The patient may benefit from a cast for two to three weeks at that time.[28]

Complications

- There are few long-term adverse effects of nursemaid's elbow.
- The recurrence rate is 27–39%.[25,29]
- In the setting of failed reductions, be sure to consider occult fractures or cartilage injuries.

Pediatric Considerations

- Nursemaid's elbow is primarily a pediatric condition.

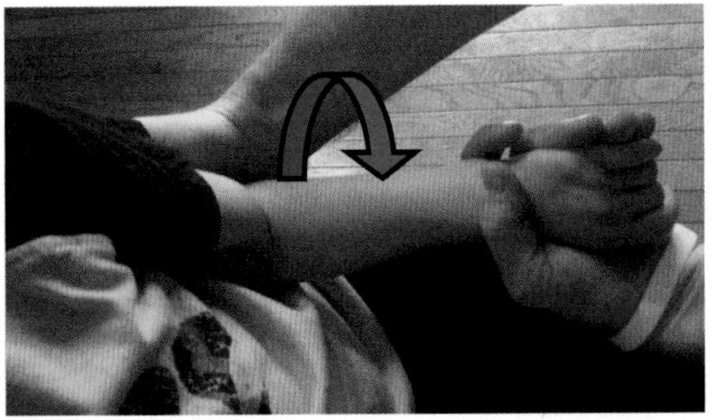

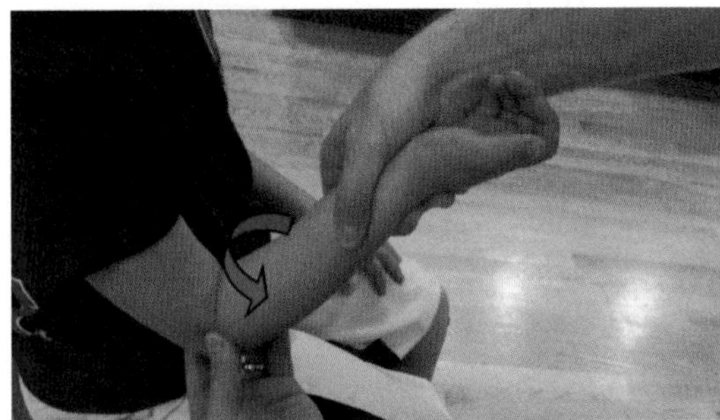

Figure 2.12. Hyperpronation reduction and supination/flexion reduction of nursemaid's elbow.

Pearls and Pitfalls

- In children less than 6 months old, consider child abuse.
- If the diagnosis is strongly suspected, try to incorporate a reduction into the physical examination to keep the patient at ease and to promptly alleviate his/her symptoms.
- Be sure to observe the patient after reduction to ensure a full return to function.

Radial Head Fractures

General Description

- Radial head fractures are the most common elbow fracture in adults, representing 30% of such fractures.[30]
  - Such fractures represent up to 5.4% of adult fractures.[31]
  - They are uncommon in children, representing only 1% of all fractures.[32]
- Most radial head fractures are not associated with concomitant injuries.
  - However, this should not preclude further evaluation based on the provider's clinical suspicion.

Mechanism

- The most common mechanism of injury is a FOOSH injury.
  - This results in a direct axial load to the elbow.
  - The forearm is usually pronated.
- A posterior lateral rotary force can cause a radial head fracture, which is often present in an elbow dislocation.
- A direct blow can also result in this type of fracture, although this mechanism is uncommon and should prompt consideration of other types of elbow fractures.

Presentation

- Be sure to elicit the specific mechanism of injury, asking specifically about a FOOSH.
- The typical presentation involves a patient holding the affected arm in abduction near the chest with the elbow flexed.
- Movement at the elbow (e.g., flexion, extension, supination, and pronation) typically aggravates the patient's pain.

Physical Exam

- Observe carefully for ecchymosis and/or swelling over the lateral elbow.
- Tenderness to palpation over the radial head (distal to the lateral epicondyle) should localize the pain.
  - Passively rotating the elbow in either direction should worsen pain.
  - Crepitance may also be present.
- Diligently observe and document the patient's ROM at the elbow (including flexion, extension, supination, and pronation).
  - Be sure to compare to the unaffected elbow, if necessary.
  - Preservation of ROM is up to 97% specific for the absence of a radial head fracture.[33]
- It is essential to palpate both the wrist and the forearm.
  - An Essex–Lopresti fracture could be present, which involves a proximal radial fracture in addition to disruption of the radioulnar joint and/or interosseous membrane. (Figure 2.13)
  - This injury results in instability of the forearm.
- Pay close attention to the stability of the UCL.
  - Perform *moving valgus stress testing* and/or the *modified milking maneuver*. (See Figure 2.7 earlier in chapter)

Essential Diagnostics

- Plain films of the elbow are critical in evaluating for this injury.
- A valid clinic decision rule (East Riding Elbow Rule, or ER2) exists to help determine if plain films are necessary.[34]
  - The absence of the following excludes an acute elbow fracture:
    - Inability to flex the elbow
    - Tenderness over the radial head, olecranon, and/or medial epicondyle
    - Presence of bruising
  - The specificity is poor (24%), but the sensitivity is 100%.
- AP and lateral radiographs are usually sufficient to make the diagnosis.

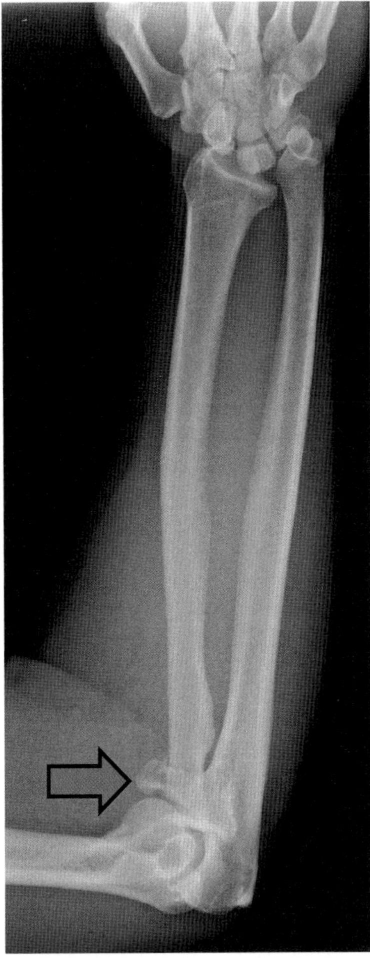

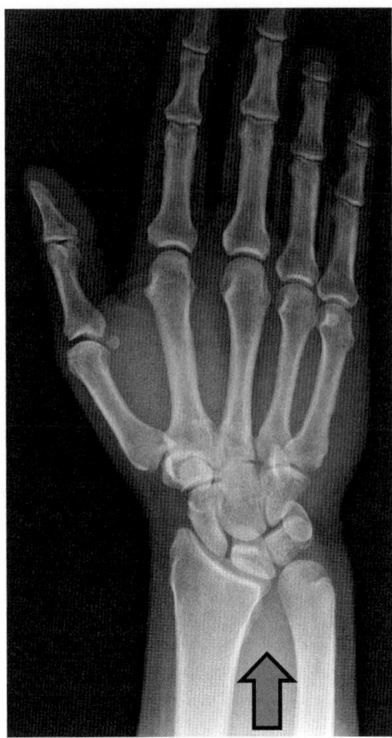

Figure 2.13 An Essex-Lopresti fracture showing a fracture of the proximal radial head (left) and disruption of the radioulnar joint (right).

  - Radial head views should be obtained if an abnormal fat pad sign (detailed next) is appreciated on standard imaging.
- Assess the plain films for the fat pad signs. (Figure 2.14)
  - Either the anterior or posterior fat pad sign can be indicative of a fracture in the absence of an obvious cortical disruption.
  - These fat pad signs are the result of a joint effusion and should be considered the result of an intra-articular fracture.
  - The anterior fat pad, also known as the "sail sign," may represent an occult fracture, especially when it is elevated and resembles a sail, but it is not always abnormal.
  - The posterior fat pad sign is always abnormal and suggests an underlying fracture.
- The Mason classification, which has been modified over time by Johnston and Morey, may help categorize these injuries based on radiographic findings and guide further management.[35]
  - Type I: A nondisplaced or minimally displaced fracture.
    - Includes less than 2-mm intra-articular displacement of the fracture.
    - The fragment size must be less than or equal to 30% of the articular surface.
  - Type II: A displaced fracture of the radial head and/or neck
    - The fracture is displaced more than 2 mm.
    - There also must be more than 30% of the articular surface visible.

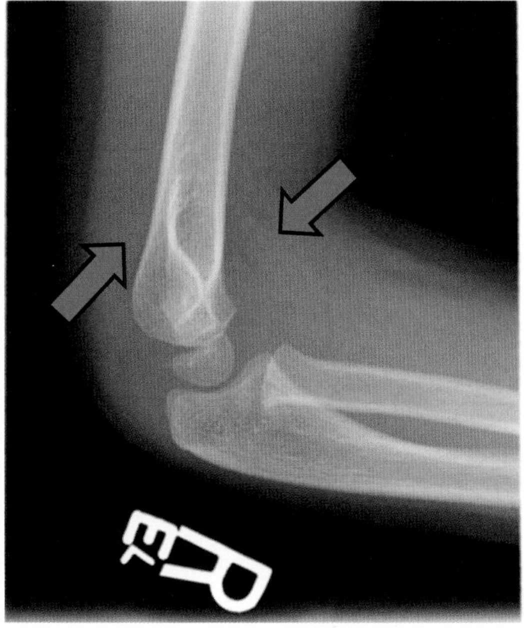

Figure 2.14. Anterior ("sail sign") and posterior fat pad signs in the setting of a radial head fracture.

- Type III: Severely comminuted fracture of the radial head and/or neck. (Figure 2.15)
- Type IV: Radial head fracture in the setting of an elbow dislocation.
  - Type IV injuries combined with a coronoid fracture result in the "terrible triad" of the elbow.

- To gain insight into the size of a fracture fragment, a CT of the elbow may be beneficial.
- Plain films of the wrist and/or forearm should be considered if clinically indicated (e.g., to evaluate for an Essex-Lopresti fracture).

ED Treatment

- Elbow aspiration may decrease pain and increase ROM. (Figure 2.16)
  - There is no benefit of anesthetic injection with aspiration vs. aspiration alone for Mason type I fractures.[36]
- Treatment in the ED should be guided by the Mason classification.
  - Type I: Treatment with a shoulder sling for up to three to four days with active ROM as soon as possible.[37]
    - These are treated nonoperatively.

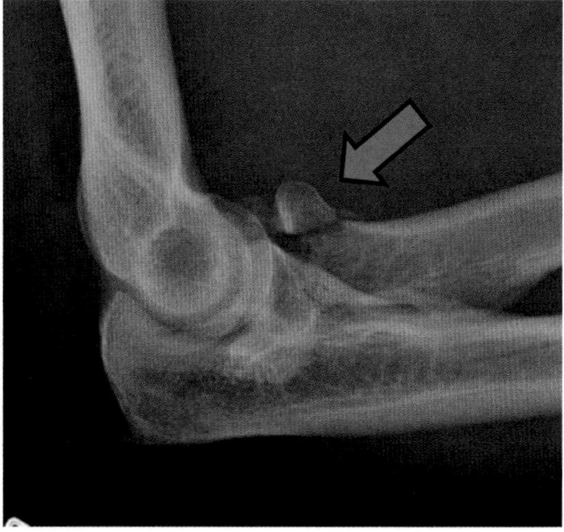

Figure 2.15. A Mason type III comminuted fracture of the radial head.

    - Advise the patient to perform ROM to the point of pain.
    - Ice, acetaminophen, and/or oral opiates are reasonable for pain control.
  - Type II: These patients can be splinted with a posterior splint if neurovascularity is otherwise intact.
    - These patients should follow-up with an orthopedic surgeon within two to three days to be assessed for surgical evaluation.
    - While controversial, the literature currently trends to favoring a surgical repair of these injuries.[38]
    - However, if no mechanical block exists, Mason type II fractures may be treated conservatively.[30]
  - Type III: Orthopedic consultation is recommended for surgical intervention (open reduction internal fixation, or ORIF, resection, or resection with arthroplasty).[39]
  - Type IV: Reduction of the dislocation is essential.
    - Treatment of the fracture will then require the assistance of an orthopedic surgeon.
    - The timing of orthopedic consultation depends on the type of fracture (Mason type II vs. Mason type III).

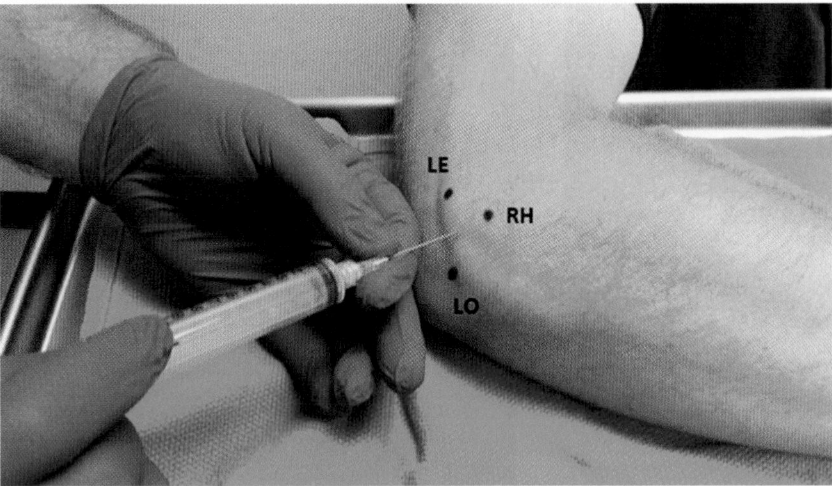

Figure 2.16. Elbow aspiration/injection technique. Place the elbow flexed at approximately 90°. Identify the three key bony landmarks: LE = Lateral Epicondyle; RH = Radial Head; LO = Lateral Olecranon. After prepping the elbow in a sterile fashion, use an 18- or 20-gauge needle to enter the elbow joint through the recess in the center of the triangle created by the noted bony landmarks.

Disposition

- Type I fractures can follow-up with a primary care or sports medicine provider in one to two weeks.
  - Be certain to counsel the patient to initiate ROM as soon as possible.
  - A subsequent referral to orthopedics can be made if a complication surfaces.
- Type II fractures should have orthopedic surgery follow-up within two to three days of presenting to the emergency department.
- Type III radial head fractures warrant orthopedic evaluation in the ED, especially in the setting of neurovascular compromise.
- Type IV: If successfully reduced, with no other fractures or ligamentous injuries present, these patients may follow-up with orthopedics within one week.
  - The rules for follow-up of these injuries plus either type II or type III fractures is noted earlier.

Complications

- Failure of the ROM to progress weekly should raise concern for an intra-articular mechanical block and warrant further investigation.
- Minimal restriction of extension, supination, and pronation should be present at six weeks following a type I injury.
- Patients may have increased cold sensitivity for one year.[40]
- Partial ulnar nerve and/or posterior interosseous nerve injuries may occur.[41]
- Long-term pain is infrequent.

Pediatric Considerations

- Occult radial head fractures (e.g., type I fractures) in children may require longer splinting/casting to protect the fracture from displacement.
- Consider imaging the contralateral side in patients whose growth plates are not fused.

Pearls and Pitfalls

- The literature suggests that normal full elbow extension, lack of radial head/olecranon/medial epicondyle tenderness, and the absence of bruising excludes fracture in the adult elbow and eliminates the need for imaging.
  - This clinical decision rule does not apply to children.
- Remember to palpate the wrist and the forearm to avoid missing concomitant injuries such as Essex–Lopresti fractures and Monteggia fractures.
- Initiate ROM in these patients as soon as can be tolerated to prevent contractures/loss of motion.

- When to intervene surgically for radial head fractures remains a controversial topic; a low threshold for contacting orthopedics is appropriate if there is concern.

Supracondylar Fractures

General Description

- Supracondylar fractures are most common in the pediatric population, with a peak age of 5–6.[42]
  - Skeletally mature patients tend to suffer more elbow dislocations and intercondylar fractures.
- Pediatric supracondylar fractures are described according to the Gartland classification.[42] (Figure 2.17)
  - Type I: Nondisplaced and typically diagnosed based upon the presence of the posterior fat pad sign
  - Type II: Partially displaced but maintaining some degree of cortical continuity
  - Type III: Fully displaced with no continuity; high frequency of neurovascular injury

Mechanism

- Supracondylar fractures typically occur from two different mechanisms: extension type (98%) and flexion type (2%).[42]
- Extension-type fractures typically occur due to a FOOSH mechanism.
  - The distal fragment is displaced posteriorly.
- Flexion-type fractures occur with a fall on a flexed elbow.
  - The distal fragment is displaced anteriorly.

Presentation

- Patients present with complaints of elbow pain and/or swelling.
- Extension-type injuries are often held in extension.
- Flexion-type injuries are frequently held in flexion.

Physical Exam

- There will be diffuse tenderness of the elbow and limited ROM.
- A thorough neurovascular exam is essential.
  - Radial nerve and anterior interosseous nerve (median) injuries are most common.
  - Assess thumb extension (radial), finger abduction (ulnar), and the ability to make OK sign (anterior interosseous branch of median).
  - Two-point discrimination of more than 6 mm is abnormal.[42]
- Assess for other ipsilateral fractures in the upper extremity.

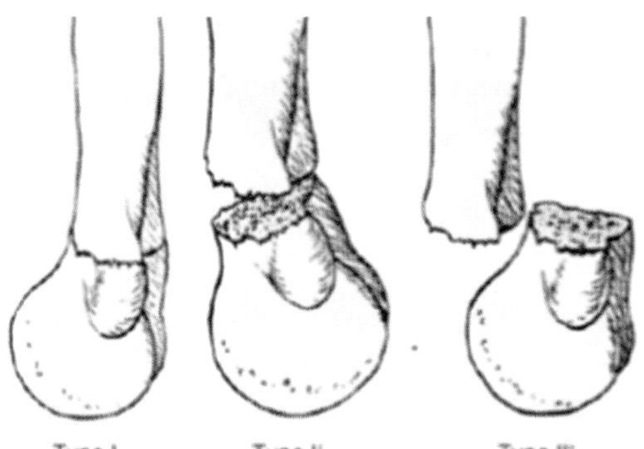

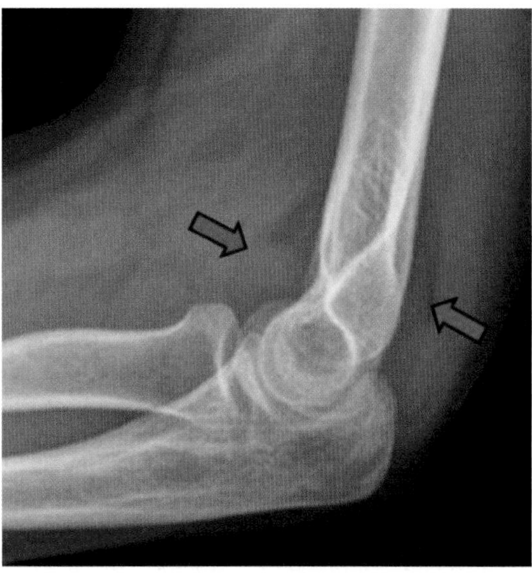

Figure 2.17. The Gartland classification of pediatric supracondylar fractures (Left) and a lateral radiograph depicting a type II injury with anterior and posterior fat pad signs (Right).

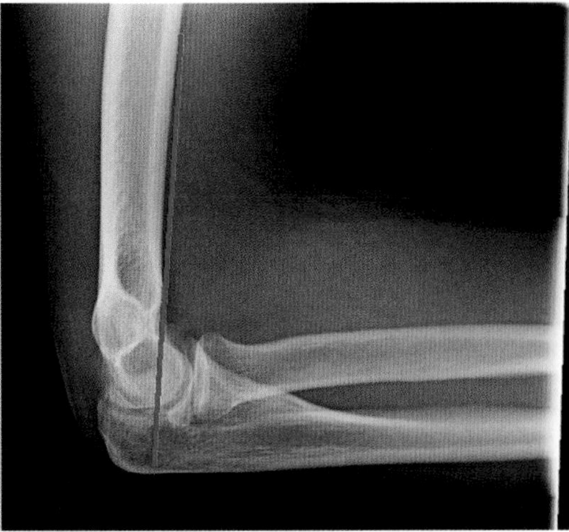

Figure 2.18. Lateral view of the elbow depicting an appropriate anterior humeral line.

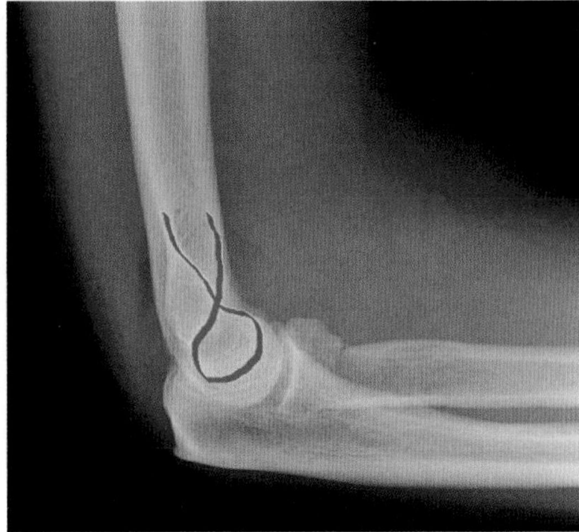

Figure 2.19. Lateral view of the elbow displaying a proper figure-of-eight (hourglass) sign.

- Evaluate for evidence of compartment syndrome.

Essential Diagnostics

- AP and lateral radiographs of the elbow should be obtained.
  - The posterior fat pad sign is much more reliable than the anterior fat pad sign.[43]
  - Obtain additional radiographs based upon concern for ipsilateral fractures of the upper extremity.
  - The anterior humeral line should pass through the middle third of the capitellum.[43] (Figure 2.18)
- Evaluate the lateral plain film for a figure–of-eight (or hourglass) sign. (Figure 2.19)
  - This shape is present in the distal humerus when a true lateral radiograph is secured.
  - Absence of this sign suggests an imperfect lateral view or a supracondylar fracture.

ED Treatment

- Type I fractures that are closed and neurologically intact should be immobilized at 60–90° of flexion in a full arm posterior splint and neutral forearm rotation.[42,43]
  - The patient needs outpatient follow-up with an orthopedic surgeon in twenty-four to forty-eight hours.
- Type II fractures are largely managed with closed reduction and percutaneous pinning, although there is some variability in practice pattern.[27,42-44]
  - Splint the fracture at 20–40° of flexion.
  - Avoiding extremes of extension/flexion helps preserve blood flow.[42]
- Type III fractures require operative fixation, usually with closed reduction and percutaneous pinning.[27,42-44]
- All open fractures and fractures associated with neurovascular compromise require emergent orthopedic consultation.

Disposition

- Closed, neurovascularly intact type I fractures can be splinted, with outpatient orthopedic follow-up in one to two days.[27,42-44]
- Type II and type III fractures need emergent orthopedic consultation and admission for monitoring of neurovascular status.[43]

Return to Work/Sports

- Due to the length of immobilization (three to six weeks), an additional four to eight weeks may be needed for ROM and strengthening exercises.[43]
- The patient may return to work at any time, depending upon the ability to perform work duties with a splinted and/or weak upper extremity.
- Physical therapy is recommended for those seeking accelerated return to work or sports, with a focus on ROM and strengthening.

Complications

- Compartment syndrome should be considered in a patient refusing to open their hand, pain with passive extension, and/or severe forearm swelling and tenderness.
- Anterior interosseous nerve (median) injury manifests as an inability to make "OK" sign (opposing distal phalanx of thumb and index finger).
- Weakness with thumb extension and/or numbness at base of thumb may reflect a radial nerve injury.
- Vascular injury (especially to the brachial artery) can lead to Volkmann's contracture (forearm muscle wasting and weakness).
- The most common long-term complication is elbow stiffness and loss of ROM.
  - A mild deficit of extension (10–15°) is common but does not typically affect function.[45]

Pediatric Considerations

- The absence of a radial pulse is common in children, likely secondary to spasm.
  - Assess for other signs of ischemia/compartment syndrome is noted earlier.
  - Reduction of the fracture usually restores the pulse; reduction should not be delayed to obtain an angiographic study.

Pearls and Pitfalls

- Supracondylar fractures may be mistaken for a posterior elbow dislocation on physical exam.
- A supracondylar fracture may be confused with lateral/medial condyle fractures and transphyseal fractures.
- When reducing the fracture avoid exaggerating the deformity to achieve anatomic alignment (e.g., applying additional valgus stress to a valgus deformity); this can result in damage to the brachial artery.
- When the posterior fat pad sign is present in an adult, the differential diagnosis should also include a radial head fracture.

Monteggia Fractures

General Description

- Monteggia fractures involve a fracture of the proximal third of the ulna with dislocation of the radial head.
- The Bado classification system (type I–IV) describes the fracture-dislocation pattern based on the direction of ulnar angulation and direction of the radial head dislocation.[46] (Figure 2.20)

Mechanism

- The injury most commonly occurs due to a FOOSH mechanism.
  - The impact hyperpronates the forearm, resulting in the defining fracture/dislocation.
  - The fracture may also occur subsequent to a direct blow to the posterior ulna.

Presentation

- Signs and presentation of a Monteggia fracture vary based upon the subtype of the lesion.
- Patients present with pain, swelling, and a possible deformity.
- Patients may complain of weakness with thumb extension and paresthesias in the radial nerve distribution due to injury to the posterior interosseous nerve.[43]

Physical Exam

- The radial head may be palpable in the antecubital fossa.
- The forearm may appear shortened.
- A thorough neurovascular exam is essential, as the radial nerve is frequently injured with these fractures.
  - Assess the sensation over dorsum of the base of the thumb and thumb extension.

Essential Diagnostics

- AP and lateral views are usually sufficient, but they must completely visualize the ulna, radius, elbow, and wrist.
- McLaughlin's line (or the radiocapitellar line) is helpful to assess for occult radial head dislocation.
  - This is a line drawn through radial shaft and head that should bisect the capitellum.[47] (Figure 2.21)
  - This line should intersect the capitellum regardless of the degree of elbow flexion or extension.
  - If the ulna fracture is angulated, the apex will point in the same direction as the radial head dislocation.[47]

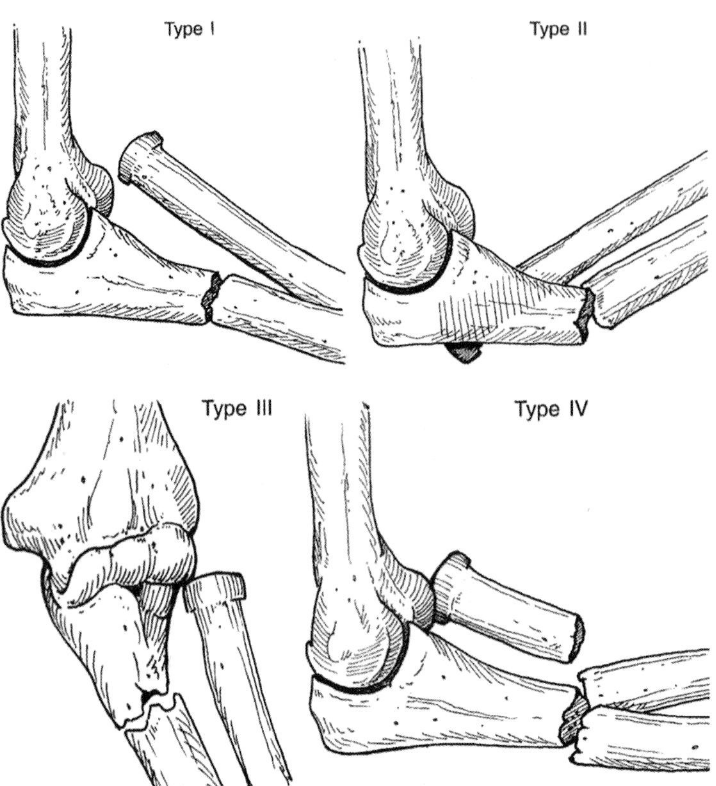

Figure 2.20. The Bado classification system for Monteggia fractures. Courtesy of Mike Cadogan.

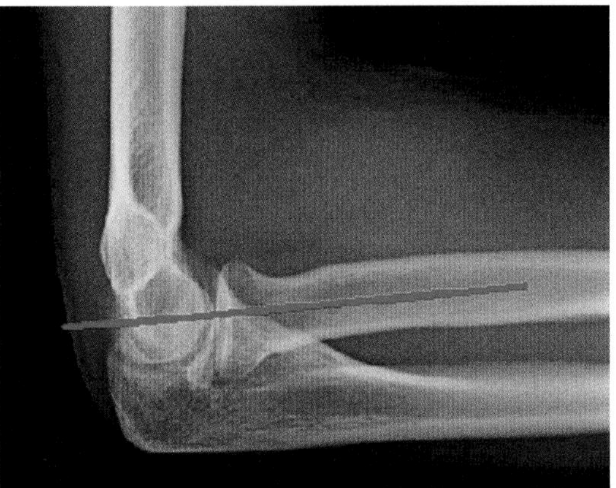

Figure 2.21. A lateral radiograph of the elbow depicting McLaughlin's line properly bisecting the capitellum.

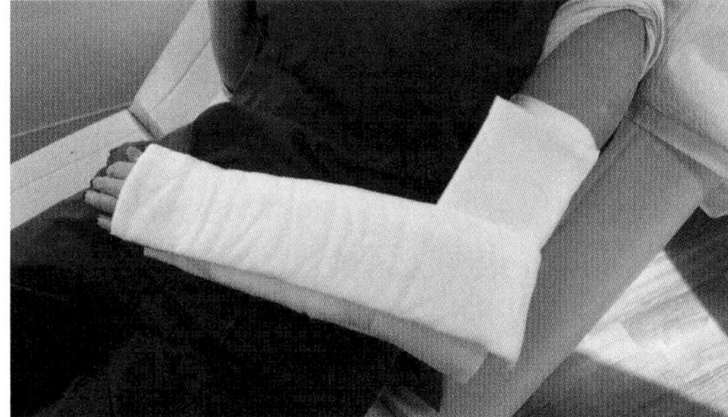

Figure 2.22: A double sugar-tong splint.

ED Treatment

- Monteggia injuries have high potential for complications and merit consultation with an orthopedic surgeon in the ED.[45,47]
  - Prompt reduction of the radial head is necessary to minimize risk of injury to the posterior interosseous nerve (radial nerve).
  - The radial head relocates as a result of reducing the ulna fracture.
- The patient should be immobilized in a double sugar-tong splint. (Figure 2.22)
  - After open reduction and internal fixation (ORIF) of the ulna, the elbow is supported with a removable splint.
  - Active ROM is initiated within the first two weeks.[48]
  - Pediatric fractures treated with closed reduction are casted for approximately six weeks.[45,47,48]

Disposition

- These patients warrant immediate consultation with an orthopedic surgeon in the ED.

Return to Work/Sports

- Return to activity can be considered when ROM is near normal and strength is 80%.[45]
  - For patients treated with ORIF, ROM is initiated within the first two weeks.
  - Full return to work/recreational activity may take up to three to four months.[49]
  - Return to play is possible in four to six months.[49]

Complications

- Radial nerve injuries are most common (posterior interosseous nerve).
- Nonunion can occur.
  - The incidence for nonunion in forearm fractures is less than 2%.[50]
  - This rate is considerably higher for Monteggia lesions, particularly type IV injuries, as compared to other forearm fractures.[50]
- Chronic radial head dislocations are more likely if the radial head dislocation is missed initially, resulting in limited pronation and supination.[45]

Pediatric Considerations

- Orthopedic consultation in the ED is paramount.
- Closed reduction is the treatment of choice for pediatric Monteggia fractures.[45,47,48]
- Consider imaging the unaffected arm if a radial head dislocation is uncertain.

Pearls and Pitfalls

- Concomitant distal forearm fractures may be missed.
- The neuropraxia of the radial nerve often improves spontaneously and does not require surgical exploration.[50]
- Prolonged immobilization increases risk of posttraumatic elbow stiffness.[50]

Little Leaguer's Elbow/Osteochondritis Dissecans (OCD) Lesions

General Description

- Elbow pain in the pediatric population (Little Leaguer's elbow) is generally caused by repetitive valgus overload.
- Little Leaguer's elbow includes: medial epicondylar avulsion, medial humeral overgrowth (when chronic), ulnar neuritis, and OCD lesions of the capitellum. (Figure 2.23)
  - In the ED, the workup and treatment of the disease processes comprising Little Leaguer's elbow is similar.
- OCD lesions entail avascular necrosis of the subchondral bone and overlying articular cartilage.[19]
  - OCD is most common in adolescent males.[19]

Mechanism

- The exact pathophysiology of OCD lesions is unknown.
- Repetitive trauma or overuse, especially through throwing, is thought to lead to microfracture and compromised circulation of the subchondral bone.
  - This causes separation of the articular surface and formation of loose bodies.

Presentation

- A skeletally immature patient with complaints that may include: [19,45]

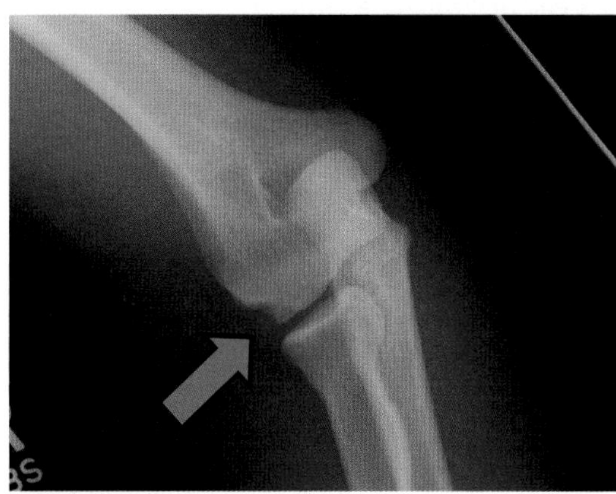

Figure 2.23. An OCD lesion of the right capitellum in a high school pitcher.

- The gradual onset of pain
  - Pain that is dull and aching
  - Loss of full elbow extension
  - Intermittent swelling
  - Decreased throwing effectiveness
  - Catching
  - Locking
  - Clicking
- There is generally a history of repetitive trauma or sports-related activities.

Physical Exam

- ROM of the elbow may be restricted, especially if a loose body is present.
- The capitellum is the most common site of involvement, and a joint effusion may be present.[19]

Essential Diagnostics

- Plain films of the elbow should include a minimum of three views (AP, lateral, and oblique). (Figure 2.24)
  - An osteochondral fragment in the joint or the lucency of the fracture may be visualized.
  - To delineate if there is a loose body present, contralateral elbow films may be obtained for comparison of the ossification centers.

ED Treatment

- Definitive management of OCD lesions is controversial and may be treated both operatively and nonoperatively.[51]
- The first line of treatment is to cease the offending activity (especially throwing) and control pain.
  - Sufficient pain control may be obtained with NSAIDs.
- Some recommend treatment by immobilization with a sling or cast.
  - However, rest and cessation of activities are the mainstays of treatment.

Disposition

- Patients with OCD and/or Little Leaguer's elbow may be safely discharged from the ED.
- Outpatient orthopedic surgery or sports medicine follow-up is indicated.

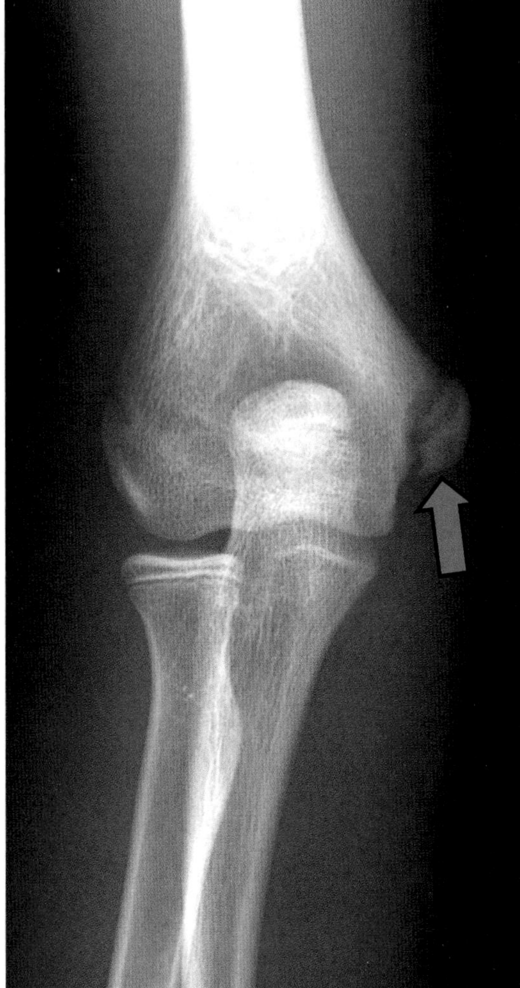

Figure 2.24. AP radiographs of a patient with Little Leaguer's elbow.

  - Such a referral is especially important in cases with loose bodies, as they may require surgical excision.
  - Many of these injuries may be treated conservatively with relative rest, pain control, and a rehabilitation program.
- The patient should not be cleared for return to sports from the ED.
  - Return to play without a brace may occur when there is resolution of the lesion by plain films or MRI.[45]
  - Return to play with a brace is appropriate when the patient has pain-free and full ROM.[45]
  - Time to radiographic healing is variable, ranging from six weeks to two years.[51]

Complications

- In cases where surgical interventions have been performed, 10–20% of athletes fail to return to sports at the pre-injury level.[45]
- Larger lesions are associated with increased risks of ongoing pain, stiffness, and arthritis.

Pediatric Considerations

- OCD and Little Leaguer's elbow are primarily disorders of the skeletally immature.

Pearls and Pitfalls

- Plain films of the elbow (and possibly the contralateral elbow) are indicated to evaluate for fractures and/or loose bodies within the joint.
- The first line of treatment is to cease the activity that causes pain (especially throwing).
- Orthopedic surgery or sports medicine outpatient referral is indicated in all cases.

Ligamentous Injuries (UCL/RCL)

General Description

- Valgus instability is caused by disruption of the medial collateral ligament complex (also referred to as the UCL complex or the "Tommy John" ligament).
- The lateral ligament complex (also referred to as the RCL complex) prevents rotational instability between the distal humerus and the proximal radius and ulna.
- Medial ligamentous instability is much more common than lateral instability.[52]

Mechanism

- Valgus instability
  - Chronic instability commonly results from overhead throwing, particularly baseball.
  - It is due to repetitive microtrauma secondary to overload during the throwing process.
  - Dislocation of the elbow is the most likely etiology of acute instability.
  - The differential diagnosis includes medial epicondylitis, flexor/pronator injuries, ulnar neuropathy, and Little Leaguer's elbow.
- Rotational instability
  - Most commonly occurs secondary to trauma (e.g., an elbow dislocation) and involves an avulsion of the ligamentous origins from the lateral epicondyle.[52]
  - Other etiologies include iatrogenic injury during surgical intervention for lateral epicondylitis or operative interventions to the radial head.
    - It has also been described as a sequela of nonoperative treatment of lateral epicondylitis.[53]

Presentation

- Valgus instability
  - Acute injury
    - In throwing athletes, a popping sensation may be reported in addition to the sudden onset of pain.
    - Direct trauma, including dislocation of the elbow, may cause this injury.
  - Chronic injury
    - Patients often describe vague elbow pain or localized medial elbow pain, generally gradual in onset.
    - It may be accompanied by ulnar nerve symptomatology.[45]
    - Throwing athletes report a decline in throwing velocity and accuracy, pain during the throwing motion, and/or pain following an episode of heavy throwing.[54]
- Rotational instability
  - Common complaints include:
    - Pain
    - Locking
    - Snapping
    - Clicking
    - A feeling of instability
  - These complaints may be worse with activity.
  - Typically a history of trauma or elbow dislocation may be elicited.
  - If noted following a surgical intervention to the elbow an iatrogenic cause should be suspected.

Physical Exam

- The elbow should be in 15–30° degrees of flexion for evaluation of ligamentous instability.

- Only very subtle differences in laxity may be present, therefore requiring a very detailed examination.
- Valgus instability
  - In acute injuries, an area of ecchymosis may be present over the medial elbow.
  - Tenderness to palpation may be present over the medial epicondyle.
    - Tenderness may subside following a period of rest and may not be present in chronic injuries.
  - Several of the special tests related to valgus instability are detailed in the "Focused Physical Examination" section earlier in this chapter and in Figure 2.7.[45,55]
    - The *valgus stress test* may be performed in either the prone or seated position.
      - With the elbow in approximately 20° of extension, palpate the medial joint line.
      - Stabilize the distal humerus with the other hand and apply a valgus stress to the elbow.
      - A positive test results in pain or excessive laxity.
    - *Modified milking maneuver.*
    - *Moving valgus stress test.*
    - Examination of the contralateral elbow should be performed to aid in the differentiation between physiologic versus pathologic laxity.
- Rotational instability
  - It is difficult to demonstrate instability, although provocative testing may reproduce the instability on clinical examination.[52,53]
  - The lateral ligaments are tested with the *varus stress test* (Figure 2.7) and internal rotation of the arm.
  - The *posterolateral rotary instability test* may assess for rotational instability.
    - With the patient in the supine position place the affected arm overhead.
    - The elbow should be in full extension and the forearm supinated.
    - Apply a valgus force with axial compression as the elbow is slowly flexed.
      - This may cause dislocation of the radiocapitellar joint.
      - Pronation and continued flexion reduces the joint.
      - Apprehension is also considered a positive test.

Essential Diagnostics

- Valgus instability
  - Radiographs including a minimum of three views of the elbow (AP, lateral, and oblique views) should be obtained.
  - Additionally, valgus stress radiographs may be obtained.
    - Stress radiographs should be taken of both elbows for comparison.
    - There are no cutoff values for abnormal stress radiographs, although increased opening of 0.5 mm is indicative of injury.[55]
    - The most common abnormal findings are olecranon osteophytes and calcifications within the UCL.[54]
  - Additional studies may include MRI, CT arthrogram, and/or ultrasound. (Figure 2.25)
    - Imaging aside from radiographs is generally not indicated in the ED.
- Rotational instability
  - Plain and stress radiographs are the most useful diagnostic tools aside from the physical examination.
    - Subtle abnormalities in chronic instability may be present, most notably a defect in the posterolateral margin of the capitellum.[53]

ED Treatment

- Valgus instability
  - Acute injuries associated with elbow dislocation necessitate reduction of the elbow, splinting, and careful evaluation for neurovascular compromise.
  - If neurological or vascular compromise is noted, emergent consultation with orthopedic surgery and/or vascular surgery is indicated.

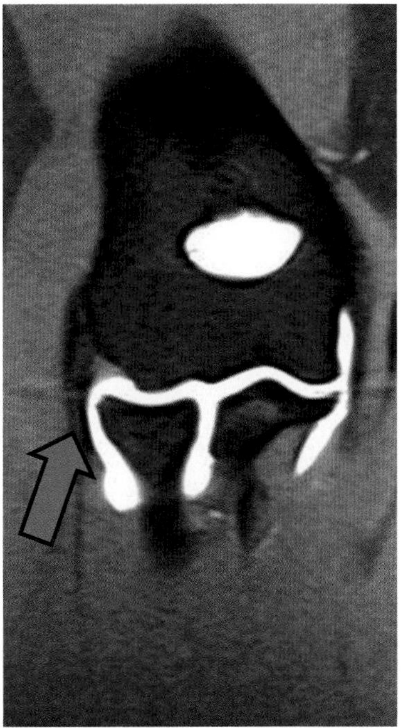

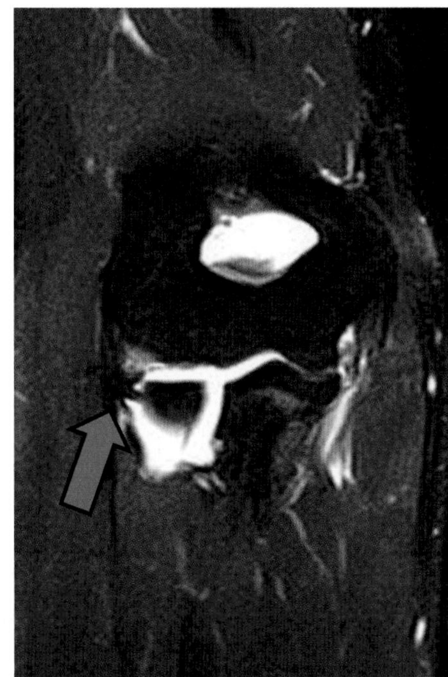

Figure 2.25. Contrast-enhanced MRI imaging of a high school pitcher with a UCL tear.

- A trial of supportive, nonsurgical treatment is appropriate in isolated UCL injuries.[54,55]
  - Cease throwing activities and activities that provoke pain.
  - Provide pain control with NSAIDs.
- Rotational instability
  - Halt activities that provoke the symptoms.
  - Provide pain control as needed.

Disposition

- Valgus instability
  - In the setting of an acute injury with an associated elbow dislocation, disposition is dependent on neurovascular status and the availability of close follow-up.
  - Isolated acute and chronic injuries may be safely discharged from the ED.
    - Follow-up with an orthopedic surgeon or sports medicine provider within one week for reassessment and initiation of a rehabilitation program is advised.
    - Athletes should not be cleared for return to play from the ED.
    - The following patients are surgical candidates:[55]
      - Throwing athletes with a complete UCL tear
      - Failed rehabilitation of partial tears
      - Symptomatic, non-throwing athletes following a minimum of three months of rehabilitation
- Rotational instability
  - These patients may be safely discharged from the ED.
  - There are no absolute indications for surgical repair.[53]
  - Follow-up with an orthopedic surgeon or sports medicine provider in approximately one week.

Complications

- While rare, an associated medial epicondyle fracture may require surgical intervention.[54]
- Following a surgical intervention, transient neuropraxia of the ulnar nerve may be present.[54]

Pediatric Considerations

- The pediatric considerations for similar elbow pain are discussed in detail in "Little Leaguer's Elbow/OCD Lesions" earlier in this chapter.

Pearls and Pitfalls

- In acute injuries associated with an elbow dislocation, the neurovascular status of the extremity should be reassessed frequently.
- Plain radiographs, including stress views, are the most useful diagnostic tool aside from the physical examination.
- For chronic injuries, activity modification, especially ceasing activities that provoke the symptoms, is the first-line treatment.

Biceps Tendon Ruptures

General Description

- The distal biceps inserts at the bicipital tuberosity of the radius.
  - The brachial artery and median nerve sit just medial to the biceps insertion.
- Primarily, the biceps serves as a forearm supinator.
  - Its secondary role is as an elbow flexor.
- These ruptures represent only 10% of all biceps ruptures (90% are proximal).[56]
- Distal biceps ruptures are more prevalent in males between the ages of 40 and 60.[57]
- The dominant arm is affected 80% of the time.[58]
- A classification for the extent of injury exists (Ramsey Classification), but it is not practical for use in the ED.[59]
  - A component of the classification, chronicity of injury, is relevant.
  - Acute injuries are those that occur within four weeks of presentation.

Mechanism

- The most common mechanism of injury involves an eccentric force (lengthening contraction under tension) with the elbow flexed at 90°.[60]
- Older patients may have a more innocuous mechanism secondary to an underlying degenerative distal biceps tendon.

Presentation

- Most patients will describe an acute incident associated with a "snap" sound or a tearing sensation.
- A significant decrease in strength with forearm supination and elbow flexion will often be detailed.
  - However, for chronic injuries (longer than four weeks), flexion strength may increase significantly, although likely not back to baseline.[61]
  - Forearm supination weakness will remain prominent.

Physical Exam

- Important visual signs at the flexion crease of the elbow associated with a distal biceps rupture include:
  - Swelling
  - Loss of the fullness of the anterior elbow
  - Ecchymosis
- A palpable defect is usually appreciated.
  - The *hook test* can assist in assessing a potential distal biceps defect. (Figure 2.5)
    - Continuity of the tendon on palpation may suggest a partial distal biceps tear.
- Prominence at the mid- or proximal humerus is often seen, known as the "*reverse Popeye sign*." (Figure 2.26A)
  - Active biceps flexion may produce retraction of the muscle belly proximally.
  - This can also be seen with proximal biceps tendon ruptures (referred to as a "Popeye sign" with the prominent biceps muscle typically located more distally towards the elbow. Please see further discussion in the Shoulder chapter).
- Observe for lack of and/or weakness with supination and/or flexion at the elbow.
- Perform the *biceps squeeze test.* (Figure2.26B)
  - Hold the elbow in 60–80° of flexion with the wrist slightly pronated.
  - With one arm stabilizing the elbow, the other hand should squeeze across the biceps brachii.
  - A positive test is a failure to observe supination.
  - This test has a sensitivity of 96%.[62]

Essential Diagnostics

- A distal biceps rupture is a clinical diagnosis; no imaging is essential in the ED to make this diagnosis.
- Plain films of the elbow (AP and lateral) should be considered to rule out an avulsion fracture. (Figure 2.27)

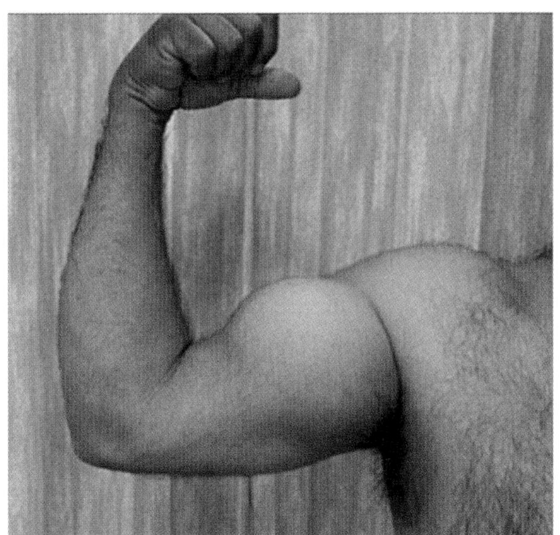

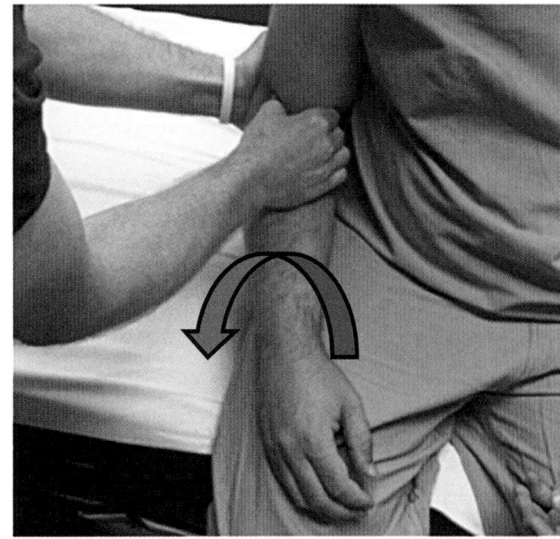

Figure 2.26A and B. **A,** A positive "reverse Popeye sign" due to a distal biceps tendon rupture. Courtesy of Francis Lam. The biceps squeeze test.

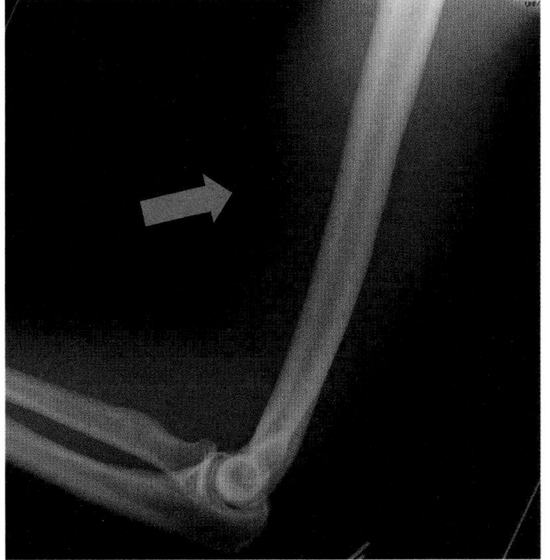

Figure 2.27. "Reverse popeye sign" as seen on plain films.

- Ultrasound may be beneficial, but MRI is the imaging modality of choice to confirm the diagnosis.
  - MRI has a sensitivity of 92% with a specificity of 85% for these injuries.[13]
  - Neither ultrasound nor MRI is indicated in the ED.

ED Treatment

- Acute management in the ED revolves around pain control.
- ROM, without resistance, is encouraged to prevent a loss of motion.
- No splinting or immobilization is indicated.
  - A shoulder sling may be used for comfort.
- Caution patients against significant lifting or repetitive supination/pronation activities.

Disposition

- Follow-up with an orthopedic surgeon is recommended within two to three days.
  - Surgical outcomes are optimal if the repair occurs within two weeks, although up to four weeks is acceptable.[63]
  - The goal with early surgery is to prevent scarring of the tendon.
- Patients may elect for nonoperative treatment.
  - This is more appropriate in the elderly, sedentary, or otherwise poor surgical candidates.
- Studies have shown that patients undergoing an operative repair may regain up to 97% flexion strength and 95% supination strength.[64]
- The typical postoperative recovery period for full return to work or sport following surgery is six to seven months.[45]

Complications

- Nonoperative treatment may result in 30% less flexion strength, 40% less supination strength, and up to 86% less supination endurance.[64,65]
- Depending upon where the tendon scars, there may be decreased flexion in patients who refrain from operative repair.

- There are some complications associated with surgery (radial nerve injury, loss of rotation, heterotopic ossification, etc.).
  - 3–4% of patients will have persistent nerve lesions.[66]
- Complications tend to occur more often in chronic distal biceps ruptures (lasting more than four weeks).[67]
- Re-rupture is an uncommon occurrence, but has been reported (2%).[68]

Pediatric Considerations

- This is an extremely rare condition in the pediatric population; no special considerations exist.

Pearls and Pitfalls

- Pay particular attention to a patient's supination strength at the elbow, as that may prove more insightful than flexion strength.
- Use the *hook* and *biceps squeeze tests* to better delineate the patient's pathology.
- Refrain from advanced imaging in the ED.
- Ensure prompt orthopedic follow-up to avoid the sequelae of decreased ROM, strength, and endurance at the elbow.

Distal Triceps Tendon Ruptures

General Description

- The distal triceps inserts at the olecranon, forming both deep and superficial attachments.
  - The radial nerve innervates the triceps muscle.
- It is the only major elbow extender.
  - Its secondary role is as an elbow flexor.
- These injuries were once thought to be extremely rare, but their prevalence has been increasing.
  - The injury is twice as likely to occur in men.[69]
  - There is no clear predilection to dominant or nondominant sides.[70]

Mechanism

- Most frequently, distal triceps tears are the result of a fall on an outstretched hand with a concomitant eccentric contraction of the triceps upon impact.[71]
- Another possible mechanism of injury involves a direct below to the elbow.
  - An associated avulsion fracture of the olecranon may also be present.

Presentation

- A specific inciting event or traumatic injury is often noted.
- A tearing sensation is frequently reported.
- Inquiring about a loss of elbow extension might be beneficial in making the diagnosis.
- Particular activities have a higher reported risk of causing distal triceps ruptures.
  - Weightlifting, football, baseball pitching, and javelin throwing are associated with these injuries.[72-75]
- There are other pre-disposing risk factors that warrant consideration.[72,76-79]
  - Hyperparathyroidism
  - Osteogenesis imperfecta
  - Marfan syndrome
  - Systemic lupus erythematous
  - Steroid use (local and systemic; anabolic or otherwise)

Physical Exam

- A palpable depression may be appreciated just proximal to the olecranon.
  - This may be subtle in the setting of acute swelling or an individual with significant muscle mass.
- Ecchymosis might be present, but it may also take several days to surface.
- The key to the diagnosis is assessing the ability to extend the elbow and the associated strength.
  - Start by assessing the patient's ability to extend the elbow against gravity.
  - Marked weakness suggests a complete triceps tear.
  - Utilize the contralateral extremity for comparison.
- The *Thompson triceps test* also has some utility. (Figure 2.28)
  - Hold the arm in flexion against gravity.
  - Compress the triceps.
  - A positive test will result in no extension of the elbow with compression.

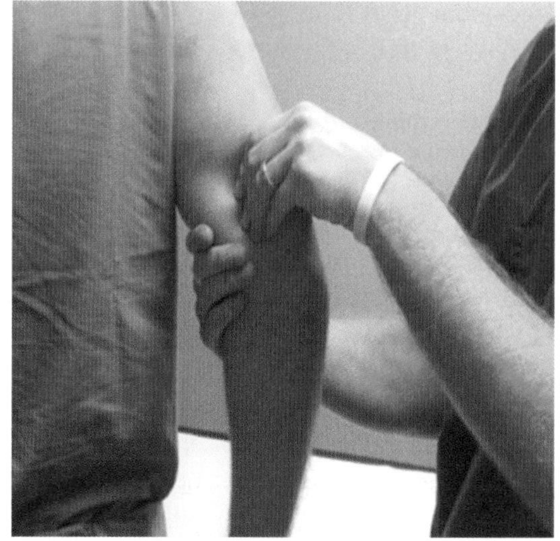

Figure 2.28. The Thompson triceps test.

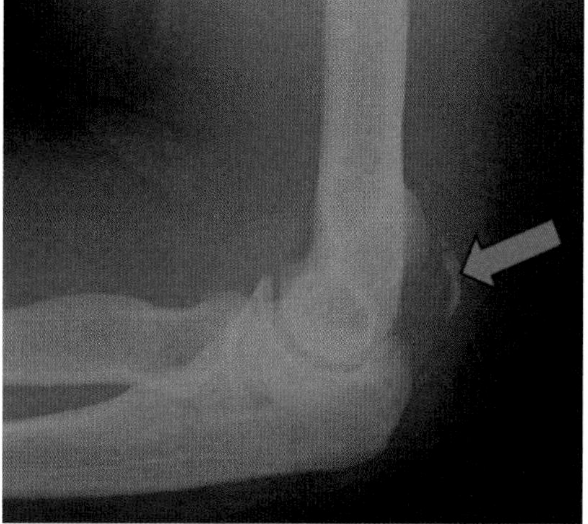

Figure 2.29. "Flake sign" on plain films resulting from a triceps rupture.

- Other physical exam findings associated with a distal triceps rupture include:
  - Cubital tunnel syndrome: irritation, entrapment, or compression of the ulnar nerve.
  - Snapping elbow: may be due to the ulnar nerve or the medial head of the triceps snapping across the medial epicondyle.

Essential Diagnostics

- Plain films are important in the evaluation of potential triceps ruptures given the concern for an associated avulsion injury of the olecranon.
  - AP, lateral, and radial head imaging should be secured.
  - Look for a "flake sign," reflective of an avulsion fracture resulting in a triceps rupture. (Figure 2.29)
  - Be sure to look for associated injuries; radial head fractures have been associated with triceps rupture.
- Unclear or atypical presentations may warrant further imaging via outpatient MRI.
  - MRI may also detail the extent of a partial tear.
  - Some orthopedists contend that a tear of greater than 50% warrants surgical repair.[80]

ED Treatment

- No emergent intervention is needed in the ED.
- Pain control should be emphasized, along with rest, ice, and elevation in an attempt to reduce swelling.
- No splinting or immobilization is indicated in the ED, however a sling may be utilized for comfort.

Disposition

- Follow-up with an orthopedic surgeon or sports medicine specialist is recommended within twenty-four to forty-eight hours.
- Nonoperative treatment is appropriate for partial tears.
  - These patients may be splinted in 30° of extension for four to six weeks.
- Operative treatment is recommended for complete distal triceps ruptures.
  - A major contraindication (e.g., systemic illness) would make a repair unlikely.
  - Patients who may have low functional status but require their upper extremities for transferring are still considered surgical candidates.
- Surgical repair within three weeks results in the best outcomes.[70]
- Postoperatively, studies suggest a return to 92% extension strength compared to the unaffected extremity.[81]

- By four months following surgery patients should resume eccentric muscle contractions.[45]

Complications

- Aside from weakness and/or persistent loss of extension, complications from the distal triceps rupture itself are rare.[82]
- Posterior compartment syndrome has been reported with distal triceps ruptures.
    - Postoperatively, patients may experience a flexion contracture of 5–20°.[83]
- Olecranon bursitis, ulnar neuritis, and re-rupture are all postsurgical complications that have been reported.

Pediatric Considerations

- This is an extremely rare condition in the pediatric population; no special considerations exist.

Pearls and Pitfalls

- Be sure to ask about risk factors and predisposing conditions, which should increase suspicion for a distal triceps rupture.
- Focus on the patient's ability to extend the elbow, comparing the relative strength to the opposite extremity.
- Plain films of the elbow are recommended; be certain to look for concomitant injuries (e.g., a radial head fracture).
- Referral to an orthopedic surgeon is indicated for complete distal triceps ruptures.

Lateral/Medial Epicondylitis

General Description

- Medial and lateral epicondylitis are overuse syndromes.
- Medial epicondylitis (golfer's elbow) involves the common flexor tendon originating at the medial epicondyle.
- Lateral epicondylitis (tennis elbow) involves the radiohumeral joint or the lateral epicondyle.[51]
    - It may be thought of as a wrist extensor tendinopathy.
- There is equal incidence in men and women.[45]
- The most common age of presentation is between 40 and 60, although cases from ages 12 to 80 have been reported.[45]

Mechanism

- Though they occur in athletes, medial and lateral epicondylitis are most common in adults with occupations requiring repetitive rotary motion (e.g., grasping and twisting).[51]
- Lateral epicondylitis consists of degeneration of the common extensor tendons through microtears/microtrauma.
    - This most commonly involves the extensor carpi radialis brevis tendon.[45,84]
- Medial epicondylitis is less common and less debilitating than lateral epicondylitis.[84]
    - This involves the common flexor origin, namely the flexor carpi radialis.

Presentation

- Lateral epicondylitis features a dull ache over the lateral elbow radiating down the forearm, usually gradual in onset.[19,45]
    - Pain may occur with simple tasks, such as shaking hands and lifting objects with handles.
- Medial epicondylitis involves tenderness and pain along the medial epicondyle, also usually of gradual onset.[45]

Physical Exam

- Lateral epicondylitis
    - Tenderness may be localized either directly over the lateral epicondyle or slightly anterior and 1–2 cm distal to the lateral epicondyle.[45,84]
    - *Tennis elbow and Cozen's test*s are useful in helping to make the diagnosis. (Figure 2.26)
    - Middle finger resistance test (*Maudsley's test*) reproduces pain with resisted extension of the middle finger.
    - Pain may also be reproduced with resisted supination of the forearm.
    - There is usually full active and passive ROM.
        - Pain may be present with full elbow extension and forearm pronation.[85]
    - Remember that the differential diagnosis includes radicular pain and ligamentous pathology.

- An examination of the entire upper extremity, including provocative testing (e.g., Spurling's test, which is discussed in the Cervical Spine chapter), is indicated to rule out radicular pain mimicking lateral epicondylitis.
- If crepitus, clicking, joint effusion, or elbow flexion contractures are observed, elbow joint or ligamentous pathology should be suspected.[45]

- Medial epicondylitis
  - Tenderness is localized to the medial aspect of the elbow and medial epicondyle.
  - Pain is exacerbated with resistance to wrist flexion and forearm pronation.[45,84]
  - *Golfer's elbow test* (supination of the forearm along with extension of the wrist and elbow) can reproduce pain at the medial epicondyle.
  - Normal strength, sensation, and ROM are typical.
    - Decreased hand grip strength may be present.
  - The differential diagnosis includes ligamentous instability or primary ulnar neuropathy.
    - The *moving valgus stress testing* (Figure 2.27 middle picture) produces pain and laxity if ligamentous instability is present.
    - The *elbow flexion test* (maximal elbow flexion and wrist extension for 3 minutes) will produce pain and numbness if ulnar neuropathy is present.[45]
      - This test has a sensitivity of 75% with a specificity of 99%.[86]
      - Compressing the nerve increases the sensitivity to 98%.[86]

Essential Diagnostics

- A thorough physical examination is key; epicondylitis is a clinical diagnosis.
- Radiographs should be obtained to exclude a fracture.
  - Calcifications may be seen over epicondyle in chronic epicondylitis.[19] (Figure 2.30)

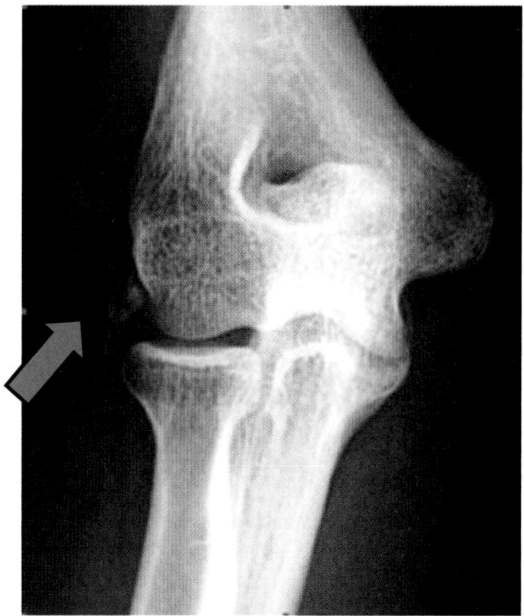

Figure 2.30. Calcification of the common extensor tendon(s) in lateral epicondylitis.

- Bedside ultrasound may be used by practitioners proficient in musculoskeletal ultrasound to aid in confirmation of the diagnosis.

ED Treatment

- Treatment is aimed at behavior modification to prevent forearm musculature overuse.
  - Limiting activities that include wrist flexion and extension will decrease strain on the flexion and extensor tendons attaching at the epicondyles.
- Heat, ice, and NSAIDs aid in symptom control.[84]
  - The initial duration of parenteral NSAID use is ten to fourteen days if there are no medical contraindications.[45]
- Topical NSAIDs may reduce pain in the short term.
- Bracing may be beneficial.
  - Counterforce bracing (sometimes termed tennis elbow braces or forearm straps) may be used to decrease the force experienced by the musculature and tendons proximal to the brace.[45,87]

- Wrist extensor splinting allows for increased immobilization of the wrist extensors compared to the counterforce bracing.
  - It has been shown to provide greater pain relief than counterforce bracing.
  - The wrist brace may be more cumbersome and interfere with activities related to work or daily living.[87]
- Both counterforce bracing and wrist extensor splinting have superior pain relief when compared to placebo bracing.[85]
  - There are no absolute indications for bracing or splinting.[85]

- Routine immobilization of the elbow is not recommended.
- The role of local injections is debatable.
  - Local corticosteroids have been shown to be superior to NSAIDs at four weeks.
  - However, no long-term differences have been found.[85]
    - Injections have been falling out of favor due to recent studies showing no benefit over placebo.[45]
  - Local corticosteroid injections may be considered after failed trials of conservative therapies.[45]
    - Yet, a recent study found that corticosteroid injections for chronic epicondylitis resulted in worse clinical outcomes after one year vs. placebo.[88]
  - While not a first-line therapy, there is emerging evidence that alternative therapies such as local platelet rich plasma (PRP), polidocanol, prolotherapy and/or autologous whole blood injections may be beneficial in the treatment of lateral epicondylitis.[89, 90]
    - The long-term outcome of lateral epicondylitis treated with alternative injections is unknown when compared to conservative management and corticosteroid injections, however initial evidence is promising.
    - There may be barriers to patient access, including relative lack of experienced providers performing this therapy as well as financial burdens.
    - For the emergency medicine provider, knowledge of this therapy may be beneficial for counseling purposes if a patient presents with chronic lateral epicondylitis following the aforementioned management.

Disposition

- Patients with medial or lateral epicondylitis may be safely discharged from the emergency department.
- Lateral epicondylitis is a self-limiting process that may last twelve to eighteen months.[85]
  - Patients should be counseled regarding the expected time period for complete recovery.
- All patients should receive routine follow-up with a primary care provider or a sports medicine provider.
- Rehabilitation includes wrist flexor and forearm pronator stretching and isometric exercises.
  - As flexibility, strength, and endurance improve, eccentric and concentric resistive exercises are added.[45]
  - A sport or job simulation is then performed, followed by a gradual return to normal activity.

Complications

- Failure of conservative treatment for greater than six months with resultant continued debilitating pain prompts consideration of surgical debridement.[45]
  - About 4–11% of patients who seek medical attention may require surgical intervention after failed conservative therapy.[91]

Pediatric Considerations

- Medial elbow pain is the chief concern in most cases of Little Leaguer's elbow.
  - See the section on OCD/Little Leaguer's elbow for further information.

Pearls and Pitfalls

- Plain films of the elbow may be helpful in identifying avulsion fractures or calcifications.

- Initial treatment is aimed at activity modification to prevent overuse of the forearm musculature.
- Routine corticosteroid injections are falling out of favor and alternative injections (whole blood, PRP, etc.) may prove to be more beneficial.

Cubital Tunnel Syndrome (Ulnar Neuritis)

General Description

- Cubital tunnel syndrome is also often referred to as ulnar neuritis.
- Due to entrapment, irritation, and/or traction of the ulnar nerve, it is the most common elbow neuropathy.[92]
  - Overall, it is the second most common compressive neuropathy (following carpal tunnel syndrome).[92]
- This condition is far more common in men than women (up to 8:1).[25]

Mechanism

- The act of throwing may result in cubital tunnel syndrome.
  - There is strain on the ulnar nerve during all phases of throwing.[93]
  - Additionally, elbow flexion during late cocking requires the ulnar nerve to elongate.[94]
  - Located next to the ulnar nerve, the medial collateral ligament may become inflamed during throwing, resulting in ulnar nerve impingement.
- Other mechanisms/causes of cubital tunnel syndrome include:
  - Fascial/muscle hypertrophy (e.g., medial head of the triceps)
  - Anomalous muscles
  - Soft tissue mass (e.g., lipoma)
  - UCL instability/tear
  - Osteophytes
  - Ulnar nerve subluxation
  - Fractures/dislocations (affecting the movement of the ulnar nerve)

Presentation

- Symptoms generally start as paresthesias of the little finger and medial half of the ring finger.

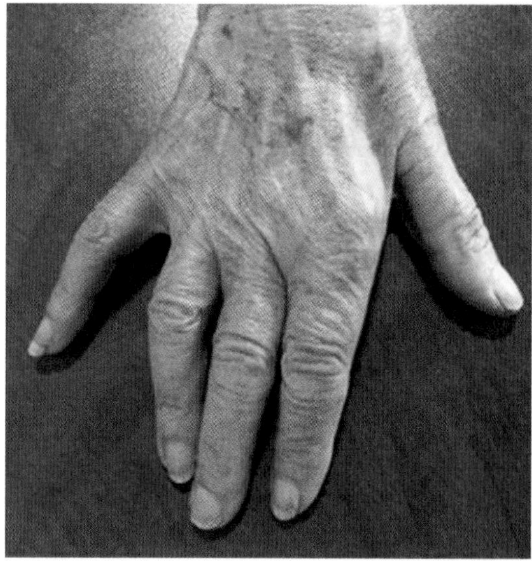

Figure 2.31. Wartenberg sign with the little finger abducted.

- Prolonged paresthesias may result in intrinsic hand muscle weakness and resulting dysfunction.
  - Extrinsic muscle function (e.g., flexor carpi ulnaris and flexor digitorum profundus) is generally preserved.[95]
- If severe, patients may have muscle paralysis, claw hand deformity, and/or weak pinching/grasping ability.
  - Severe abduction or claw deformity of the little finger only is known as the *Wartenberg sign.* (Figure 2.31)
- Pain may be noted both proximally and distally along the medial elbow.
  - The patient may need to throw/stress the elbow to reproduce the pain.

Physical Exam

- A thorough neurologic examination focusing on the little and ring fingers is essential, assessing for both sensory and motor differences relative to the contralateral side.
- Flexion and extension of the elbow may result in ulnar nerve subluxation.
  - Look and listen for a snapping or popping sensation, which is often painful.
- *Tinel's sign* may be used to assess for ulnar neuritis, but it may be falsely negative.

- The test entails tapping over the ulnar nerve along the medial elbow.
- A positive test reproduces the patient's symptoms.
- The sensitivity and specificity of this test are 62% and 53%, respectively.[96]

- The *elbow flexion test* may be used to reproduce the patient's symptoms.
  - Fully flex the elbow and extend the wrist for one minute.
  - Numbness and/or tingling in the ulnar nerve distribution suggests compression at the elbow.
  - This test has a sensitivity of 61%, with a specificity of 40%.[97]
- The *scratch test* should be performed as well.[97]
  - The patient should adduct both arms, flex the elbows to 90°, and keep the wrists neutral.
  - While the examiner applies internal rotation at the forearm the patient should resist this pressure.
  - The examiner should then scratch over the cubital tunnel.
  - Immediately, internal rotation is then applied to the patient's forearms again.
  - A positive test results in immediate loss of external rotation resistance.
    - This resolves within five seconds.

Essential Diagnostics

- Plain films of the elbow (AP and lateral) should be considered to rule out a fracture or other anatomic irregularities.
  - A cubital tunnel (or sulcus) view may be secured to better assess this region. (Figure 2.32)
- MRI or ultrasound modalities may be considered as an outpatient to evaluate the ulnar nerve and/or for soft tissue masses but are not essential in the emergency department.
- Electromyography (EMG) and nerve conduction velocity (NCV) testing can be performed as an outpatient to confirm the diagnosis.

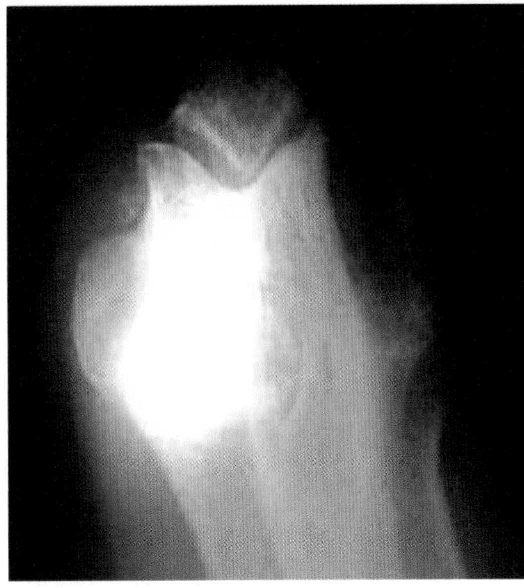

Figure 2.32. A cubital tunnel radiograph view.

ED Treatment

- No emergent emergency department treatment is necessary for cubital tunnel syndrome.
- NSAIDs may be administered for pain control.
- Emphasize behavior modification.
- A night splint to keep the elbow extended may be offered to limit movement and decrease irritation/pain.

Disposition

- Patients with cubital tunnel syndrome do not require orthopedic consultation in the emergency department and may be discharged to home safely.
- Individuals should be counseled on avoiding symptom-provoking, repetitive activity until re-evaluated.
- NSAIDs may be used for pain control.
- Padding of the elbow may help to reduce irritation of the ulnar nerve.
- A referral to a sports medicine provider or an orthopedic surgeon is warranted within one to two weeks.
  - Physical therapy focusing on nerve-gliding exercises may be recommended at that time.
  - Up to 90% of patients may respond to conservative therapy.[98]

- Patients are generally not considered surgical candidates until symptoms have persisted for more than three months or if the symptoms are recurrent for throwing athletes.[99,100]

Complications

- Delayed presentation or diagnosis may result in the significant complications of claw hand and/or intrinsic hand muscle wasting.

Pediatric Considerations

- This condition is uncommon in the pediatric population; no special pediatric considerations exist.

Pearls and Pitfalls

- Be sure to assess for UCL instability/tears as a causative factor, especially in overhead throwing athletes.
- Consider tumors in the differential diagnosis.
- Emphasize the importance of minimizing repetitive activity to patients; conservative treatment is generally quite effective for cubital tunnel syndrome.

Pronator Syndrome

General Description

- Pronator syndrome (or pronator teres syndrome) may involve the median nerve or its distal branch, the anterior interosseous nerve.
- Affected patients present with symptoms similar to carpal tunnel syndrome (e.g., hand pain and/or paresthesias on the volar aspects of the thumb, index, middle, and lateral half of the ring fingers).
- Overall an uncommon entity, it typically arises in patients in their 50s.[14]
  - Females are four times more likely to develop this condition than males.[101]

Mechanism

- Most frequently, pronator syndrome is the result of compression of the median nerve between the heads of the pronator teres.
  - If the area of compression is more distal the anterior interosseous nerve may be affected.
- Specific potential causes of this condition include:
  - Repetitive occupational activity involving supination/pronation.
    - Fast-pitch softball and race car driving have a predilection toward this condition.[45]
  - Muscle hypertrophy (e.g., weight lifters)
  - A sudden, forceful event involving forearm pronation
  - Anatomic variations (e.g., anomalous supracondyloid process)
  - Vascular abnormalities (e.g., a persistent median artery) also reported.[102]

Presentation

- Patients with this condition often have well-developed upper extremity musculature, particularly in the forearm.
- Generally, the pain is insidious in onset, although acute precipitating events may occur.
- The associated pain is typically reported in the proximal, anterior forearm/elbow.
- When the proximal median nerve is compressed the motor symptoms are minimal.
  - If the anterior interosseous nerve is affected, patients may report hand weakness and/or difficulty with pinching.
- Activity will often be cited as worsening symptoms.
- The pain associated with pronator syndrome typically does not occur at night (which can differentiate this condition from carpal tunnel syndrome).[103]

Physical Exam

- Visual inspection of the forearm might reveal a pronator muscle mass.
- Sensation should be assessed, particularly involving the palmar aspect of the thumb, index, and middle fingers and the medial aspect of the ring finger.
  - Decreased sensation over the thenar eminence suggests a proximal lesion of the median nerve (as opposed to carpal tunnel syndrome).
- *Tinel's sign* may be present, which may be elicited by tapping the anterior forearm over

the pronator region, with reproduction of symptoms in the aforementioned distribution of the hand.
  - *Tinel's sign* should not be present over the wrist.
- Weakness of the following muscles may be appreciated on physical examination:
  - Intrinsic hand muscles (lumbricals, opponens pollicis, flexor pollicis brevis, etc.)
  - Extrinsic finger flexors
  - Wrist flexors
  - Pronator quadratus

Essential Diagnostics

- Plain films of the elbow (AP and lateral) should be considered to rule out anatomic abnormalities (e.g., supracondyloid process).
- No other emergent imaging is necessary in the emergency department.
  - MRI is generally not recommended in making the diagnosis of pronator syndrome secondary to difficulties appreciating the median nerve with this modality.
  - While the evidence validating its efficacy is lacking, ultrasound is recommended by some as the first imaging modality in evaluating for pronator syndrome.[104]
  - EMG is beneficial in confirming the diagnosis, but again such testing is not germane to the emergency department.
    - Positive findings generally only result after four to six weeks of symptoms.[14]

ED Treatment

- No emergent emergency department treatment is necessary for pronator syndrome.
- NSAIDs may be administered for pain control.
- Emphasize behavior modification.
- A splint may be offered to limit excessive elbow flexion, although this may prove to be cumbersome for the patient.

Disposition

- Patients with pronator syndrome do not require orthopedic consultation in the emergency department and may be discharged to home safely.
- Individuals should be counseled on avoiding symptom-provoking, repetitive activity until re-evaluated.
- NSAIDs may be used for pain control.
- A referral to a sports medicine provider or an orthopedic surgeon is warranted within one to two weeks.
  - Conservative management (including activity avoidance, rest, and NSAIDs) has been shown to be 50–70% effective.[105]
  - Corticosteroid injections into the pronator muscle, avoiding the median nerve, may be beneficial.
  - There is no clear delineation as to when to consider conservative management a failure and progress to surgical intervention.[106]

Complications

- Complications typically stem from delayed presentation/diagnosis.
- Axon loss and muscular atrophy may arise as complications, although these may improve if decompression of the median nerve is achieved.

Pediatric Considerations

- This condition is uncommon in the pediatric population; no special pediatric considerations exist.

Pearls and Pitfalls

- This diagnosis has been shown to be delayed by up to two years in some patients; keep pronator syndrome in differential for patients with carpal tunnel-like symptoms.
- A key symptom in making this diagnosis is the absence of night pain in pronator syndrome, which is not the case in carpal tunnel syndrome.
- Also evaluate for decreased sensation over the thenar eminence, suggesting a more proximal neuropathy involving the median nerve.

Olecranon Bursitis and Septic Bursitis

General Description

- Olecranon bursitis is inflammation of the bursa overlying the olecranon process at the proximal aspect of the ulna.[19]

- In septic bursitis, *Staphylococcus aureus* is the most commonly identified organism (80–90% of cases).[19,107]
  - *Streptococcus, Nocardia asiatica, Brucella abotrus, Mycobacterium kansasii,* fungi, and algae have also been reported as causes of septic bursitis.[107]
- The evidence regarding septic olecranon bursitis evaluation and treatment is limited to retrospective case series studies, accounting for the variation in evaluation and treatment.[108]

Mechanism

- Inflammation of the bursa may be caused by several mechanisms, including:[19]
  - Acute trauma
  - Chronic friction due to overuse; common associated occupations involving repetitive movements or leaning on the elbow, such as plumbers and computer workers
  - Crystal deposition (gout and pseudogout)
  - Infection
  - Systemic disease (e.g., rheumatoid arthritis, scleroderma, uremia)

Presentation

- Focal pain and swelling over the posterior elbow (Figure 2.33) that may radiate proximally or distally are often present.
- The pain may range from mild to severe, and may be sharp or dull.
- Patients with septic bursitis may have systemic symptoms, including fever and/or chills.

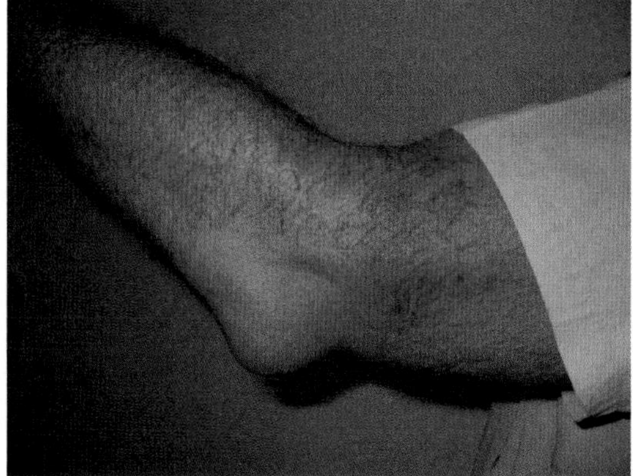

Figure 2.33. Olecranon bursitis with overlying redness.

Physical Exam

- Focal warmth and tenderness over the posterior elbow are frequently appreciated.
  - This is not a reliable determinant of etiology, as these may be present in infectious as well as other pathologies.[19,107]
- Swelling of the olecranon bursa will be present.
- Elbow flexion may be limited due to skin tightening over the inflamed area.
- There may be overlying erythema or cellulitis present.

Essential Diagnostics

- A thorough physical examination is essential.
- Aspiration of the bursa and fluid analysis is controversial.
  - Concerns regarding routine aspiration include seeding bacteria in a noninfected bursa and potential formation of a fistula at the site of aspiration.[108]
  - Aspiration is relatively contraindicated if there is an overlying cellulitis, as this may introduce bacteria into a noninfected bursa.
  - Aspiration is not recommended if the patient has already been on antibiotics, as the likelihood of identifying an organism is low.[108]
  - A posterolateral approach should be used to avoid the ulnar nerve.[19] (Figure 2.16)
- If performed, fluid analysis studies should include:[19]
  - Cell count and differential
  - Crystal analysis
  - Gram stain
  - Culture
- There are several important considerations regarding the interpretation of the fluid aspirate.
  - There is considerable overlap within inflammatory, noninflammatory, and infectious etiologies.
  - Cell count results should be interpreted in light of the clinical picture and the other fluid analysis studies.[19]

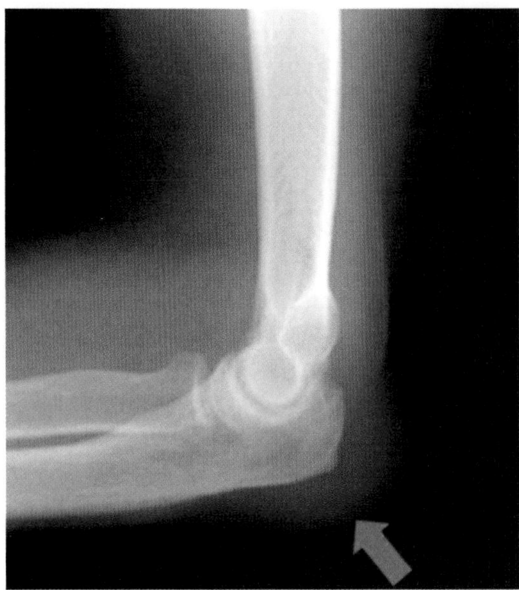

Figure 2.34. Posterior soft tissue swelling on plain film due to olecranon bursitis.

- Predominance of polymorphonuclear cells (PMN) and a white blood cell (WBC) count of greater than 50,000 are strongly suspicious for an infectious etiology.[19]
    - However, the WBC in septic bursitis may be as low as 1,500.[45]
- WBC count in noninfectious bursitis may range from 50 to more than 10,000.
    - There is usually a predominance of mononuclear cells.[45]
- The Gram stain and culture are critical when the cell count is indeterminate, which can be the case particularly in an early infection.[19]

- Plain films (a minimum of two views, AP and lateral) should be obtained to rule out fracture, dislocation, and/or signs of osteomyelitis. (Figure 2.34)
    - The sensitivity for detecting osteomyelitis on plain films is 43% to 75%, while the specificity is 75% to 83%.[109]
- In patients with an elevated serum WBC count (>10,000/mm^3) and an elevated C-reactive protein (CRP) (>0.5mg/dl), septic bursitis should be assumed until proven otherwise.[107]

ED Treatment

- Aspiration has both diagnostic and therapeutic utility as detailed earlier.
    - However, the literature is not clear as to whether aspiration should be routinely performed; clinical judgment should be used in making this decision.
    - Aspiration, compression, and protection from trauma are usually sufficient to resolve the condition when due to a noninfectious etiology.[84]
    - Serial aspirations (after twenty-four to forty-eight hours) have been utilized and are effective in conjunction with parenteral antibiotics for curing septic bursitis.[108]
- In otherwise healthy patients, perform aspiration and fluid analysis followed by treatment with culture-specific antibiotics.[108]
    - Antibiotics (including coverage for *S. aureus)* should be initiated while awaiting culture results if there is strong suspicion for infection.[19]
        - The antibiotic may be changed to a culture-specific antibiotic once this information is available.
    - If there is a contraindication for aspiration, antibiotics should be initiated.
- Pain control with NSAIDs and, if needed, opiate pain medication is advised.
- Treat the underlying condition(s) (e.g., gout).
- Compression of the area overlying the bursa, including following aspiration, will aid in preventing further accumulation of fluid within the bursa.[19,107]
- Patients with septic olecranon bursitis and specific signs/symptoms/risk factors (listed here) require consideration for intravenous antibiotics and orthopedic surgery consultation for possible drainage.[110]
    - Fever (>38°C)
    - Chills
    - Signs of SIRS/sepsis
    - Persistent/worsening cellulitis after twenty-four to forty-eight hours of antibiotic treatment
    - Immunocompromised patients

Disposition

- In the absence of systemic signs of infection, patients with olecranon bursitis and septic olecranon bursitis may be discharged from the ED.
  - If there are systemic signs of infection (SIRS), consideration of intravenous antibiotics, hospital admission, and surgical consultation is warranted.
  - There should be a low threshold for hospital admission in immunocompromised patients with septic bursitis.
- Follow-up with a primary care provider, sports medicine physician, or orthopedic surgeon in one to two days is advised.
  - Athletes should not be cleared for return to sport from the ED.
- Symptoms may be recurrent.
  - Failure of aspiration and antibiotics to resolve septic olecranon bursitis might necessitate open incision and drainage (I&D).
  - In refractory cases of noninfectious bursitis, surgical excision of the bursa may be performed.[19]

Complications

- Seeding of a noninfected bursa by aspirating through an overlying cellulitis has been reported.[107,110,111]
  - There is insufficient data to support corticosteroid injections into the bursa, and an infection rate of up to 10% has been noted when performed.[110,111]
- Recurrence of symptoms may require serial aspiration, open I&D, and/or excision of the bursa.
- Osteomyelitis of the olecranon may occur secondary to chronic septic bursitis.[19]

Pediatric Considerations

- Posterior elbow complaints are quite uncommon in the pediatric population.[45]
- The differential diagnosis should include irregular ossification of the olecranon ossification center, avulsion of the olecranon, and osteophyte formation.[45]
  - An outpatient orthopedic surgery or sports medicine referral should be made for these cases.

Pearls and Pitfalls

- In immunocompromised patients, cell counts for septic bursitis may be lower than expected.
  - Maintain a high index of suspicion for infectious etiology in this population.
- Recognize that focal warmth, tenderness, and swelling are not reliable in differentiating infectious vs. noninfectious etiologies of olecranon bursitis.
- Keep septic arthritis in the differential.
  - Septic arthritis is discussed in more detail later; the diagnosis and treatment of septic arthritis is similar to that for other major joints, including the knee.

Septic Arthritis (Infectious Arthritis)

General Description

- Septic arthritis is a medical emergency associated with significant morbidity.[112,113]
- It is defined as an infection within a joint space.
- A delay in presentation and/or diagnosis significantly increases morbidity and mortality.[114]
- The most common location of septic arthritis is the knee, followed by the hip, shoulder, and elbow.[114]
- The most common causative organism is *Staphylococcus aureus* (50–60% of cases).[115]
  - Streptococci (20%) and gram-negative bacilli (5–10%) are the other most common pathogens.[115]

Mechanism

- The most common mechanism of joint infection is hematogenous spread.[114]
- Other causes include direct inoculation, operative contamination, and spread from a contiguous infection.[115]

Presentation

- Up to 85% of cases present with joint pain, swelling, warmth, and decreased ROM.[112]
- A monoarticular pattern is usually present.
- The symptoms are typically acute in onset.
- Patients may report systemic symptoms such as fevers and chills, although these are not always present.

- A total of 10–27% of atraumatic acutely swollen joints may be due to septic arthritis.[112]
  - The differential diagnosis includes gout, pseudogout, rheumatoid arthritis, Lyme disease, lupus, disseminated *Neisseria gonorrhoeae*, reactive arthritis, and/or osteoarthritis exacerbation.[112,114,115]
- Septic arthritis may occur in otherwise healthy individuals, but risk factors include:[115,116]
  - Advanced age
  - Rheumatologic disease
  - Immunodeficiency
  - Diabetes mellitus
  - Coexisting infections
  - Alcohol and drug abuse
  - Internal fixation devices

Physical Exam

- Visual inspection often reveals a joint effusion with associated warmth at the elbow.
- Moderate to severe monoarticular joint pain with ROM is appreciated.
  - Pain with ROM is the most sensitive examination finding.[114]
- ROM is often severely reduced, often due to pain.
- The physical examination does not significantly change the post-test probability of septic arthritis.[114]

Essential Diagnostics

- Plain films of the elbow (AP and lateral) should be obtained to rule out a fracture, dislocation, foreign bodies, evidence of joint prostheses, and/or evidence of osteomyelitis.
- Joint aspiration is an essential aspect of the workup for septic arthritis.
  - See Figure 2.16 for a description of performing an elbow arthrocentesis.
  - Arthrocentesis may be performed on patients on therapeutic warfarin anticoagulation.
    - The risk of clinically significant hemorrhage is less than 10%.[114]
- Laboratory analysis of the joint aspirate should include:
  - Cell count with differential
  - Gram stain
  - Culture
  - LDH
  - Crystal analysis
- When analyzing the results of the joint aspirate consider the following:
  - A negative Gram stain does not rule out septic arthritis.[114]
  - A culture should still be obtained if crystals are identified.[114]
  - WBC counts may vary greatly in septic arthritis; however, a value of greater than 50,000 with more than 90% PMNs is highly suggestive of infection.[112–114]
    - Since there is overlap between WBC counts in septic arthritis and inflammatory arthritis a diagnosis cannot be made solely on the joint aspirate WBC count.
  - In patients with prosthetic joints, the synovial fluid WBC count may be significantly lower than in those with native joints.[116]
  - A synovial lactate of greater than 10mmol/L is highly suggestive of septic arthritis.[114]
    - There are no studies evaluating point-of-care synovial lactate in the diagnosis of septic arthritis.[114]
  - One trial reports that a synovial lactate dehydrogenase (LDH) of less than 250 U/L may be sufficient to rule out septic arthritis.[114]
    - Synovial testing for Lyme disease and/or *Neisseria gonorrhoeae* should be considered when possible exposure exists.
- Serum laboratory markers may be of some utility.
  - No serum laboratory marker is diagnostic for septic arthritis.
  - Elevated WBC and ESR values are commonly used markers to suggest an infectious source.[112]
  - A CRP of greater than 10.5 mg/dL is highly concerning for septic arthritis.[112]
  - Blood cultures should be considered, especially in patients with systemic symptoms (fevers, chills, etc.).

- In patients with prosthetic joints, a rise in CRP after a postoperative decline in CRP is suggestive of infection.[116]
- Ultimately, the diagnosis of septic arthritis in the emergency department relies upon clinician judgment.[112]

ED Treatment

- Prompt evaluation and diagnosis is critical in the setting of septic arthritis.
- Evaluate and treat systemic symptoms, including signs of sepsis.
- Cultures (joint aspirate and blood) should be obtained prior to the administration of antibiotics.
- When selecting antibiotic coverage for septic arthritis, consider the following:
  - Coverage of *Staphylococcus* and *Streptococcus* is essential as they are the most common causative organisms.
  - In patients with prosthetic joints, fluoroquinolones are the initial treatment of choice and should be combined with rifampin for staphylococcal infections.[116]
- Emergent orthopedic consultation should be pursued.
  - Open, arthroscopic, and/or needle drainage of the infected joint may be necessary.[114]

Disposition

- Septic joints require hospital admission for intravenous antibiotics and likely an emergent surgical intervention.
- The patient will likely require eight to ten weeks of antibiotic therapy following diagnosis.[114]

Complications

- The main complications of septic arthritis are related to delayed diagnosis and/or treatment.
- Specific complications may include cartilage destruction and permanent loss of ROM.

Pediatric Considerations

- Septic arthritis is associated with recent infections, including respiratory infections.[117]
- The elbow is not a common site of septic arthritis.[117]
- Presentation may be slowly progressive.

Pearls and Pitfalls

- Prompt evaluation and treatment of septic arthritis is essential.
- Septic arthritis must always be considered in the differential diagnosis of joint pain.
- It is important to accurately diagnose the cause of a painful, swollen joint, as treatment for the potential causes varies considerably.

Table 2.2: Key diagnosis, History, Physical Exam Findings and Treatment

Key Diagnosis	History	Physical Exam Findings	ED Treatment
Elbow Dislocations	FOOSH; rarely posterior elbow trauma; a rotational component may be present	Posterior dislocation = prominent olecranon Anterior dislocation = extended, lengthened forearm	Immediate reduction +/− splinting; prompt orthopedic or sports medicine referral (two to three days)
Nursemaid's Elbow	Occur in children < 5 years old secondary to a longitudinal force applied to the forearm	An unused elbow without deformity; flexion/extension may be preserved with limited supination	Reduction, most often without analgesia and/or imaging
Radial Head Fractures	FOOSH injury; rarely due to a posterior lateral rotary force; can occur with an elbow dislocation	Radial head tenderness with decreased range of motion; be sure to also evaluate the wrist (Essex-Lopresti lesion)	Type I (nondisplaced) = early range of motion Type II (displaced) = splint and refer to orthopedics

Table 2.2: *(cont.)*

Key Diagnosis	History	Physical Exam Findings	ED Treatment
			Type III (comminuted): surgical repair
Supracondylar Fractures	FOOSH (98%) vs. a direct fall on a flexed elbow (2%)	Elbow swelling; reduced ROM; radial and anterior interosseous nerve injuries do occur	Type I fractures (nondisplaced)= splint with orthopedic follow-up Type II-III fractures = orthopedic consultation in the ED
Monteggia Fractures	FOOSH injury with hyperpronation most common	Radial head may be palpable in the antecubital fossa; radial nerve injury is possible	The radial head relocates with reduction of ulna fracture; requires prompt orthopedic referral
OCD Lesions	Pediatric population with a history of sports (e.g., pitching) or direct trauma; gradual onset aching pain	Possible decreased ROM due to a loose body; an effusion may be present	Cease offending activity; orthopedic/sports medicine referral for all; loose bodies may need surgical removal
Ligamentous Injuries	May be acute or chronic; acute associated with elbow dislocation; chronic most common in overhead throwers	Evaluate with the elbow in 15–30° of flexion; evaluate both elbows for subtle differences	Acute = reduce dislocation and verify neurovascular status Chronic = Cease exacerbating activities and follow-up in one week with orthopedics or sports medicine
Distal Biceps Ruptures	Eccentric loading of the biceps tendon with the elbow flexed at 90°	Prominence at the mid-humerus; swelling and ecchymoses; lack of strength with flexion/supination	No acute ED treatment is necessary; follow-up with orthopedics in two to three days
Distal Triceps Ruptures	FOOSH with concomitant eccentric contraction of the triceps	Lack of the ability to extend or significant weakness with elbow extension; Thompson triceps test is also valuable	No acute ED treatment is necessary; a surgical repair for complete tears is advised within three weeks
Lateral/Medial Epicondylitis	Ache/tenderness along medial or lateral epicondyle; gradual onset; worse with activity	Normal strength, sensation, and ROM; tenderness focused over epicondyle; lateral = pain with resisted wrist extension	Behavior modification; heat, ice, and NSAIDs; consider counterforce bracing and wrist splinting
Olecranon/ Septic Bursitis	Warmth, tenderness, pain, and swelling focused over the posterior elbow	Focal warmth and erythema do not differentiate infectious from noninfectious etiologies	Antibiotics if concern for septic bursitis; consider aspiration; use compression and NSAIDs; follow-up in 24–48 hours
Cubital Tunnel Syndrome	Medial arm pain proximal and/or distal to the elbow; numbness/tingling of the ring and little fingers of the affected extremity	Paresthesias of the ring and little fingers; intrinsic hand muscle weakness; clawed hand with delayed presentation	NSAIDs for pain control; behavior modification; night splint/padding as necessary

Table 2.2: (cont.)

Key Diagnosis	History	Physical Exam Findings	ED Treatment
Pronator Syndrome	Pain/paresthesias on the volar aspect of the thumb, index, and middle fingers and lateral half of the ring finger; absence of night pain	Intrinsic hand muscle weakness; positive Tinels sign over the anterior forearm; +/- decreased sensation over the thenar eminence	NSAIDs for pain control; behavior modification; +/- corticosteroid injections; splinting if tolerated
Septic Arthritis	Generally monoarticular joint pain, swelling, warmth, and decreased range of motion	Painful and often decreased range of motion; elbow effusion with warmth	Arthrocentesis should be performed; antibiotics and orthopedic consultation for consideration of a surgical intervention are warranted

Table 2.3: Indications for Orthopedic Surgery Consultation in the Emergency Department

Indication/Sign/Symptom
Neurovascular compromise
Inability to reduce an elbow dislocation
Grossly unstable elbow fracture/dislocation
Concern for compartment syndrome
Open fractures
Septic arthritis/septic bursitis with systemic signs of infection

Recommended Readings

Arundel D, Williams P, Townend W. Deriving the east riding elbow rule (ER2): A maximally sensitive decision tool for elbow injury. *Emergency Medicine Journal.* 2014; 31(5): 380–383.

Eiff M, Hatch R. *Fracture Management for Primary Care.* Saunders-Elsevier. Philadelphia. 2012.

Ladenhauf HN, Schaffert M, Bauer J. The displaced supracondylar humerus fracture: Indications for surgery and surgical options, a 2014 update. *Current Opinion in Pediatrics.* 2014; 26(1): 64–69.

DeLee JC, Drez D, Miller MD. *Delee and Drez's Orthopaedic Sports Medicine,* 3rd Edition. Saunders-Elsevier. Philadelphia. 2010.

Sears BW, Spear LM. Evaluation and management of adult elbow dislocations in the emergency department. *Emergency Medicine.* 2014; 4(2): 175.

References

1. Sheehan SE, Dyer GS, Sodickson AD, Ketankumar IP, Khurana B. Traumatic elbow injuries: What the orthopedic surgeon wants to know. *Radiographics.* 2013; 33(3): 869–889.
2. Freed HA, Shields NN. Most frequently overlooked radiographically apparent fractures in a teaching hospital emergency department. *Annals of Emergency Medicine.* 1984; 13(10): 900–904.
3. Harrast MA, Finnoff JT. Elbow and forearm. In *Sports Medicine Study Guide and Review for Boards.* Demos Medical. New York. 2012; 245.
4. Beals, RK. The normal carrying angle of the elbow: A radiographic study of 422 patients. *Clinical Orthopaedics and Related Research.* 1976; 119: 194–196.
5. Hoppenfeld, S. *Physical Examination of the Spine and Extremities.* Prentice-Hall. Upper Saddle River. 1976; 37.
6. Tullos HS, Erwin W, Woods GW, et al.. Unusual lesions of the throwing arm. *Clinical Orthopaedics.* 1972; 88: 169.
7. O'Driscoll SW, Goncalves LB, Dietz P. The hook test for distal biceps tendon avulsion. *American Journal of Sports Medicine.* 2007; 35(11): 1865–1869.
8. O'Driscoll SW, Lawton RL, Smith AM. The "moving valgus stress test" for medial collateral ligament tears of the elbow. *American Journal of Sports Medicine.* 2005; 33(2): 231–239.
9. Josefsson PO, Nilsson BE. Incidence of elbow dislocation. *Acta Orthopaedica Scandinavica.* 1986; 57(6): 537–538.
10. Cohen MS, Hastings H. Acute elbow dislocation: Evaluation and management. *Journal of the*

American Academy of Orthopaedic Surgeons. 1998; 6: 15–23.

11. Konya MN, Aslan A, Sofu H, Yildirim. Biepicondylar fracture dislocation of the elbow joint concomitant with ulnar nerve injury. *World Journal of Orthopedics*. 2013; 4(2): 94–97.
12. Stoneback JW, Owens BD, Sykes J, Athwal GS, Pointer L, Wolf JM. Incidence of elbow dislocations in the United States population. *Journal of Bone and Joint Surgery*. 2012; 94(3): 240–245.
13. Linscheid Rl, Wheeler DK. Elbow dislocations. *JAMA*. 1965; 194: 1171–1176.
14. Bracker MD, Achar SA, Pana AL, Taylor KS. *Elbow dislocations. The 5-Minute Sports Medicine Consult,* 2nd Edition. Lippincott, Williams, and Wilkins. Philadelphia. 2011.
15. Miller M, Hart J, MacKnight J. Elbow dislocations. In *Essential Orthopaedics*. Saunders-Elsevier. Philadelphia. 2010; 258.
16. Sparks SR, De La Rosa J, Bergan JJ, Hoyt DB, Owens EL. Arterial injury in uncomplicated upper extremity dislocations. *Annals of Vascular Surgery*. 2000; 14: 110–113.
17. Stanley D, Trail IA. Elbow dislocations. In *Operative Elbow Surgery*. Churchill Livingstone Elsevier. Philadelphia. 2012; 361.
18. Marcheix B, Chaufour X, Ayel J, Hollington L, Mansat P, Barret A, Bossavy JP. Transection of the brachial artery after closed posterior elbow dislocation. *Journal of Vascular Surgery*. 2005; 42(6): 1230–1232.
19. Wolfson AB, Hendey GW, Harwood-Nuss A, et al.. *Harwood-Nuss' Clinical Practice of Emergency Medicine,* 5th Edition. Lippincott, Williams, and Wilkins. Philadelphia. 2010: 270.
20. O'Driscoll SW. Classification and evaluation of recurrent instability of the elbow. *Clinical Orthopaedics and Related Research*. 2000; 370: 34–43.
21. Douglas K, Cannada LK, Archer KR, Dean DB, Lee S, Obremskey W. Incidence and risks factors of heterotopic ossification following major elbow trauma. *Orthopaedics*. 2012; 35(6): e815–e822.
22. Baird EO, Kang QK. Prophylaxis of heterotopic ossification: An updated review. *Journal of Orthopaedic Surgery and Research*. 2009; 4(12): 1–8.
23. Korus L, Morhart M, Jarman A, Olson J. Median nerve reconstruction after entrapment in the elbow. *Canadian Journal of Plastic Surgery*. 2009; 17(4): 130–132.
24. Mehta, JA, Bain GI. Elbow dislocations in adults and children. *Clinics in Sports Medicine*. 2004; 23(4): 609–627.
25. Schunk JF. Radial head subluxation: Epidemiology and treatment of 87 episodes. *Annals of Emergency Medicine*. 1990; 19(9): 1019–1023.
26. Macias CG, Bothner J, Wiebe R. A comparison of supination/flexion to hyperpronation in the reduction of radial head subluxations. *Pediatrics*. 1998; 102(1): e10.
27. Schaider JJ, Barkin RM, Hayden SR, Wolfe RE, Barkin AZ, Shayne P, Rosen P. *Rosen and Barkin's 5-Minute Emergency Medicine Consult,* 5th Edition. Lippincott, Williams, and Wilkins. Philadelphia. 2011.
28. Kaplan RE, Lillis KA. Recurrent nursemaid's elbow (annular ligament displacement) treatment via telephone. *Pediatrics*. 2002; 110(1): 171–174.
29. Illingworth DM. Pulled elbow: A study of 100 patients. *British Medical Journal*. 1975; 2: 672–675.
30. Roidis NT, Papadakis SA, Rigopoulos N, Basdekis G, Poultsides L, Karachalios T, Malizos K, Itamura J. Current concepts and controversies in the management of radial head fractures. *Orthopedics*. 2006; 29(10): 904–916.
31. Calfee R, Madom I, Weiss APC. Radial head arthroplasty. *Journal of Hand Surgery*. 2006; 31(2): 314–321.
32. Papageorgiou TG, Panos NE, Gigis IP, Samoladas EP, Beslikas TA, Christoforidis IE. Treatment of a late presenting displaced radial neck fracture in a 10 years-old girl. *Journal of Medical Cases*. 2011; 2(6): 252–254.
33. Darracq MA, Vinson DR, Panacek EA. Preservation of active range of motion after acute elbow trauma predicts absence of elbow fracture. *American Journal of Emergency Medicine*. 2008; 26 (7): 779–782.
34. Arundel D, Williams P, Townend W. Deriving the east riding elbow rule (ER2): A maximally sensitive decision tool for elbow injury. *Emergency Medicine Journal*. 2014; 31(5): 380–383.
35. Iannuzzi NP, Leopold SS. In brief: The mason classification of radial head fractures. *Clinical Orthopaedics and Related Research*. 2012; 470(6): 1799–1802.
36. Chalidis BE, Papadopoulos PP, Sachinis NC, Dimitriou CG. Aspiration alone versus aspiration and bupivacaine in the treatment of undisplaced radial head fractures: A prospective randomized study.

Journal of Shoulder and Elbow Surgery. 2009; 18(5): 676–679.

37. Hammacher ER, van der Werken C. Radial head fracture: Operative or conservative treatment? The Greek temple model. *Acta Orthopaedica*. 1996; 62 (Suppl. 1): 112–115.
38. Guido, Z, Galli S, Marchese M, Mascio L, Pazzagliz UE. The surgical treatment of isolated Mason type 2 fractures of the radial head in adults: Comparison between radial head resection and open reduction and internal fixation. *Journal of Orthopaedic Trauma*. 2012; 26(4): 229–235.
39. Janssen RP, Vegter J. Resection of the radial head after Mason type-III fractures of the elbow: Follow-up at 16 to 30 years. *Journal of Bone and Joint Surgery*. 1998; 80: 231–233.
40. Hotchkiss RN, Green DP. Fractures and dislocations of the elbow. In *Rockwood and Green's Fractures in Adults,* 3rd Edition. Lippincott-Raven. Philadelphia. 1991: 805–825.
41. Pappas N, Bernstein J. Fractures in brief: Radial head fractures. *Clinical Orthopaedics and Related Research*. 2010; 468(3): 914–916.
42. Omid R, Choi PD, Skaggs DL. Supracondylar humeral fractures in children. *Journal of Bone and Joint Surgery*. 2008; 90 (5): 1121–1132.
43. Eiff M, Hatch R. Elbow fractures. In *Fracture Management for Primary Care.* Saunders-Elsevier. Philadelphia. 2012; 130–153.
44. *The treatment of pediatric supracondylar humerus fractures: evidence-based guideline and evidence report.* American Academy of Orthopaedic Surgeons. 2011; 1-249. Available at: www.aaos .org/research/guidelines/ SupracondylarFracture/ SupConFullGuideline.pdf.
45. DeLee JC, Drez D, Miller MD. *Delee and Drez's Orthopaedic Sports Medicine,* 3rd Edition. Saunders-Elsevier. Philadelphia. 2010.
46. Baldo J. The Monteggia lesion. *Clinical Orthopaedics*. 1967; 50: 71–76.
47. Perron AD, Hersh RE, Brady WJ, et al.. Orthopaedic pitfalls in the ED: Galeazzi and Monteggia fracture-dislocation. *American Journal of Emergency Medicine*. 2001; 19(3): 225–228.
48. Ring D, Jupiter J, Waters P. Monteggia fractures in children and adults. *Journal of the American Academy of Orthopaedic Surgery*. 1998; 6: 215–224.
49. Chhabra, AB. ORIF forearm fractures. In *Sports Medicine Conditions: Return to Play: Recognition, Treatment, and Planning*. Lippincott, Williams, and Wilkins. Philadelphia. 2014.
50. Eathiraju S, Dorth D, Mudgal C, Jupiter J. Monteggia fracture-dislocations. *Hand Clinics*. 2007; 23(2): 165–177.
51. Edmonds EW, Polousky J. A review of knowledge in osteochondritis dissecans: 123 years of minimal evolution from Konig to the ROCK Study Group. *Clinical Orthopaedics and Related Research*. 2013; 471: 1118–1126.
52. Cohen MS, Bruno RJ. The collateral ligaments of the elbow anatomy and clinical correlation. *Clinical Orthopaedics and Related Research*. 2001; 383: 123–130.
53. Reichel LM, Milam GS, et al.. Elbow lateral collateral ligament injuries. *Journal of Hand Surgery*. 2013; 38: 184–201.
54. Bruce JR, Andrews JR. Ulnar collateral ligament injuries in the throwing athlete. *Journal of the American Academy of Orthopaedic Surgeons*. 2014; 22: 315–325.
55. Langer P, Fadale P, Hulstyn M. Evolution of the treatment options of ulnar collateral ligament injuries of the elbow. *British Journal of Sports Medicine*. 2006; 40: 499–506.
56. Sutton KM, Dodds SD, Ahmad CS, Sethi PM. Surgical treatment of distal biceps rupture. *Journal of the American Academy of Orthopaedic Surgeons*. 2010; 18: 139–148.
57. El Maraghy A, Devereaux M, Tsoi K. The biceps crease interval for diagnosing complete distal biceps tendon ruptures. *Clinical Orthopaedics and Related Research*. 2008; 466(9): 2255–2262.
58. Bauman GI. Rupture of the biceps tendon. *Journal of Bone and Joint Surgery*. 1934; 16: 966–967.
59. Ramsey, ML. Distal biceps tendon injuries: Diagnosis and management. *Journal of the American Academy of Orthopaedic Surgeons*. 1999; 7 (3): 199–207.
60. Safran MR, Graham SM. Distal biceps tendon ruptures: Incidence, demographics, and the effect of smoking. *Clinical Orthopaedics and Related Research*. 2002; 404: 275–283.
61. Lee HG. Traumatic avulsion of tendon of insertion of biceps brachii. *American Journal of Surgery*. 1951; 82: 290–292.
62. Virk MS, DiVenere J, Mazzocca AD. Distal biceps tendon injuries: Treatment of partial and complete tears. *Operative Techniques in Sports Medicine*. In press.
63. American Academy of Orthopaedic Surgeons. Biceps tendon tear at the elbow. *OrthoInfo*. 2009. Available at: orthoinfo.aaos.org/topic.cfm?topic=a00376.
64. Morrey BF, Askew LJ, An KN, Dobyns JH. Rupture of the distal tendon of the biceps brachii: A

biomechanical study. *Journal of Bone and Joint Surgery*. 1985; 67: 418–421.

65. Baker BE, Bierwagen D. Rupture of the distal tendon of the biceps brachii: Operative versus non-operative treatment. *Journal of Bone and Joint Surgery*. 1985; 67: 414–417.
66. Klonz A, Loitz D, Wohler P, Reilmann H. Rupture of the distal biceps brachii tendon: Isokinetic power analysis and complications after anatomic reinsertion compared with fixation of the brachialis muscle. *Journal of Shoulder and Elbow Surgery*. 2003; 12: 607–611.
67. Kelly EW, Morrey NF, O'Driscoll SW. Complications of repair of the distal biceps tendon with the modified two-incision technique. *Journal of Bone and Joint Surgery*. 2000; 82A: 1575–1581.
68. Cain RA, Nydick JA, Stein MI, Williams BD, Polikandrioitis JA, Hess AV. Complications following distal biceps repair. *Journal of Hand Surgery*. 2012; 37(10): 2112–2117.
69. Bach BR, Warren RF, Wickiewicz. Triceps rupture: A case report and literature review. *American Journal of Sports Medicine*. 1987; 15: 285–289.
70. Kokkalis ZT, Mavrogenis AF, Spyridonos S, Papagelopoulos PJ, Weiser RW, Sotereanos DG. Triceps brachii distal tendon reattachment with a double row technique. *Orthopedics*. 2013; 36(2): 110–116.
71. Yeh PC, Dodds SD, Smart LR, Mazzocca AD, Sethi PM. Distal triceps rupture. *Journal of the American Academy of Orthopaedic Surgery*. 2010; 18 (1): 31–40.
72. Sollender JL, Rayan GM, Barden GA. Triceps tendon rupture in weight lifters. *Journal of Shoulder and Elbow Surgery*. 1998; 7: 151–153.
73. Sherman OH, Snyder SJ, Fox JM. Triceps tendon avulsion in a professional body builder: A case report. *American Journal of Sports Medicine*. 1984; 12: 328–329.
74. Mair SD, Isbell WM, Gill TJ, et al.. Triceps tendon ruptures in professional football players. *American Journal of Sports Medicine*. 2004; 32: 431–434.
75. Slocum DB. Classification of elbow injuries from baseball pitching. *Journal of Texas Medicine*. 1968; 64: 48–53.
76. Match RM, Corrylos EV. Bilateral avulsion fracture of the triceps tendon insertion from skiing with osteogenesis imperfect tarda: A case report. *American Journal of Sports Medicine*. 1983; 11: 99–102.
77. Preston FS, Adicoff A. Hyperparathyroidism with avulsion at three major tendons. *New England Journal of Medicine*. 1961; 266: 968.
78. Farrar EL, Lipper FG. Avulsion of the triceps tendon. *Clinical Orthopaedics*. 1981; 161: 242–246.
79. Stannard JP, Bucknell AL. Rupture of the triceps tendon associated with steroid injections. *American Journal of Sports Medicine*. 1993; 21: 482–485.
80. Strauch RJ, Rosenwasser MP. Single incision repair of distal biceps tendon rupture. *Techniques in Hand and Upper Extremity Surgery*. 1998; 2: 253–261.
81. van Riet RP, Morrey BF, Ho E, O'Driscoll SW. Surgical treatment of distal triceps ruptures. *Journal of Bone and Joint Surgery*. 2003; 85: 1961–1967.
82. Pantazopoulos T, Exarchou E, Stavrou Z, Hartofilakidis-Garofalidis G. Avulsion of the triceps tendon. *Journal of Trauma*. 1975; 15: 827–829.
83. Tarsney FF. Rupture and avulsion of the triceps. *Clinical Orthopedics of North America*. 1972; 83: 177–183.
84. Goldman L, Schafer A. *Goldman's Cecil Medicine*, 24th Edition. Philadelphia. 2012; 1676–1681.
85. Ahmad Z, Siddiqui N, et al.. Lateral epicondylitis: A review of pathology and management. *Bone and Joint Journal*. 2013; 95B: 1158–1164.
86. Shin R, Ring D. The ulnar nerve in elbow trauma. *Journal of Bone and Joint Surgery*. 2007; 89(5): 1108–1116.
87. Rishi G, Adamson G, et al.. A prospective randomized study comparing a forearm strap brace versus a wrist splint for the treatment of lateral epicondylitis. *Journal of Shoulder and Elbow Surgery*. 2010; 19: 508–512.
88. Coombes BK, Bisset L, et al.. Effect of corticosteroid injection, physiotherapy, or both on clinical outcomes in patients with unilateral lateral epicondylalgia: A randomized controlled trial. *Journal of the American Medical Association*. 2013; 309(5): 461–469.
89. Ahmad Z, Brooks R, Kang SN, et al.. The effect of platelet-rich plasma on clinical outcomes in lateral epicondylitis. *Arthroscopy*. 2013; 29(11): 1851–1862.
90. Rabago D, Best TM, Zgierska AE, et al.. A systematic review of four injection therapies for lateral epicondylosis: Prolotherapy, polidocanol, whole blood and platelet-rich plasma. British Journal of Sports Medicine. 2009; 43 (7):471-481.
91. Calfee RP, Patel A, et al.. Management of lateral epicondylitis: Current concepts. *Journal of the American Academy of Orthopaedic Surgeons*. 2008; 16(1): 19–29.

92. Bozentka, DJ. Cubital tunnel syndrome pathophysiology. *Current Orthopaedics and Related Research*. 1998; 351: 90–94.

93. Aoki M, Takasaki H, Muraki T, et al.. Strain on the ulnar nerve at the elbow and wrist during throwing motion. *Journal of Bone and Joint Surgery*. 2005; 87 (11): 2508–2514.

94. Buehler MJ, Thayer DT. The elbow flexion test: A clinical test for the cubital tunnel syndrome. *Clinical Orthopaedics*. 1988; 233: 213–216.

95. Morrey BF. *The Elbow and Its Disorders*. WB Saunders. Philadelphia. 1985; 497–501.

96. Beekman R, Schreuder AH, Rozeman CA, Koehler PJ, Uitdehaag BM. The diagnostic value of provocative clinical tests in ulnar neuropathy at the elbow is marginal. *Journal of Neurology, Neurosurgery, and Psychiatry*. 2009; 80(12): 1369.

97. Cheng CJ, Mackinnon-Patterson B, Beck JL, et al.. Scratch collapse test for evaluation of carpal and cubital tunnel syndrome. *Journal of Hand Surgery*. 2008; 33: 1518–1524.

98. Szabo RM, Kwak C. Natural history and conservative management of cubital tunnel syndrome. *Hand Clinics*. 2007; 23: 311–318, v-vi.

99. Keefe DT, Lintner DM. Nerve injuries in the throwing elbow. *Clinical Sports Medicine*. 2004; 23: 723–742, xi.

100. Charles YP, Coulet B, Rouzaud JC, et al.. Comparative clinical outcomes of submuscular and subcutaneous transposition of the ulnar nerve for cubital tunnel syndrome. *Journal of Hand Surgery*. 2009; 34: 866–874.

101. Stål M, Hagert C, Moritz U. Upper extremity nerve involvement in Swedish female machine milkers. *American Journal of Industrial Medicine*. 1998; 33(6): 551–559.

102. Jones NF, Ming NL. Persistent median artery as a cause of pronator syndrome. *Journal of Hand Surgery*. 1988; 13(5): 728–732.

103. Hartz CR, Linscheid RL, Gramse RR, Daube JR. The pronator teres syndrome: Compressive neuropathy of the median nerve. *The Journal of Bone and Joint Surgery*. 1981; 63(6): 885–890.

104. Klauser As, Tagliafico A, Allen GM, et al.. Clinical indications for musculoskeletal ultrasound: A delphi-based consensus paper of the European society of musculoskeletal radiology. *European Radiology*. 2012; 22(5): 1140–1148.

105. Johnson RK, Spinner M, Shrewsbury MM. Median nerve entrapment syndrome in the proximal forearm. *Journal of Hand Surgery*. 1979; 4(1): 48–51.

106. Dang AC, Rodner CM. Unusual compression neuropathies of the forearm, part II: Median nerve. *Journal of Hand Surgery*. 2009; 34(10): 1915–1920.

107. Baumbach SF, Lobo CM, et al.. Prepatellar and olecranon bursitis: Literature review and development of a treatment algorithm. *Archives of Orthopaedic and Trauma Surgery*. 2014; 134: 359–370.

108. Abzug JM, Chen NC, Jacoby SM. Septic olecranon bursitis. *Journal of Hand Surgery*. 2012; 37A; 1252–1253.

109. Pineda C, Vargas A, Rodriquez AV. Imaging of osteomyelitis: Current concepts. *Infectious Disease Clinics of North America*. 2006; 20(4): 789–825.

110. Maxwell DM. Nonseptic olecranon bursitis management. *Canadian Family Physician*. 2011; 57: 21.

111. Herrera FA, Meals RA. Chronic olecranon bursitis. *Journal of Hand Surgery*. 2011; 36A: 708–709.

112. Roberts J, Schaefer E, Gallo RA. Indicators for detection of septic arthritis in the acutely swollen joint cohort of those without joint prostheses. *Orthopedics*. 2014; 37(2): 98–102.

113. Mehta P, Schnall SB, Zalavras CG. Septic arthritis of the shoulder, elbow, and wrist. *Clinical Orthopaedics and Related Research*. 2006; 451: 42–45.

114. Carpenter CR, Schuur JD, Everett WW, Pines JM. Evidence-based diagnostics: Adult septic arthritis. *Academic Emergency Medicine*. 2011; 18(8): 781–796.

115. Muñoz-Egea MC, Blanco A, Fernández-Roblas R, et al.. Clinical and microbiological characteristics of patients with septic arthritis: A hospital-based study. *Journal of Orthopaedics*. 2014; 11(2): 87–90.

116. Trampuz A, Zimmerli W. Diagnosis and treatment of implant-associated septic arthritis and osteomyelitis. *Current Infectious Disease Reports*. 2008; 10(5): 394–403.

117. Bowakim J, Marti R, Curto A. Elbow septic arthritis in children: Clinical presentation and management. *Journal of Pediatric Orthopedics*. 2010; 19 (3): 281–284.

Chapter 3

Wrist

Christopher R. Pruitt

Background

- The wrist represents the region from the distal radius and ulna to the carpometacarpal joints.
- It is one of the most complex and dynamic joints in the human body, and yet also one of the most commonly injured regions.
- Spectrum of disease varies greatly, ranging from simple sprains to complex fracture/dislocation patterns with associated neurologic compromise.
- This provides for a vast array of potential pathology, making the evaluation and diagnosis of injury quite difficult.
- Making things even more complex, even subtle injury patterns can have dramatic and longstanding complications if not properly diagnosed and treated at initial presentation.
- Consequences from injury and delay in diagnosis include:[1]
  - Rising medical costs
  - Decreased school attendance
  - Lost work hours
  - Loss of independence
  - Chronic pain
  - Lasting functional disability
- A thorough knowledge of anatomy, mechanism of injury, injury patterns, radiographic findings, and appropriate treatment and follow-up are imperative for optimal patient care.

Epidemiology

- Wrist injuries are one of the most common presentations in the ED, accounting for 2.5% of all ED visits.[2]
- Incidence appears to be increasing worldwide, likely multifactorial:[3]
  - Advancing age and changes in bone metabolism
  - Increasing sports activity in children
  - Increasing obesity rates
- The most common fracture is the distal radius fracture, which accounts for one-sixth of all fractures seen and treated in US emergency departments.[4]
  - Colles fracture is the most common fracture in all persons less than 75 years old
- Carpal fractures account for 20% of fractures to wrist and hand.[5]
- Injury patterns tend to be bimodal in distribution, affecting youth and elderly populations primarily.
  - Younger patients tend to present with higher mechanism injuries.
    - Motor vehicle accidents
    - Sports injuries
  - Elderly patients present after low mechanism falls.
- The vast majority of wrist pathology occurs via a fall on outstretched hand (FOOSH) (fall on an outstretched hand) mechanism.

Anatomic Considerations / Pathophysiology

- The wrist is composed of the distal radius and ulna, as well as eight carpal bones that are arranged in two transverse rows (Figure 3.1).
  - Proximal carpal row (radial to ulnar) – scaphoid, lunate, triquetrum, pisiform.
  - Distal carpal row (radial to ulnar) – trapezium, trapezoid, capitate, hamate.
  - The carpal rows form three "arcs," which are key to identifying injury on PA radiograph.
    - Proximal border of the scaphoid, lunate, and triquetrum

  - Distal border of the proximal carpal row
  - Proximal border of the capitate and hamate
  - These arcs should be smooth and continuous
  - Each of the carpal bones is separated by a uniform 1–2 mm.
- Principle movements of the wrist are flexion, extension, radial deviation, and ulnar deviation.
- The radius articulates directly with the proximal carpal row.
  - Articular surface is both concave and tilted.
    - Concavity "cups" the scaphoid and lunate

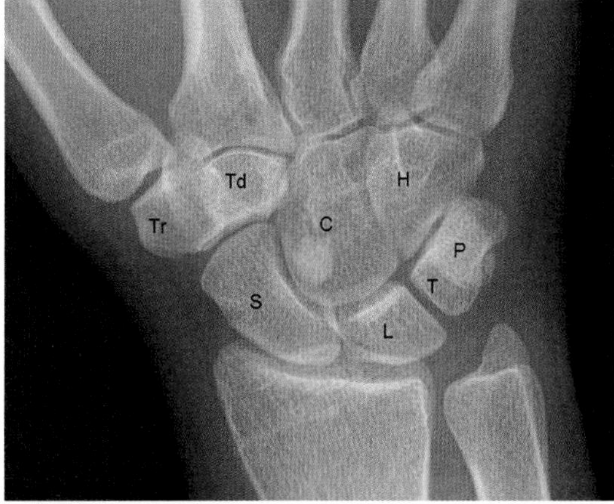

Figure 3.1. PA view of the carpal bones.S = Scaphoid, L = Lunate, T = Triquetrum, P = PisiformTr = Trapezium, Td = Trapezoid, C = Capitate, H = Hamate.

    - Normal volar tilt of 0–22° (lateral radiograph)
    - Normal radial tilt ("or radial inclination") of 15–30° (PA radiograph)
- The ulna has no direct bony articulations.
  - Ulna has a nonosseous fibrocartilage union with the radius, triquetrum, and lunate, called the triangular fibrocartilage complex (TFCC). (Figure 3.2)
- The ulna articulates with the radius at the distal radioulnar joint (DRUJ).
  - Stability of this joint is maintained by the TFCC, interosseous membrane, and both dorsal and volar radioulnar ligaments.
  - Pronation and supination are accomplished through articulations at the proximal and distal radioulnar joints.
- There are two classifications of ligaments in the wrist: extrinsic and intrinsic.
  - Extrinsic ligaments connect carpal bones to the radius, ulna, or metacarpals.
  - Intrinsic ligaments connect carpal bones to one another.
- Extrinsic ligaments are further characterized as dorsal or volar.
  - Volar ligaments are relatively stronger than dorsal counterparts, which plays a role in injury pattern and associated carpal instability.
- There is dual vascular supply to the wrist with the radial and ulnar arteries.

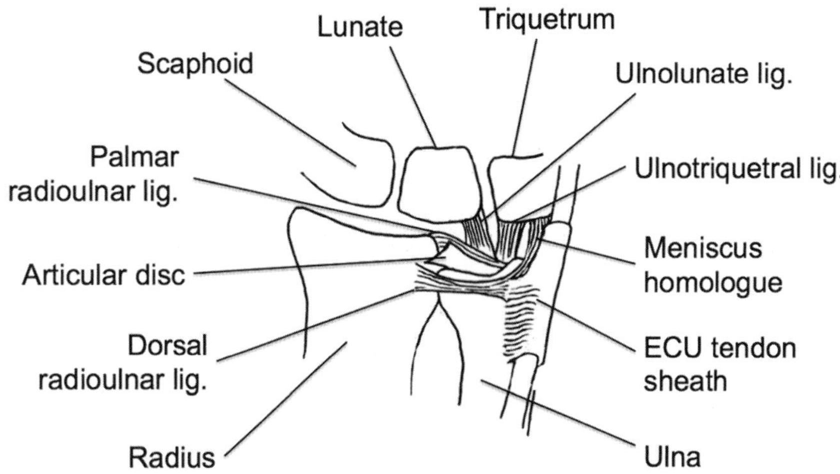

Figure 3.2. Triangular Fibrocartilage Complex (TFCC). Illustration by Yvonne Chow.

- Radial artery runs lateral (radial) to the flexor carpi radialis.
- Ulnar artery is just radial to the flexor carpi ulnaris.

- Many of the carpal bones have solitary vascular supply, paradoxically running in a distal to proximal course. This has significant impact on fracture healing, depending on anatomic location of the lesion, which is described later in more detail.
- Motor and sensory inputs are from radial, ulnar, and median nerves:
  - Radial nerve courses dorsally, supplying motor function to wrist extension and finger extension; sensory input is to the dorsum of the hand.
  - Median nerve runs within the carpal tunnel on the volar aspect of the wrist, supplying motor function to wrist flexion, finger flexion, thumb flexion, extension, and abduction; sensory input is to the volar aspect of the hand for the first three digits.
  - Ulnar nerve runs parallel to the ulnar artery and passes through Guyon's canal, consisting of the pisiform and hook of the hamate; it controls hypothenar muscles, interossei, and the fourth and fifth digit lumbricals; sensory input is to the ulnar side of the palm and fourth and fifth digits.
- Each of these nerves is susceptible to injury with certain fracture patterns, to be discussed later in the chapter.

Focused History and Physical Examination

History

- As with any medical presentation, a good history is paramount.
- Key features include:
  - Mechanism of injury
  - Timing and duration or pain
  - Alleviating and aggravating features
  - Neurovascular changes
  - History of prior injury or surgery
  - Baseline motor and sensory function prior to injury
  - Hand dominance
  - Special attention to baseline activity and occupation

Physical Examination

- Physical examination begins with appearance and comparison to the opposite extremity.
  - Note swelling, ecchymosis, deformity, and distal perfusion
  - Point of maximal tenderness, referred pain
  - Passive and active ROM, noting pain and limitations
- Palpable landmarks:
  - Dorsal (radial to ulnar) (Figure 3.3):
    - Radial Styloid
      - Distal end of the radius, easily palpable and usually visible on inspection
    - Snuff box (Figure 3.4)
      - Bordered proximally by the radial styloid, radially by the abductor pollicis longus and extensor pollicis brevis, and ulnarly by the extensor pollicis longus tendon
      - Scaphoid resides within the snuff box, more prominent with ulnar deviation

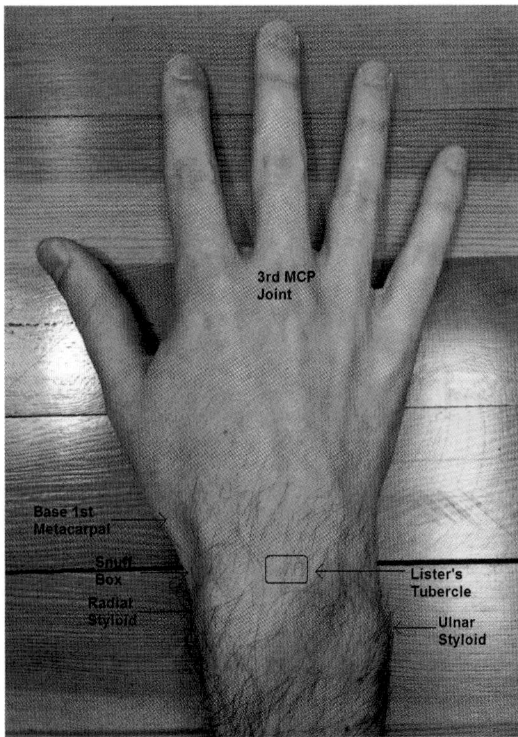

Figure 3.3. Dorsal landmarks of the wrist.

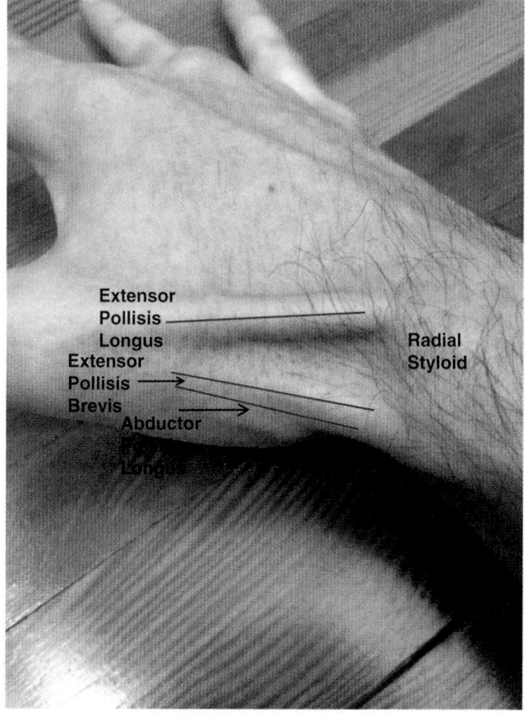

Figure 3.4. Anatomic snuff box landmarks. The radial styloid forms the base, and both the scaphoid and trapezium may be palpated within the snuff box.

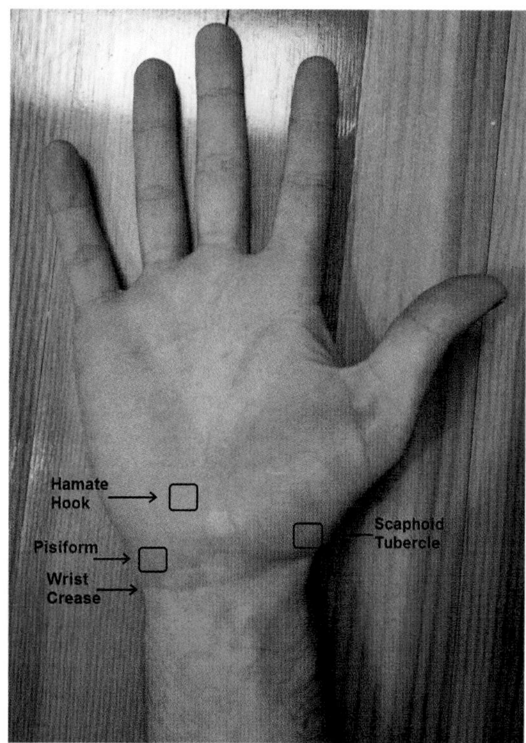

Figure 3.5. Volar landmarks of the wrist.

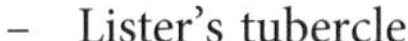

- Lister's tubercle
  - Depression felt just ulnar to the radial styloid
  - Landmark for the scapholunate joint
  - Capitate is palpated just distal with the wrist in neutral position
  - Lunate is palpable with the wrist in flexion
- Ulnar styloid
  - Bony prominence on the dorsal ulnar aspect, easily visible
- Triquetrum
  - Palpable just distal to the ulnar styloid

- Volar (radial to ulnar)(Figure 3.5):
  - Scaphoid Tubercle
    - Just distal to the radial styloid, at the thenar muscle base
  - Pisiform
    - At the base of the hypothenar muscles, just distal to the ulnar styloid and distal wrist crease
  - Hook of the hamate
    - Approximately 1 cm distal and radial to the pisiform

- Range of motion:
  - Test range of motion of the wrist in all directions and compare to the contralateral side.
  - Range of motion at the wrist includes:
    - Flexion
    - Extension
    - Pronation
    - Supination
    - Radial deviation
    - Ulnar deviation
- Special tests:
  - *Finkelstein test* (De Quervain's tenosynovitis) (Figure 3.6)
    - Patient places the thumb in flexion within the palm, and examiner deviates the wrist ulnarly.
    - Positive = pain
  - *Tinel's sign* (carpal tunnel syndrome) (Figure 3.7)

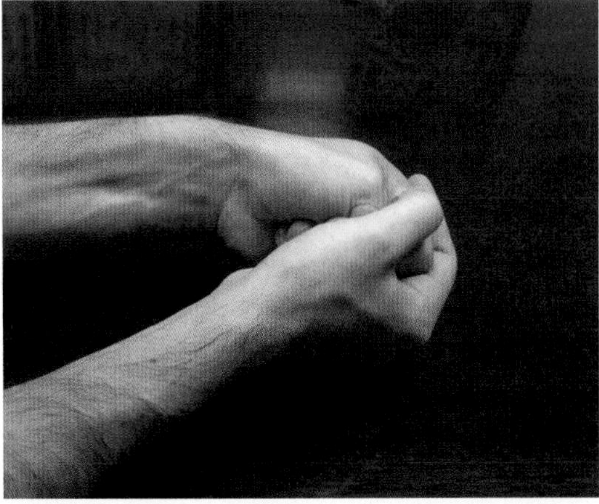

Figure 3.6. Finkelstein test.

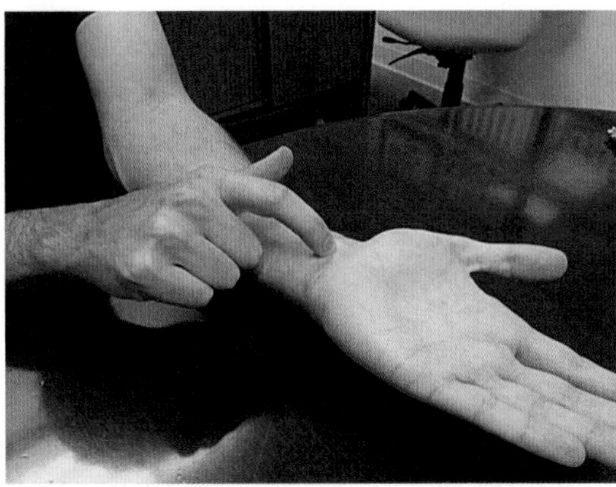

Figure 3.7. Tinel's sign.

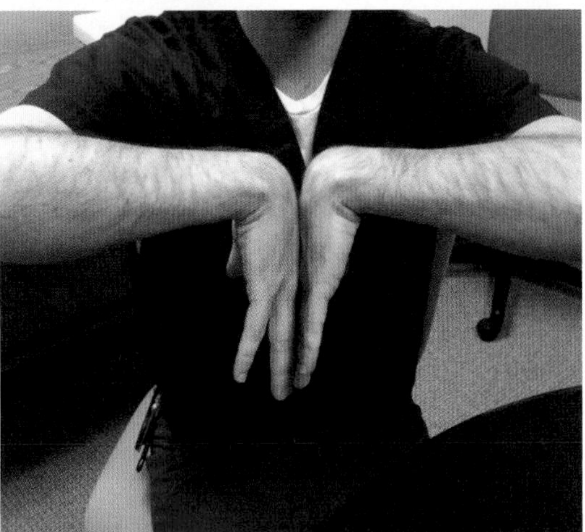

Figure 3.8. Phalen's test.

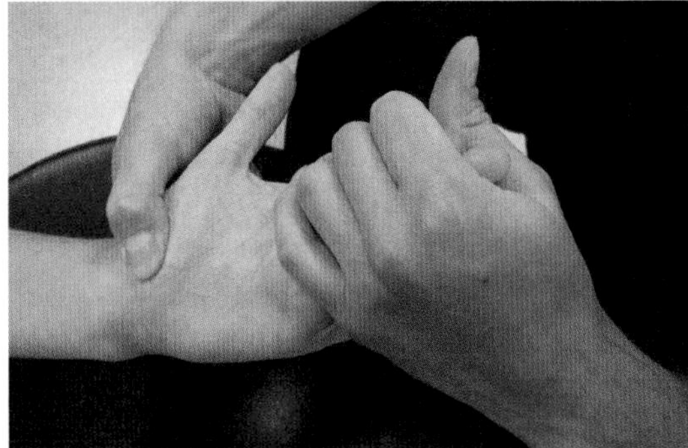

Figure 3.9. Scaphoid shift test.

  - Tapping the volar wrist over the carpal tunnel
  - Positive = paresthesias in median nerve distribution

- *Phalen's test* (carpal tunnel syndrome) (Figure 3.8)
  - Dorsiflexion of the wrist for upwards of 60 seconds
  - Positive = paresthesias in median nerve distribution

- *Scaphoid shift test* (scapholunate dissociation) (Figure 3.9)
  - Examiner's thumb presses on the base of the thenar eminence, over the scaphoid, while the hand wraps around the wrist.
  - Examiner's opposite hand holds the patient's hand at the level of the MCP joints.
  - The wrist is held in extension and mild ulnar deviation.
  - While applying thumb pressure over the scaphoid, the wrist is gently flexed and radially deviated.
  - Positive = if the scaphoid shifts dorsally
  - While releasing pressure on the scaphoid, examiner or patient may feel or hear a "click" as the scaphoid returns to its normal position.

- *TFCC compression test* (TFCC tear) (Figure 3.10)
  - Axial load the wrist and then deviate wrist to ulnar side.
  - Test is positive if it creates a click and reproduces the patient's pain.

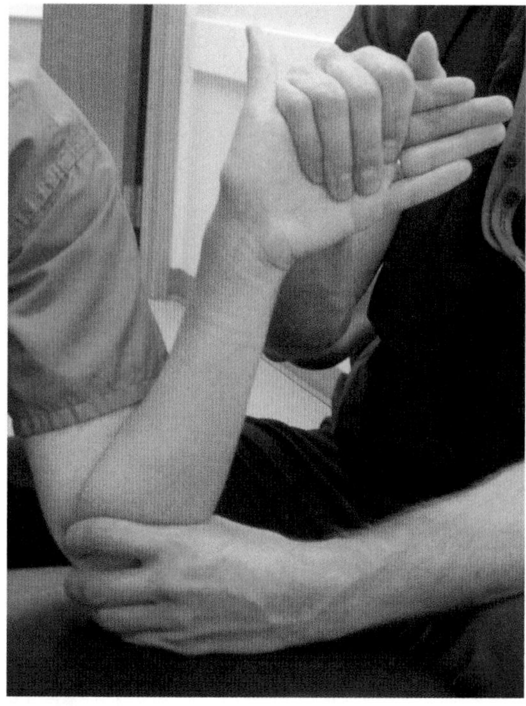

Figure 3.10. Triangular fibrocartilage complex (TFCC) compression test.

- *Piano key test*
  - Assesses the stability of the DRUJ.
  - With the wrist in pronation, volar pressure is placed on the distal ulna.
  - Test is positive if pain or instability is elicited compared to contralateral side.
- *Shuck test* (Figure 3.11)
  - Also tests stability of DRUJ
  - The distal radius is held with one hand, and the distal ulna with the other.
  - The distal radius is moved dorsally.
  - This test is positive if it elicits pain or instability compared to the contralateral side.

- Neurovascular exam:
  - Two-point discrimination is the most sensitive test for sensory function of the nerves.
  - Compare to uninjured hand
    - Volar
      - Distinguish two blunt points that are 2–5 mm apart on the fingertips, 7–10 mm at the base of the palm[6]

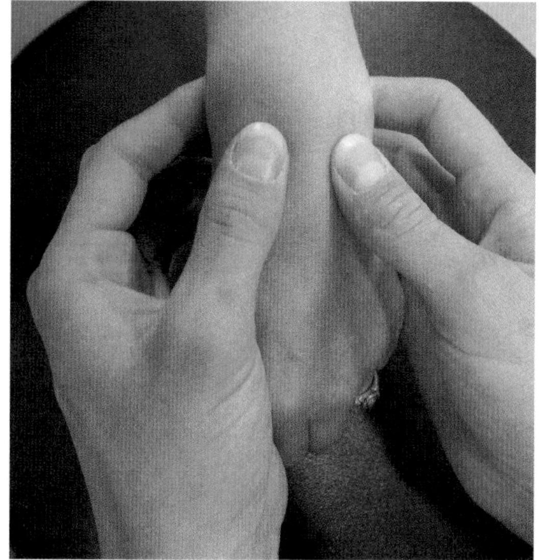

Figure 3.11. Shuck test.

    - Dorsal
      - Distinguish two blunt points at 7–12 mm
  - Median nerve
    - Sensory – sensation to the index fingertip
    - Motor – thumb abduction
  - Ulnar nerve
    - Sensory – sensation to little fingertip
    - Motor – abduction of fingers, or thumb adduction
  - Radial nerve
    - Sensory – sensation to dorsum of thumb/webspace
    - Motor – extension of wrist and MCPs
- Vascular exam:
  - Radial pulse
  - Ulnar pulse
  - Capillary refill

Radiographic Considerations

- Evaluation begins with PA, lateral, and oblique radiographs of the wrist.
  - PA radiograph provides detailed information for both obvious and subtle injury patterns (Figure 3.12).

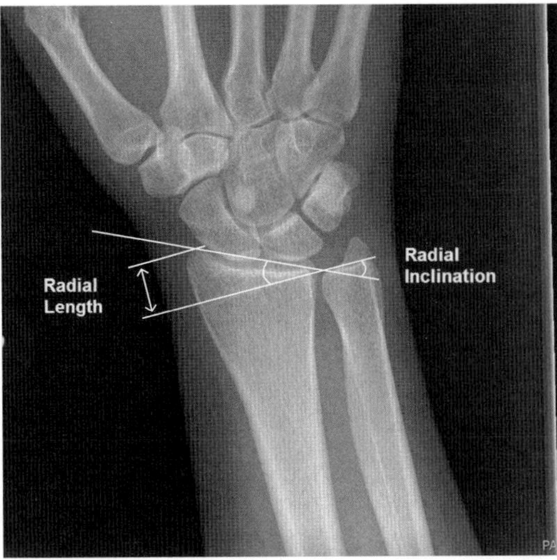

Figure 3.12. Normal radial length and inclination on PA radiograph.

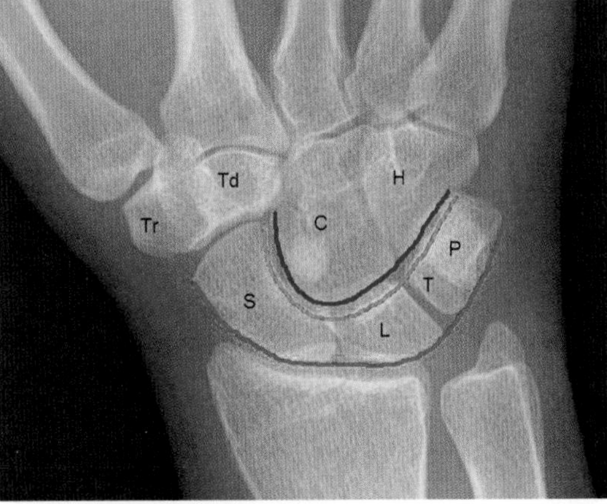

Figure 3.13. Carpal arcs on PA view.

- Radial length (height) – measurement from the ulnar articular surface to the tip of the radial styloid
    - Normal is 9–12 mm
    - Shortening is suggestive of distal radial fracture
- Radial tilt (inclination) – measurement of ulnar slant of the radial articular surface
    - Normal is 15–30°
    - Decrease is suggestive of fracture or DRUJ disruption
- Carpal arcs (Figure 3.13)– three smooth lines drawn between carpal bones
    - Proximal – proximal border of scaphoid, lunate and triquetrum
    - Middle – distal border of proximal carpal row
    - Distal – proximal border of capitate and hamate
    - Disruption of these lines is suggestive of fracture, dislocation, or both
- Carpal distance – the space between each of the carpal bones
    - Normal is 1–2 mm, equal distance between each bone
    - Pathologic is greater than 3 mm

- Lateral radiograph evaluates the fracture line, volar or dorsal displacement, intra-articular extension, and carpal alignment.
    - Lateral radiograph should have no more than 2 mm of the ulna projecting beyond the radius
    - Pronator quadratus fat pad – normal radiolucent linear line just volar to the radius and ulna
        - Volar displacement, bowing, or loss of fat pad suggests radius or ulna fracture
    - Volar tilt of radius (Figure 3.14) – the natural angle of the radiocarpal joint
        - Normal is 0–22° volar angulation
        - Measured by the angle formed by a line perpendicular to the long axis of the radius and a line along the surface of the distal radius
        - Fractures with dorsal angulation need to be reduced to neutral or + volar tilt for good functional outcome
    - Straight line should exist between central axis of the radius, lunate, capitate and the third metacarpal. (Figure 3.15)
        - Normal variance up to 10°
        - Disruption is suggestive of fracture or carpal dislocation
    - Scapholunate angle (Figure 3.16) – angulation between intersecting lines drawn through the central axis of the scaphoid and lunate
        - Normal is 30–60°
        - Angulation greater than this suggests rotary subluxation of the scaphoid, or fracture

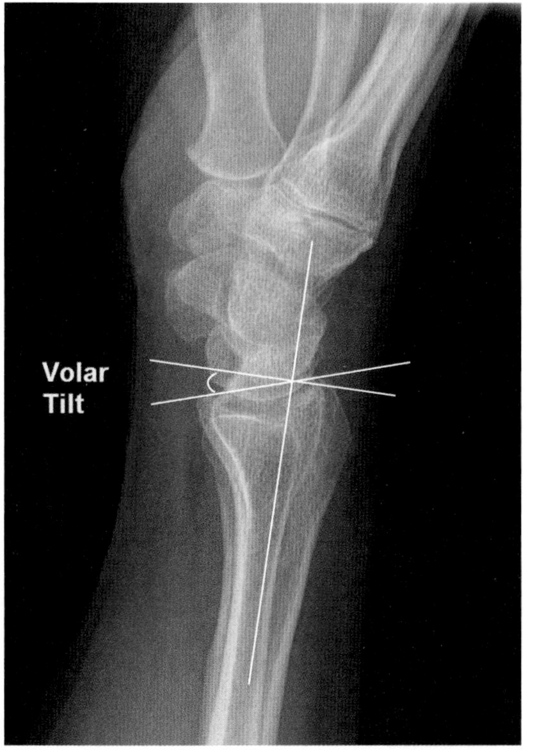

Figure 3.14. Normal volar tilt on lateral radiograph.

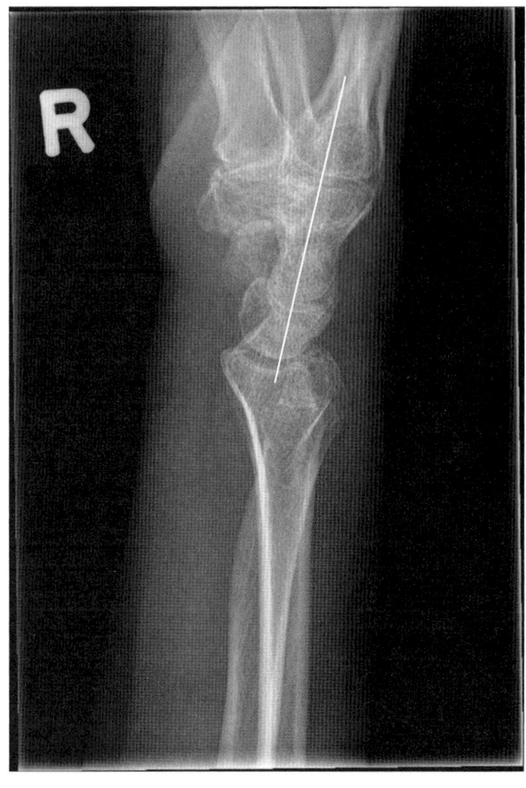

Figure 3.15. Straight line through radius, lunate, capitate, and metacarpal.

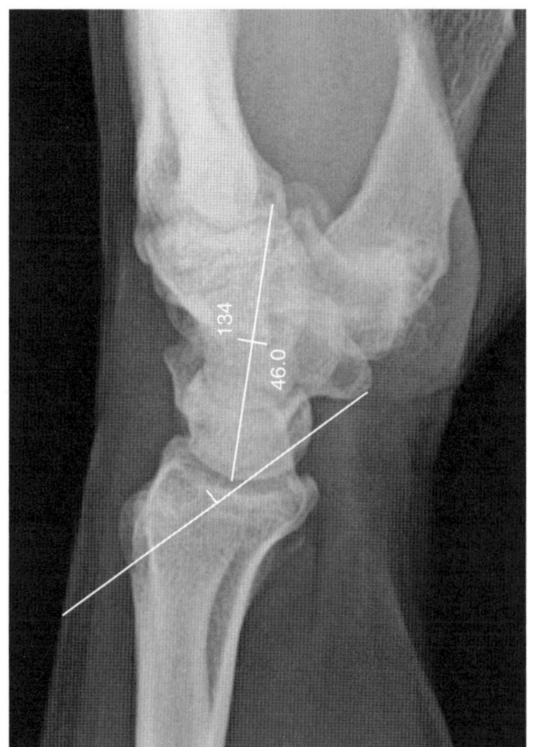

Figure 3.16. Normal scapholunate angle.

- Capitolunate angle – angulation between central axis lines through capitate and lunate
  - Normal is 0–30°
  - Greater than 30° suggests carpal dislocation

- Oblique radiograph is best for assessing the most radial carpal bones.
  - Scaphoid, trapezoid, trapezium more clearly seen in this view compared to the PA
  - Also helpful for assessing intra-articular extension of distal radius fractures

- Dedicated views may be obtained with suspicion for certain injuries.
  - Scaphoid view – PA radiograph with the wrist held in ulnar deviation
    - Exposes the scaphoid
    - Enhances detection of subtle fractures

- Carpal tunnel view – wrist is held in hyperextension, radiograph is directed across the volar wrist.
  - Good for detection of hamate and pisiform fractures
- Clenched fist view – AP radiograph with patient clenching the fist forcefully
  - Accentuates potential scapholunate dissociation

Differential Diagnosis-Emergent and Common Diagnoses

Scaphoid Fractures

General Description

- Most common fractured carpal bone, accounting for 62–87% of all carpal fractures[7]
- Scaphoid serves as a link between the carpal rows.
  - Bulk of it is articular surface
  - Acts to stabilize the carpal rows
- Also one of the most frequently missed carpal fractures
  - Misdiagnosed as "wrist sprain"
  - Delay in diagnosis increases chance for poor outcome
- High incidence of AVN and nonunion due to poor vascular supply

Table 3.1 Emergent and Common Diagnoses in the Emergency Department

Emergent Diagnoses	Common Diagnoses
Perilunate dislocation	Scaphoid fracture
Lunate dislocation	Distal radius fracture
Displaced distal radius fracture	Carpal tunnel syndrome
Any open fracture	De Quevain's tenosynovitis
Any injury associated with neurovascular compromise	Ganglion cyst
Any unstable fracture or dislocation	

  - Blood enters the dorsal cortex near the tubercle waist
  - Proximal bone has no direct blood supply
- Fractures are characterized by anatomic location:
  - Proximal pole – 10–20%
  - Scaphoid waist – vast majority at 70–80%[8]
  - Distal pole – majority are pediatric[9]
  - Tubercle

Mechanism

- Injury occurs with forced hyperextension and axial load of the wrist, described as FOOSH
- Radial deviation impinges the scaphoid against the radius
- Approximately 3% occur with flexion injury[10]

Presentation

- Typically seen in young adults, age 15–30
  - Rare in children, as the carpus is primarily cartilaginous until adolescent years
- Dorsal wrist pain just distal to the radial styloid
- Complaint of pain with wrist and thumb movement
- Swelling and ecchymosis is variable

Physical Examination

- Overall excellent sensitivity, but poor specificity at 74–80%
  - Tenderness directly over the scaphoid, both volar and dorsal
  - Tenderness in anatomic snuff box – 90% sensitive, 40% specific
  - Axial load of thumb in line with first metacarpal
  - Resisted supination
  - Flexion and radial deviation

Essential Diagnostics

- Standard PA, oblique, and lateral x-ray views will pick up many fractures (Figures 3.17 and 3.18).
  - Look for displaced scaphoid fat stripe as subtle finding[11]
- If the exam is suggestive of injury, a scaphoid view increases sensitivity.

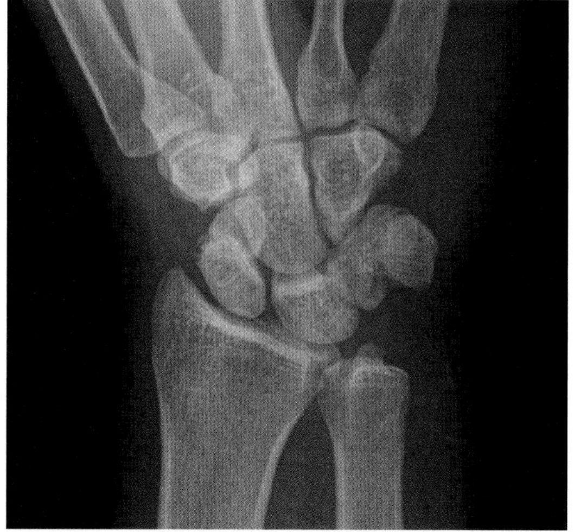

Figure 3.17. Displaced and angulated scaphoid fracture.

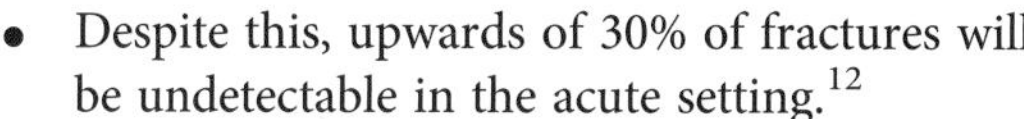

- Despite this, upwards of 30% of fractures will be undetectable in the acute setting.[12]
- CT scan is very sensitive for fracture, but cases of false negatives have been reported.
- Wrist MRI has been reported as 100% sensitive in multiple studies, but is not readily available in most EDs.

ED Treatment and Disposition

- Based on suspicion for injury and x-ray findings

Clinically Suspected Injury, XR Normal

- Splint in short arm thumb spica
- Re-examine in seven to ten days, repeat x-ray
  - If negative but continued clinical suspicion, reapply splint and re-evaluate again in seven to ten days, consider bone scan, CT, or MRI
  - If positive for nondisplaced fracture, thumb spica cast for six weeks

Nondisplaced Scaphoid Fracture

- Thumb spica splint in the ED
  - Debate over long vs. short arm splints, no clear correct answer
- Follow-up with thumb spica casting
  - Period of immobilization varies depending on anatomic location of fracture; more proximal fracture = longer
  - Average immobilization is twelve weeks

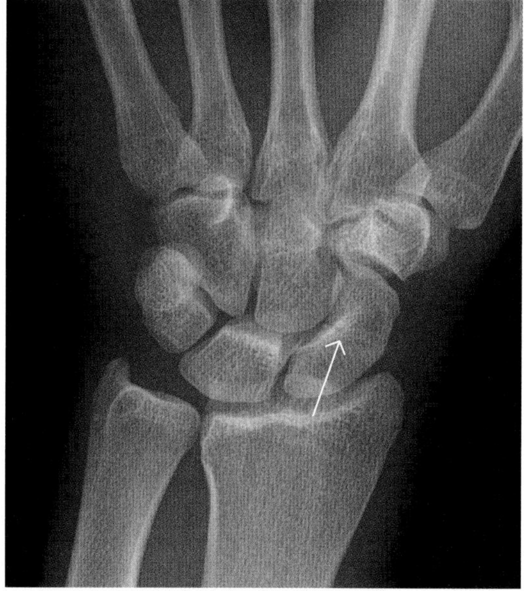

Figure 3.18. Abnormal fat pad in subtle scaphoid fracture.

Displaced Scaphoid Fracture

- Thumb spica splint in the ED
- Significant displacement, comminution, and/or angulation require hand surgeon consultation and urgent referral
  - Such injuries require open reduction and internal fixation
  - Absolute indications: $\geq$1-mm displacement, $\geq$ 15-mm angulation

Return to Play

- Most athletes will undergo surgical fixation to allow for earlier return to athletic activity.
  - If screw fixation with satisfactory union is achieved, patients may begin athletics within a few weeks while remaining in cast with appropriate paddling
- After the cast has been removed, early ROM and strengthening with physical therapy are essential to restore function.
- The wrist should remain in rigid bracing with activity until:
  - Radiographic evidence of union
  - Strength and ROM are similar to the uninjured extremity
  - Pain subsides

Complications

- Given the tenuous blood supply, scaphoid fractures have a high rate of nonunion and avascular necrosis (AVN).
  - Incidence of AVN 13–40%[13,14]
  - Nonunion rates vary according to injury pattern and treatment:
    - Displaced fractures, 50% rate of nonunion
    - Nondisplaced and immobilized, 15% nonunion rate[15]
    - Proximal > waist > distal > tubercle
- Delayed union and nonunion are directly related to premature discontinuation of immobilization.
- There is a high incidence of chronic pain and radiocarpal arthritis.

Pediatric Considerations

- Low likelihood of carpal injury until adolescence
- High incidence in teenage athletes

Pearls and Pitfalls

- 90% of scaphoid injuries occur in isolation.
- If there is suggestion of injury on examination, treat as such despite normal x-rays.
  - Up to 30% of initial x-rays read as normal
  - Place in thumb spica and arrange for follow-up within one week
- Hesitate to diagnose "wrist sprain," truly a diagnosis of exclusion.
- Any injury to the proximal scaphoid warrants consultation, as some surgeons will elect for operative stabilization vs. conservative therapy.

Triquetrum Fractures

General Description

- Second most common carpal fracture
- Two general types:
  - Dorsal chip – most common
  - Triquetral body
- Excellent vascular supply, thus low risk for AVN and nonunion

Mechanism

- Dorsal chip – typical mechanism with FOOSH, in ulnar deviation
  - Hamate forces triquetrum against radius or ulnar styloid
- Body – direct impact on dorsal hand, usually high mechanism
  - Association with perilunate dislocations

Presentation

- Variable presentation
  - Possible pain, swelling, and ecchymosis on dorsum of the hand

Physical Examination

- Tenderness and edema to the dorsum of the hand, just distal to the ulnar styloid
- Limited ROM with both flexion and extension

Essential Diagnostics

- Dorsal chip – best seen on lateral radiograph
- Body – standard PA or oblique views

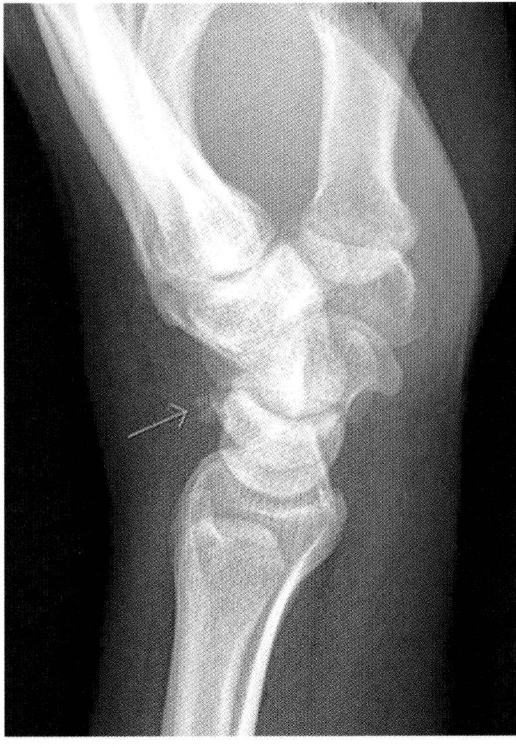

Figure 3.19. Dorsal chip fracture of the triquetrum.

ED Treatment and Disposition

- Treat with volar splint in the ED, followed by short arm cast.
- Four to six weeks usually results in complete healing.

Return to Play

- Athletes can return to sports while casted provided that there is adequate padding.
- After cast removal, athletes should remain in a semi-rigid brace until there is no further tenderness.

Complications

- Rarely ulnar nerve injury
- Limited AVN due to good vascular supply

Pediatric Considerations

- None

Pearls and Pitfalls

- In patients with perilunate fracture/dislocation, make sure to search for triquetral body fractures.

Lunate Fractures

General Description

- Account for 1.4–6% of carpal fractures[16,17]
- Lunate lies between the radius and the distal capitate
- Two general fracture patterns:
  - Dorsal avulsion
  - Lunate body
- Like the scaphoid, vascular supply runs distal to proximal and predisposes the lunate to AVN
- Posttraumatic AVN, referred to as Keinbock's disease, results from approximately 20% of lunate fractures

Mechanism

- Dorsal avulsion fractures usually result from forced hyperextension, FOOSH
- Lunate body fractures typically occur from axial loading

Presentation

- Pain and swelling on the dorsum of the hand

Physical Examination

- Tenderness on the dorsum of the hand, just distal to Lister's tubercle
- Exacerbated by axial load on the third metacarpal

Essential Diagnostics

- Standard PA, oblique, and lateral radiographs frequently miss nondisplaced lunate fractures.
- Cone-down views may enhance sensitivity, but still frequently miss fractures.
- CT and MRI both offer excellent sensitivity, and may be obtained in follow-up for those with high suspicion.

ED Treatment and Disposition

- Immobilize in thumb spica splint.
- Refer to hand surgeon for casting for roughly six to eight weeks.
- Fractures with displacement of more than 1 mm, angulation, or instability warrant urgent orthopedic referral for operative intervention.

Return to Play

- Aggressive rehabilitation with ROM and strengthening should be pursued after cast removal.
- Rigid bracing should be employed until strength and ROM are similar to the uninjured side, typically at least three months.

Complications

- Much like the scaphoid, lunate fractures are prone to AVN and nonunion due to poor vascular supply, especially with proximal injury.

Pediatric Considerations

- Lunate fractures generally fair better in adolescents when compared to adults.

Pearls and Pitfalls

- Even if x-rays are negative, if clinical suspicion is high for injury, splint the patient and refer to hand surgeon for follow-up and x-rays in seven to ten days.
- Isolated lunate fractures are uncommon, necessitating a search for associated distal radius, carpal, or metacarpal injuries.

Capitate Fractures

General Description

- Largest of the carpal bones
- Centrally located in the distal carpal row
  - Articulations with proximal scaphoid and lunate, adjacent trapezoid and hamate, and the three middle metacarpals
- Given location, rarely fractured
  - Isolated fractures occur in less than 0.3% of all carpal injuries[18]
  - Frequently associated with scaphoid fracture and perilunate dislocation
  - Fractures are usually transverse in nature

Mechanism

- Two general mechanisms:
  - FOOSH, forced hyperextension
  - Direct blow to dorsum of the hand

Presentation

- Pain and swelling to the dorsum of the hand

Physical Examination

- Direct palpation on the dorsum of the hand, over the capitate, reproduces the greatest pain.
- Pain with axial loading of the third metacarpal
- Swelling and ecchymosis to the dorsum of the hand
- Rarely may have associated median neuropathy.

Essential Diagnostics

- Standard PA, lateral, and oblique views usually identify fracture
- If x-ray is negative and high clinical suspicion, CT is very sensitive.

ED Treatment and Disposition

- Nondisplaced fractures
  - Immobilization in thumb spica splint
  - Follow-up thumb spica or short arm casting for six to eight weeks
- Displaced or associated carpal instability
  - Splint and urgent hand surgeon referral for operative intervention

Return to Play

- Nonsurgical fractures may return to play once casted.
- Surgical fractures may not return to play while still in cast for approximately four to six weeks.
  - Selective return to play with protective splinting for next three months.
  - May return to play without protective splinting once full range of motion, strength, and function have been restored.

Complications

- Like scaphoid fractures, associated with AVN and nonunion, especially if proximal fracture
- High incidence of perilunate ligamentous injury and dislocation
- Median neuropathy or acute carpal tunnel syndrome

Pediatric Considerations

- Rare

Pearls and Pitfalls

- Capitate fractures rarely occur in isolation. If found, it is imperative to search for associated pathology.
  - Distal radius and scaphoid fracture
  - Perilunate instability
- Err on the side of caution and splint if there is clinical concern for fracture.

Hamate Fractures

General Description

- Most ulnar of the distal carpal bones
- Fractures are uncommon, accounting for 1–4% of carpal fractures
- Three general types:
  - Hook (or hamulus) – most common
  - Body or proximal articular surface
  - Distal articular surface

Mechanism

- Overlapping mechanisms with the different fracture patterns:
  - Hook
    - Direct impact on the palmar surface, usually from repetitive vibratory forces (hammer, racquet sports)
    - FOOSH
  - Body

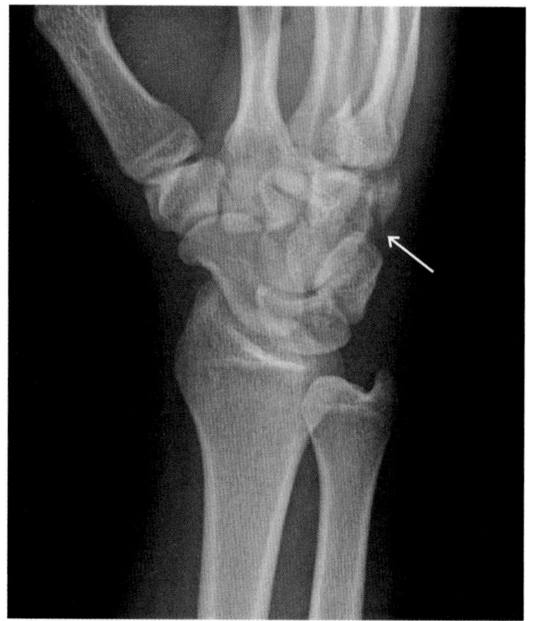

Figure 3.20. Hamate fracture on oblique radiograph.

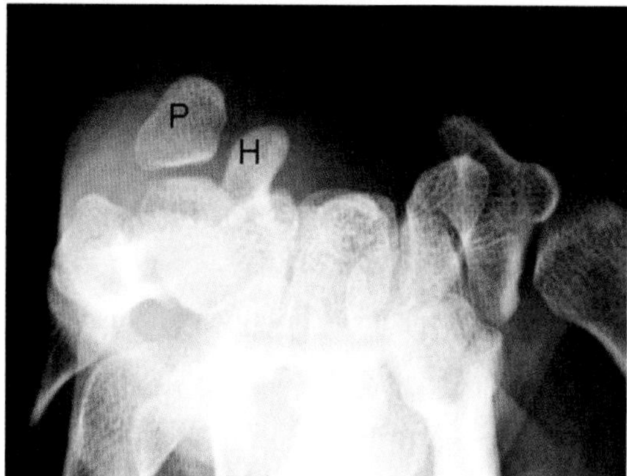

Figure 3.21. Hook of hamate on carpal tunnel view P = Pisiform, H = Hamate.

  - High impact direct force or axial load
  - FOOSH
- Distal articular surface
  - Direct blow or axial load on the fifth metacarpal

Presentation

- Pain and swelling to the hypothenar eminence
- Paresthesias in the ulnar distribution

Physical Examination

- Tenderness over the hamate, approximately 1 cm distal and radial to the pisiform
- Proximal injuries exhibit pain with wrist ROM
- Distal injuries with pain on axial load of the fifth metacarpal
- Assess for ulnar neuropathy

Essential Diagnostics

- PA, oblique, and lateral views will likely pick up significant body fractures (Figure 3.20), but frequently miss factures of the hook.
- Carpal tunnel views (Figure 3.21) and reverse oblique radiographs are best for hook fractures.
- If mechanism and exam are consistent with injury, CT can be obtained and is reportedly 100% sensitive.[19]

ED Treatment and Disposition

- Immobilize in ulnar gutter splint
- Nondisplaced fractures managed with routine follow-up in seven to ten days for casting for total of six to eight weeks.
- Displaced fractures or ulnar neuropathy: urgent follow-up and likely operative intervention

Return to Play

- Nondisplaced body fractures may return to sport immediately with semi-rigid synthetic cast.
- After operative repair, may return to sport approximately four to six weeks after function is restored.

Complications

- Ulnar neuropathy and nonunion is common with Hook fractures.
  - Usually require operative excision of the hook
- Ulnar artery injury can also occur, as it courses alongside the nerve
- Fifth MCP arthritis

Pediatric Considerations

- Rare in children.

Pearls and Pitfalls

- Pain in the hypothenar region and history of repetitive vibratory force (hammer, racket sports) should prompt search for hamate injury.
  - Obtain carpal tunnel view to search for fracture
- Ulnar neuropathy is common in hamate hook fractures.

Pisiform Fractures

General Description

- Unique as the only carpal sesamoid bone
- Only articulation is with the triquetrum.
- Flexor carpi ulnaris attaches to the volar aspect of the pisiform.
- Forms part of Guyon's canal (with hamulus) through which both ulnar artery and nerve pass
- Fractures are rare, generally carry a good prognosis
  - Avulsion
  - Transverse body
  - Comminuted

Mechanism

- Two general injury patterns
  - FOOSH or forced hyperextension
  - Direct blow to hypothenar eminence
- Avulsion fractures result from hyperextension/traction on flexor carpi ulnaris

Presentation

- Pain and swelling to the hypothenar region
- Ulnar paresthesias
- Complaint of hand weakness

Physical Examination

- Pain and swelling over the pisiform, exacerbated by wrist flexion and ulnar deviation.
- Assess for possible ulnar neuropathy

Essential Diagnostics

- Standard PA radiograph will sometimes demonstrate fracture.
- Reverse oblique and carpal tunnel views are far more sensitive.[16]

ED Treatment and Disposition

- Immobilization in volar splint
- Routine follow-up in one week with casting for total of four to six weeks
- Cases of ulnar neuropathy require urgent consultation
- Nonunion could necessitate operative excision

Return to Play

- May return to sport once casted as long as pain free

Complications

- Ulnar neuropathy as detailed earlier
- Flexor carpi ulnaris injury
- Nonunion, although rare

Pediatric Considerations

- As with other carpal injuries, pisiform fracture is rare in young children

Pearls and Pitfalls

- Ensure complete assessment and documentation of ulnar nerve function and distal perfusion with any pisiform or hamate injury.
- If you suspect injury, obtain carpal tunnel or reverse oblique films.

Trapezium Fractures

General Description

- Most radial bone of the distal carpal row
- Articulates with the scaphoid, trapezoid, and first metacarpal
- Fractures are rare, accounting for 1–4% of carpal fractures.
- Two general fracture types:
  - Trapezial ridge – serves as attachment for transverse carpal ligament
  - Trapezial body – vertical or comminuted fractures

Mechanism

- Trapezial body
  - Axial load on the adducted thumb
  - Forced hyperextension and abduction of thumb
    - Trapezium is wedged between first MCP and the radial styloid

- Trapezial ridge
  - FOOSH with direct impact on ridge
  - Avulsion by the transverse carpal ligament

Presentation

- Pain and swelling at the thenar eminence, worse with thumb movement.

Physical Examination

- Limited ROM in thumb due to pain
- Pain with axial load on first metacarpal
- Tenderness in distal snuff box

Essential Diagnostics

- Routine oblique views usually adequate, however additional views may be needed to rule out other injuries
- Carpal tunnel radiograph best for trapezial ridge[21]
- Follow-up CT highly sensitive

ED Treatment and Disposition

- Thumb spica splint in the ED
  - Nondisplaced fractures
    - Routine follow-up in one week and casting for six weeks
  - Displaced fracture of greater than 1 mm
    - Urgent hand surgery follow-up for operative intervention

Return to Play

- May return to play after six weeks of immobilization and near normal strength and range of motion. Use of a protective orthosis for an additional four weeks is recommended.

Complications

- First metacarpal joint arthritis
- Tendonitis and/or rupture of flexor carpi radials
- Concurrent radius, scaphoid, and first metacarpal fracture
- Radial artery injury

Pediatric Considerations

- None

Pearls and Pitfalls

- Pain in the snuff box and axial load on the thumb may represent more than just scaphoid injury.
- Ensure good assessment of wrist flexion due to possible flexor carpi radialis injury (primarily with trapezial ridge fracture).

Trapezoid Fractures

General Description

- Least common fracture of the carpal bones ($< 1\%$)
- Well protected and stabilized by surrounding ligaments
- Like the scaphoid, prone to AVN and nonunion[22]

Mechanism

- Two general mechanisms:
  - High energy axial load to a flexed second metacarpal
  - Dorsal crush

Presentation

- Pain to the dorsum of the hand

Physical Examination

- Reproducible tenderness to the dorsum of the hand, proximal to the base of the second metacarpal
- Pain exacerbated by movement of the second metacarpal and axial compression

Essential Diagnostics

- Fracture is usually seen with standard oblique views
- Carpal tunnel view increases sensitivity

ED Treatment and Disposition

- Thumb spica splint in the ED
  - Nondisplaced fractures
    - Routine referral for casting, total of six weeks
  - Displaced fractures/dislocations
    - Urgent hand surgery referral for reduction and fixation

Return to Play

- May return to sport once full function is restored after period of immobilization and rehabilitation

Complications

- High incidence of AVN and nonunion with fractures
- Trapezoid fractures rarely occur in isolation
  - Look for fractures at the metacarpal base
  - Potential trapezoid dorsal dislocation

Pediatric Considerations

- No specific differences

Pearls and Pitfalls

- Trapezoid fracture is exceedingly rare, but if it occurs it is usually associated with other fractures or dislocations.
- Obtain carpal tunnel view if there is clinical concern.

Carpal Instability – Scapholunate Dissociation, Perilunate and Lunate Dislocation

- Carpal instability represents a progression of ligamentous injury, first characterized by Mayfield in cadaver studies,[23] with forceful hyperextension of the wrist leading to four distinct and progressive phases of instability:
  - Stage I: scapholunate dissociation
  - Stage II: perilunate dislocation
  - Stage III: Stage II + progression to triquetral dislocation/fracture
  - Stage IV: lunate dislocation

Stage I: Scapholunate Dissociation

General Description

- Rupture of the scapholunate interosseous ligament
  - Widening of the scapholunate joint
- Possible rupture of radioscapholunate ligament
  - Rotary subluxation of scaphoid

Mechanism

- High mechanism FOOSH or forced hyperextension and ulnar deviation, as in motor vehicle accident

Presentation

- Pain with movement at the wrist, both radial and ulnar deviation
- "Crunching or clicking" sounds
- Pain usually reported on the dorsum of the hand

Physical Examination

- Variable and depending on the degree of instability
- Possible swelling and ecchymosis over the dorsum of the hand
- Reproducible tenderness over the scapholunate region (Lister's tubercle)
- *Positive scaphoid shift test* (important to compare to opposite wrist)
- Possible snuff box tenderness

Essential Diagnostics

- Begin with PA, oblique, and lateral films
  - PA will show widening on scapholunate joint space greater than 3 mm – "Terry Thomas" sign (Figure 3.22)
  - If there is rotary subluxation of scaphoid, PA will show "signet ring" sign. (Figure 3.23)
  - Lateral will reveal increased scapholunate angle (Figure 3.24)
- Clenched fist view – if suspicion for ligamentous injury
  - More sensitive for ligamentous injury at scapholunate joint

ED Treatment and Disposition

- Place in thumb spica splint in the ED
- Routine referral to hand surgeon in seven to ten days as these injuries often need operative repair

Return to Play

- Athletes may return to play after definitive treatment and normal function and strength are regained.
- This usually takes approximately three months.

Complications

- Chronic instability and further weakening of surrounding carpal ligaments if delay in diagnosis or improper treatment

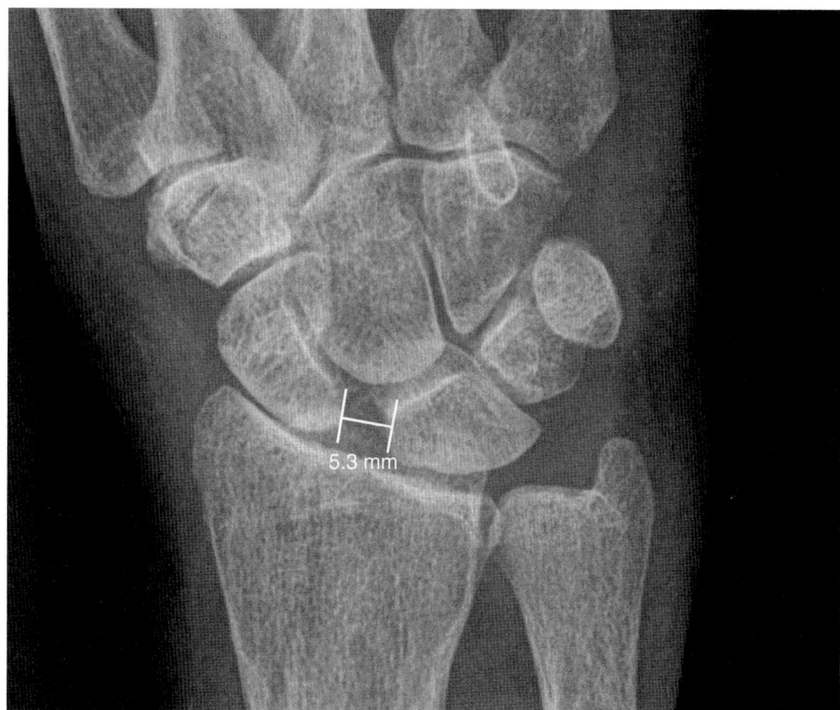

Figure 3.22. Scapholunate dissociation with widening of the intercarpal space.

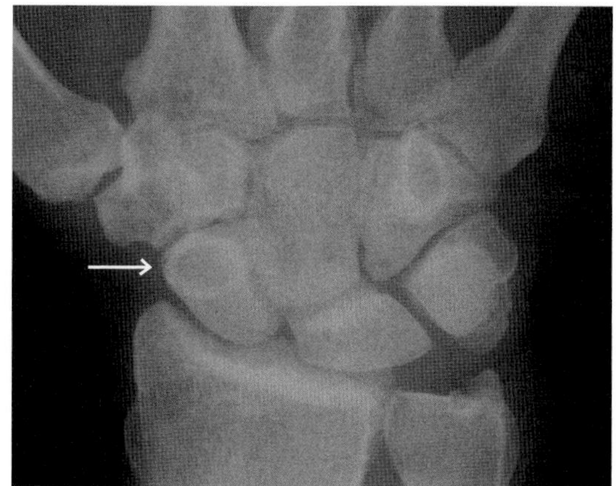

Figure 3.23. "Signet ring" sign with rotary subluxation of the scaphoid.

- Primary cause of scapholunate advanced collapse (SLAC)
- Associated with scaphoid fracture and distal radius fracture
- Chronic pain and arthritis

Pediatric Considerations

- Rare until adolescence

Pearls and Pitfalls

- Frequently missed on routine exam and x-ray
  - 5% prevalence in ED radiographs where no fracture is detected [24]
  - Hesitate before diagnosing "wrist sprain"
- If suspicious, obtain clenched fist view and err on side of splinting, with follow-up in seven to ten days

Stage II: Perilunate Dislocation

General Description

- Tear of the volar capitolunate ligament
  - Instability of the scaphoid and capitate
  - Capitate dislocates dorsally in relation to the lunate
  - Lunate retains its articulation with the radius

Mechanism

- FOOSH, forced hyperextension with ulnar deviation

Presentation

- Pain and swelling to the dorsum of the hand
- Worsened with ROM

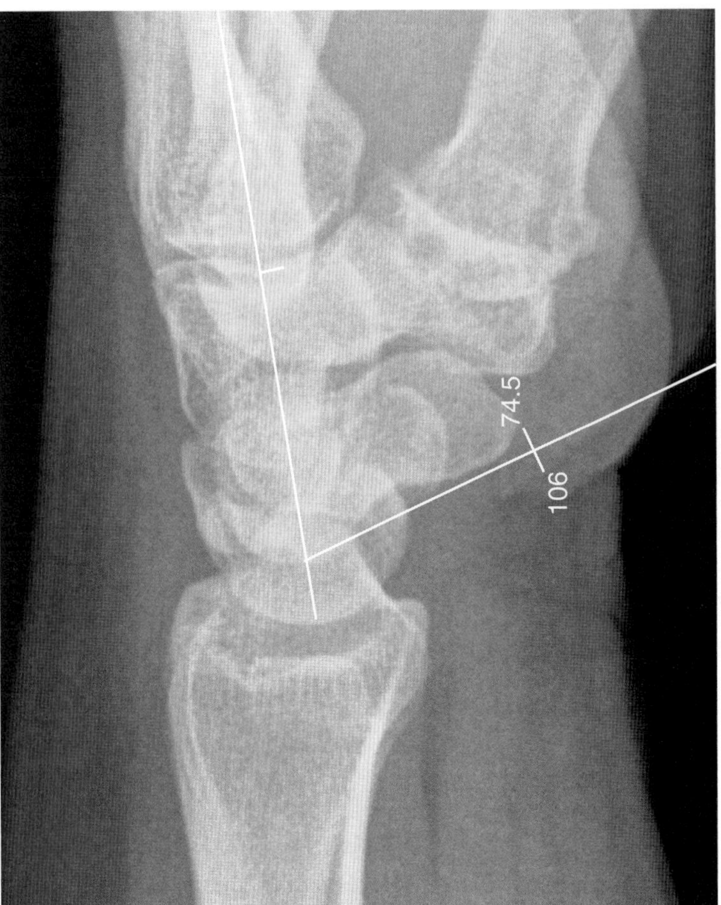

Figure 3.24. Increased scapholunate angle in scapholunate dissociation.

Physical Examination

- Reproducible tenderness on dorsum of hand
- Limited ROM secondary to pain, especially with wrist flexion
- Palpable deformity/bulge to dorsum of hand

Essential Diagnostics

- PA radiograph shows overlap of lunate and capitate
  - Disruption of normal carpal arcs (Figure 3.25)
- Lateral radiograph reveals dorsal dislocation of capitate in relation to lunate, while the lunate retains its articulation with the radius
  - "Empty teacup" sign (Figure 3.26)

ED Treatment and Disposition

- Attempts at reduction in the ED and *emergent* hand surgery consultation for stabilization

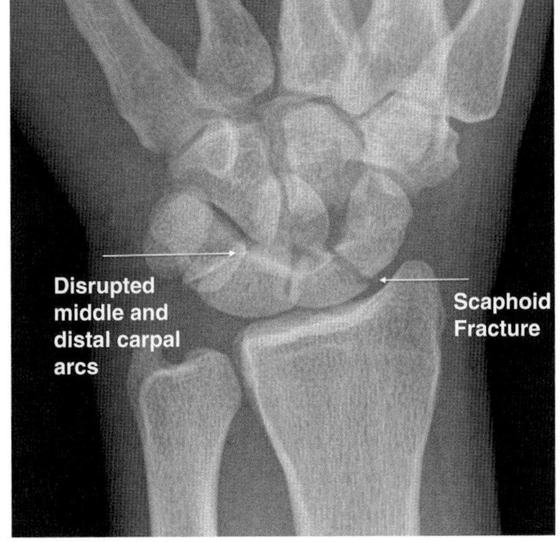

Figure 3.25. Perilunate dislocation with "jumbled carpus" appearance, with disruption of the normal carpal arcs (only the proximal arc is preserved). Note the associated scaphoid fracture.

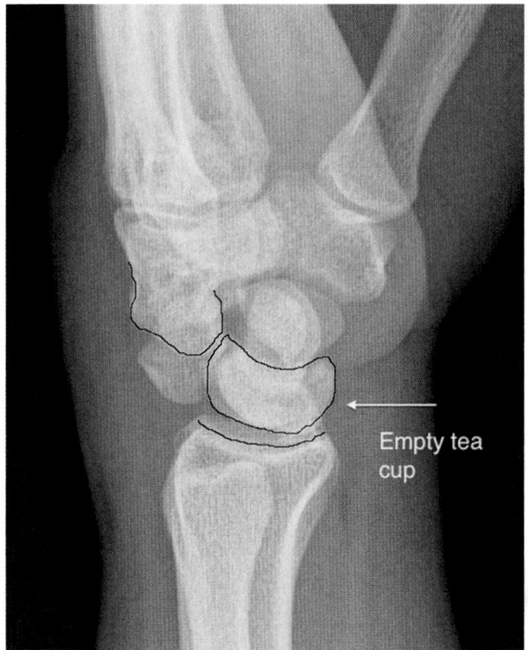

Figure 3.26. Perilunate dislocation with the capitate dislocated dorsally, showing "empty teacup" sign.

- Nerve block, hematoma block, and/or conscious sedation are required for successful reduction
- Finger traps with 10 pounds of in-line traction for at least 10 minutes to fatigue muscles and overcome spasm
- While traction is maintained, the wrist is placed into extension; with a thumb placed over the volar lunate to prevent lunate dislocation, the wrist is then flexed with mild pressure over the dorsal aspect of the capitate.
- An audible "clunk" is typically detected
- If closed reduction fails, open reduction will be required.
- Even if successfully reduced, may require surgical fixation.
- Splint in volar splint in neutral position

Complications

- Associated with scaphoid fracture and radial styloid and ulnar styloid fracture
- 60% of perilunate dislocations occur with scaphoid fractures, termed "trans-scaphoid perilunate dislocation"

Pediatric Considerations

- Rare in pediatrics

Pearls and Pitfalls

- Even if successful reduction in the ED, warrants emergent consultation given the ligamentous instability
- Look out for associated fractures

Stage III: Perilunate Dislocation with Triquetral Dislocation and/or Fracture

General Description

- Stage II + tear of the lunotriquetral interosseous ligament and volar lunotriquetral ligament
  - Dislocation of the triquetrum, and/or avulsion fracture

Mechanism

- FOOSH, forced hyperextension

Presentation

- Same as stage II

Physical Examination

- Same as stage II

Essential Diagnostics

- PA radiograph shows overlap of triquetrum with lunate or hamate.
- Lateral radiograph reveals perilunate dislocation

ED Treatment and Disposition

- Same as Stage II – emergent consultation and reduction
  - Reduction should be attempted as early as possible using the same technique described earlier.
  - Temporary placement in volar splint
- Likely need for operative intervention and stabilization

Return to Play

- Return to sports is not recommended until after definitive treatment and rehabilitation.
- Even with prompt treatment, recovery is usually prolonged and often there is a permanent limitation in range of motion.

Complications

- Same as stage II
- Volar triquetral avulsion fracture

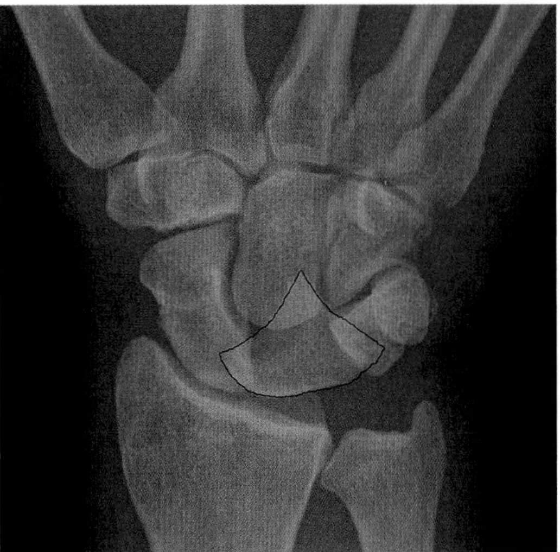

Figure 3.27. Lunate dislocation revealing a triangular appearance, referred to as "piece of pie" sign.

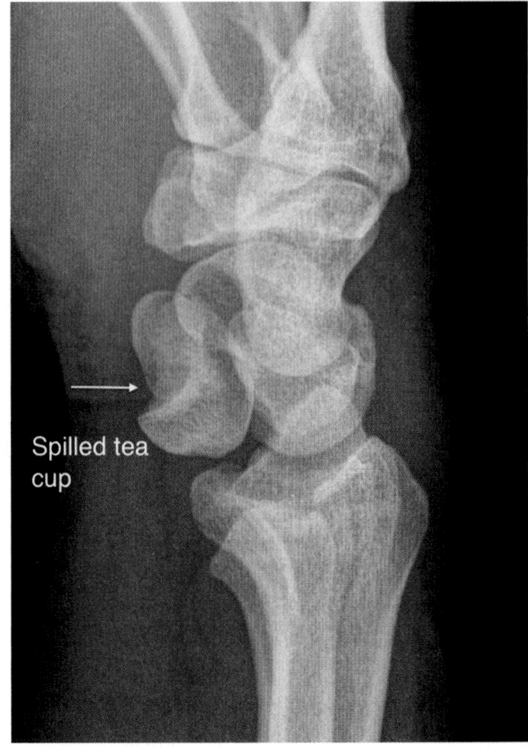

Figure 3.28. Lunate dislocation on lateral radiograph showing "spilled teacup" sign.

Pediatric Considerations

- Rare injury

Pearls and Pitfalls

- Any perilunate dislocation requires emergent consultation and reduction
- Look for associated fractures

Stage IV: Lunate Dislocation

General Considerations

- Final and most severe carpal dislocation
- Disruption of the dorsal radiocarpal ligament
  - Lunate dislocates volar to capitate
  - Capitate migrates proximal and may rest against the radius

Mechanism

- FOOSH, forced hyperextension with ulnar deviation

Presentation

- Pain, swelling, and limited ROM

Physical Examination

- Limited ROM secondary to pain
- Likely fullness to the volar aspect of hand, indicating dislocation
- Assess for possible median neuropathy

Essential Diagnostics

- PA radiograph shows lunate as triangular in appearance, "piece of pie" sign (Figure 3.27) (normally lunate is quadrangular in appearance)
- Lateral radiograph shows volar-displaced lunate in relation to radius and capitate.
  - Volar tilt, "spilled teacup" sign (Figure 3.28)
- Look for associated fractures

ED Treatment and Disposition

- *Emergent* hand surgery consultation
- Attempts at reduction as described earlier with slight modification:
  - Finger traps with 10 pounds countertraction for 10 minutes to overcome muscle spasm
  - Wrist is initially flexed to relax the volar ligaments and assist with manipulation of the lunate back into its fossa.
  - While inline traction in maintained, the wrist is then extended and operators thumb is pressed on the lunate volarly.

- While pressure is maintained on the lunate, the wrist is flexed while continuing inline traction.
- An audible "clunk" is typically detected with reduction.
- Close assessment for median neuropathy
- Temporary splinting in volar splint

Return to Play

- Patients are typically cast immobilized for twelve weeks after surgical fixation and repair of Stage II–IV injuries, thus necessitating vigorous physical therapy after cast removal.
- Resumption of activity in not recommended until strength and ROM are restored to near baseline levels, typically four to five months post injury.

Complications:

- Acute carpal tunnel syndrome
- Scaphoid fracture, radial and ulnar styloid fracture, triquetral fracture
- Midcarpal dislocation – dislocation of both lunate and capitate

Pediatric Considerations

- Rarely seen in pediatrics

Pearls and Pitfalls

- Even if adequately reduced in the ED, most require operative intervention
- High incidence of acute carpal tunnel syndrome

Injuries to distal radius and ulna

- Wrist fractures represent one of the most common injuries in all patient age groups
- Usual mechanism of injury is a FOOSH
- Discussion will focus on five distal radius injury patterns:
  - Colles fracture
  - Smith fracture
  - Barton fracture
  - Hutchinson fracture
  - DRUJ dislocation
- Separate discussion on unique pediatric fractures
  - Torus fracture
  - Greenstick fracture
  - Growth plate injuries – Salter–Harris classification

Colles Fracture

General Considerations

- Most common distal radius fracture
- Most common fracture in persons less than 75 years old
- Classified as distal radial metaphyseal fracture with dorsal angulation and/or displacement

Mechanism

- FOOSH

Presentation

- Pain and swelling to the dorsal wrist

Physical Examination

- Notable tenderness and edema to the dorsum of the wrist
- Possible angulation, with classic "dinner fork" deformity (Figure 3.29)
- Assess complete neurovascular exam, as acute median neuropathy is a known complication
- Complete exam of flexor tendon function

Essential Diagnostics

- PA and lateral radiograph of the wrist are usually adequate
  - PA – reveals fracture line, loss of radial height, possible comminution or intra-articular extension (Figure 3.30)
  - Lateral – demonstrates degree of angulation and displacement, loss of volar tilt (Figure 3.31)

ED Treatment

Nondisplaced Fractures

- Sugar-tong splint
- Outpatient follow-up in one week for reevaluation and casting for four to six weeks

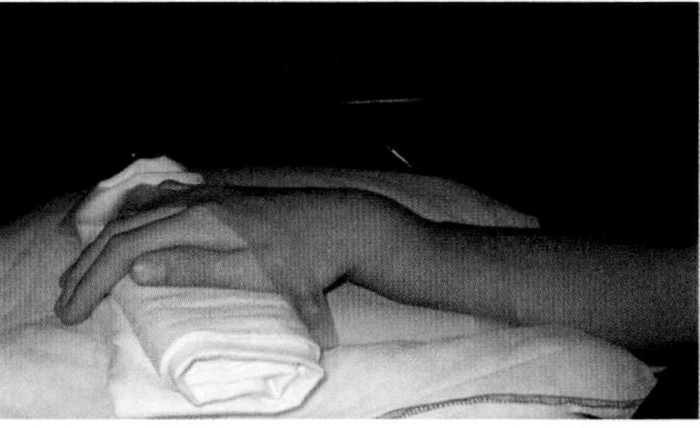

Figure 3.29. Classic "dinner fork" appearance in Colles fracture.

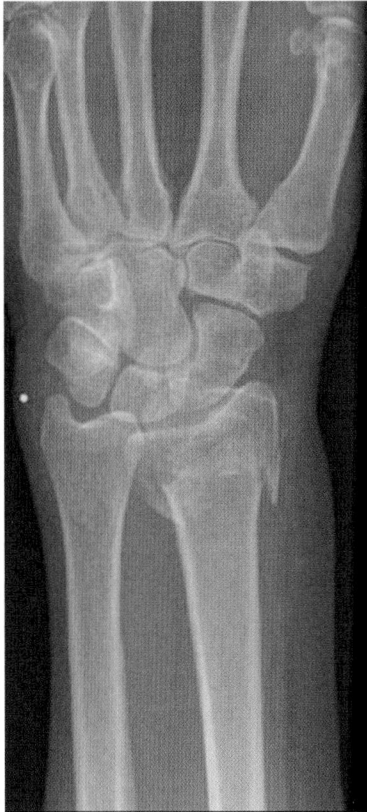

Figure 3.30. PA radiograph of Colles fracture. There is loss of radial length and inclination.

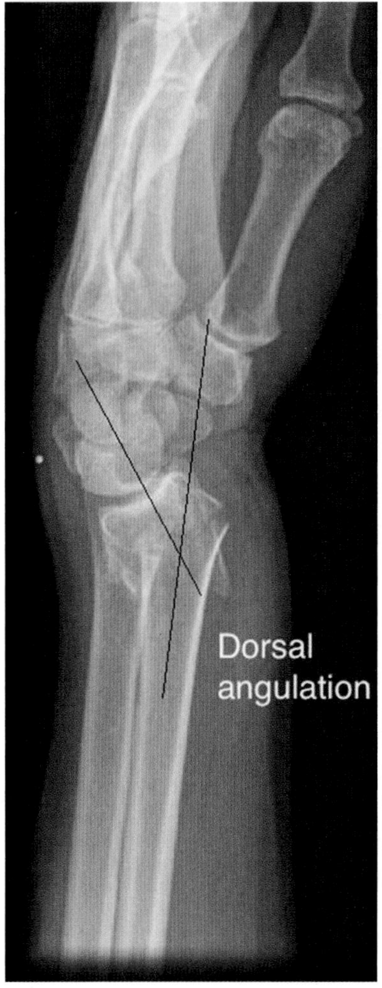

Figure 3.31. Lateral radiograph of Colles fracture with dorsal angulation and displacement. Note the loss of normal volar tilt.

Displaced and/or Angulated Fractures

- Need for closed reduction to restore functional alignment
  - Hematoma block or regional anesthesia, possible conscious sedation required
  - Finger traps with inline traction and weighted countertraction for 10–15 minutes
  - To reduce fracture, dorsiflex the wrist to recreate injury pattern, then realignment with volarly directed pressure
  - Imperative to correct radial height, radial tilt and volar tilt for functional recovery
  - Splint in sugar-tong with 15° flexion and ulnar deviation using three point molding technique.
  - If proper reduction, recommend outpatient follow-up in two to three days for re-evaluation to ensure stability
  - Casting will occur at seven days if able to maintain reduction, for a total of six to eight weeks.
  - Urgent orthopedic referral for complex or inadequate reduction, instability, or severe comminution as will likely need operative intervention
  - Emergent referral for neurovascular compromise

Return to Play

- Decision is based upon evidence of both radiographic and clinical healing, with a minimum of four to six weeks required.
- For certain sports with high dependence on wrist and forearm movement, or high propensity for direct impact, patients should not return to activity until strength and range of motion are close to baseline.

Complications

- Acute median neuropathy from fracture fragments in carpal tunnel or stretching of median nerve
- Lower incidence of ulnar nerve injury and compartment syndrome
- Associated ulnar styloid and neck injuries, carpal injuries, and DRUJ dislocation
- Flexor tendon injuries
- Chronic complications include degenerative arthritis, chronic pain and malunion, reflex sympathetic dystrophy.[25]

Pediatric Considerations

- Common injury in pediatric population
- Usually heal with minimal complications provided adequate reduction
- Close follow-up for any intra-articular extension injuries

Pearls and Pitfalls

- While Colles fracture is a common injury, be careful not to miss subtle associated pathology such as DRUJ dislocation and carpal injury which portend greater complications with delayed diagnosis
- Carefully assess and document neurovascular exam pre and post reduction and splinting
- Assess adequate reduction of radial length, radial tilt, and ulnar tilt
- Urgent consultation for significant displacement, intra-articular injury, instability

Smith Fracture

General Considerations

- Distal radial metaphysis fracture with volar displacement and/or angulation
- Referred to as "reverse Colles"
- Less common, occurring 10% as often as Colles fracture

Mechanism

- Three general mechanisms:
  - Direct impact to dorsal wrist
  - Fall on flexed wrist with hyperflexion
  - Fall on supinated forearm with wrist dorsiflexed

Presentation

- Pain and swelling to the wrist

Physical Examination

- Tenderness and edema to the volar wrist, worse with movement
- Notable volar fullness referred to as "garden spade" deformity
- Neurovascular exam for median neuropathy and radial pulse (neuropathy less common than with Colles)

Essential Diagnostics

- PA and lateral radiographs are usually adequate
  - PA reveals fracture location, possible intra-articular extension (Figure 3.32)
  - Lateral is best view to evaluate angulation and displacement (Figure 3.33)

ED Treatment and Disposition

- Reduction is necessary and sometimes difficult due to fracture impaction
- Hematoma block and possible conscious sedation may be required
- Inline traction with finger traps and 10 pounds counterweight

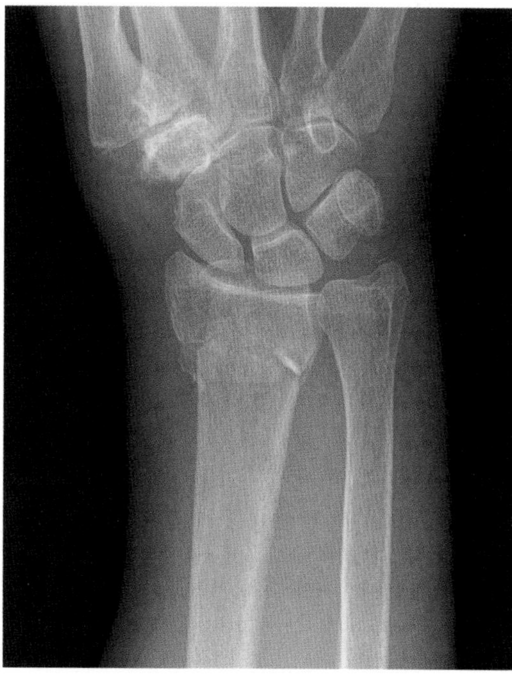

Figure 3.32. Smith fracture on PA radiograph. Note loss of radial length and inclination.

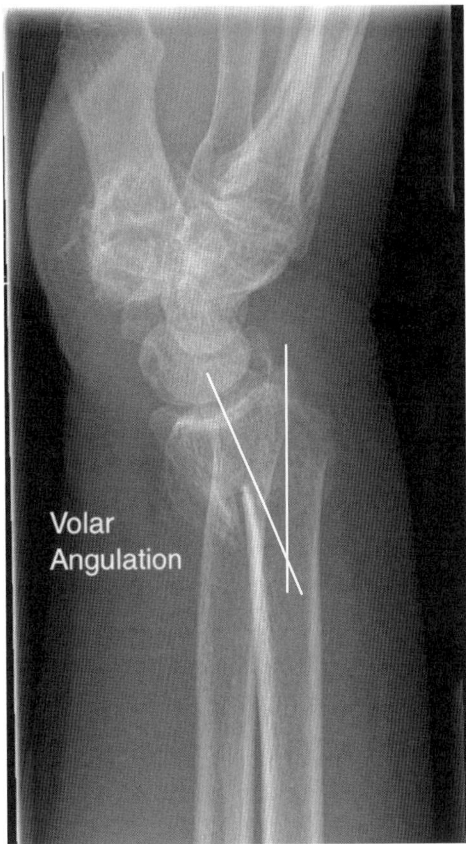

Figure 3.33. Smith fracture showing volar angulation and displacement.

- To dislodge impacted fragments, slight hyperflexion to recreate injury pattern, then realignment with dorsally directed pressure
- Immobilize in sugar-tong splint
- If reduction is successful, orthopedic follow-up in seven days for casting
- Low threshold for ED orthopedic consultation for reduction

Return to Play

- Same as Colles fracture

Complications

- Overall, much lower complication rate when compared to Colles fracture
- Concurrent ulnar or carpal bone injury
- Chronic arthritis, median nerve injury, and malunion
- Most require operative stabilization

Pediatric Considerations

- Same as adult

Pearls and Pitfalls

- Some authorities recommend orthopedic consultation for reduction, unless operator is very familiar with Smith fracture reduction.
- Close documentation of neurovascular status pre and post reduction

Barton's Fracture

General Considerations

- Oblique, intra-articular facture of the rim of the distal radius
  - Can be either volar or dorsal rim fracture
    - Volar fracture sometimes referred to as "reverse Barton's"
  - Carpal bones are subluxed along with the fracture fragment.
- Rare fracture pattern, seen in only 0.5–1.6% of distal radius fractures

Mechanism

- High mechanism blow to the radiocarpal joint in either flexion or extension:
  - Volar flexion: volar rim fracture with volar carpal subluxation
  - Dorsiflexion: dorsal rim fracture with dorsal carpal subluxation

Presentation

- Pain and swelling to the wrist, worse with movement

Physical Examination

- Tenderness and edema to the wrist
- Limited ROM secondary to pain
- Deformity noted on either volar or dorsal surface
- Note any paresthesias or motor weakness

Essential Diagnostics

- PA and lateral radiographs are usually adequate.
  - Lateral most helpful for identification of fracture type and degree of angulation/displacement (Figure 3.34)

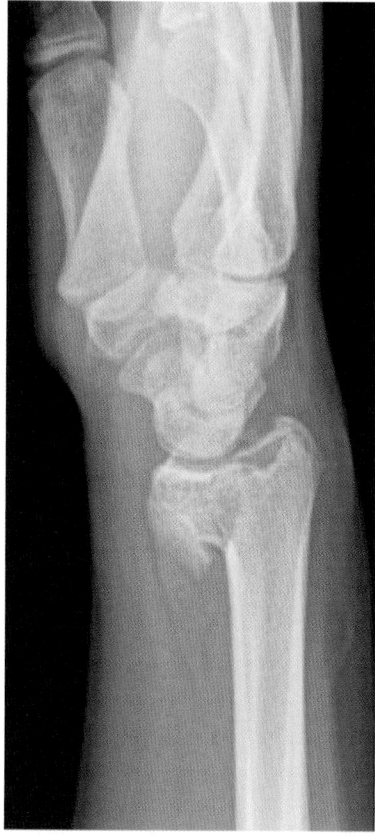

Figure 3.34. Volar Barton's fracture, showing intra-articular extension and displacement of carpal bones.

ED Treatment and Disposition

- Reduction with restoration of normal anatomic lines imperative
- Similar technique as with Colles fracture for dorsal Barton's fracture
- Place in sugar-tong splint, forearm neutral position
- Given intra-articular injury, urgent consultation with orthopedic surgery is recommended as some will prefer early operative correction

Return to Play

- Given how rare this injury is, all return to play decisions should be made in consultation with orthopedic surgery.

Complications

- Most arise from failed initial reduction and delayed presentation
- Arthritis, carpal instability are most common.
- Rarely radial nerve injury

Pediatric Considerations

- Same as adult

Pearls and Pitfalls

- Injury is inherently unstable and likely requires ORIF
- Proper restoration of radiocarpal joint is imperative; thus low threshold for orthopedic consultation for reduction

Hutchinson Fracture

General Considerations

- Intra-articular fracture of the radial styloid
- Termed "chauffeur's fracture," as it was originally noted to be associated with hand crank motors.

Mechanism

- Direct impact to the radial aspect of the distal radius
  - Force can impact directly on the radius or from transmission through the scaphoid

Presentation

- Pain and swelling to the radial aspect of the wrist

Physical Examination

- Tenderness over the radial styloid, worse with radial deviation
- Associated swelling and ecchymosis
- Possible pain with axial load of the thumb
- Assess for possible scaphoid tenderness or scapholunate instability

Essential Diagnostics

- PA and lateral radiographs are usually adequate. (Figure 3.35)
- If suspicion for concurrent scaphoid injury, get scaphoid view

ED Treatment and Disposition

- Sugar-tong splint application in the ED, with follow-up for casting for six weeks
- If the fracture is significantly displaced or unstable, urgent orthopedic consultation is required.
  - Styloid is the primary attachment for many wrist ligaments, thus malalignment or nonunion has deleterious consequences.
  - Many surgeons prefer early operative stabilization

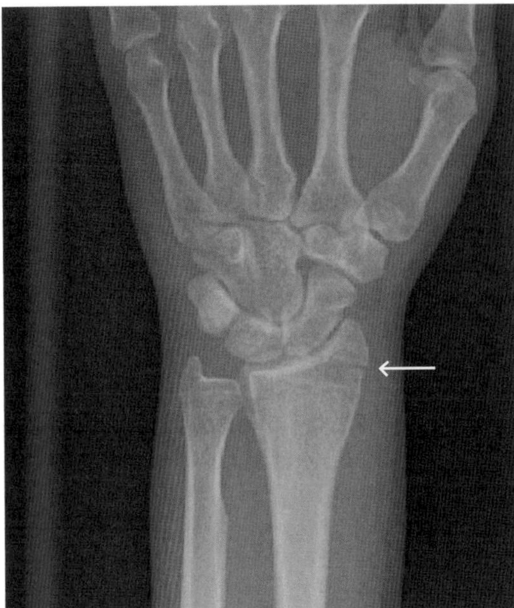

Figure 3.35. Hutchinson fracture of the radial styloid. Despite benign appearance, this is an inherently unstable fracture.

Return to Play

- Given the rarity of this injury, all return to play decisions should be made in consultation with orthopedic surgery.

Complications

- Concurrent scaphoid fracture or scapholunate dissociation
- Chronic post-traumatic arthritis

Pediatric Considerations

- Same as adult

Pearls and Pitfalls

- Radial styloid fracture is inherently unstable despite its relatively unimpressive XR appearance; thus urgent referral to orthopedics.

DRUJ Dislocation

General Considerations

- DRUJ disruption can occur in isolation or more commonly in conjunction with distal radius or ulnar head fracture.
  - Most common with Galeazzi fractures (radius fracture at junction of distal and middle third of radius with associated disruption of the DRUJ)
- Injury is frequently missed as radiographs can appear "normal."
- Ulnar styloid may dislocate in either direction.
  - Dorsal – more common
  - Volar
- Clinically, this is an important injury as complications are frequent.

Mechanism

- Fall with FOOSH mechanism
  - Injury caused by hypersupination or hyperpronation at the wrist
    - Supination – volar dislocation
    - Pronation – dorsal dislocation

Presentation

- Pain to the ulnar aspect of the wrist
- Patient reports "popping" sound upon injury

Physical Examination

- Asymmetric appearance of the ulnar styloid compared to uninjured extremity
  - Can either be an excessive or decreased prominence of the styloid, depending on volar or dorsal displacement
    - Excessive prominence = dorsal dislocation
    - Loss of prominence = volar dislocation
- Pain with supination and pronation
- Crepitus with ROM over the ulnar styloid
- *Positive piano key test*
- *Positive shuck test* (Figure 3.11)

Essential Diagnostics

- PA and lateral radiographs are typically read as "normal" in the absence of associated fracture (distal radius, ulnar styloid).
  - True lateral radiograph is difficult to obtain due to pain
- Note dorsal prominence of ulna head (normal is < 2mm)

ED Treatment and Disposition

- If there is an associated bony injury, fracture reduction will likely reduce the DRUJ.
- Reduction can be difficult as the ulnar head may be lodged against the radius.
- Splint in long arm splint in supination

- Urgent orthopedic consultation and follow-up
  - Operative intervention is likely needed as there is usually a tear in the TFCC.
  - Immobilization in long arm cast for an average of six weeks

Return to Play

- Athletes may return to play after appropriate definitive management and rehabilitation program.
- A protective orthosis may be worn until full strength is regained.

Complications

- Chronic pain, decreased ROM

Pearls and Pitfalls

- Most DRUJ dislocations occur in association with distal radius fractures.
- Proper reduction is necessary, with a low threshold for orthopedic consult.
- Many occur in the setting of "normal" radiographs.

Pediatric Distal Radius Factures

General Considerations

- While there are many similarities with adult injuries, certain anatomic differences yield unique pathology in the pediatric population
- Fractures are first characterized as involving the radial metaphysis or the physis (growth plate).
  - *Growth Plate* – injuries are characterized by the Salter–Harris nomenclature, ranging from grade I to grade V, which will dictate treatment and prognosis. Injuries involving the growth plate can lead to growth retardation and poor functional outcome.
    - Grade I – suspected disruption of the epiphyseal and metaphyseal junction (x-rays are usually normal)
    - Grade II – fracture through the metaphysis and physis
    - Grade III – fracture through the epiphysis and physis
    - Grade IV – fracture from the epiphysis through the physis and extending to the metaphysis
    - Grade V – severe force transmitted through the physis, with "crush"-type injury
  - *Metaphyseal Fractures* – the periosteum is relatively strong and thus displays a progression of injury
    - Torus – a "buckling" of the cortex, without evidence of displacement or angulation
    - Greenstick – partial or incomplete fracture of the metaphysis, with disruption of the cortex on one side
      - By definition, there is associated bowing or angulation of the bone
    - Complete – disruption of both cortices, as with adult fractures

Mechanism

- Most pediatric distal radius fractures occur via FOOSH
- Occasionally via direct impact on the dorsal wrist

Presentation

- Pain and swelling to the wrist

Physical Examination

- Can vary from an essentially normal-appearing wrist (Salter I or torus fracture) to significant swelling and deformity to the distal radius
- Exam is the same as with adults.
  - Compare with uninjured extremity
  - Ensure no injury to proximal and distal joints
  - Good neurovascular exam

Essential Diagnostics

- Routine PA and lateral radiographs usually suffice

ED Treatment and Disposition

- Growth Plate Fractures:
  - Salter Harris I – short-arm splint, routine follow-up in one week, casting for three to four weeks

- Salter Harris II – if there is displacement then will require reduction in ED; sugar-tong splint and routine orthopedic follow-up for casting.
- Salter Harris III – depending on amount of displacement, could require operative intervention and orthopedic reduction; sugar-tong splint and urgent follow-up.
- Salter Harris IV – urgent orthopedic consultation, as will likely need operative intervention
    - Place sugar-tong splint in ED
- Salter Harris V – potential for severe growth retardations, thus urgent orthopedic consultation

- Metaphyseal Fractures:
    - Torus – short-arm splint and routine referral
    - Greenstick – will need reduction to improve angulation to less than 10°; sugar-tong splint and follow-up in five to seven days
    - Complete – reduction in ED, sugar-tong splint

Return to Play

- Athlete may return to sport after appropriate period of immobilization, evidence of fracture healing, and return to normal strength and full range of motion.

Complications

- Any injury involving the growth plate may arrest development.

Pearls and Pitfalls

- Have a high level of suspicion for Salter-Harris injury in pediatrics, as missed injuries may have drastic consequences later.
- Salter-Harris I and V injuries may appear radiographically normal on first inspection, thus err on the side of caution and immobilize, with close orthopedic follow-up.
    - Look for subtle pronator quadratus fat pad displacement
- Pediatric injuries require earlier follow-up than adults, as the fractures heal faster and if improperly aligned can make operative intervention more difficult.

Soft Tissue Injuries

Carpal Tunnel Syndrome

General Considerations

- Carpal tunnel syndrome (CTS) is a median neuropathy caused by compression of the median nerve within the carpal tunnel.
    - Carpal tunnel:
        - Formed by the volar aspect of the carpal bones and the transverse carpal ligament
        - Compartment contains nine flexor tendons and the median nerve
- Lifetime incidence is 5.8% in women and 0.6% in men.[26]
- Numerous causes and risk factors for CTS
    - Distal radius fracture
    - Carpal bone dislocation – lunate
    - Repetitive wrist strain
    - Systemic conditions:
        - Rheumatoid arthritis
        - Diabetes mellitus
        - Collagen vascular disease
        - Hypothyroidism
        - Congestive heart failure
        - Hormonal – pregnancy and menopause

Mechanism

- Anything that increases pressure within the carpal tunnel, thus compressing the median nerve
    - Acute bony entrapment within carpal tunnel
    - Hematoma from associated fracture
    - Flexor synovial thickening
    - Fluid retention

Presentation

- Numbness, paresthesias, and pain to the volar hand
    - Prominent in thumb, index, and middle fingers
    - Sparing the fifth digit
- Worse at night and early morning

Physical Examination

- General inspection of the wrist compared to the opposite extremity, looking for symmetry, deformities, edema

- Detailed neurologic exam of radial, ulnar, and median nerves
  - Decreased sensation over median distribution
- Assess proximally as well, as cervical radiculopathy and thoracic outlet syndrome may mimic symptoms
- *Phalen's test* – wrist flexion for 60 seconds that reproduces symptoms
  - Sensitivity 76%, specificity 80%[27]
- *Tinel's sign* – tapping over carpal tunnel reproduces symptoms
  - Sensitivity 42–85%, specificity 54–98%[27]
- *Durkan's test* – compression over carpal tunnel
  - Sensitivity 87%, specificity 90% [28]

Essential Diagnostics

- If acute symptoms and associated with trauma, standard radiographs as detailed in prior sections for assessment of fracture/dislocation
- Chronic symptoms are evaluated with nerve conduction studies.

ED Treatment and Disposition

- If associated with fracture or dislocation, emergent reduction and consultation with orthopedics
- Chronic or not associated with trauma
  - Initial treatment is conservative.
    - Splint in neutral position
    - Nonsteroidal anti-inflammatory drugs
    - Cortisone injections
  - Surgery with carpal tunnel release
    - Predictors of need for surgery – more than 50 years old, symptoms more than ten months, constant symptoms, +*Phalen's test* at less than 30 seconds, stenosing flexor tenosynovitis
  - Majority of patients respond to conservative therapy, yet 80% of symptoms recur within one year[29]

Return to Play

- Usually athletes do not need sports restrictions unless associated with an acute injury or there is significant weakness
- Athletes may continue sports participation through treatment as long as normal strength and pain-free range of motion

Complications

- Permanent median neuropathy

Pearls and Pitfalls

- Acute carpal tunnel syndrome requires emergent consultation.
  - High level of suspicion for distal radius fractures and carpal dislocations
- Chronic carpal tunnel syndrome is managed as an outpatient.

De Quervain's Tenosynovitis

General Considerations

- Tenosynovitis is an inflammation to the tendon synovial sheath.
- De Quervain's represents the most common form
  - Affects extensor pollisis brevis and abductor pollisis longus
- Greater prevalence in females by factor of 10:1
- Some association with rheumatoid arthritis and postmenopausal states

Mechanism

- Either overuse injury or idiopathic

Presentation

- Pain over the radial styloid, with radiation to the thumb and distal forearm

Physical Examination

- Reproducible tenderness over the radial styloid and the tendon sheaths
- *Positive Finkelstein test* (Figure 3.6)

Essential Diagnostics

- No acute imaging needed

ED Treatment and Disposition

- First-line treatment is conservative
  - Rest, ice, NSAIDs, and thumb splint
  - Usually enough to relieve symptoms
- Can attempt steroid injection into the tendon sheath
  - 50:50 mix of local anesthetic and steroid

  - Success rate reported of up to 90%[30]
  - Ultrasound guidance increases successful placement
- Surgery recommended if continued symptoms despite two injections within one year

Return to Play

- Usually only short-term sports restrictions are needed, if any
- Athlete may return to play upon regaining pain-free range of motion and normal strength

Complications

- Chronic pain

Pearls and Pitfalls

- Not a common ED complaint
- Consider alternative diagnosis such as carpometacarpal arthritis

TFCC Injury

General Considerations

- TFCC is a multiunit structure serving as major stabilizer of DRUJ.
- Composed of:
  - Ulnar-carpal ligaments
  - Radioulnar ligaments
  - Ulnar meniscus homolog
  - Articular disc
  - Ulnar collateral ligament
  - Extensor carpi ulnaris tendon sheath
  - (Figure 3.2)
- Located between the ulna, lunate and triquetrum, thus its "triangular" appearance
- TFCC is responsible for the dynamic mobility and stability of the wrist, ensuring range of motion and fluidity in all directions.
- TFCC injury may be a cause for both acute and chronic ulnar sided wrist pain, although commonly misdiagnosed and undertreated.
- Injury is frequently seen in gymnasts and tennis players, as well as with lower impact but repetitive use such as by bowlers and construction workers.

Mechanism

- Majority of TFCC injuries are due to traumatic overloading of the wrist, with forced hyperextension (FOOSH) and ulnar deviation.
- Given its underlying mechanics, excessive pronation and supination may also serve as etiology for injury.

Presentation

- Hallmark of TFCC injury is ulnar-sided wrist pain.
- Some patients will point to the region just distal to the ulnar styloid.
- Many times there is preceding trauma, or a story of a "wrist sprain that never fully healed."
- Frequently associated with distal radius and ulnar styloid fracture

Physical Examination

- Tenderness localized to space between ulnar styloid and pisiform, sometimes referred to as the "fovea sign"
- Pain is usually exacerbated by resisted extension and ulnar deviation.
- Clicking or crepitus may be elicited by resisted supination/pronation, yet is not specific for injury.
- Often positive *TFCC compression test* (Figure 3.10)

Essential Diagnostics

- X-rays in the ED are generally used to rule out associated fracture or dislocation, as TFCC injuries will not be detected on plain films
  - Positive ulnar variance (ulna is longer than radius) predisposes to TCFF injury
- MRI may be performed on an outpatient basis.
  - Sensitivity of 60%, high specificity at 90%[31]

ED Treatment and Disposition

- Conservative treatment with splinting/immobilization
- Early referral to physical therapy for range of motion and strengthening
- Persistent pain or subluxation may be followed up with orthopedics for possible arthroscopy.

Return to Play

- Patients treated conservatively with range of motion and strengthening may return to athletics once symptoms have subsided.

- Surgically repaired TFCC injuries typically require a minimum of four weeks of cast immobilization, followed by two to four weeks of physical therapy to restore strength and ROM.
- Return to full activity is dependent upon the demands of the sport.

Complications

- Improper treatment may lead to premature degenerative changes, as well as chronic instability at the DRUJ.

Pearls and Pitfalls

- High index of suspicion for TFCC injury with ulnar sided wrist pain, especially in young athletes with repetitive extension/pronation mechanism
- Hesitate to diagnose "wrist sprain"

Ganglion Cyst

General Considerations

- The most common soft tissue tumor of the hand and wrist
- Ganglion is a cystic structure of gelatinous fluid formed by synovial tissue at a joint or tendon sheath.
- Most common location on the dorsal wrist, but also volar wrist and flexor tendons
- Cysts are usually 2 cm or less in diameter.

Mechanism

- In most cases patient do not recall any inciting trauma
- Cause is unknown, but possibly due to minimal trauma or repetitive irritation.

Presentation

- Patients complain of swelling and possible pain at the site of the mass, typically dull and "achy" and worse with direct pressure or repetitive activity
- Insidious in onset

Physical Examination

- Notable fluid-filled nodule, sometimes tender to palpation, without overlying erythema or induration.
  - Most common location at the dorsal scapholunate joint
- Transilluminates with light

Essential Diagnostics

- No imaging is required for diagnosis, but ultrasound is the modality of choice and can aid in aspiration.
- If the diagnosis is unclear, MRI may be used to differentiate from other types of masses

ED Treatment and Disposition

- No emergent treatment is required, as most resolve spontaneously.
- Reassure patient of benign nature
- For chronic symptoms or worsening pain, aspiration may be performed.
- Corticosteroid injection may help with symptom management.
- Frequently recur, and thus may undergo operative excision

Return to Play

- Generally, no sports restrictions are required.
- If significant pain or swelling, may be reasonable to restrict participation for a couple of weeks to allow swelling to subside.

Complications

- Recurrence

Pearls and Pitfalls

- Most common benign growth on the wrist, commonly the dorsal aspect
- Ultrasound may be very useful for identification and patient reassurance

Tables: Key diagnoses, history and physical exam findings, treatment, and indications for Orthopedic consultation in the ED.

Table 3.2 Distal Radius Fractures

Radius Fractures	History and Physical Exam Findings	Treatment	Disposition	Key Points
Colles (Extension)	"Dinner folk deformity," dorsal displacement/ angulation Median nerve exam	Reduce to volar tilt > 0, Sugar-tong splint 15° flexion and ulnar deviation with three-point mold	R – normal alignment, 7–10 d U – difficult reduction, poor alignment, intra-articular E – median neuropathy, open	Most common fracture Acute median neuropathy Chronic arthritis
Smith (Flexion)	"Garden spade deformity," volar displacement/ angulation	Reduce in ED, low threshold for ortho reduction Sugar-tong in slight extension	R – normal alignment, 7–10 d U – difficult reduction, poor alignment, intra-articular E – open	1/10th as common as Colles Neuropathy less common Complicated reduction
Barton's	Intra-articular rim, either volar or dorsal with carpal displacement	Reduce in ED Sugar-tong in neutral	U – unstable joint, likely need for ORIF E – median neuropathy	Rare fracture, but unstable and likely needing ORIF
Hutchinson	Radial styloid	Reduce in ED Sugar-tong in neutral	R – good reduction, no DRUJ involvement U-unstable or significant displacement	Unstable and likely needing ORIF Associated with scaphoid fx and scapholunate dissociation

Abbreviations: R = Routine; U = Urgent; E = Emergent; ORIF = operative reduction, internal fixation.

Table 3.3 Carpal Fractures

Carpal Fracture	History and Physical Exam Findings	Treatment	Disposition	Key Points
Scaphoid	Snuff box, first metacarpal axial load, thumb movement	S – thumb spica ND – thumb spica D – thumb spica	S – f/u 1 week for XR ND – f/u 1 week for casting D – U referral, ORIF	Most common carpal fracture High risk injury for AVN and chronic OA Seen best on Scaphoid XR Treat conservatively if injury suspected
Lunate	Lister's tubercle, dorsum of hand, axial load third MC	Thumb spica	ND – routine D(>1mm) – U, ORIF	Rare fracture High risk for AVN

Table 3.3 (cont.)

Carpal Fracture	History and Physical Exam Findings	Treatment	Disposition	Key Points
Capitate	Just distal to Lister's tubercle, axial load third metacarpal	Thumb spica	Routine	Rare fracture, but high risk for AVN Rarely occurs in isolation
Triquetrum	Dorsum of hand, distal to ulnar styloid	Dorsal Chip – volar splint Transverse – volar splint	Routine	Second-most common fracture Good prognosis
Hamate	Volar hand, just distal and radial to pisiform Ulnar nerve exam	Ulnar gutter	ND – routine D – urgent Hook – U, possible need for excision	Ulnar neuropathy Seen best on carpal tunnel XR
Pisiform	Volar hand, distal to ulnar styloid Ulnar nerve exam	Ulnar gutter	Routine	Ulnar neuropathy Flexor carpi ulnaris injury Carpal tunnel XR
Trapezoid	Dorsal hand, base of second metacarpal and axial load	Thumb spica	Routine	Least common fracture Prone to AVN
Trapezium	Thumb movement, first metacarpal axial load, distal snuff box	Thumb spica	Routine	Associated with scaphoid and radius fracture Rare radial artery injury

Abbreviations: R = Routine; U = Urgent; E = Emergent; ORIF = operative reduction, internal fixation; S = Suspected; ND = Nondisplaced; D = Displaced; AVN = avascular necrosis.

Table 3.4 Carpal Instability

Injury	Diagnosis	Treatment	Disposition	Key Points
Scapholunate dissociation	Scapholunate space > 3 mm "Terry Thomas," possible "signet ring" sign	Volar splint	Routine	#1 cause of SLAC and OA
Perilunate dislocation	Dorsally displaced capitate on lateral XR, "empty teacup"	Volar splint	Emergent, ORIF	Unstable 60% association with scaphoid fracture
Lunate dislocation	Volar displaced lunate, "spilled teacup," proximally displaced capitate	Volar splint	Emergent, ORIF	Unstable Acute carpal tunnel syndrome

Abbreviations: ORIF = operative reduction, internal fixation; SLAC = scapholunate advanced collapse; OA = osteoarthritis.

Recommended Reading

Simon's Emergency Orthopedics, Chapter 12: Wrist

Rosen's Emergency Medicine, Chapter 48: Wrist and Forearm

Netter's Sports Medicine, Chapter 45: Hand and Wrist Injuries

Fracture Management for Primary Care, Chapter 5: Carpal Fractures, Chapter 6: Radius and Ulna Fractures

Green's Operative Hand Surgery, Part III: Wrist (Chapters 15–18)

References

1. Alderman AK, Storey AF, Chung KC. Financial impact of emergency hand trauma on the

health care system. *J Am Coll Surg* 2008;206(2):233–238.

2. Larsen CF, Lauritsen J. Epidemiology of acute wrist trauma. *Int J Epidemiol* 1993; 22 (5):991–916.
3. Nellans KW, Kowalski E, Chung KC. The epidemiology of distal radius fractures. *Hand Clin* 2012; 28(2):113–125.
4. Chung KC, Spilson SV. The frequency and epidemiology of hand and forearm fractures in the United States. *J Hand Surg* 2001;26(5):908–915.
5. Welling RD, Jacobson JA, Jamadar DA, et al.. MDCT and radiology of wrist fractures: Radiographic sensitivity and fracture patterns. *Am J Roentgenol* 2008; 190(1): 10–16.
6. Hainline B. Nerve Injuries. *Med Clin North Am* 1994;78 (2):327–343.
7. Vigler M, Aviles A, Lee SK. Carpal fractures excluding the scaphoid. *Hand Clin* 2006; 22 (4):501–516.
8. Cooney WP, Linscheid RL, Robyns JH: Fractures and dislocations of the wrist. In: Rockwood, CA, Green DP, Bucholz RW, ed. *Fractures in Adults*, vol 1. 4th ed. Philadelphia: Lippincott-Raven; 1996:563–678.
9. Kozin SH. Incidence, mechanism and natural history of scaphoid fractures. *Hand Clin* 2001;17(4):515–524.
10. Barton, NJ. Twenty questions about scaphoid fractures. *J Hand Surg Br* 1992; 17(3):289–310.
11. Gumucio CA, Fernando B, Young VL, et al.. Management of scaphoid fractures: A review and update. *South Med J* 1989;82(11):1377–1388.
12. Perron, AD, Brady WJ, Keats TE, et al.. Orthopedic pitfalls in the ED: Scaphoid fracture. *American Journal of Emergency Medicine* 2001; 19(4):310–316.
13. Pao V, Chang J. Scaphoid nonunion: Diagnosis and treatment. *Plast Reconstr Surg* 2003; 112(6):1666–1676.
14. Botte MJ, Pacelli LL, Gelberman RH. Vascularity and osteonecrosis of the wrist. *Orthop Clin North Am* 2004; 35 (3):405–421.
15. Slade JF III, Jaskwhich D. Percutaneous fixation of scaphoid fractures. *Hand Clin* 2001;17(4):553–574.
16. Teisen H, Hjarbaek J. Classification of fresh fractures of the lunate. *J Hand Surg* 1988; 13(4):458–462.
17. Brach P, Goitz R. An update on the management of carpal fractures. *J Hand Ther* 2003; 16(2):152–160.
18. Garcia-Elias M. Carpal bone fractures. In: Watson HK, Weinzweig J, eds. *The wrist.* Philadelphia: Lipincott, Williams, and Wilkins 2001; 173–186.
19. Steinberg B. Acute wrist injuries in the athlete. *Orthop Clin North Am* 2002; 33 (3):535–545.
20. Lacey JD, Hodge JC. Pisiform and hamulus fractures: easily missed wrist fractures diagnosed on a reverse oblique radiograph. *J Emerg Med* 1998; 16 (3):445–452.
21. Cohen MS. Fractures of the carpal bones. *Hand Clin* 1997; 13(4): 587–599.
22. Jeong GK, Kram D, Lester B. Isolated fractures of the trapezoid. *Am J Orthop* 2001; 30 (3):228–230.
23. Mayfield JK, Johnson RP, Kilcoyne RK. Carpal dislocations: Pathomechanics and progressive perilunar instability. *J Hand Surg Am* 1980; 5(3):226–241.
24. Jones WA. Beware the sprained wrist: The incidence and diagnosis of scapholunate instability. *J Bone Joint Surg Br* 1998;70 (2):293–297.
25. Kozin SH, Wood MB. Early soft-tissue complications after fractures to the distal part of the radius. *J Bone Joint Surg Am* 1993;75 (1):144–153.
26. Bland JD. Carpal tunnel syndrome. *Curr Opin Neurol* 2005; 18(3):581–585.
27. Kuschner SH, Ebramzadeh E, Johnson D, et al.. Tinel's sign and Phalen's test in carpal tunnel syndrome. *Orthopedics* 1992:15 (11):1297–1302.
28. Wiesler ER, Chloros GD, Cartwright MS, et al.. The use of diagnostic ultrasound in carpal tunnel syndrome. *J Hand Surg Am* 2006:31 (5):726–732.
29. Viera AJ. Management of carpal tunnel syndrome. *Am Fam Physician* 2003; 68 (2):265–272.
30. Witt J, Pess G, Gelberman RH. Treatment of de Quervain tenosynovitis: A prospective study of the results of injection of steroid and immobilization in a splint. *J Bone Joint Surg Am* 1991; 73 (2):219–222.
31. De Smet L. Magnetic resonance imaging for diagnosing lesions of the triangular fibrocartilage complex. *Acta Orthop Belg* 2005;71(4):396–398.

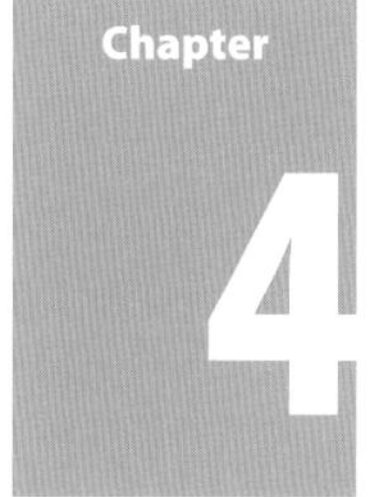

Hand

Yvonne C. Chow and Amanda Akin
Illustrations by Yvonne Chow

Background/Epidemiology

- Injuries to hand and digits common
- Estimated 5–30 percent of ED injuries[1,2]
- Up to 18 percent of all fractures
- Up to 9 percent of all sports-related injuries
- 1.7:1 male-to-female ratio[3]
- 60 percent injuries between 16–32 years of age[3]
- Typical mechanisms of injury include fall on outstretched hand or direct blow
- Mortality exceedingly rare
- Morbidity major concern; severe or poorly managed injuries may affect long-term function of hand and wrist
    - Digit laceration accounts for third most common reason for lost workdays in United States (following back and leg strain)[4,5]

Anatomical Considerations/ Pathophysiology

- Dorsal (extensor) surface
- Volar (flexor) surface
- Radial (lateral) border
- Ulnar (medial) border
- Five metacarpal bones (Figure 4.1)
    - Second and third metacarpal bones are relatively immobile
    - Intrinsic movements of the hand are dependent on stability of the above.[6]
- Thumb consists of proximal and distal phalanges, with two sesamoids at metacarpophalangeal (MCP) joint.
- Fingers consist of proximal, middle, and distal phalanges.
- Metacarpal and proximal phalanx articulate at MCP joint.
- Proximal and middle phalanges articulate at proximal interphalangeal (PIP) joint.
- Middle and distal phalanges articulate at distal interphalangeal (DIP) joint.
- Thumb only has single interphalangeal (IP) joint.
- Pediatric physes located at base of all phalanges and first metacarpal, and at heads of second to fifth metacarpals (Figure 4.2).
- Nine finger flexor tendons (Figure 4.3).
    - Four superficial flexors attach to middle phalanx of fingers – flex PIP
    - Five deep flexors pass through split in superficial tendons to attach to distal phalanx of thumb and fingers – flex DIP
    - Anchored by annular ligaments ("pulleys") to prevent bowstringing
    - Course through flexor tendon sheaths
- Extensor tendons (Figure 4.4)
    - Common extensor tendon attaches to middle phalanx via central slip – extends PIP.
    - Lateral extensor bands form terminal extensor tendon, which attaches to distal phalanx – extends DIP.
    - Course through extensor expansion complex (extensor hood).
- Joint capsule of IP and MCP joints thickened at volar aspect to form dense fibrous structure called volar plate.[7]
- Digit collateral ligaments provide medial/ lateral stability.
    - Maximally lengthened when digit flexed at 70° at MCP, 30° at PIP, 15° at DIP.[8]
    - Immobilization should occur at above angles to prevent contractures.[9]
- The hand is innervated by the median, radial, and ulnar nerves
- Median nerve
    - Motor to thumb abduction, flexion, opposition

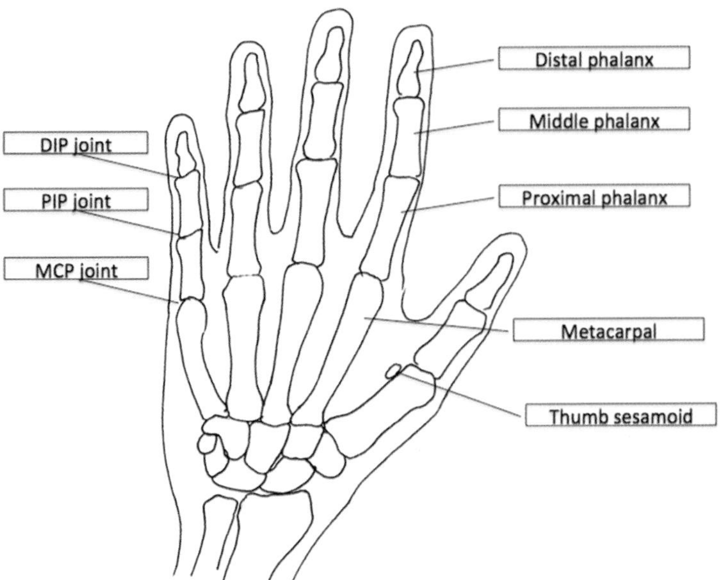

Figure 4.1. Bony anatomy of hand.

  - Sensation to volar hand from thumb to radial (lateral) half of ring finger (including dorsal tips) (Figure 4.5A)
- Radial nerve
  - Motor to thumb extension/abduction, MCP extension, and wrist extension
  - Sensation to dorsal hand from thumb to radial (lateral) half of ring finger (excluding dorsal tips) (Figure 4.5B)
- Ulnar nerve
  - Motor to thumb adduction, little finger abduction, finger adduction/abduction
  - Sensation to dorsal and volar hand from little finger to ulnar half of ring finger (Figure 4.5c)
- Vascular supply from radial and ulnar arteries
- Lymphatic and venous drainage located on dorsum of hand[6]

Focused History and Physical Exam

- Important history elements:
  - Hand dominance
  - Sport, position, or occupation
  - Mechanism of injury
  - Position of hand during injury
  - Prior hand injury or surgery
- General physical exam elements:
- Inspection
  - Soft tissue swelling

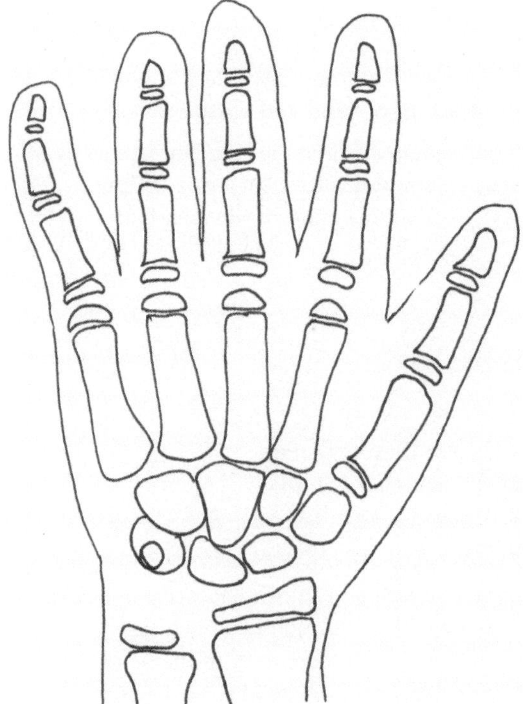

Figure 4.2. Locations of pediatric growth plates. Note the physis of the first metacarpal is located at the metacarpal base, rather than at the metacarpal head as in the rest of the metacarpals.

  - Obvious gross deformity (mallet finger, boutonnière)
  - Finger posture
  - Muscle wasting
  - Skin discoloration

Table 4.1 Key Anatomic Structures and Associated Functions

Structure	Function	Notes
Flexor digitorum profundus tendon	DIP flexion	Disruption causes Jersey finger Ulnar innervation
Flexor digitorum superficialis tendon	PIP flexion	Median innervation
Terminal extensor tendon	DIP extension	Disruption cases mallet finger Radial innervation
Central extensor slip	PIP extension	Disruption causes boutonnière deformity Radial innervation
Volar plate	Prevents IP hyperextension	Associated with dorsal dislocations
Collateral ligaments	Provide medial and lateral stability at MCP and IP joints	Radial collateral ligament commonly injured in finger dislocations 1st MCP ulnar collateral ligament injured in Skier's/Gamekeeper's thumb
Lumbrical muscles	MCP flexion	2nd and 3rd – ulnar innervation 4th and 5th – median innervation
Interosseous muscles	Finger abduction and adduction	Ulnar innervation
Thenar eminence (muscle bellies of abductor pollicis brevis, flexor pollicis brevis, opponens pollicis)	Thumb flexion, opposition	Atrophy suggests median nerve injury
Hypothenar eminence (muscle bellies of abductor digiti minimi, flexor digiti minimi brevis, opponens digiti minimi)	Little finger abduction, MCP flexion, and opposition	Atrophy suggests ulnar nerve injury

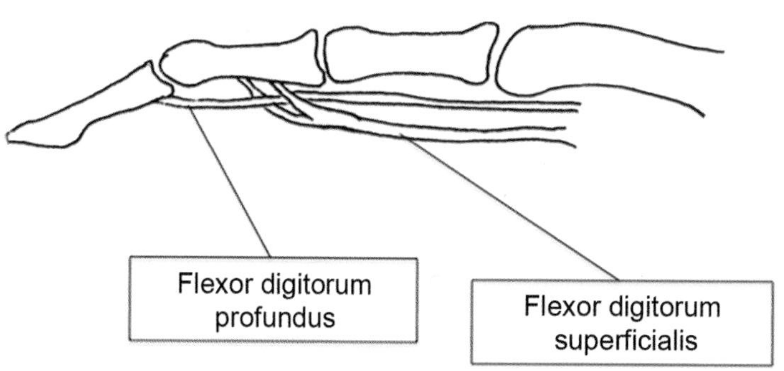

Figure 4.3 Flexor tendon anatomy.

- Wounds
- Nail avulsion or hematoma
- Compare with contralateral side

- Palpation
  - Point of maximal tenderness
  - Bony crepitus
  - Nodules along flexor tendon
- Range of motion (ROM)
  - Full extension of digits
  - Full flexion of digits into clenched fist
    - Phalanges should be parallel and pointing towards scaphoid bone, with all nails positioned in same plane (Figure 4.6A and Figure 4.6B).

- Special tests
  - Collateral ligament testing:
    - Hold phalanx proximal and distal to joint being tested, and attempt to open joint by applying both radial and ulnar stress (Figure 4.7A).
    - Stabilize first metacarpal and apply radial stress to proximal phalanx of thumb (Figure 4.7B).
    - Test at 0° and 30° (point of maximal tautness)
  - Test tendon function against resistance
    - Full ROM preserved with 90 percent laceration if no resistance.[6,10]
    - Pain along tendon during resistance testing suggests partial laceration[10]
  - Deep flexor tendon: flex DIP with PIP/MCP held in extension (Figure 4.8)
  - Superficial flexor tendon: flex PIP with other digits held in extension (Figure 4.9)
- Neurovascular (NV) exam
  - Palpate regional pulses and assess capillary refill.
  - Doppler useful for assessing digital arteries
  - Test sensory using two-point discrimination with paperclip ends 5 mm apart.
  - Median nerve
    - Touch tip of thumb to tip of index finger ("OK" sign) and resist pulling through the ring (Figure 4.10A)
    - Touch tip of thumb to tip of little finger and resist pulling apart (Figure 4.10B)
    - Test sensation over eponychium of index and middle fingers (Figure 4.10C)
  - Radial nerve
    - Extend wrist and digits at MCP against resistance (Figure 4.11A)
    - Test sensation at dorsum of thumb web space (Figure 4.11B)
  - Ulnar nerve
    - Spread fingers against resistance (Figure 4.12A)
    - Push fingers together against resistance
    - Test sensation over little finger tip (Figure 4.12B)

Differential Diagnosis-Emergent and Common Diagnoses

Table 4.2 Emergent and Common Diagnoses in the Emergency Department

Emergent Diagnoses	Common Diagnoses
Severe crush injury	Finger sprain
Vascular injury with signs of ischemia or compromise	Finger dislocation
High pressure injection injury	Collateral ligament rupture (gamekeeper's thumb)
Flexor tenosynovitis	Volar plate injury
Compartment syndrome	Phalanx fracture
	Jersey finger
	Mallet finger
	Central slip rupture (boutonniere deformity)
	Metacarpal fracture
	Boxer's knuckle
	Fight bite
	Tendon laceration
	Trigger finger
	Subungal hematoma
	Nailbed laceration

Acute Tendon and Ligament Injuries

Jersey finger

General Description

- Avulsion injury of flexor digitorum profundus (Figure 4.13)
- May include bony avulsion.

Mechanism

- Forceful extension of flexed DIP joint
- Commonly occurs when athlete grabs opponent's jersey

Presentation

- Pain and swelling at the DIP

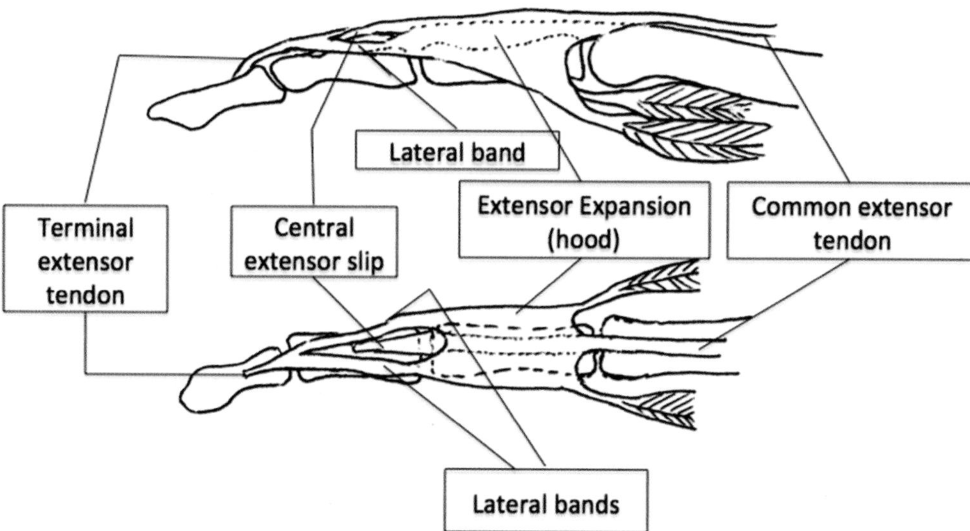

Figure 4.4. Extensor tendon complex anatomy.

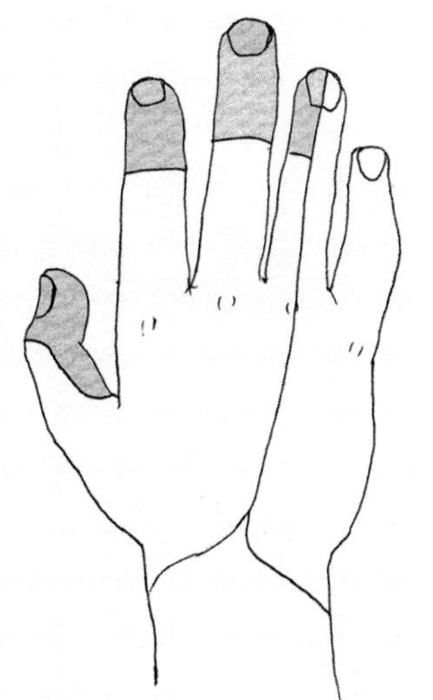

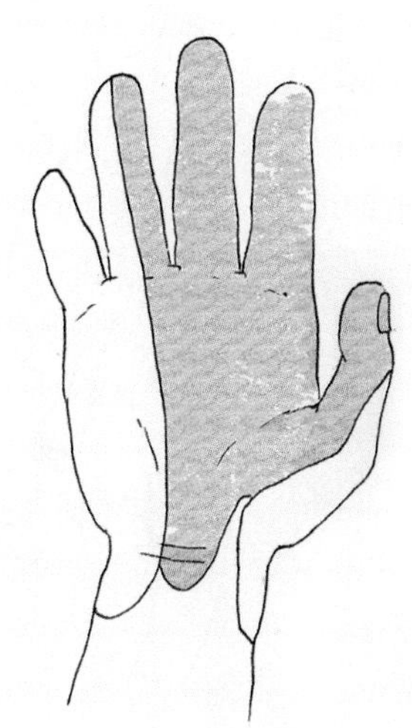

Figure 4.5a. Sensory distribution of median nerve.

Physical Exam

- Unable to actively flex isolated DIP on exam
- Volar tenderness at DIP and palm (due to retracted tendon)

Essential Diagnostics

- Digit x-rays to include AP, lateral, and oblique views.
- X-ray may show avulsion fracture at volar base of distal phalanx.

ED Treatment

- Dorsal splint is placed with slight flexion of MCP and IP joints.
- Urgent orthopedic referral for surgical repair [11,12]

Disposition

- Discharge
- Orthopedic referral in 1–2 days for surgical repair

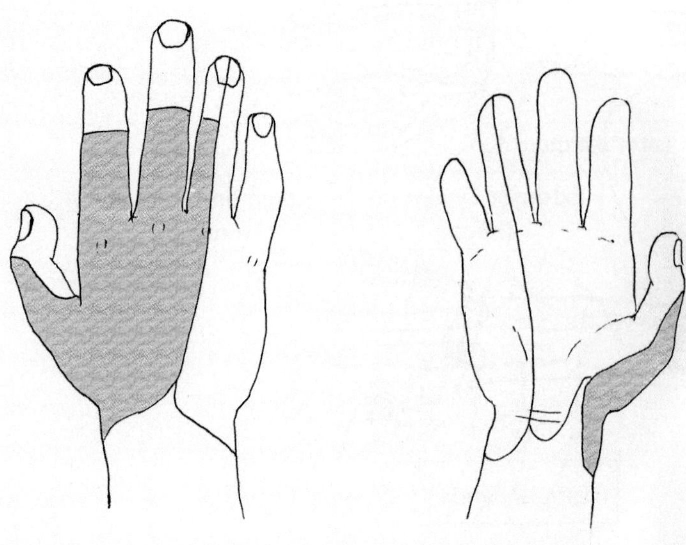

Figure 4.5b. Sensory distribution of radial nerve.

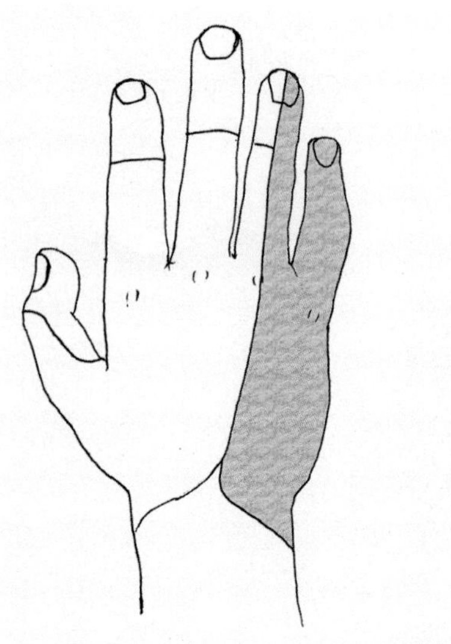

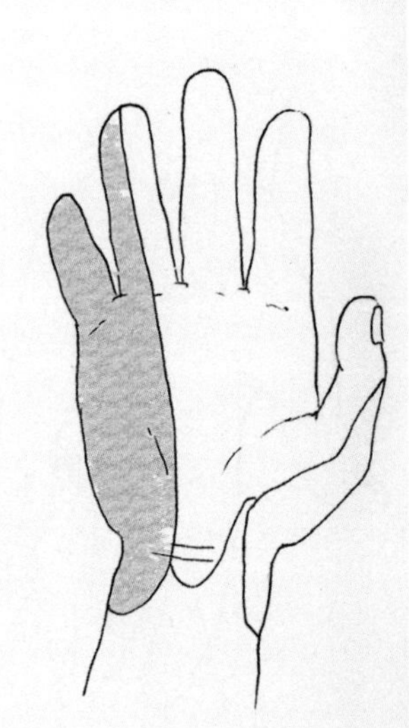

Figure 4.5c. Sensory distribution of ulnar nerve.

- Return to sports requires clearance following surgical repair.
  - Early return in mitten-type splint/cast possible for sports with no grasping motion[11]
  - Full return with grasping motion usually takes four to six months[11]

Complications

- Loss of deep flexor function if unrepaired or treatment delayed

Pediatric Considerations

- None

Pearls and Pitfalls

- Poor outcome if repair delayed more than seven days[12]

Central Slip Rupture

General Description

- Avulsion injury of central extensor slip (Figure 4.14)

Mechanism

- Deep contusion to PIP
- Forceful flexion of extended PIP
- Volar dislocation of PIP

Presentation

- Pain and swelling at PIP

Physical Exam

- Dorsal tenderness at PIP
- Weak active extension of PIP
- Classic boutonnière deformity (flexion deformity of PIP with hyperextension of DIP) rarely seen in acute setting[13]

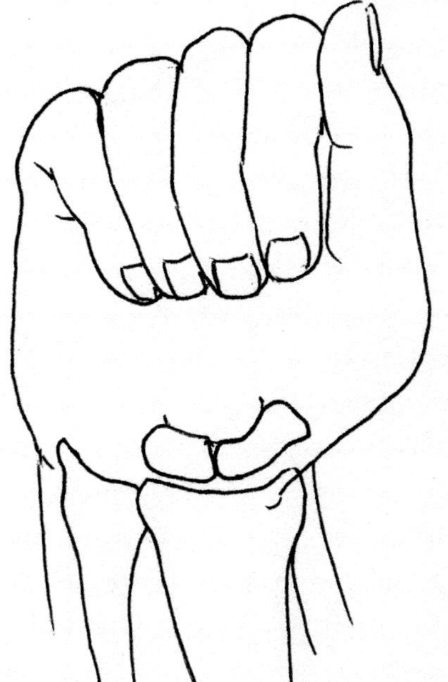

Figure 4.6A. Normal alignment of digits pointing to scaphoid.

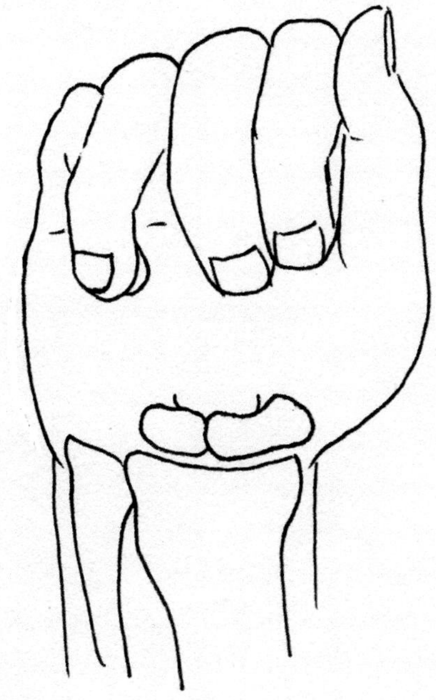

Figure 4.6B. Malrotation causing misaligned digit.

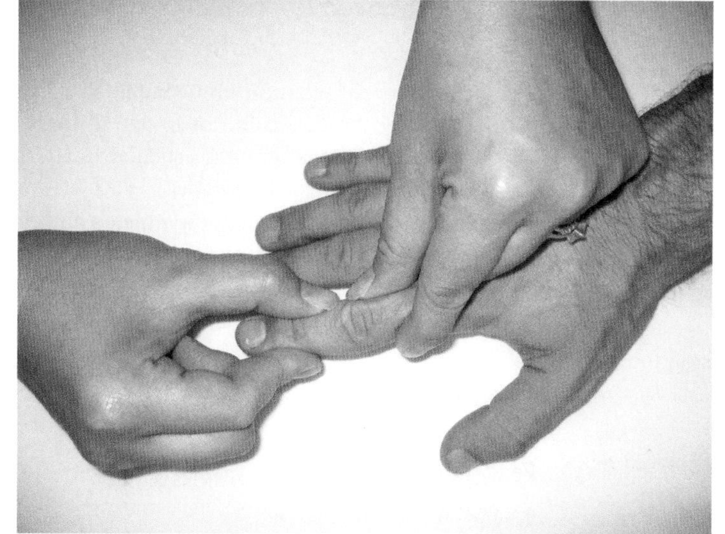

Figure 4.7A. Collateral ligament testing of the PIP joint.

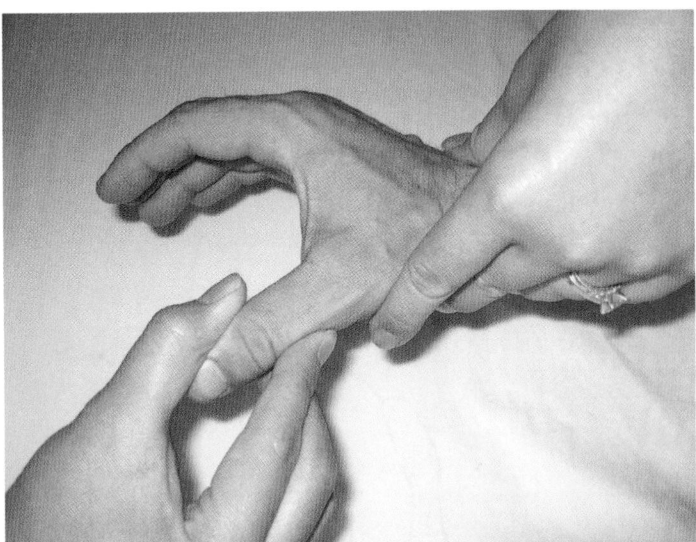

Figure 4.7B. Ulnar collateral ligament testing of the thumb.

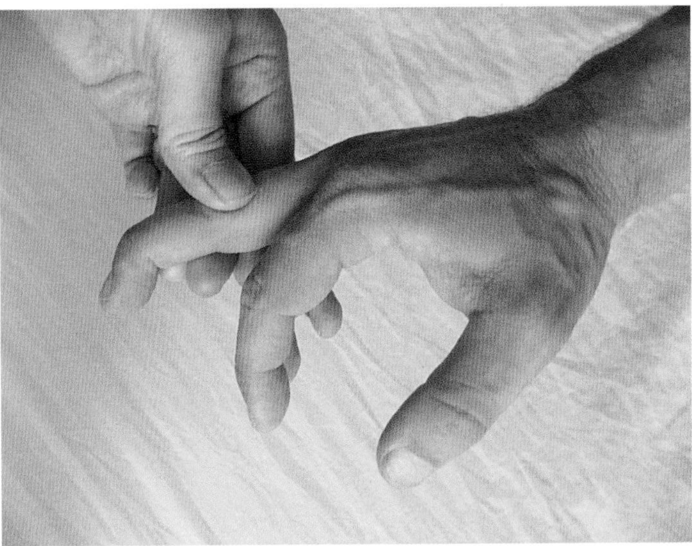

Figure 4.8. Test deep flexor tendon function by isolating DIP flexion.

Essential Diagnostics

- Digit x-rays to include AP, lateral, and oblique views.
- X-ray may show avulsion fracture at dorsal base of middle phalanx.
- Ultrasound may be useful for diagnosis.

ED Treatment

- Splint PIP joint in complete extension for four to six weeks
- Leave DIP free

Disposition

- Discharge
- Orthopedic consultation immediately if irreducible PIP dislocation or in two to three days if large, displaced, intra-articular fracture at base of middle phalanx[10,13]
- Return to sports dependent on athlete's ability to participate with PIP immobilized in extension.

Complications

- May cause boutonnière deformity if left untreated

Pediatric Considerations

- None

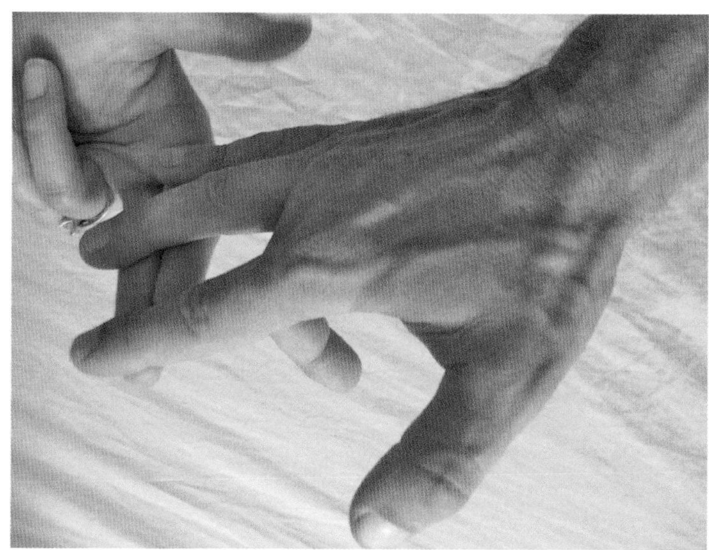

Figure 4.9. Test superficial flexor tendon function by isolating PIP flexion of each digit individually.

Pearls and Pitfalls

- Treat injured PIP joint with weak extension and dorsal tenderness empirically as central slip rupture, even without boutonnière deformity.[13]

Mallet finger

General Description

- Terminal extensor tendon injury with associated loss of extensor function of the DIP
- May occur as intra-articular avulsion fracture (Figure 4.15A) or as isolated tendon rupture (Figure 4.15B).

Mechanism

- Forced flexion of distal phalanx with finger in extension

Presentation

- Loss of DIP extension

Physical Exam

- Distal phalanx in partially flexed position at rest
- Swelling and tenderness over dorsal aspect of digit
- Unable to actively extend DIP

Essential Diagnostics

- Digit x-rays to include AP, lateral, and oblique views.

ED Treatment

- If nondisplaced fracture or isolated tendon injury, splint with DIP in extension continuously for six to eight weeks[14,15]
- Leave PIP free

Disposition

- Discharge
- Orthopedic consultation in one week if associated avulsion fracture displaced more than 50 percent of articular surface or volar subluxation – may need ORIF.
- Recommend follow-up visits at two week intervals to monitor compliance with continuous splint.
  - Patient compliance most important factor in success of nonoperative management[15]
- Return to sports dependent on athlete's ability to participate while DIP is splinted in full extension.
- Consider extension splinting during sports for additional eight weeks after continuous splinting has been completed.[16]

Complications

- If improperly treated patient will develop swan-neck deformity – flexion of DIP with hyperextension of PIP.

Pediatric Considerations

- Salter–Harris type II fracture mimics mallet finger or DIP joint dislocation on exam, even though this is an extra-articular fracture.[16,17]

- Splint in slight DIP hyperextension for up to six weeks.[16]
- Require close follow-up with weekly x-rays for two weeks to ensure alignment is stable.[17]
- Pediatric hand surgeon referral if open or irreducible fracture.

Pearls and Pitfalls

- DIP must remain in strict extension for six to ten weeks for proper healing.
- Patient should be shown how to change splint while keeping DIP extended against a hard surface.
- Any flexion that occurs at DIP requires starting treatment over at day one.[17]
- Extension lag may persist following treatment, but usually does not lead to functional deficit.[16]

Boxer's knuckle

General Description

- Rupture of sagittal band on radial aspect of the extensor hood.[6,18]

Mechanism

- Traumatic blow to MCP

Presentation

- Pain and swelling over dorsal MCP joint

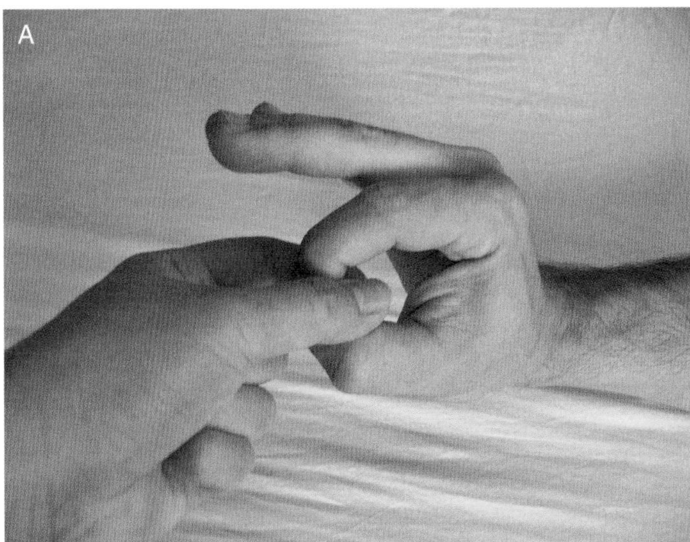

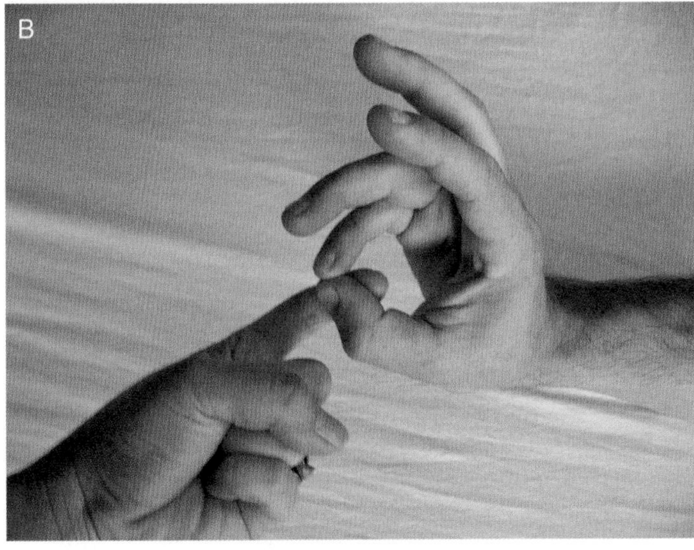

Figures 4.10A and B. Median nerve motor testing.

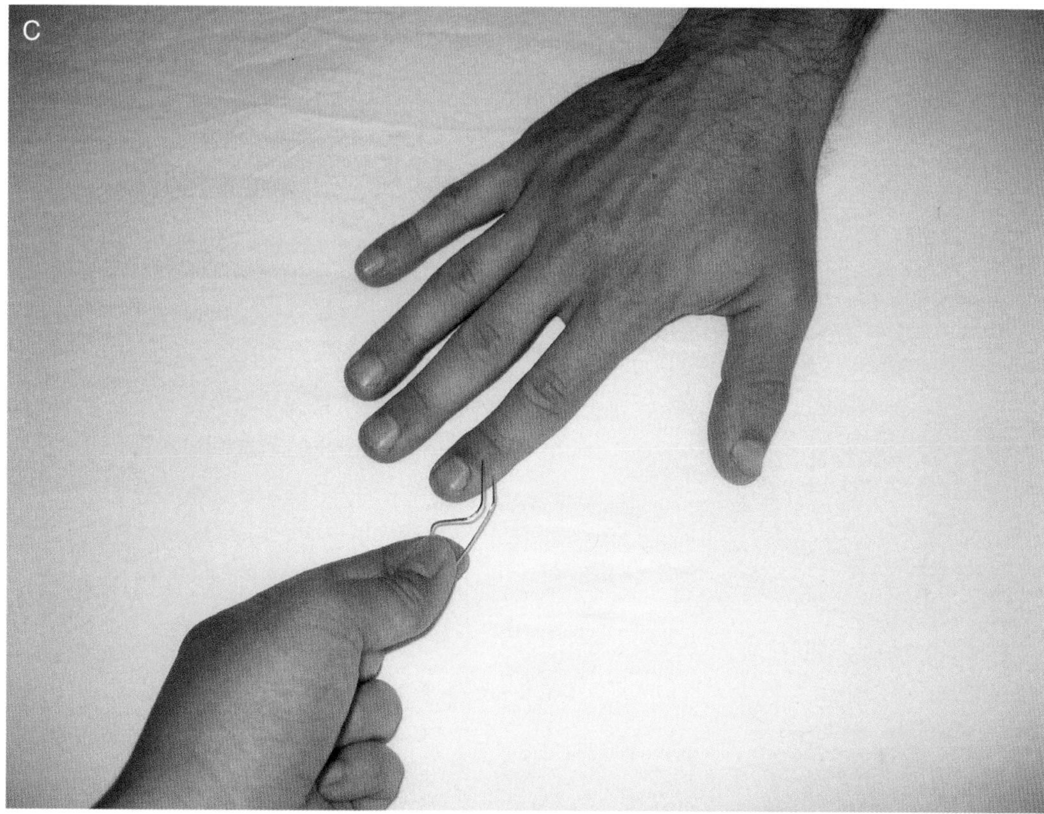

Figures 4.10C. Median nerve sensory testing.

Physical Exam

- Ulnar subluxation of extensor tendon during MCP flexion
- Patient unable to actively extend MCP joint
- Painful relocation of extensor tendon with passive MCP extension

Essential Diagnostics

- Hand/digit x-rays to include AP, lateral, and oblique views

ED Treatment

- Passively extend to relocate tendon.
- Splint placed with MCP in extension.
- If punctures wounds/fight bites are present:
  - Prescribe antibiotics to cover oral flora, update tetanus.
  - Do not primarily close wounds
  - Irrigate wounds copiously prior to any splint placement.

Disposition

- Discharge
- Hand surgeon follow-up in one week
- May return to sports with MCP splinted in extension, as limited by pain

Complications

- Deep space infection may occur with fight bites (see "Fight bite" for further details)

Pediatric Considerations

- None

Pearls and Pitfalls

- None

Tendon Laceration

General Description

- Injury to flexor or extensor tendons
- May be open or closed
- May be partial or complete
- See "Jersey finger," "Central slip rupture," and "Mallet finger" for injuries to specific tendons

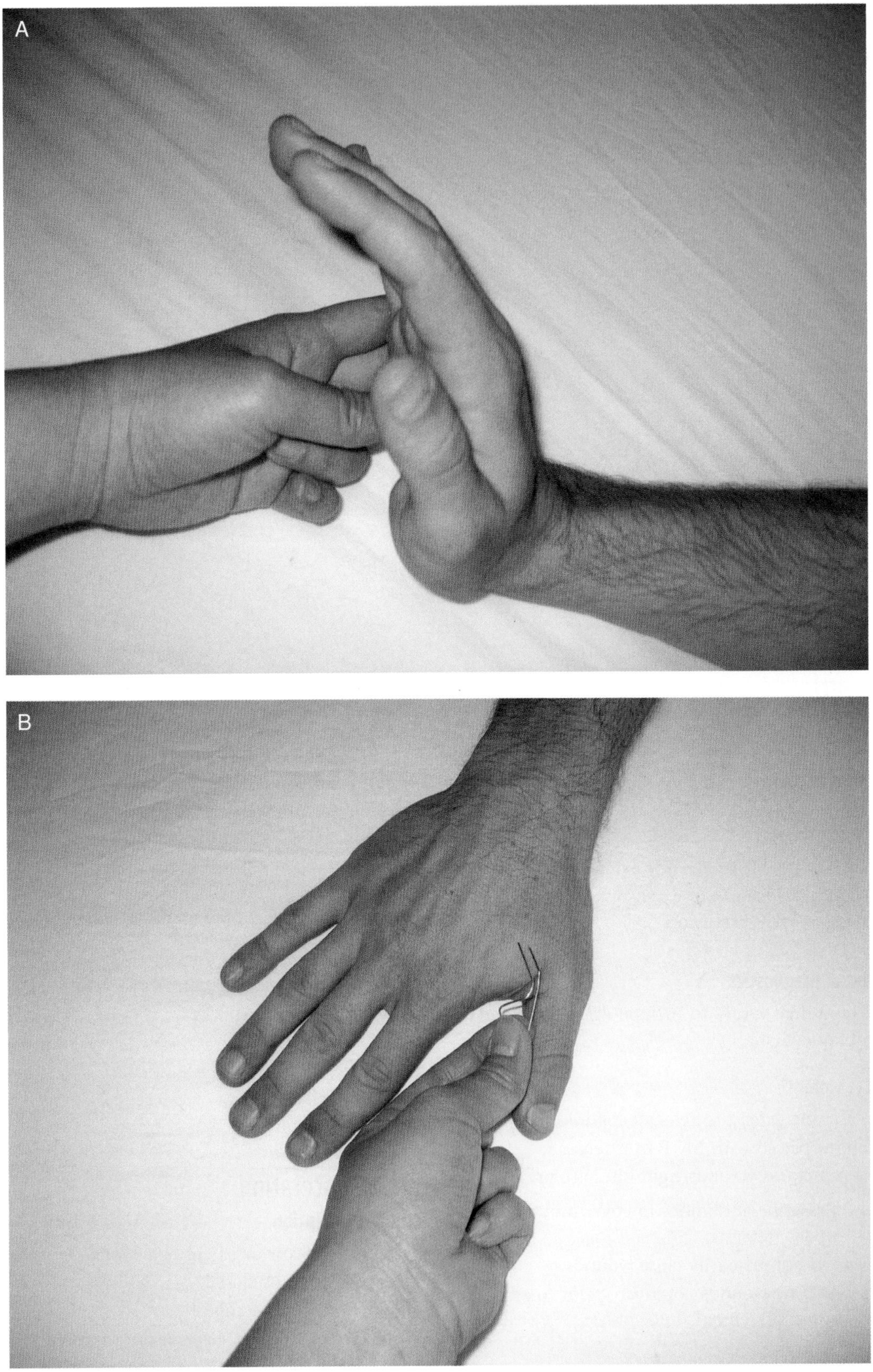

A

B

Figures 4.11A and B. Radial nerve (A) motor and (B) sensory testing.

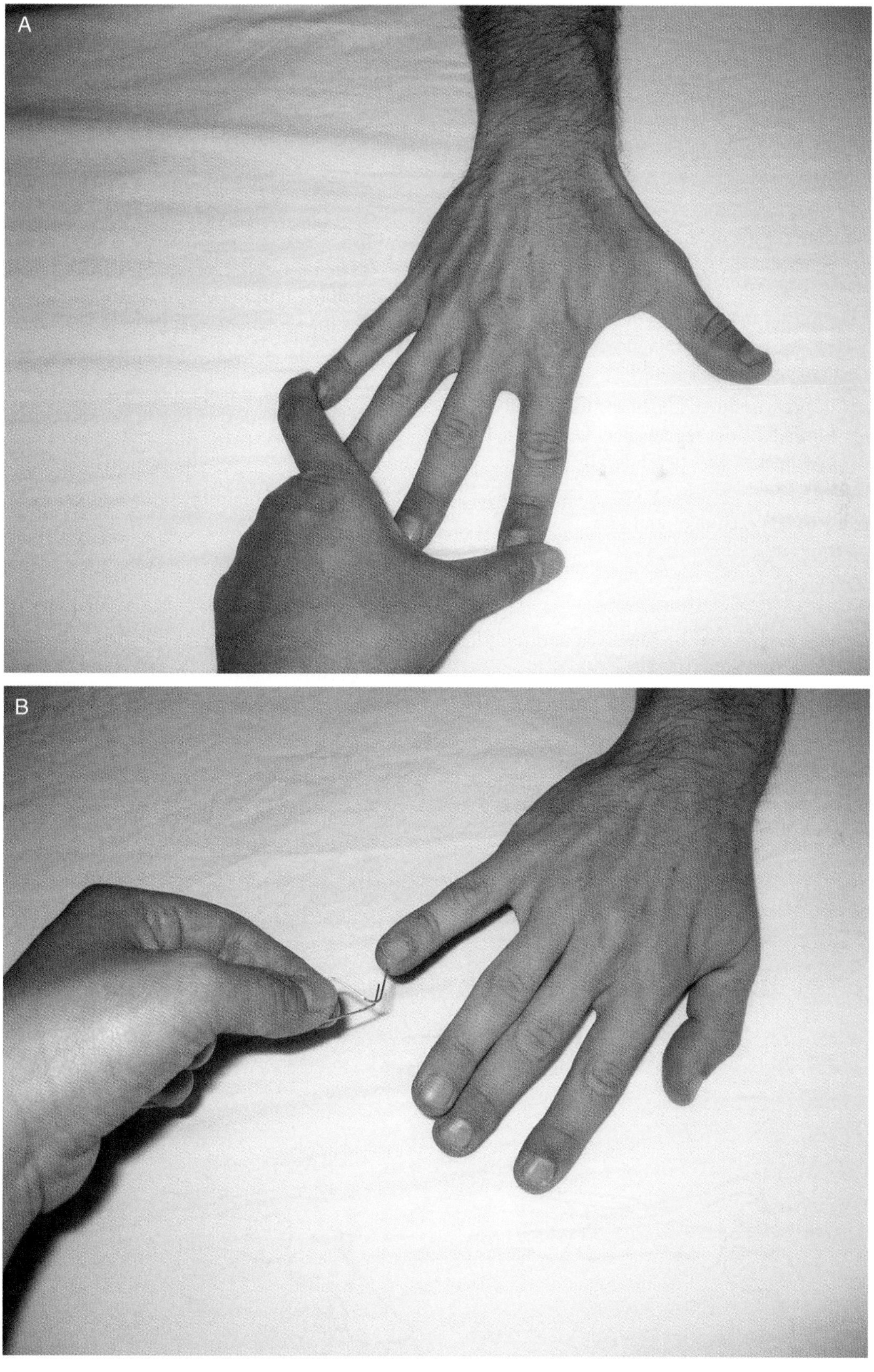

A

B

Figures 4.12A and B. Ulnar nerve (A) motor and (B) sensory testing.

Mechanism

- Most commonly caused by sharp object lacerating skin and underlying tendon.
- Direct blunt force
- Opposing force to tendon during contraction

Presentation

- Pain and swelling to affected area
- May have acute deformity

Physical Exam

- Skin wound may be present
- Determine position of hand when injury occurred
  - Inspect visible tendon during full digit ROM
  - Injured area of tendon may be retracted proximal to, or extend distally past, skin wound.
- Must isolate each digit and joint for appropriate testing.
- Test active ROM
- Test strength against resistance
  - Full motion may be preserved with only 10 percent tendon intact[6,10]
  - Pain along tendon during resistance testing suggests partial laceration[10]

Essential Diagnostics

- Hand/digit x-rays to include AP, lateral, and oblique views

ED Treatment

- Irrigate wound if contaminated.
- No definitive recommendations for treatment of partial lacerations:[6,19]
  - Consult with orthopedics regarding appropriate follow-up
  - Partial flexor lacerations: apply dorsal splint in position of function for three to four weeks
  - Partial extensor lacerations: apply splint with MCP in full extension (to reduce tension on tendon) for three to four weeks
- Complete flexor tendon lacerations:
  - Require urgent hand surgeon consultation, preferably within twelve to twenty-four hours.[6]
  - Avoid excessive manipulation of transected tendon (promotes adhesions)[6]
  - Apply dorsal splint in position of function.
- Complete extensor tendon lacerations
  - If located over proximal phalanx or dorsum of hand, may be repaired by experienced ED physician using figure-of-eight or horizontal mattress sutures.[6,10,20]

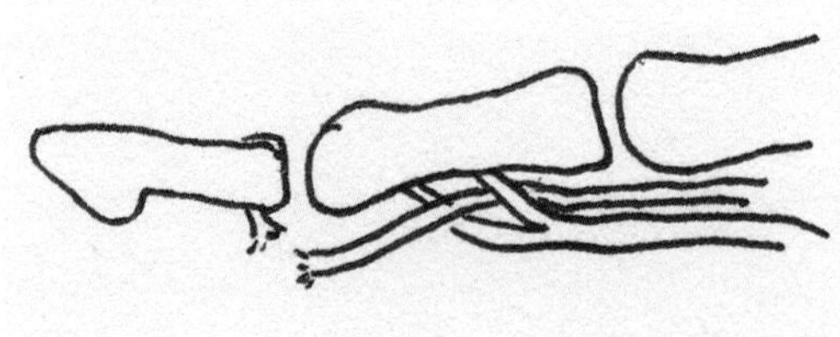

Figure 4.13. Flexor digitorum profundus rupture in jersey finger injury.

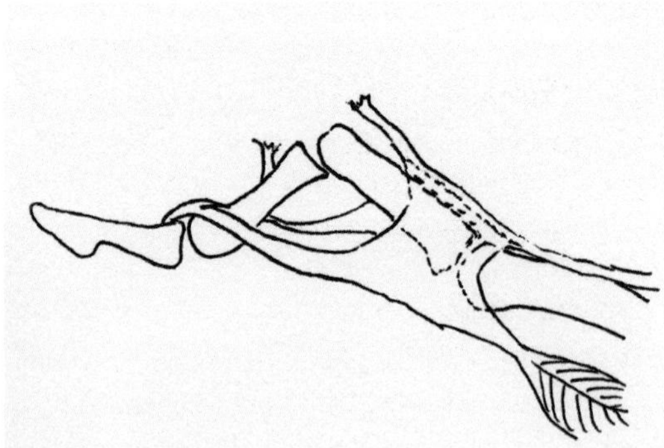

Figure 4.14. Schematic of a boutonnière deformity following central extensor slip rupture.

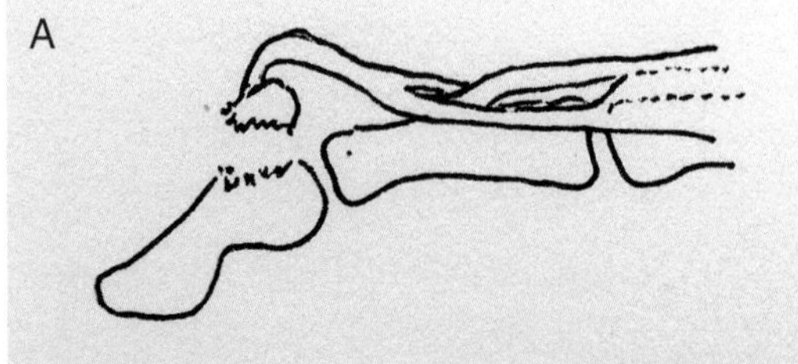

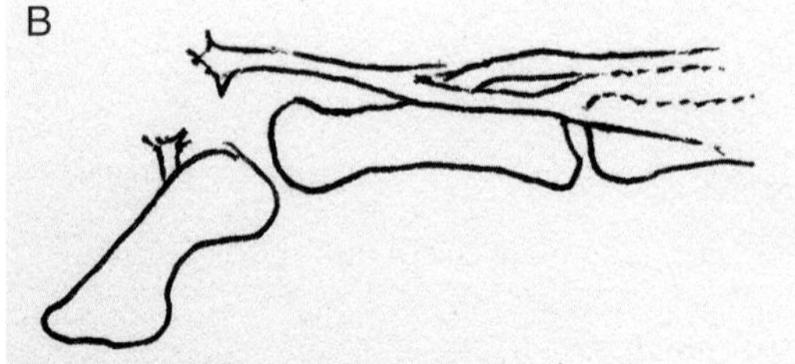

Figures 4.15 A and B. Mallet finger injury (A) with and (B) without avulsion fracture of distal phalanx.

- Otherwise refer to hand surgeon for immediate primary or delayed primary (within one week) repair.[6,20]
- Lacerations resulting from fight bites should have delayed repair following course of antibiotics; may need IV antibiotics and intraoperative washout.

Disposition

- Discharge
- Urgent orthopedic referral within one day for complete flexor lacerations[6]; within one to two days for complete extensor lacerations.[6,20]
- Orthopedic referral in one week for partial lacerations.
- May be reasonable to return to play as soon as one to two weeks for partial lacerations, may be limited by ability to participate while wearing protective splint.
- Return to sports requires clearance following surgical repair
  - Full return to play with normal strength and ROM may take several months

Complications

- Loss of flexion or extension function
- Entrapment and triggering of finger from partial flexor tendon rupture

Pediatric Considerations

- Urgent referral within twenty-four hours to pediatric hand surgeon recommended for all flexor and extensor tendon injuries.[10]

Pearls and Pitfalls

- Closed injuries may be easily missed and untreated, resulting in chronic deformities.
- Open injuries may be missed if tendon not inspected during full digit ROM.

Skier's/Gamekeeper's Thumb

General description

- Sprain or rupture of ulnar collateral ligament (UCL) of thumb (Figure 4.16)

Mechanism

- Forced abduction of thumb at MCP joint

Presentation

- Pain and swelling over ulnar aspect of thumb MCP

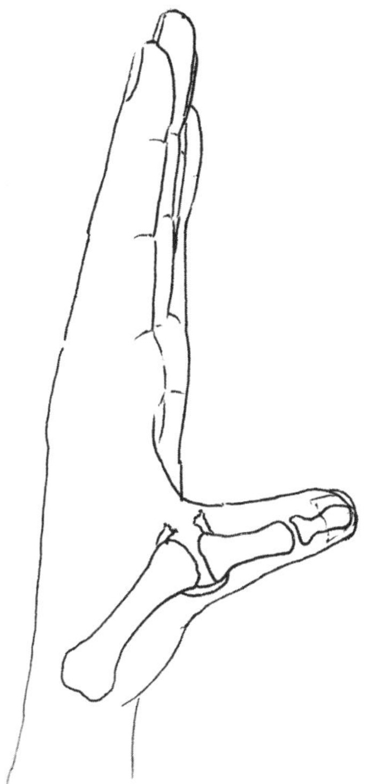

Figure 4.16. Rupture of the ulnar collateral of the thumb.

Physical Exam

- Tenderness over ulnar aspect of thumb MCP
- Unable to resist adduction stress to thumb (Figure 4.7b)
  - Lack of endpoint on stress testing indicates complete rupture
- Weakness with pinching

Essential Diagnostics

- Obtain x-rays prior to stress testing
- Thumb x-rays to include AP, lateral, and oblique views
- "Sag sign" caused by volar subluxation of proximal phalanx suggests UCL injury

ED Treatment

- Thumb spica splint[21]
- Urgent referral to orthopedics if complete rupture or associated fracture

Disposition

- Discharge
- Orthopedic referral in two to three days for surgical repair if complete rupture or

associated fracture, otherwise follow-up in one week.[10,21]
- Partial tears with limited laxity may be treated with thumb spica cast for four to six weeks.
- Return to sports dependent on severity of injury and athlete's ability to participate with protective thumb spica splint in place.
- Full return to sports without splint once ROM and strength have returned to normal, usually six to eight weeks for nonoperative cases and twelve weeks for operative treatment.[21]

Complications
- Long-term instability will result in difficulty with pinching motion.

Pediatric Considerations
- Prompt pediatric hand surgeon referral in one to two days for ORIF if avulsion fracture at insertion of UCL present.[22]

Pearls and Pitfalls
- Base of adductor pollicis aponeurosis may interpose between ends of UCL in complete rupture (Stener lesion) and inhibit healing; will require surgical repair.

Volar Plate Rupture

General Description
- Injury to volar plate at MCP, PIP, or DIP joint
- Most commonly at PIP

Mechanism
- Hyperextension of joint
- Dorsal dislocation

Presentation
- Pain and swelling at the affected joint

Physical Exam
- Tenderness at volar aspect of affected joint
- Test collateral ligaments for concomitant injury (Figure 4.7A)
- Unstable injury if joint able to be hyperextended or dorsally subluxed with passive ROM.
- Joint may be "locked" in extension if volar plate becomes caught between articular surfaces.

Essential Diagnostics
- Digit x-rays to include AP, lateral, and oblique views.
- X-ray may show avulsion fracture at volar base of middle phalanx.

ED Treatment
- If stable: buddy tape alone to prevent hyperextension, or dorsal block splint with PIP at 30° flexion for one to two weeks followed by buddy tape and early ROM.[23,24]
- If unstable but reducible: dorsal block splint as above for four weeks with weekly decreases in amount of flexion to reach full extension over one month.[23,24]
- If irreducible: emergent consultation with hand surgeon.

Disposition
- Discharge
- Immediate orthopedic consultation from ED if irreducible
- Orthopedic referral in two to three days if unstable or intra-articular avulsion fracture fragment – may require operative treatment[10]
- Stable injuries treated with dorsal block splint should have weekly follow-up to gradually decrease amount of flexion in splint until full extension is reached.
- Return to sports dependent on athlete's ability to participate with dorsal block splint or buddy tape in place.[23]

Complications
- May cause swan-neck deformity (hyperextension of PIP and flexion of DIP) if untreated

Pediatric Considerations
- None

Pearls and Pitfalls
- Identification of injury important for appropriate treatment and avoidance of swan-neck deformity.

Fractures and Dislocations

Finger Dislocation

General Description
- May occur at DIP, PIP, or MCP
- Most commonly dorsally dislocated
- Associated with volar plate rupture
- Volar DIP dislocations highly associated with terminal extensor tendon rupture[25]

- Volar PIP dislocations highly associated with central slip rupture[26]

Mechanism

- Hyperextension
- Varus or valgus forces

Presentation

- Pain and swelling over affected joint
- Obvious deformity
- May have spontaneously reduced (usually with lateral dislocations).

Physical Exam

- Tenderness and swelling over affected joint
- Deformity may be subtle, but is usually obvious and will indicate direction of dislocation.
- Following closed reduction, assess:
  - Flexor tendon function (Figures 4.8, 4.9)
  - Extensor tendon function
  - Collateral ligaments and volar plate with stress testing (Figure 4.7A)

Essential Diagnostics

- Digit x-rays to include AP, lateral, and oblique views prior to reduction.
- Consider stress views if suspect collateral ligament rupture or questionable exam.

ED Treatment

- DIP dislocations:
  - Reduce with longitudinal traction and gentle manipulation.
  - Simple, reducible dorsal dislocation: splint DIP in 20° flexion for one to two weeks.[25]
  - Simple, reducible volar dislocation: splint DIP in full extension for eight weeks (due to high association with terminal extensor tendon rupture).[25]
- PIP dislocations:
  - Reduce with longitudinal traction and gentle manipulation.
  - Simple, reducible dorsal dislocations: buddy tape for three to six weeks[25]
  - Simple, reducible volar dislocations: splint PIP in full extension for six weeks (due to high association with central slip rupture).[25]
- MCP dislocations:
  - Reduce by placing wrist and IP joints in flexion to relax flexor tendons, then apply pressure to base of proximal phalanx and push distally over metacarpal head.[10,27]
  - Simple, reducible MCP dislocations: apply dorsal blocking splint for two to three weeks.[27]
  - First MCP dislocations: apply short arm thumb spica splint for four to six weeks[27]

Disposition

- Discharge
- Emergent orthopedic consultation if irreducible
- Orthopedic consultation within one week if unstable[6,25,26] (see volar plate rupture), associated deep flexor tendon rupture (see jersey finger), associated fractures, volar MCP dislocations[27], complete UCL rupture in thumb MCP dislocation (see Skier's thumb).
- Orthopedic follow-up in one week for all MCP dislocations.[27]
- If no indications for orthopedic referral, may return to play immediately following reduction with buddy tape or other protective splint as tolerated.[25,26]

Complications

- Restricted joint flexion due to thickened capsule.
- Joint instability due to volar plate or collateral ligament injury.

Pediatric Considerations

- Image unaffected contralateral side to adequately assess for physeal injuries.

Pearls and Pitfalls

- Attempting to reduce MCP dislocations with longitudinal traction and hyperextension may turn simple dislocation into complex (irreducible) dislocation.[27]
- MCP dislocations are often irreducible due to interposition of volar plate between articular surfaces, and require open reduction.
- Finger and hand swelling may take months to resolve.

Distal Phalanx Fracture – Tuft Fracture

General Description

- Extra-articular fracture of distal phalanx
- May be longitudinal, transverse, or comminuted

Mechanism

- Usually by direct blow

Presentation

- Pain and swelling of distal phalanx

Physical Exam

- Tenderness and swelling of distal phalanx
- May have associated subungual hematoma or nailbed injury

Essential Diagnostics

- Digit x-rays to include AP, lateral, and oblique views

ED Treatment

- Rest, ice, elevate, and compress
- Drain hematoma if greater than 50 percent involvement[17]
- Repair nailbed laceration if present (see "Nailbed injury" for further details)
- Simple molded aluminum hairpin finger splint for protection against further injury for up to three weeks.[6,17]

Disposition

- Discharge
- Repeat x-rays unnecessary
- Orthopedic referral within one week if open or significantly displaced comminuted fracture
- If simple nondisplaced tuft fracture, may return to sports immediately in protective splint as tolerated.

Complications

- Malunion may occur, but usually does not affect function if soft tissues heal appropriately.

Pediatric Considerations

- Consider Salter–Harris type I fracture if tender over open physis at base of distal phalanx

Pearls and Pitfalls

- None

Middle and proximal phalanx fractures

General Description

- Typically transverse fracture through shaft
- Rotational abnormalities may be present

Mechanism

- Direct blow
- Traction or axial load
- Twisting, grabbing jersey

Presentation

- Pain and swelling to phalanx

Physical Exam

- Tenderness and swelling to phalanx
- Assess for dorsal or volar angulation
- Assess for rotational malalignment (all digits should point to scaphoid when folded into palm) (Figures 4.6A and 4.6B).

Essential Diagnostics

- Digit x-rays to include AP, lateral, and oblique views.

ED Treatment

- If nondisplaced fracture, buddy tape for two to four weeks[28,29]
- If displaced, perform closed reduction with digit block, then immobilize with gutter splint or Burkhalter splint for four to six weeks.[28,29]
- Appropriate antibiotics for open fractures

Disposition

- Discharge
- Follow-up for repeat x-rays in one to two weeks
- Immediate orthopedic consultation for open fractures
- Orthopedic consult within one week for unstable (comminuted, spiral, fail to maintain reduction) fractures.
- Return to sports as early as one to two weeks with buddy taping for nondisplaced fractures, up to six weeks for more complex fractures.[28,29]

Complications

- Deformity or loss of function from no treatment or improper reduction
- Stiffness from overtreatment (prolonged or unnecessary immobilization)

Pediatric Considerations

- Consider Salter–Harris type I fracture if tender over open physis at base of phalanx
- The following fractures often require prompt ORIF and should be referred to

pediatric hand specialist within one to two days[22]:

- Phalangeal neck or condyle (malunion may limit digit flexion)
- Malrotation
- Widely displaced, irreducible base of proximal phalanx (due to entrapped soft tissue)
- Avulsion at insertion of first MC ulnar collateral ligament (pediatric skier's thumb)

Pearls and Pitfalls

- Make sure to assess for rotational deformity, as these may be subtle
- Ensure appropriate follow-up to ensure that the patient does not stay in the splint for too long and have persistent joint stiffness.

Metacarpal Fractures

General Description

- Neck fractures occur at the weakest point of metacarpal
  - Boxer's fracture: fifth metacarpal neck fracture
- First metacarpal base fractures of note:
  - Bennett fracture: intra-articular fracture with subluxation/dislocation of carpometacarpal joint (Figure 4.17A)
  - Rolando fracture: intra-articular comminuted fracture (Figure 4.17B)

Mechanism

- Direct blow or crush

Presentation

- Pain and swelling to dorsal hand
- Difficulty making fist

Physical Exam

- Tenderness and swelling over dorsal aspect of metacarpal
- Assess for rotational malalignment (all digits should point to scaphoid when folded into palm) (Figures 4.6A and 4.6B)
- Assess flexor (Figures 4.8, 4.9) and extensor tendon function

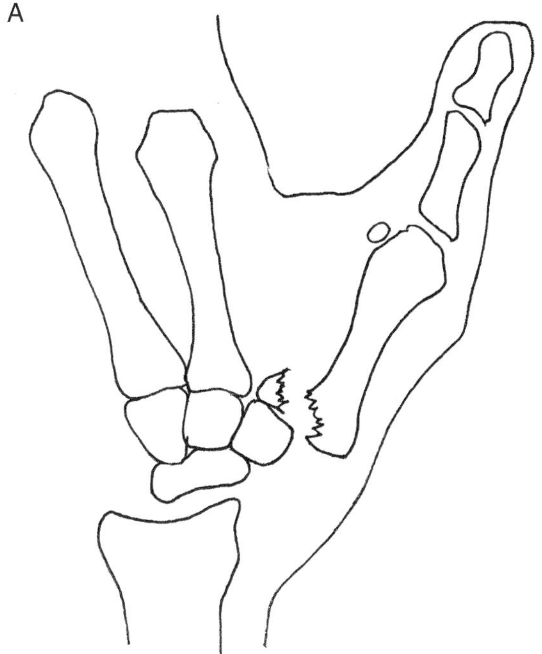

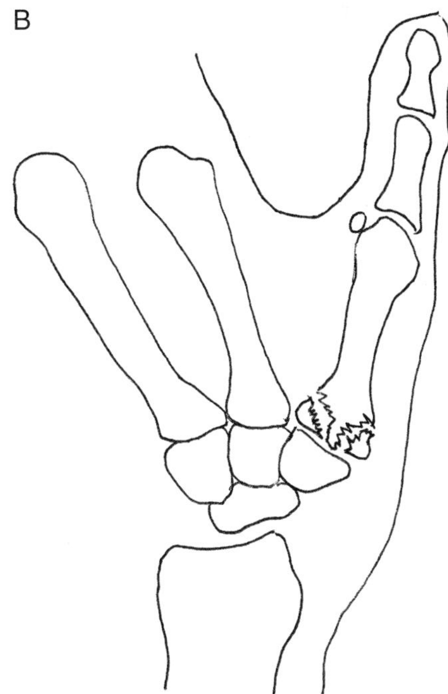

Figures 4.17A and B. Intra-articular base of first metacarpal fractures: (A) Bennett and (B) Rolando fractures.

- Assess ulnar nerve motor and sensory function (may be injured with base of fourth or fifth metacarpal fractures) (Figures 4.12A and 4.12B).

Essential Diagnostics

- Hand x-rays to include AP, lateral, and oblique views

ED Treatment

- Closed reduction of neck fractures: with MCP and PIP joints flexed to 90°, apply volar directed pressure to fracture site while applying dorsal directed pressure to proximal phalanx to push distal fracture fragment into position.
- Closed reduction of shaft/base fractures: longitudinal traction and volar directed pressure at fracture site.
- If acceptable alignment, immobilize in splint for three to four weeks[6,30,31]:
  - Thumb spica splint for first metacarpal fractures
  - Radial gutter splint for second or third metacarpal fractures
  - Ulnar gutter splint for fourth or fifth metacarpal fractures
  - Volar splint is acceptable alternative to gutter splint for second through fifth metacarpal fractures[6]
- Acceptable limits of angulation at NECK:[6,10,30]
  - Less than 15° for second or third metacarpal
  - Less than 20° for fourth metacarpal
  - Less than 30–50° for fifth metacarpal; no published consensus exists[30]
- Acceptable limits of angulation at BASE: [6,10,31]
  - Less than 10° for second or third metacarpal
  - Less than 20° for fourth or fifth metacarpal
  - Less than 30° for first metacarpal
- Appropriate antibiotics for open fractures
- If fight bite is present:
  - Prescribe antibiotics to cover oral flora, update tetanus
  - Do not primarily close wound
  - Irrigate wound copiously prior any splint placement

Disposition

- Discharge
- Follow-up for repeat x-rays in one week
- Immediate orthopedic consultation for open fractures
- Orthopedic consultation within one week for malrotated, displaced, or intra-articular base fractures (two to three days for Bennett and Rolando fractures[10]), angulation over acceptable limits above, or concomitant nerve or tendon injury.
- Return to sports conservatively after two to four weeks of splinting, as limited by patient's ability to participate with splint/orthotic protection in place.[30]
- Some hand surgeons may allow immediate return to play with protective cast orthosis.[30]

Complications

- Impaired grip if malunion due to malrotation
- Chronic carpometacarpal joint arthritis with intra-articular base fractures
- Rarely may cause compartment syndrome

Pediatric Considerations

- Consider Salter–Harris type I fracture if tender over open physis
- Physes located at second through fifth metacarpal heads and at base of first metacarpal.

Pearls and Pitfalls

- Any untreated malrotation may lead to impairment of normal hand function
- Remove rings to avoid constriction from soft tissue swelling

Soft Tissue Injuries and Infections

Subungual Hematoma

General Description

- Bleeding under nail due to nailbed injury

Mechanism

- Direct blow or crush

Presentation

- Pain to nailbed with discoloration of nail

Physical Exam

- Obvious blood pooling under nail
- Tenderness to nailbed

Essential Diagnostics

- Digit x-rays to include AP, lateral, and oblique views to evaluate for associated distal phalanx fracture.

ED Treatment

- Trephination with electrocautery device or 18-gauge needle if symptomatic or more than 50 percent of nailbed affected.

Disposition

- Discharge
- No follow-up necessary
- May return to sports immediately, with precautions on proper wound care after trephination such as avoiding swimming or hot tub use.[32]

Complications

- Uncommonly may develop infection following trephination
- Recurrent subungual hematoma to same nailbed may predispose nail to onychomycosis

Pediatric Considerations

- None

Pearls and Pitfalls

- Consider melanoma if history and exam not consistent with simple subungual hematoma (atraumatic; nontender)

Nailbed Injury

General Description

- Disruption of nail from nailbed or laceration of nailbed
- May occur with or without subungual hematoma

Mechanism

- Direct blow or crush

Presentation

- Pain and deformity to nail area

Physical Exam

- Laceration through nail
- Tenderness to nailbed area

Essential Diagnostics

- Digit x-rays to include AP, lateral, and oblique views to evaluate for associated distal phalanx fracture.

ED Treatment

- All nailbed lacerations should be primarily repaired:[6]
  - Anesthetize with digital block
  - Sterilely prepare hand
  - Dissect nail plate from nailbed bluntly with fine scissors
  - Repair nailbed laceration with 5-0 absorbable suture
  - Replace nail or place Xeroform gauze under nail fold and suture in place in two places laterally
  - If replacing nail, trephinate holes at lateral borders of nail plate to thread sutures through
  - Apply protective hairpin splint and dressing
- Prophylactic antibiotics if grossly contaminated wound or associated distal phalanx fracture.

Disposition

- Discharge
- Orthopedic referral in one week if associated fracture
- Follow-up in ten days to remove material under nail fold
- May return to sports immediately as tolerated by pain and ability to participate with protective splint and dressing in place

Complications

- Regrowth of deformed nail may occur if nailbed is not appropriately separated from the dorsal roof matrix under nail fold.

Pediatric Considerations

- None

Pearls and Pitfalls

- None

Compartment Syndrome

General Description

- Elevated tissue pressure within hand compartment, restricting blood flow and tissue perfusion

Mechanism

- Crush injury
- Fractures
- Iatrogenic due to cast or compressive dressing

Presentation

- Severe pain and swelling

Physical Exam

- Disproportionate pain to exam
- Pain worse with passive stretch
- Paresthesias may not occur in hand compartment syndromes[10]

Essential Diagnostics

- Compartment pressure testing is difficult and often inexact[10]

ED Treatment

- Removal of restrictive cast or compressive dressing
- Immediate orthopedic consultation

Disposition

- Admit for serial exams
- Immediate orthopedic consultation for possible fasciotomy
- Return to sports requires clearance following surgical intervention

Complications

- If untreated, muscle necrosis and fibrosis
- Severe contracture deformities limiting hand function

Pediatric Considerations

- None

Pearls and Pitfalls

- Diagnosis typically made on clinical basis due to unreliability of compartment pressure testing in the hand.

Bowler's Thumb

General Description

- Overuse injury causing perineural fibrosis of ulnar digital nerve of thumb

Mechanism

- Repetitive compression to ulnar digital nerve of thumb

Presentation

- Tingling and hypoesthesia at pulp of thumb

Physical Exam

- Tender nodule may be palpable on ulnar side of thumb

Essential Diagnostics

- None indicated

ED Treatment

- Rest, ice, compression, elevation
- Activity modification with temporary rest from bowling[6,33,34]

Disposition

- Discharge
- Follow-up in four to six weeks
- Orthopedic consultation if failure of conservative management or desire to return to play more quickly[33]
- Return to sports dependent on resolution of symptoms; usually by four months[34]
- Successful return often necessitates:
  - Use of commercial bowling thumb guard or splint
  - Increase size or change position of thumb hole
  - Alteration to grip

Complications

- Recurrent or persistent symptoms if attempt to continue bowling, or no alterations are made upon return to play

Pediatric Considerations

- None

Pearls and Pitfalls

- None

Trigger Finger (Stenosing Tenosynovitis)

General Description

- Overuse injury causing thickened nodule in flexor tendon
- Nodule catches behind A1 pulley in flexion, causing digit to become stuck in flexed position (Figure 4.18)

Mechanism

- Repetitive trauma with compression to flexor tendon at MCP

Presentation

- Pain at volar base of affected digit
- Painful catching or clicking with digit ROM
- Digit may be locked in flexion

Physical Exam

- Tender palpable nodule along flexor tendon
- Active flexion reproduces locking or catching

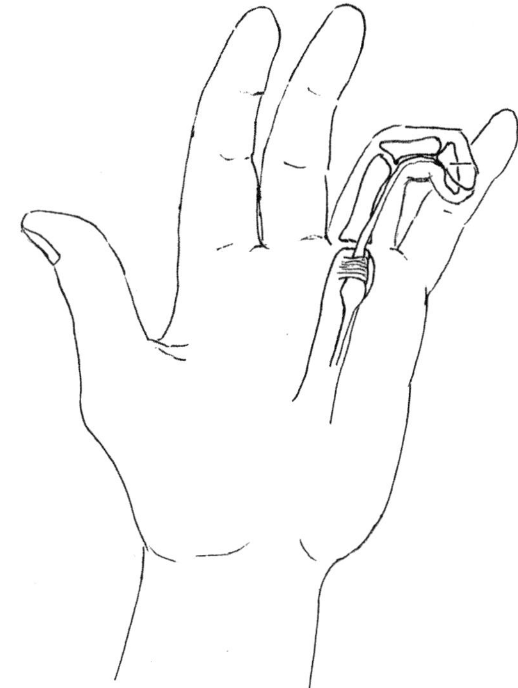

Figure 4.18. Trigger finger: thickened nodule on flexor tendon becomes caught on A1 pulley causing locking and catching during digit extension.

Essential Diagnostics

- None indicated

ED Treatment

- Ice friction massage
- Splint MCP at 15° of flexion to reduce tendon motion for six to ten weeks[35]
- Activity modification
- Consider lidocaine/corticosteroid injection into tendon sheath

Disposition

- Discharge
- Follow-up in four to six weeks
- Orthopedic consultation if failure of conservative management; may require surgical release of A1 pulley
- Return to sports dependent on resolution of symptoms or ability to participate with modifications or splinting

Complications

- If untreated, may result in PIP flexion contracture or distal triggering of DIP

Pediatric Considerations

- Almost exclusively seen in thumb in children
- Up to 63 percent of pediatric trigger digits may resolve spontaneously

Pearls and Pitfalls

- Higher incidence in patients with diabetes, rheumatoid arthritis, and connective tissue disorders; these patients are less likely to respond to steroid injection therapy.

Fight Bite

General Description

- Laceration over dorsal MCP sustained due to human bite

Mechanism

- Closed fist striking against tooth of opponent during fist fight

Presentation

- Pain and swelling surrounding wound over dorsal MCP joint

Physical Exam

- Tenderness and swelling over dorsal MCP joint with overlying laceration
- Associated wound may be small (<5 mm)
- Explore wound to assess for tendon or joint involvement

Essential Diagnostics

- Hand x-rays to include AP, lateral, and oblique views to evaluate for foreign body, fracture, or osteomyelitis

ED Treatment

- Copious irrigation
- Leave wound open to heal by secondary intention
- Full course of oral antibiotics to cover human oral flora
- IV antibiotics and orthopedic consultation for operative debridement if wound appears infected

Disposition

- Admit if wound appears infected, otherwise discharge
- ED or PCP follow-up in one to two days for wound check
- Orthopedic referral for tendon/joint involvement or evidence of infection
- Return to sports within one week with protective dressing if uncomplicated (no deep structure involvement or evidence of infection); otherwise return to play dependent on postoperative clearance

Complications

- Septic arthritis of MCP or tendon sheath infection if unrecognized and untreated

Pediatric Considerations

- None

Pearls and Pitfalls

- Treat all lacerations overlying dorsal MCP joints as fight bites unless proven otherwise

Flexor Tenosynovitis

General Description

- Infection along flexor tendon sheath

Mechanism

- Extension of infection from overlying wound such as laceration or animal bite

Presentation

- Pain and swelling to affected digit and palmar hand

Physical Exam

- Erythema and obvious wound may be present
- Kanavel's signs:
  - Fusiform swelling of digit
  - Partial flexion of digit at rest
  - Tenderness along flexor tendon sheath
  - Pain with passive extension of digit

Essential Diagnostics

- Hand and digit x-rays to include AP, lateral, and oblique views to evaluate for foreign body or subcutaneous emphysema due to gas producing infection

ED Treatment

- Prompt broad spectrum IV antibiotics
- Immediate consult for intraoperative debridement

Disposition

- Admit
- Emergent orthopedic consultation for intraoperative debridement

Complications

- Rapid spread to communicating deep spaces
- Chronic tendon scarring

Pediatric Considerations

- None

Pearls and Pitfalls

- Extend digit without applying pressure to flexor surface by lifting up on nail distally[6]
- Consider disseminated gonorrhea in sexually active patients without history of trauma/ wounds[36]

Table 4.3 Key Diagnosis, History, Physical Exam Findings, and Treatment

Diagnosis	History	Physical exam	Treatment
Jersey finger (flexor digitorum profundus disruption)	Forceful extension of flexed DIP, e.g. pulling away of object being grasped by tip of finger	Unable to flex DIP joint	Dorsal splint with slight flexion of MCP and IP joints and urgent referral within 1–2 days for surgical repair
Mallet finger (terminal extensor tendon disruption)	Forceful flexion of extended DIP	Unable to extend DIP joint; distal phalanx partially flexed while at rest	Splint DIP in full extension for 6–8 weeks
Boutonnière deformity (central extensor slip rupture)	Forceful flexion of extended PIP	Weak extension of PIP; classic Boutonnière deformity may not be seen in acute setting	Splint PIP in full extension for 4–6 weeks
Trigger finger	Overuse injury associated with repetitive compressive trauma to volar MCP area	Tender nodule on flexor tendon at base of finger; locking or snapping during finger ROM	Lidocaine and corticosteroid injection is first-line therapy; alternatively may rest, splint, ice massage; may require surgical release if conservative measures fail
Skier's/Gamekeeper's thumb (ulnar collateral ligament disruption)	Forced abduction of thumb at MCP joint, e.g. falling on outstretched ski pole	Lack of endpoint on ulnar collateral ligament stress testing; weak thumb pinch	Thumb spica splint for 2–4 weeks, up to 6 weeks if associated avulsion fracture; urgent referral within 2–3 days for surgical repair if complete rupture
Finger dislocation	Hyperextension or valgus/varus force to finger	Gross deformity or laxity at joint; may have spontaneously reduced; assess carefully for tendon disruption; assess for collateral ligament or volar plate instability with stress testing	Closed reduction and buddy tape or splint for 1–3 weeks if stable; may require prolonged splinting if associated tendon disruption; may require open reduction
Finger fracture	Direct blow, axial load, traction, or rotational force to finger	Tenderness and swelling over fracture site; assess carefully for rotational deformity	Buddy tape for 2–4 weeks if simple nondisplaced fracture; closed reduction and gutter or Burkhalter splint for 4–6 weeks for displaced fractures; may require surgical fixation
Hand fracture	Direct blow or crush injury to hand	Pain and swelling to dorsal hand over fracture site; assess carefully for rotational deformity	Closed reduction and splint for 3–4 weeks (thumb spica, radial gutter, ulnar gutter, or volar splint depending on which metacarpal is involved); refer for surgical fixation for intra-articular base fractures, unacceptable amounts of angulation, or any malrotation

Table 4.3 *(cont.)*

Diagnosis	History	Physical exam	Treatment
Fight bite	Laceration over dorsal MCP caused by striking combatant's mouth	Open wound over dorsal MCP joint, may be small and innocuous; assess carefully for associated tendon injury or capsular disruption	Irrigate thoroughly, broad spectrum antibiotics to cover human oral flora, leave wound open to heal by secondary intention; if already infected, IV antibiotics and orthopedic consultation for operative washout
Nailbed injury	Direct blow or crush to nail area	Deep laceration through nail plate or disruption of nail plate from nailbed; subungual hematoma may or may not be present	Evacuate subungual hematoma if symptomatic or >50% involvement; repair nailbed lacerations primarily

Table 4.4 Indications for Orthopedic Consultation

Diagnosis	Indication for Consult	Time Frame for Referral
Jersey finger (flexor digitorum profundus disruption)	Always requires surgical repair	1 day
Boutonnière deformity (central extensor slip rupture)	Large displaced intra-articular fracture at base of middle phalanx	1–2 days
Mallet finger (terminal extensor tendon disruption)	Displacement >50% of articular surface Volar subluxation	1 week
Flexor tendon laceration	Complete lacerations Partial lacerations	Within 12–24 hours 1 week
Extensor tendon laceration	Complete lacerations Partial lacerations	1–2 days 1 week
Skier's/gamekeeper's thumb	Complete rupture Partial tear	2–3 days 1 week
Volar plate rupture	Intra-articular avulsion fracture	2–3 days
Finger dislocation	Any MCP dislocation Unstable joint post reduction Associated fractures Associated tendon disruption	1 week
Distal phalanx tuft fractures	Open fracture Significantly displaced and comminuted fractures	1 week
Middle/proximal phalanx fractures	Comminuted or spiral fractures Failure to maintain reduction	1 week
Metacarpal fractures	Bennett or Rolando fractures Concomitant nerve or tendon injury Any malrotation or displacement Angulation above acceptable limits Intra-articular base fractures (other than thumb)	2–3 days 1 week

Table 4.4 (cont.)

Diagnosis	Indication for Consult	Time Frame for Referral
Nailbed injury	Associated distal phalanx fracture (open fracture)	1 week
Compartment syndrome	Any strong clinical suspicion of compartment syndrome	Immediate
Fight bite	Evidence of active infection Associated tendon injury Associated joint capsule disruption	Immediate 1 day
Flexor tenosynovitis	Always requires intraoperative debridement	Immediate
Bowler's thumb	Failure of conservative measures Desire for more rapid return to play	1 month

Recommended Reading

A. Andrade and H. G. Hern. Traumatic hand injuries: The emergency clinician's evidence-based approach. *Emerg Med Pract* 2011; 13(6): 1–23.

D. T. Fufa and C. A. Goldfarb. Fractures of the thumb and finger metacarpals in athletes. *Hand Clin* 2012; 28(3): 379–88.

J. J. Peterson and L. W. Bancroft. Injuries of the fingers and thumb in the athlete. *Clin Sports Med* 2006; 25(3): 527–42, vii–viii.

References

1. Angerman P, Lohmann M. Injuries to the hand and wrist: A study of 50,272 injuries. *J Hand Surg Br*. 1993; 18B: 642–644.
2. DeHaven K, Lintner D. Athletic injuries: Comparison by age, sport, and gender. *Am J Sports Med*. 1986; 14: 218–224.
3. Frazier W, Miller M, Fox R, et al.. Hand injuries: Incidence and epidemiology in an emergency service. *JACEP*. 1978; 7:265–268.
4. Sorock G, Lombardi D, Courtney T, et al.. Epidemiology of occupational acute traumatic hand injuries: A literature review. *Safety Science*. 2001; 38: 241–256.
5. Courtney T, Webster B. Disabling occupational morbidity in the United States: an alternative way of seeing the Bureau of Labor Statistics data. *J Occ Env Med*. 1999; 41: 60–69.
6. R. R. Simon, S. C. Sherman, and S. J. Koenigsknecht. Hand. In: Simon R. R., Sherman S. C., and Koenigsknecht S. J. *Emergency Orthopedics*, 6th ed. McGraw-Hill, 2011. Chapter 11. Hand [accessed April 24, 2014]. Available from: accessemergencymedicine.mhmedical.com/content.aspx?bookid=460&Sectionid=40703383.
7. J. C. Thompson. *Netter's Concise Orthopaedic Anatomy*, 2nd ed. Philadelphia, Saunders, 2010. Chapter 6. Hand. 183–218.
8. A. C. Rettig. Closed tendon injuries of the hand and wrist in the athlete. *Clin Sports Med*. 1992; 11(1): 77–99.
9. W. A. Lillegard. Wrist, Hand, and Finger Injuries. In: McKeag D. B., Moeller J. L., eds. *ACSM's Primary Care Sports Medicine*, 2nd ed. Philadelphia, Lippincott Williams & Wilkins, 2007; 403–420.
10. M. Davenport and D. G. Sotereanos. Injuries to the Hand and Digits. In: Tintinalli J. E., Stapczynski J. S., et al., eds. *Tintinalli's Emergency Medicine: A Comprehensive Study Guide*, 7th ed. McGraw-Hill, 2001; 1796–1807.
11. J. E. Sprin and A. Kakimoto. Flexor Tendon Avulsion/Jersey Finger. In: Bracker M. D., Achar S. A., Pana A. L. et al., eds. *The 5-Minute Sports Medicine Consult*, 2nd ed. Philadelphia, Lippincott Williams & Wilkins, 2011; 162–163.
12. FDP Avulsion/Rupture. In: Wheeless C. R., ed. *Wheeless' Textbook of Orthopaedics [internet]*. Durham (NC): Duke University Division of Orthopaedic Surgery/Data Trace Publishing; 1996–2014 [updated May 28, 2013; accessed May 4, 2014]. Available from: www.wheelessonline.com/ortho/fdp_avulsion_rupture
13. J. Feden and R. Khaund. Central Slip Avulsion and Pseudoboutonniere Deformities. In: Bracker M. D., Achar S. A., Pana A. L. et al., eds. *The 5-Minute Sports Medicine Consult*, 2nd ed. Philadelphia, Lippincott Williams & Wilkins, 2011; 68–69.
14. D. Simpson, M. M. McQueen, and P. Kumar. Mallet deformity in sport. *J Hand Surg [Br]*. 2001; 26: 32–3.
15. H. H. Handoll and M. V. Vaghela. Interventions for treating mallet finger injuries. *Cochrane Database Syst Rev*. 2004; **(3)**: CD004574.v

16. R. A. Coel and Q. Hoang. Extensor Tendon Avulsion from the Distal Phalanx/Mallet Finger. In: Bracker M. D., Achar S. A., Pana A. L. et al., eds. *The 5-Minute Sports Medicine Consult,* 2nd ed. Philadelphia, Lippincott Williams & Wilkins, 2011; 150–151

17. T. L. Pommering. Fracture, Distal Phalanx. In: Bracker M. D., Achar S. A., Pana A. L. et al., eds. *The 5-Minute Sports Medicine Consult,* 2nd ed. Philadelphia, Lippincott Williams & Wilkins, 2011; 188–191.

18. Extensor Mechanism of Fingers. In: Wheeless C. R., ed. *Wheeless' Textbook of Orthopaedics [internet].* Durham (NC): Duke University Division of Orthopaedic Surgery/Data Trace Publishing; 1996–2014 [updated December 15, 2011; accessed April 29, 2014]. Available from: www.wheelessonline.com/ortho/ extensor_mechanism_of_fingers

19. Partial Laceration of Flexor Tendons. In: Wheeless C. R., ed. *Wheeless' Textbook of Orthopaedics [internet].* Durham (NC): Duke University Division of Orthopaedic Surgery/Data Trace Publishing; 1996–2014 [updated December 21, 2012; accessed April 29, 2014]. Available from: www.wheelessonline.com/ortho/partial_laceration_of_flexor_tendons

20. Extensor Tendon Lacerations. In: Wheeless C. R., ed. *Wheeless' Textbook of Orthopaedics [internet].* Durham (NC): Duke University Division of Orthopaedic Surgery/Data Trace Publishing; 1996–2014 [updated May 28, 2013; accessed April 29, 2014]. Available from: www.wheelessonline.com/ortho/extensor_tendon_lacerations

21. I. Shrier and D. Somogyi. Thumb Ulnar Collateral Ligament Sprain (Skier's thumb). In: Bracker M. D., Achar S. A., Pana A. L. et al., eds. *The 5-Minute Sports Medicine Consult,* 2nd ed. Philadelphia, Lippincott Williams & Wilkins, 2011; 592–593.

22. P. M. Waters. Operative carpal and hand injuries in children. *J Bone Joint Surg Am.* 2007; 89: 2064–2074.

23. J. C. Leggit and C. J. Meko. Acute finger injuries: Part I. tendons and ligaments. *Am Fam Physician* 2006; 73(5): 810–816.

24. Dorsal Fracture Dislocations of the PIP Joint. In: Wheeless C. R., ed. *Wheeless' Textbook of Orthopaedics [internet].* Durham (NC): Duke University Division of Orthopaedic Surgery/Data Trace Publishing; 1996–2014 [updated October 4, 2012; accessed May 4, 2014]. Available from: www.wheelessonline.com/ortho/dorsal_fracture_dislocations_of_the_pip_joint

25. J. J. Stacy and J. McDaniel. DIP Dislocation. In: Bracker M. D., Achar S. A., Pana A. L. et al., eds. *The 5-Minute Sports Medicine Consult,* 2nd ed. Philadelphia, Lippincott Williams & Wilkins, 2011; 122–123.

26. S. Akbar. PIP Joint Dislocations. In: Bracker M. D., Achar S. A., Pana A. L. et al., eds. *The 5-Minute Sports Medicine Consult,* 2nd ed. Philadelphia, Lippincott Williams & Wilkins, 2011; 470–471.

27. J. Stumbo. MCP (metacarpophalangeal) Dislocation. In: Bracker M. D., Achar S. A., Pana A. L. et al., eds. *The 5-Minute Sports Medicine Consult,* 2nd ed. Philadelphia, Lippincott Williams & Wilkins, 2011; 374–375.

28. M. M. Linder and A. Harcourt. Fracture, Middle Phalanx. In: Bracker M. D., Achar S. A., Pana A. L. et al., eds. *The 5-Minute Sports Medicine Consult,* 2nd ed. Philadelphia, Lippincott Williams & Wilkins, 2011; 224–225.

29. J. H. Lynch and K. deWeber. Fracture, Proximal Phalanx. In: Bracker M. D., Achar S. A., Pana A. L. et al., eds. *The 5-Minute Sports Medicine Consult,* 2nd ed. Philadelphia, Lippincott Williams & Wilkins, 2011; 241–240.

30. Q. Hoang and C. Koutures. Fracture, Metacarpal Neck: I-V. In: Bracker M. D., Achar S. A., Pana A. L. et al., eds. *The 5-Minute Sports Medicine Consult,* 2nd ed. Philadelphia, Lippincott Williams & Wilkins, 2011; 220–221.

31. T. Robbins. Fracture, Metacarpal Base/Shaft: I-V. In: Bracker M. D., Achar S. A., Pana A. L. et al., eds. *The 5-Minute Sports Medicine Consult,* 2nd ed. Philadelphia, Lippincott Williams & Wilkins, 2011; 218–219.

32. K. Weber. Subungual Exostosis and Hematoma. In: Bracker M. D., Achar S. A., Pana A. L. et al., eds. *The 5-Minute Sports Medicine Consult,* 2nd ed. Philadelphia, Lippincott Williams & Wilkins, 2011; 558–559.

33. S. Swanson, L. H. Macias, and A. A. Smith. Treatment of Bowler's neuroma with digital nerve translocation. *Hand (NY).* Sep 2009; 4(3): 323–326.

34. D. Ostrovskiy, A. Wilborn. Acute Bowler's thumb. *Neurology* 2004; 63: 938.

35. Y. Chow and R. Kapur. Trigger finger. In: Bracker M. D., Achar S. A., Pana A. L. et al., eds. *The 5-Minute Sports Medicine Consult,* 2nd ed. Philadelphia, Lippincott Williams & Wilkins, 2011; 610–611.

36. C. A. Germann and M. W. Fourre. Nontraumatic Disorders of the Hand. In: Tintinalli J. E., Stapczynski J. S., et al., eds. *Tintinalli's Emergency Medicine: A Comprehensive Study Guide,* 7th ed. McGraw-Hill, 2001; 1920–1926.

Chapter 5

Pelvis, Hip, and Thigh

Aaron J. Monseau and Brenden J. Balcik

Background / Epidemiology

- In this chapter, the vast majority of time will be devoted to injuries that are typically seen in an athletic population.
- While injuries such as a crushed pelvis or angulated femur fracture are obviously very serious and even life threatening, their management is relatively straightforward with a prompt call to the orthopedist.
- This chapter is meant to give a better understanding of the pelvis, hip, and thigh with an outline of some often overlooked, yet still important, disorders.
- Injuries to the pelvis and hip are especially important because they can affect the patient's gait and the patient's core which, in turn, can precipitate a whole host of secondary injuries.
- Pain in the hip can involve several different areas, each of which can be associated with a different set of disorders.
- The hip joint is a potential space that will fill up with fluid when there is irritation of the joint space.
- Some pain that is felt in the hip is actually referred pain from the lumbar spine.
- For those Americans who are over 60 years old, about 14 percent report significant hip pain on most days.[1]
  - A similar study in England of those over 65 years old found about 19 percent reported hip pain.[2]
  - An Italian cohort of those over 65 years old reported hip pain in about 12 percent.[3]
- As for serious complications after trauma, the pelvis and thigh can both hold enough blood for a patient to bleed out without any blood leaving the body.

Anatomical Considerations / Pathophysiology

- The pelvis (Figure 5.1) supplies an attachment point for some of the largest muscles of our body and, as such, is integral to the movement of our torso and lower extremities.
- The acetabulum is composed of portions from the ilium, ischium, and pubis which form a horseshoe shape socket for the hip.
- The femoral head is a large cylindrical mass of bone whose blood supply can be interrupted relatively easily, which makes it especially susceptible to osteonecrosis.
- Weight loss should be encouraged in all overweight individuals but especially those with hip and lower extremity pain.
  - During walking, the forces on the hip can exceed five times the patient's body weight.
  - For a patient who is 50 pounds overweight, their hips can experience over 250 extra pounds.
- The relatively deep acetabulum with the robust musculature that surrounds the hip makes it a very stable joint, especially when compared to the other ball-and-socket joint, the shoulder.
  - The stability of the hip means that the range of motion is relatively limited.
    - The relative instability of the shoulder is what gives the shoulder its incredible range of motion.
- Remember that when the knee is flexed, internal rotation of the hip is elicited by moving the foot laterally, and external rotation of the hip is elicited by moving the foot medially.

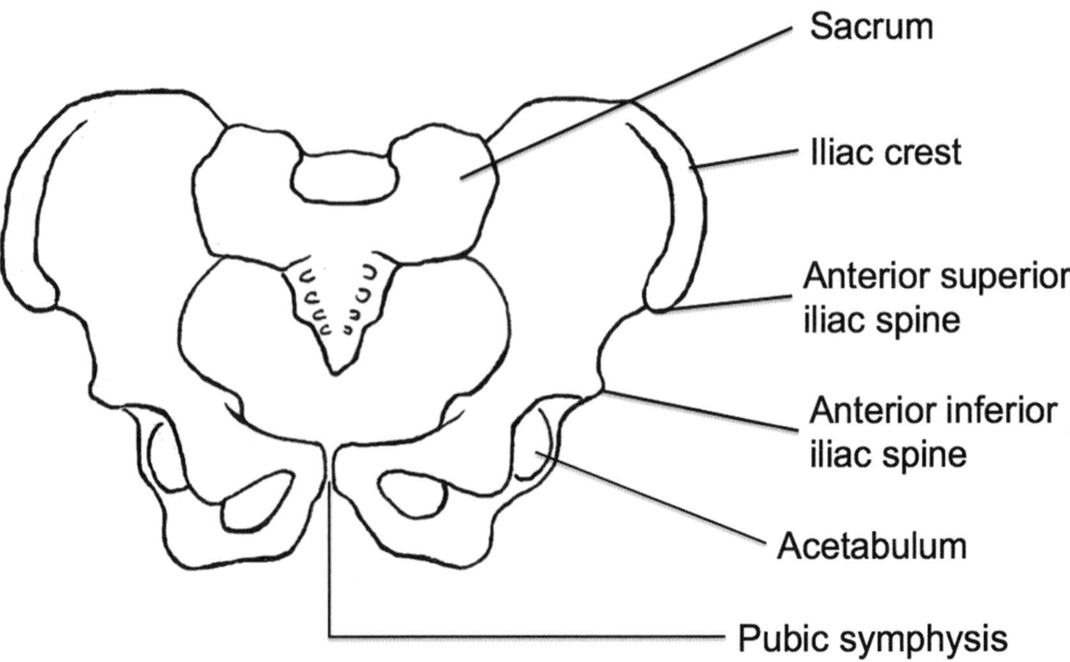

Figure 5.1. Bony anatomy of the pelvis. Illustration by Yvonne Chow.

Focused history and physical exam

History

- Location of pain is important. (see Table 5.1)
- Trauma
  - Should try to distinguish whether this is high energy, low energy, or repetitive stress.
- Timing of pain or other symptoms is important.
  - Pain occurring with running for some time that gets abruptly worse may indicate a stress fracture.
- A pop or snapping sensation may indicate a muscular or tendinous disorder.
- Resolution of pain with rest can be indicative of several disorders such as stress fracture or a vascular issue.

Physical Exam

- Pelvis/hip exam done in five positions: Standing, Seated, Supine, Lateral position, and Prone
- Physical exam will be discussed in the order of position, which is the most efficient way to do the exam.
- Normal values for hip range of motion can be found in Table 5.2.
- Standing Exam
  - Spinal alignment assessed by looking at:
    - Shoulder/iliac crest height
    - Lumbar lordosis
    - Scoliosis
  - Pelvic alignment assessed by comparing contralateral:
    - Anterior superior iliac spines and iliac crests
  - Gait
    - Watching patient walk in the room or in the hallway may provide a lot of information.
    - Antalgic gait is a sign of hip pain
    - Excessive internal or external rotation
    - Short leg limp indicates leg length discrepancy.
    - Trendelenburg gait indicates core muscle weakness.
  - *Trendelenburg test*
    - Have patient stand comfortably then stand on one leg (Figure 5.2)

Table 5.1 Differential Diagnosis Based on Location of Pain

Groin	Core muscle weakness or injury Pelvic fracture Osteitis pubis Athletic pubalgia Femoral neck stress fracture Femoroacetabular impingement Snapping hip Acetabular labral tear Slipped capital femoral epiphysis Hip fracture Hip dislocation Transient synovitis of the hip Septic arthritis Osteonecrosis of the hip Osteoarthritis of the hip
Anterior hip and upper leg	Core muscle weakness or injury Hip pointer Pelvic fracture Athletic pubalgia Femoral neck stress fracture Femoroacetabular impingement Snapping hip Acetabular labral tear Slipped capital femoral epiphysis Hip fracture Hip dislocation Transient synovitis of the hip Osteonecrosis of the hip Quadriceps hernia Quadriceps strain or tear
Posterior hip and upper leg	Core muscle weakness or injury Sacroiliac joint dysfunction Pelvic fracture Piriformis syndrome Ischial tuberosity avulsion fracture Femoroacetabular impingement Snapping hip Hip fracture Hip dislocation Osteonecrosis of the hip Hamstring strain or tear
Lateral	Core muscle weakness or injury Hip pointer Snapping hip Trochanteric bursitis Hip fracture Hip dislocation Osteonecrosis of the hip Meralgia paresthetica Iliotibial band syndrome

Table 5.2 Normal Hip Range of Motion

Flexion	0–120°
Extension	0–30°
Abduction	0–45°
Adduction	0–30°
External rotation	0–50°
Internal rotation	0–40°

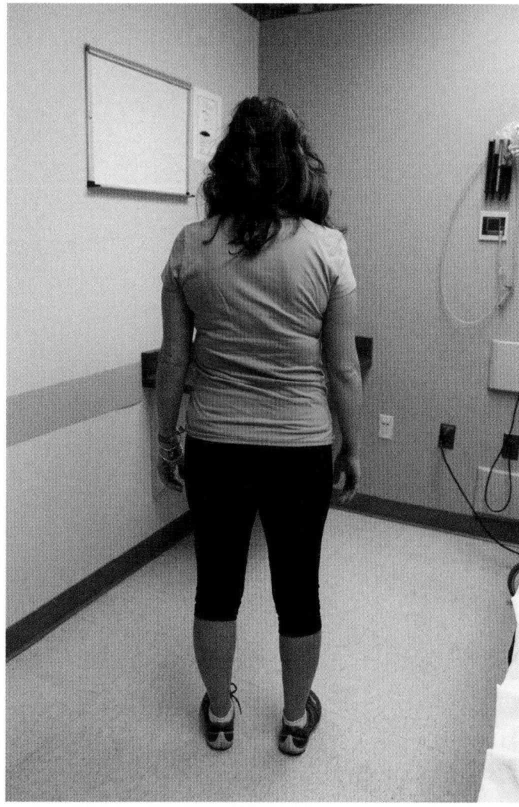

Figure 5.2. For the Trendelenberg Test, the patient should stand on the painful leg. On a normal test (Figure 5.3) the contralateral hemipelvis raises slightly or stays at the same height. On an abnormal test (Figure 5.4) the contralateral hemipelvis drops.

- When on one foot, the contralateral hemipelvis should raise slightly or at least stay at the same height (Figure 5.3).
- A drop in the contralateral hemipelvis is a sign of core muscle weakness, specifically of the gluteus medius (Figure 5.4).

- Seated Exam
  - Active internal rotation of hip (Figure 5.5)
  - Active external rotation of hip (Figure 5.6)

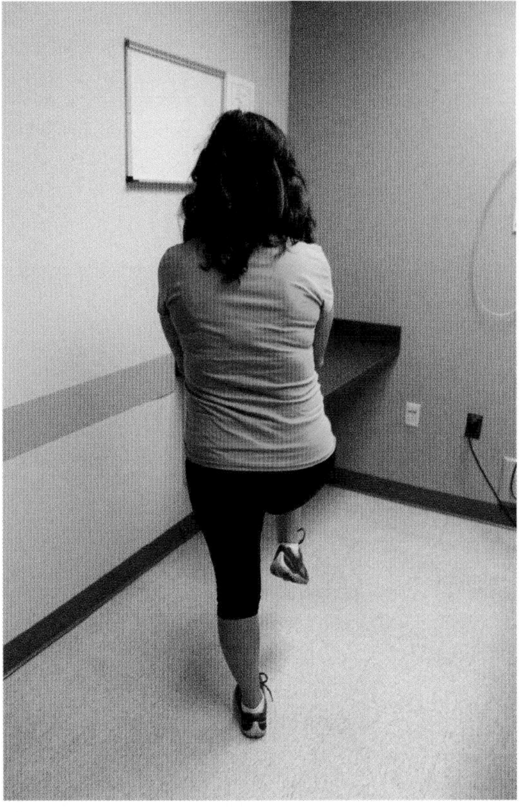

Figure 5.3.

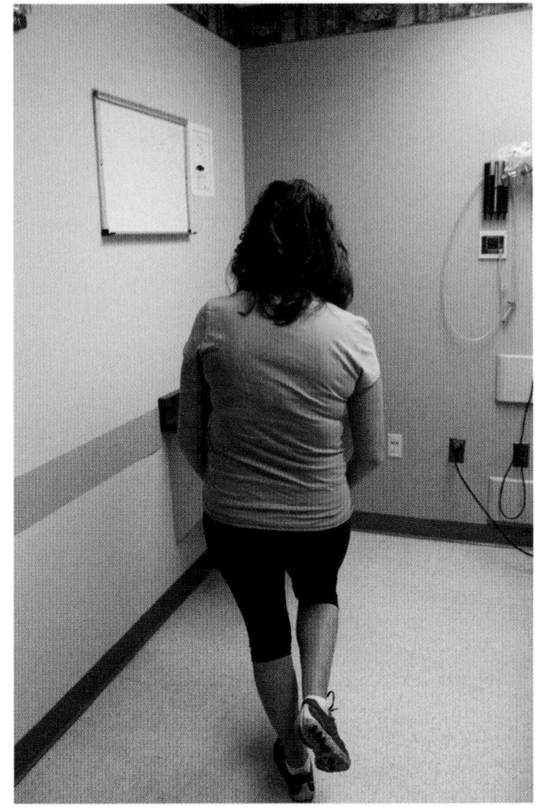

Figure 5.4.

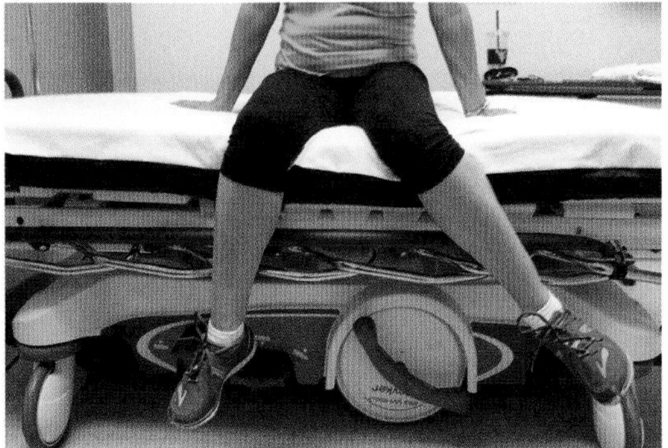

Figure 5.5. This is internal rotation of the hip. Note that the foot actually moves laterally.

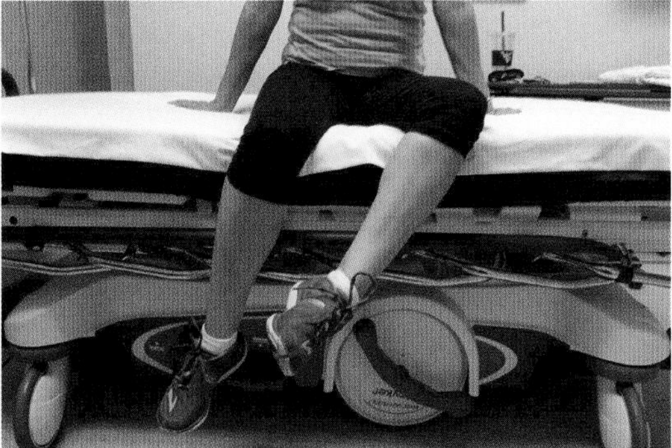

Figure 5.6. This is external rotation of the hip. Note that the foot actually moves medially.

- Resisted hip flexion
- Be sure to check passive range of motion if active range of motion is limited

- Supine Exam
  - Vascular evaluation
    - Femoral artery
    - Popliteal artery
    - Dorsalis pedis artery
    - Posterior tibial artery
    - Capillary refill
  - Neurologic evaluation
    - See Table 5.3 for central nerve roots and corresponding sensory and motor innervation.

Table 5.3 Sensory and Motor Innervations for L1-S1

Nerve Root	Sensory	Motor
L1	Just below inguinal ligament	Hip flexion
L2	Middle anterior thigh	Hip adduction
L3	Lower anterior thigh	Knee extension
L4	Medial lower leg and foot	Ankle dorsiflexion
L5	Lateral lower leg and dorsal foot	Great toe MTP and IP extension
S1	Lateral foot	Plantar flexion and eversion of the foot

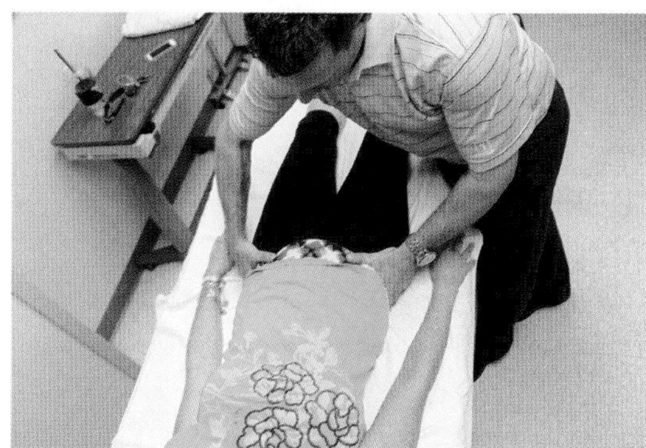

Figure 5.7. This shows the beginning position for testing for an unstable pelvic fracture or open-book pelvis. The examiner should then attempt to squeeze thumbs together. With an unstable fracture, the examiner will get his thumbs closer together when squeezing.

- Evaluation for open-book pelvis or unstable pelvis (Figure 5.7)
  - Thumbs should be placed inferior to anterior superior iliac spine with palms resting between iliac crest and greater trochanter.
  - Pelvis should be squeezed in an attempt to bring thumbs together.
  - Pelvis should NEVER be opened by attempting to separate thumbs further as this could lead to disruption of clot and precipitate massive hemorrhage
- Passive ROM
  - Log roll of leg will be painful with most intra-articular processes as well as hip fractures.

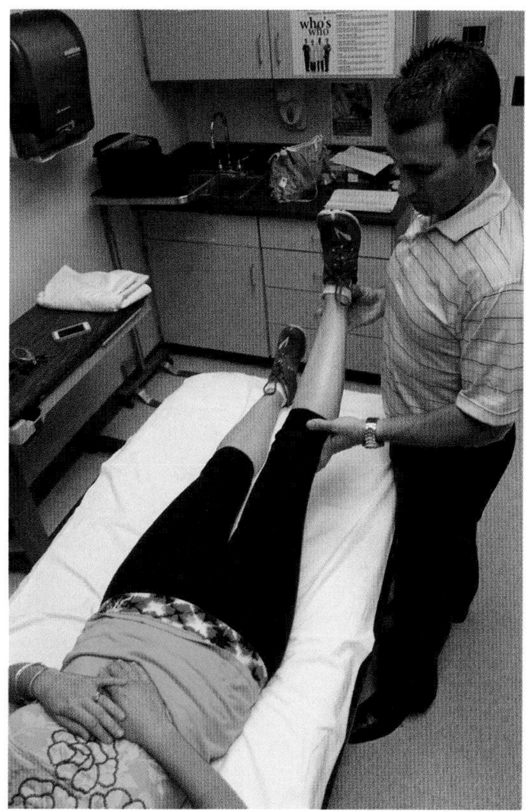

Figure 5.8. The straight leg raise test may be helpful for diagnosing sciatica.

  - Hip flexion, abduction, adduction (see Table 5.2)
- *Straight leg raise* is performed by passively flexing hip with fully extended knee (Figure 5.8).
  - Positive test for diagnosis of sciatica is pain that radiates down leg and past the knee when flexed from 15–70°.
- *Flexion Abduction External Rotation* (FABER) *test*, also called *Patrick test* (Figure 5.9)
  - Place patient in cross-legged position then apply posterior pressure to knee.
  - Posterior pain indicated sacroiliac dysfunction.
  - Groin pain may indicate intra-articular hip process or possibly adductor strain.
  - Lateral pain may indicate femoroacetabular impingement. (FAI)

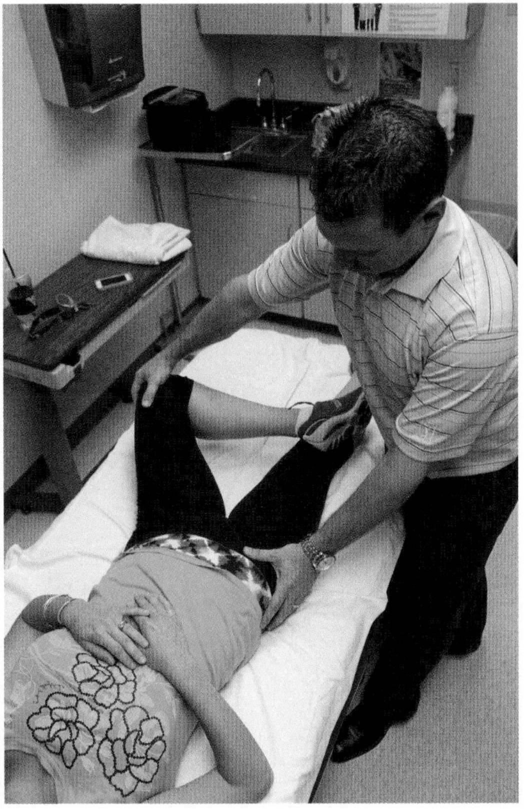

Figure 5.9. The FABER test may be helpful in the diagnosis of several disorders including sacroiliac dysfunction, femoroacetabular impingement, or intra-articular hip pain.

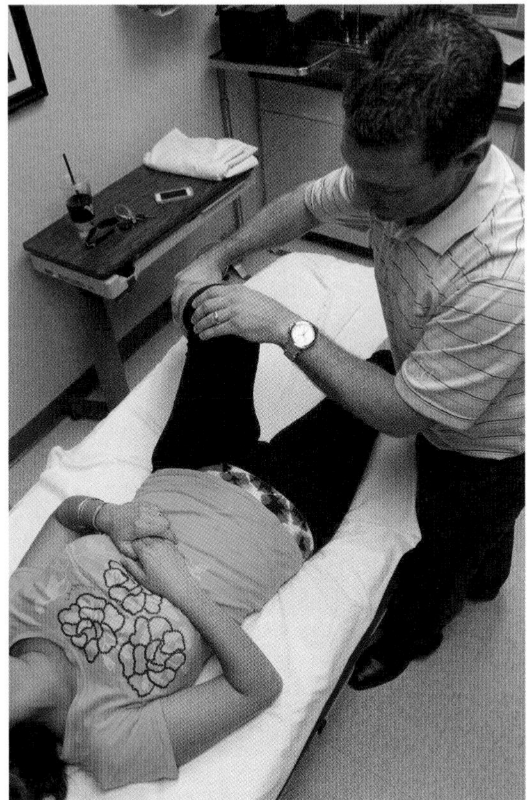

Figure 5.10. The FADDIR test is the most preferred test for femoroacetabular impingement.

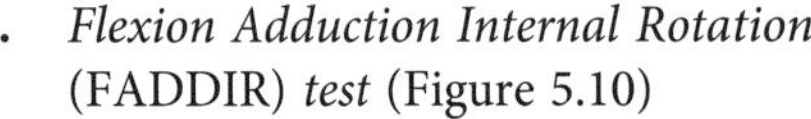

- *Flexion Adduction Internal Rotation* (FADDIR) *test* (Figure 5.10)
  - Most preferred test for FAI
  - While supine, place patient into full hip flexion, adduction, and internal rotation
  - This will cause reproducible and very uncomfortable groin pain in a positive test.
- Acetabular labrum testing
  - There are several tests for acetabular labral tears that involve passively moving the femur about the pelvis.
  - These will not be covered in detail here, but the main finding with each is a reproducible painful motion, click, or burning sensation typically felt in the groin.
- *Thomas stretch test* (Figure 5.11)
  - Nonaffected leg into extreme flexion
  - Unable to keep contralateral hip extended indicates tight iliopsoas musculature
- Strength testing
  - Hip abduction/adduction tested with hips and knees flexed
  - Iliopsoas
    - Only 15°
- Palpation
  - Abdominal fascia
  - Iliac crest
  - Anterior superior iliac spine
  - Anterior inferior iliac spine
  - Ilioinguinal ligament
  - Pubic symphysis
- *Resisted sit-up* (Figure 5.12)
  - Test for athletic pubalgia or “sports hernia”

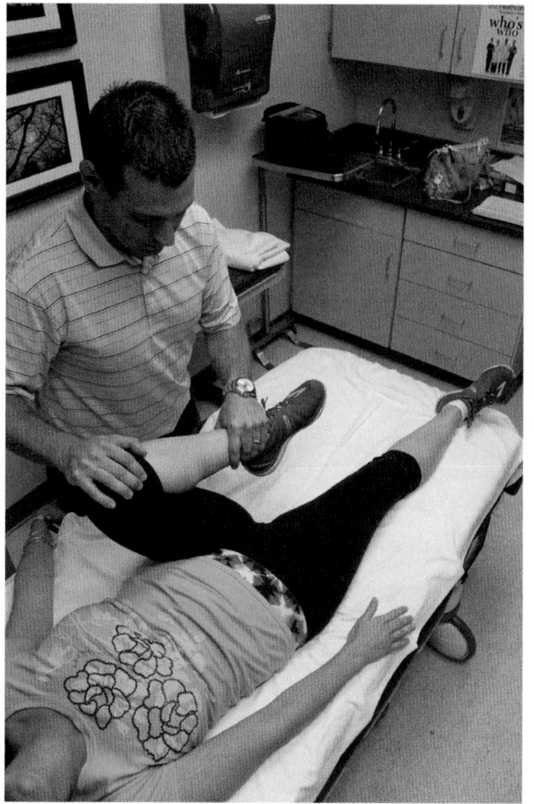

Figure 5.11. The Thomas stretch test may indicate tight iliopsoas musculature.

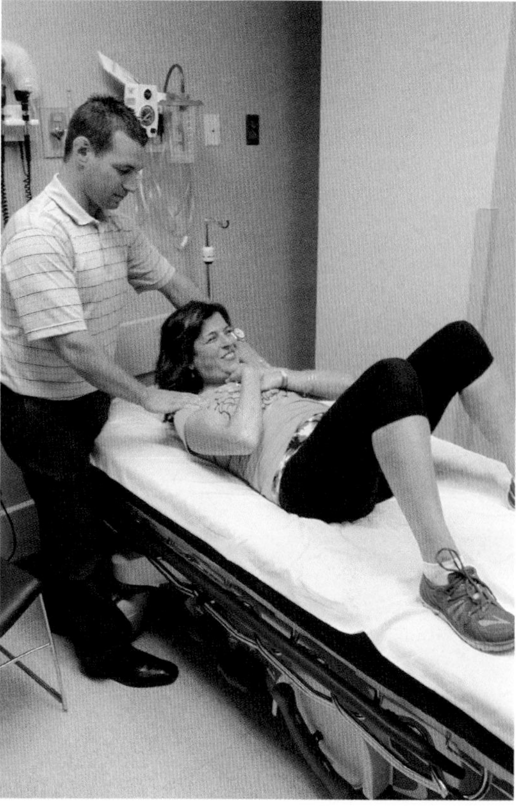

Figure 5.12. The resisted sit-up may aid the diagnosis of athletic pubalgia or "sports hernia" but may also be painful in other disorders such as osteitis pubis.

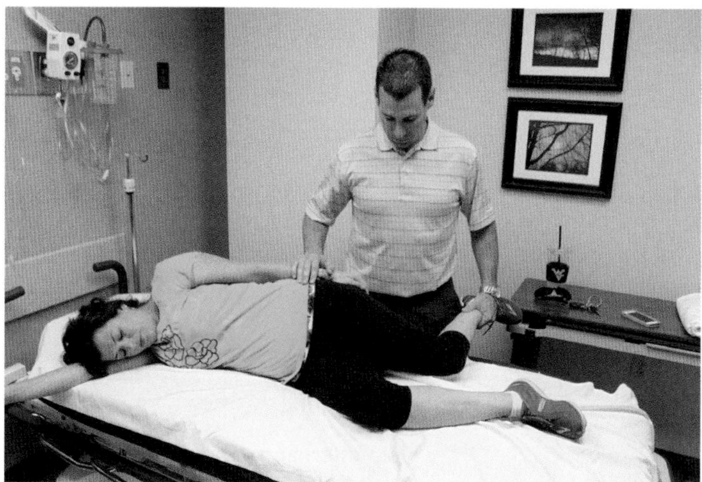

Figure 5.13. Ober's test places stress on and may indicate tightness of the iliotibial band.

  - Apply resistance while athlete is doing a sit-up.
  - Positive test is groin pain or inguinal crease pain during this maneuver.

- Lateral Exam
  - Active/Passive ROM
    - Hip extension
  - *Ober's test* (Figure 5.13)
    - Test for iliotibial band tightness
    - Adduct/extend hip with knee flexed
    - Positive test: Knee unable to drop below neutral position

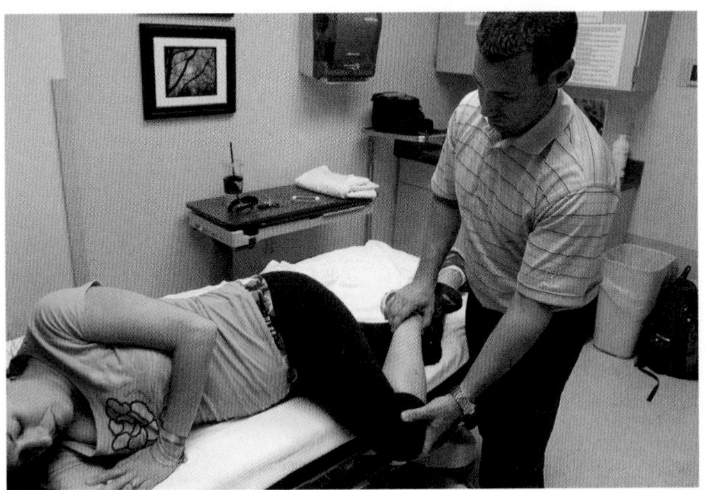

Figure 5.14. Piriformis test places stress on the piriformis muscle and may recreate the symptoms of piriformis syndrome.

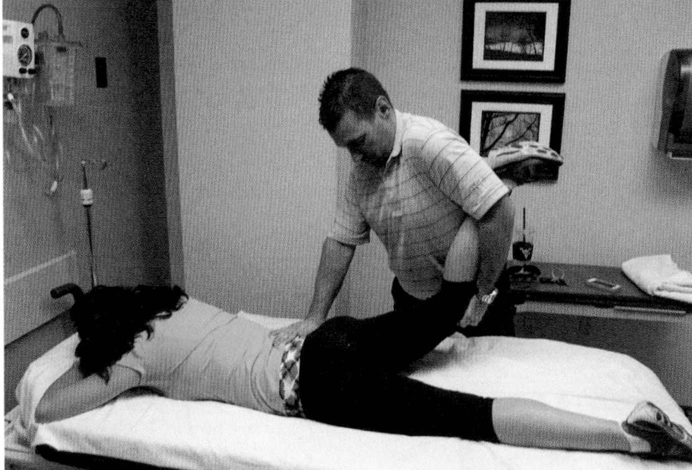

Figure 5.15. This shows the position for the femoral nerve stretch test.

- *Piriformis test* (Figure 5.14)
  - Hip and knee flexed with knee hanging off table
  - Stabilize pelvis and down on knee gives pain in buttock
- Strength testing
  - Hip abduction
- Palpation
  - Greater trochanter
  - Tensor fascia lata and iliotibial band

- Prone Exam
  - Passive ROM
    - Hip internal/external rotation
  - *Femoral nerve stretch test* (Figure 5.15)
    - Stabilize pelvis, other hand under thigh.
    - Extend hip keeping knee flexed
  - Strength testing
    - Hip internal rotation
    - Gluteus maximus isolated by extending hip with knee flexed to 90° (Figure 5.16).
    - Piriformis isolated by externally rotating hip with the hip in full internal rotation and the knee flexed to 90° (Figures 5.17 and 5.18).

- Palpation
  - Ischial tuberosity
  - Piriformis muscle
  - Sciatic nerve

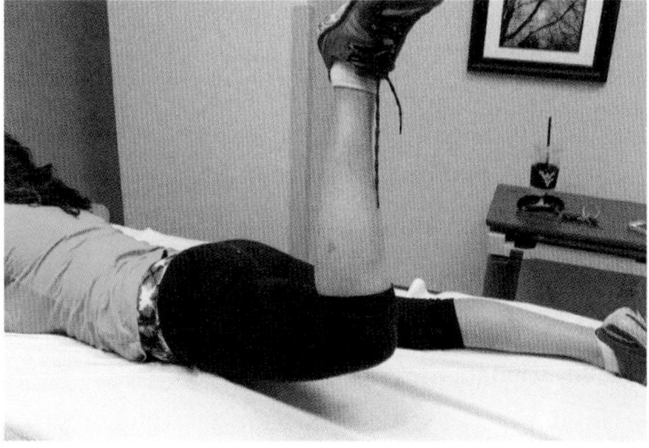

Figure 5.16. Testing strength in this position may isolate the gluteus maximus.

Differential Diagnosis – Emergent and Common Diagnoses

- Pelvis
  - Core muscle weakness or injury
  - Hip pointer
  - Sacroiliac joint dysfunction
  - Pelvic fracture
  - Piriformis syndrome
  - Osteitis pubis
  - Ischial tuberosity avulsion fracture
  - Athletic pubalgia (Sports hernia)
- Hip
  - Femoral neck stress fracture
  - FAI
  - Snapping hip
  - Acetabular labral tear

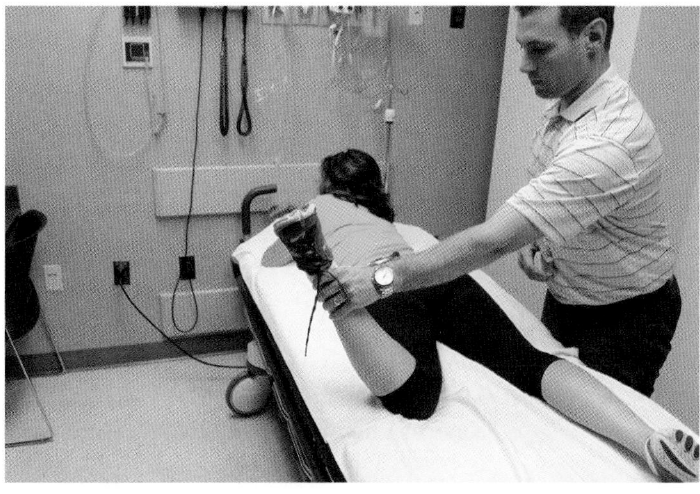

Figure 5.17. When testing the strength of the piriformis muscle, start in the position shown in Figure 5.17 and move the foot medially to the position shown in Figure 5.18.

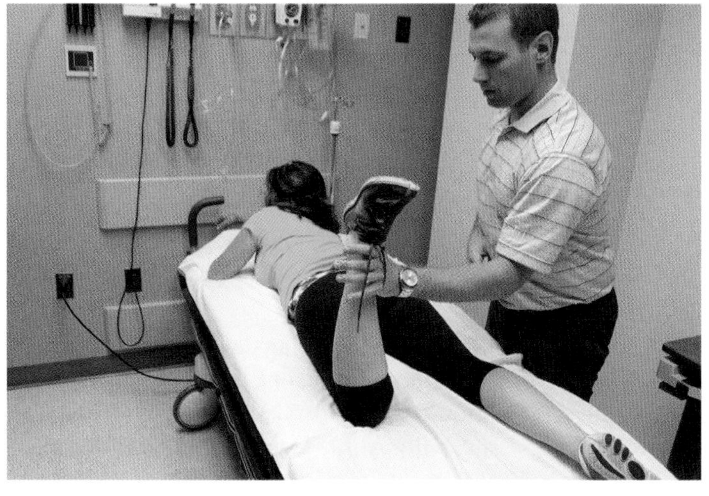

Figure 5.18.

Table 5.4 Emergent and Common Diagnoses in the Emergency Department

Emergent Diagnoses	Common Diagnoses
Unstable pelvic fracture	Core muscle weakness or injury
Slipped capital femoral epiphysis	Hip pointer
Hip fracture	Sacroiliac dysfunction
Hip dislocation	Piriformis syndrome
Septic arthritis of the hip	Trochanteric bursitis
Legg–Calve–Perthes disease	Transient synovitis of the hip
Complete hamstring or quadriceps tear	Osteoarthritis of the hip
	Iliotibial band syndrome
	Hamstring and quadriceps strain

- Slipped capital femoral epiphysis
- Trochanteric bursitis
- Hip fracture
- Hip dislocation
- Transient synovitis of the hip
- Septic arthritis of the hip
- Osteonecrosis of the hip
- Legg–Calve–Perthes Disease (LCPD)
- Osteoarthritis of the hip

- Thigh
  - Meralgia paresthetica
  - Iliotibial band syndrome
  - Quadriceps hernia
  - Hamstring strain or tear
  - Quadriceps strain or tear

Pelvis

Core Muscle Weakness or Injury

General Description

- The muscles of the abdominal wall, pelvis, buttock, and hip are generally referred to as the core muscles.
- Together, these muscles stabilize the trunk and pelvis to provide the base for coordinated movement.
- Several injuries and areas of pain are associated with core muscle weakness or abnormality.

Mechanism

- Core weakness or injury results in a derangement of the mechanics of ambulation or movement of the trunk
- This derangement typically causes overcompensation by the other muscles of the core.
- Pain may result from the initial injury or the overcompensation.

Presentation

- May present with back pain, sacroiliac pain, hip pain, groin pain, or pelvic pain.

Physical exam

- Attempt to isolate movement or movements that elicit pain since this will indicate affected muscle or muscle group.
- *Trendelenburg test* or Trendelenburg gait signifies weakness of the contralateral gluteus medius.

Essential Diagnostics

- Bone injury should be ruled out with radiographs or CT scan.
- Stress injury of pelvis or hip may need MRI or bone scan evaluation.
- Musculoskeletal ultrasound may show muscle abnormalities in the hands of an experienced operator.

ED Treatment

- Splint: None needed
- Weight-bearing status: As tolerated
  - If stress fracture strongly suspected, non-weight-bearing is appropriate
- Instructions on core strengthening exercises such as yoga poses which may be done once a day for 30–60 seconds per pose
  - High plank (Figure 5.19) and low plank (Figure 5.20)
  - Downward facing dog (Figure 5.21) and upward facing dog (Figure 5.22)
  - Chair (Figure 5.23)
  - Halfway lift (Figure 5.24) and Warrior 1 (Figure 5.25)

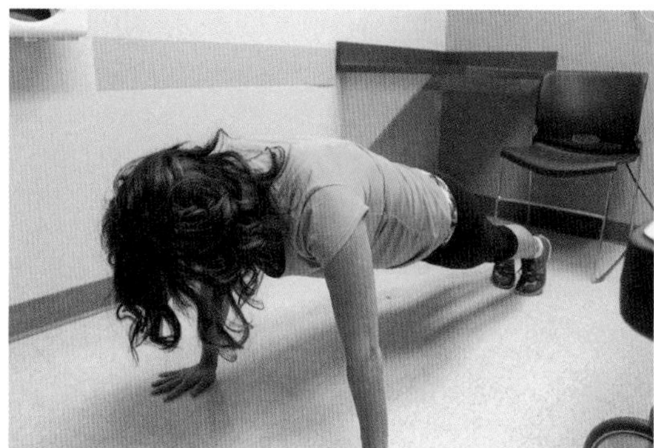

Figure 5.19. High plank position.

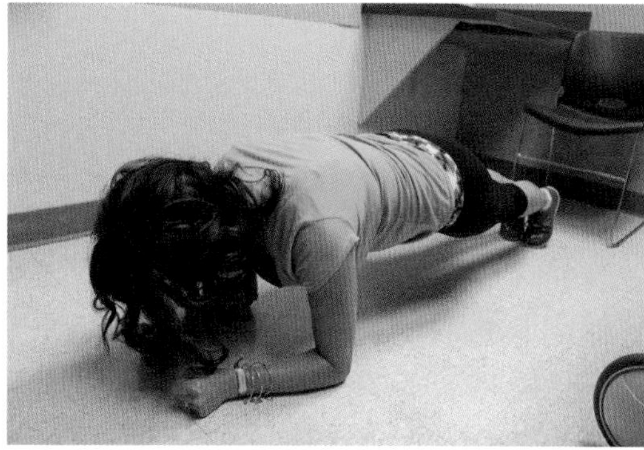

Figure 5.20. Low plank position.

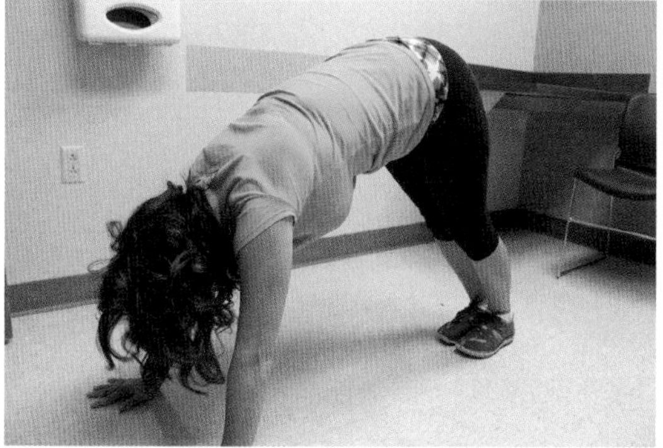

Figure 5.21. Downward facing dog position.

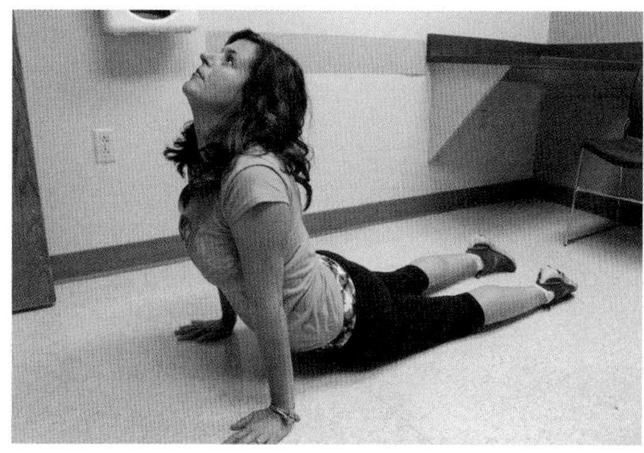

Figure 5.22. Upward facing dog position.

Disposition

- Discharge unless not safe at home due to severe limitation in ambulation
- Follow-up with primary care provider (PCP) or sports medicine physician in next one to two weeks who may order physical therapy if needed
- Return to work or sports as tolerated

Complications

- Severe chronic weakness may lead to early degenerative changes in hip due to derangement in gait.

Pediatric Considerations

- Take special care to evaluate physes on exam and with radiographs since avulsion fractures may be easily confused for muscular abnormalities.
- At times of rapid growth, core weakness or relative imbalance is common and may resolve with time alone.

Pearls and Pitfalls

- Bony injury should be ruled out.
- Simple core strengthening exercises are the treatment of choice.
- Musculoskeletal ultrasound may be helpful in the hands of an experienced operator.

Hip Pointer

General Description

- This is a contusion of the iliac crest that is often associated with a subperiosteal hematoma.
- This injury most commonly occurs in football players.

Mechanism

- This is due to a direct blow to the area usually following a collision or a fall.

Presentation

- Athlete will usually complain of pain in the area of the iliac crest.
- Often they will relate a history of trauma.

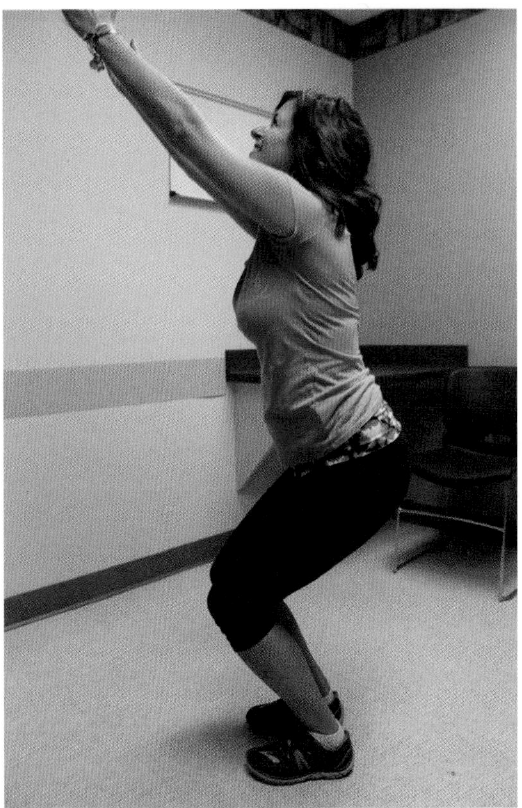

Figure 5.23. Chair position.

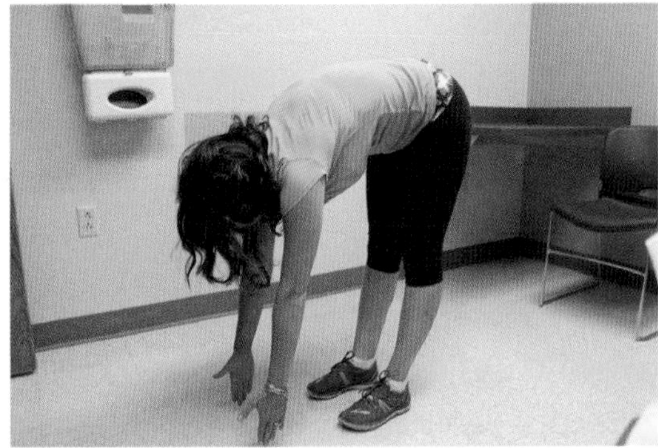

Figure 5.24. Halfway lift position.

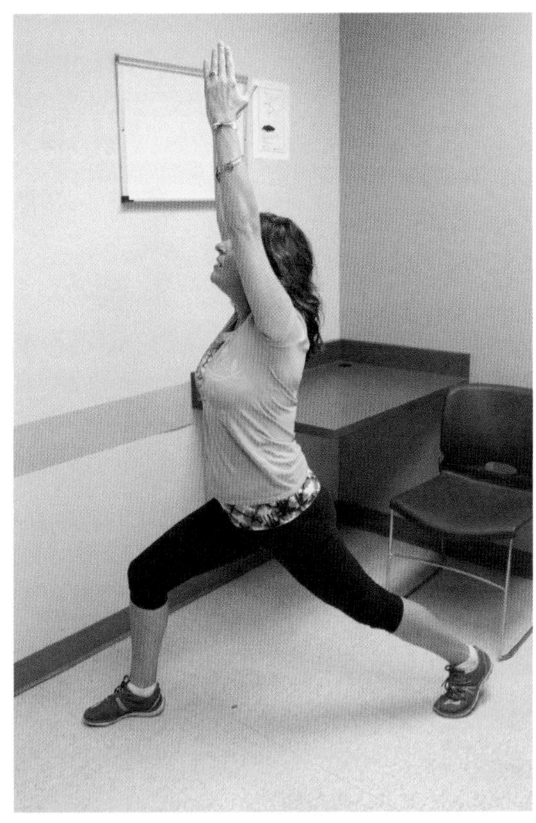

Figure 5.25. Warrior 1 position.

Physical Exam

- Tenderness, swelling, and ecchymoses at the iliac crest

Essential Diagnostics

- Anteroposterior pelvis x-ray to rule out fracture

ED Treatment

- Relative rest, ice and anti-inflammatories to reduce swelling
- May recommend gentle range of motion and strengthening exercises as tolerated

Disposition

- Discharge
- Follow-up with sports medicine or PCP in one week
- May return to sport once pain and swelling have subsided enough to allow safe return

Complications

- Usually self-limited condition
- Occasionally, significant hemorrhage into muscle may occur and lead to prolonged limitations and disability

Pediatric Considerations

- If this injury occurs in a child with open growth plates it is possible to sustain an avulsion fracture of the anterior superior iliac crest

- These are some of the last growth plates to close
- These injuries are rare and may usually be managed conservatively.
- Initial treatment is with rest, ice, and non weight-bearing with crutches for two to three weeks until able to ambulate without pain.
- Initiate stretching and strengthening program
- Athletes may usually return to sports eight to twelve weeks after injury.

Pearls and Pitfalls

- Usually a benign, self-limiting injury
- Extra caution is needed in younger patients with open growth plates who are at risk of sustaining an avulsion fracture at the anterior superior iliac spine.

Sacroiliac Joint Dysfunction

General Description

- Broad term that many view as a "wastebasket" diagnosis
- Relatively immobile joint
- High-energy pelvic injuries frequently cause fractures here, but sacroiliac joint dysfunction typically refers to low-energy disorders

Mechanism

- Arthritis in the sacroiliac joint may be caused by rheumatologic disorders or trauma.
- Septic arthritis should be considered in the appropriate clinical picture.

Presentation

- Pain attributed to the sacroiliac joint may cause buttock or posterior thigh pain

Physical Exam

- Classically, *FABER test* (Figure 5.9) used to elicit pain in this area
- Tenderness of sacroiliac joint

Essential diagnostics

- High-energy injuries require CT scan to rule out pelvic fractures which may be easily missed on plain films.
- CT scan with IV contrast or MRI may be needed to evaluate for sacroiliitis especially when infectious etiology suspected.
- When infectious etiology is being considered, labs ordered should include complete blood count (CBC), C-reactive protein (CRP), and erythrocyte sedimentation rate (ESR).
  - Basic metabolic panel is typically included as well in case intravenous antibiotics are needed.

ED Treatment

- Splint: Not needed.
- Weight-bearing status: As tolerated
- Ice and non-steroidal anti-inflammatory drugs (NSAIDs) are typically acute treatments.
- Short period of rest may also be necessary
- If infectious sacroiliitis, intravenous antibiotics should be started as early as possible.
  - If patient is being taken to the operating room for washout, consulting orthopedist may delay initial antibiotics until cultures are obtained.
  - Appropriate if patient is stable and relatively uncomplicated (i.e., no diabetes or immunosuppression).

Disposition

- Discharge typically appropriate unless being admitted for intravenous antibiotics
- Orthopedic consultation needed when infectious process is suspected.
- Follow-up in one to two weeks with PCP or sports medicine physician is typically appropriate.
- Return to work or sports as tolerated
  - May take several weeks for return to normal

Complications

- May be due to ankylosing spondylitis which includes other serious symptoms such as spine deformities, lung problems, and heart problems.
- When resulting in gait abnormalities, early degenerative changes may occur.

Pediatric Considerations

- Rheumatologic conditions should be considered in children.
- Follow-up with PCP and possibly rheumatologist will be useful since the majority of rheumatologic testing will be done as outpatient.

Pearls and Pitfalls

- Overlooked infectious etiology may result in severely disabling consequences and even sepsis.
- For noninfectious etiology, ice and NSAIDs are the typical treatments.
- Short rest period may be needed, but patient should be encouraged to get back to normal activities as soon as possible

Pelvic Fractures

General Description

- Large range of injuries typically from a high-energy impact but may result from relatively minor trauma when bones are weak such as in osteoporosis or cancer.

Mechanism

- Falls and motor vehicle crashes are common causes of pelvic fractures.
- Since the pelvis is a bony ring, once a fracture is seen great care should be taken to find a second fracture or ligamentous disruption (i.e., sacroiliac joint derangement).

Presentation

- Pain is typically localized to near the fracture.
- Groin pain may indicate acetabular or intra-articular fracture.

Physical Exam

- Pelvis palpated for tenderness.
- Evaluate for unstable pelvis by squeezing pelvis as described earlier in physical exam section (Figure 5.7).
- Log roll of leg to evaluate for intra-articular fracture or hip fracture

Essential Diagnostics

- Pelvis radiographs may show fracture but do not exclude fractures.
    - Diastasis at pubic symphysis greater than 1 cm indicates pubic instability except in women post childbirth.
    - Diastasis greater than 2.5 cm indicates sacroiliac ligamentous disruption.
- CT scan is imaging modality of choice for pelvic fractures.

ED Treatment

- If pelvis unstable, pelvic binder should be applied low on the pelvis as instructed.
    - If no binder is available, a sheet may be tied low and tight on the pelvis at the level of the greater trochanters.
- For unstable fractures, patient should be non weight-bearing.
- For stable fractures such as pubic rami fractures and many iliac crest fractures, patient may be toe-touch weight-bearing to start and progressed as pain allows, but this should be coordinated with the orthopedist who will be following the patient.
- Narcotic pain medications are typically used for the first few days to weeks after a fracture but should be phased out as soon as possible.

Disposition

- Unstable fractures are admitted.
- Emergent consult to orthopedics for unstable pelvic fracture (i.e., any time binder is applied) especially with hemodynamic instability.
- Should consult for other fractures as well
- Open reduction with internal or external fixation will be needed for unstable fractures.
- Return to work or sports to be determined by extent of fractures.

Complications

- Unstable pelvic fractures are associated with large amounts of bleeding into the pelvis that may be life threatening.
- Unstable pelvic fractures also have a high association with urethral injuries so Foley catheter should not be inserted in the ED unless a retrograde urethrogram has been performed.

Pearls and Pitfalls

- If one fracture is found, look hard for a second fracture since pelvis is a bony ring.
- Urethral catheter insertion should be deferred until retrograde urethrogram performed if unstable pelvis fracture.
- Stable fractures may be treated conservatively with crutches and outpatient follow-up.

Piriformis Syndrome

General Description

- Irritation of the sciatic nerve which runs over the piriformis muscle.
- In 20 percent of the population, the piriformis is split with the sciatic nerve actually dividing the muscle.

Mechanism

- Several etiologies have been proposed such as hyperlordosis, muscle anomalies with hypertrophy, anatomic variants of the course of the sciatic nerve or its' divisions.
- Also may be caused by external forces such as sitting for a long period of time or on an object such as a wallet.
- Foot abnormalities, such as Morton foot, may precipitate piriformis syndrome due to compensation needed by the piriformis to correct the gait abnormality.

Presentation

- Pain may be localized deep in posterior hip or buttock.
- If sciatic nerve is irritated, pain may be described as burning or may radiate down leg.

Physical Exam

- Pain precipitated by passive internal rotation and active external rotation (Figures 5.5 and 5.6).
- *Piriformis test* described earlier (Figure 5.14)

Essential Diagnostics

- Very little may be needed for this diagnosis in the emergency department.
- Testing would typically center around ruling out other causes such as cauda equina.
- Outpatient testing may include MRI of lumbar spine to exclude disc herniation.

ED Treatment

- Splint: Not needed
- Weight-bearing status: As tolerated.
- NSAIDs are used frequently.
- Steroid burst for five days may be used but typically not first line for most practitioners.
- Other medications such as gabapentin or pregabalin are prescribed for neuropathic pain but are frequently ineffective.

Disposition

- Discharge to home
- Indications to consult orthopedics (spine) would include concern for cauda equina or rapidly progressing neurologic changes.
- Follow-up in one to two weeks with PCP or sports medicine physician.
- Physical therapy is the typical first-line treatment but injections may be attempted.
- Return to work or sports as tolerated.
  - Once sciatic nerve irritated, full recovery may take a few months.

Complications

- Sciatica as a result of piriformis syndrome may be quite debilitating and painful.
- Severe and chronic piriformis dysfunction may cause gait abnormalities and early degenerative changes.

Pearls and Pitfalls

- May be easily confused for lumbosacral sciatica.
- Due to course of sciatic nerve, some patients will be predisposed to problems arising from the piriformis and should be counseled about high likelihood of future events.

Osteitis Pubis

General Description

- Inflammation of pubic symphysis seen after suprapubic surgery or in athletes.
- May be related to core weakness or a traumatic event.

Mechanism

- Likely results from repetitive microtrauma to pubic symphysis from several sources
  - Pregnancy and childbirth
  - Major trauma
  - Repeated minor trauma
  - Urologic or gynecologic surgery
  - Athletic activities that require cutting movements
- Core muscle weakness and sacroiliac joint hypermobility or hypomobility may cause additional stress on pubic symphysis.
- Infectious etiology and osteomyelitis also a possible cause.

Presentation

- Pain directly over pubic symphysis is common.
- Other possible presenting complaints:
  - Inguinal pain on one or both sides
  - Weakness and difficulty ambulating
  - Clicking or popping around pubic symphysis when standing or rolling over in bed

Physical Exam

- Tenderness over pubic symphysis
- Tenderness over superior pubic rami
- If sacroiliac dysfunction is involved, *FABER testing* (Figure 5.9) may elicit pain in sacroiliac joint.
- Pain with resisted hip adduction
- Make sure to rule out inguinal, femoral, or sports hernia

Essential Diagnostics

- Other diagnoses must be entertained such as pubic rami stress fracture.
- Radiographs of the pelvis should be obtained.
- CT scan of pelvis may be useful to rule out other pathology but is not required. This may be performed as an outpatient
- MRI may be necessary but very rarely, if ever, needed in the emergency department.
- If concerned for infectious etiology, ESR and CRP ordered in addition to CBC.

ED Treatment

- Splint: Not needed.
- Weight-bearing status: As tolerated.
- If concerned for osteomyelitis, antibiotics should be started as soon as possible.
- NSAIDs may be useful and should be started in the ED unless contraindicated.
- An oral steroid course may be useful as well but is typically reserved for protracted case.

Disposition

- Discharge unless osteomyelitis needing IV antibiotics.
- Orthopedic consult in the ED likely only needed for osteomyelitis.
- Follow-up recommended in one to two weeks.
- Activity modification
- Return to work or sports should be cautious depending on activities.

Complications

- Average time to full recovery is between seven and ten months.
- May take up to thirty-two months.
- For athletes who refuse to modify activities or rest, aggressive physical therapy and judicious use of medications may return them to prior level of activity.

Pediatric Considerations

- For young athletes, the importance of activity modification and rest should be emphasized.
- Typical duration of symptoms may significantly disrupt the young athletes' goals and success so treatment should be aggressively undertaken.

Pearls and Pitfalls

- May be a very long course with average time to resolution of seven to ten months.
- Osteomyelitis and stress fracture should be on the differential when considering osteitis pubis.
- Activity modification, rest, and anti-inflammatory medications are the typical recommendations.

Ischial Tuberosity Avulsion fracture

General Description

- Avulsion fracture of ischial tuberosity due to forceful contraction of hamstring muscle complex.
- May be final endpoint of stress fracture of ischial tuberosity.

Mechanism

- Hamstring attaches to ischial tuberosity and forceful contraction causes avulsion of bone.
- Stress reaction and stress fracture of ischial tuberosity may weaken the bone here and predispose the patient to avulsion.

Presentation

- Likely has severe pain with abrupt onset.
- Patient can usually recall the exact kick or step when it happened.
- May have been preceded by aching pain in this area in case of stress reaction/stress fracture.
- Pain localized to buttock or proximal hamstring.

Physical Exam

- Tenderness of ischial tuberosity and proximal hamstring.
- Pain aggravated by resisted knee flexion.
- May see bruising of proximal posterior leg.

Essential Diagnostics

- Radiographs are key to diagnosis.
- Musculoskeletal ultrasound may be beneficial for ruling out hamstring tear.
- CT may be necessary if clinical suspicion is high.

ED Treatment

- Splint: Not needed.
- Weight-bearing status: Non-weight bearing
- Pain control

Disposition

- Discharge likely
- Orthopedic consultation only for significantly displaced fractures to arrange early surgical intervention.
- Follow-up in next two to three days with orthopedics or sports medicine (if not significantly displaced)
- Return to work or sports will likely take several weeks for active work or sports.

Complications

- If not treated early, hamstring contracture will make repair and recovery of function much more difficult.

Pediatric Considerations

- Open physes may make this diagnosis more difficult but unequal physes should be worked up further.
- Due to relative weakness of physes compared with bone, tendon, and muscle, avulsions will likely happen directly through physes resulting in Salter–Harris I fractures.

Pearls and Pitfalls

- This is often misdiagnosed as a hamstring strain or tear which may significantly lengthen time to recovery or reduce likelihood of regaining previous level of function.

Athletic Pubalgia (aka sports hernia)

General description

- Poorly understood group of disorders with large variation of hypothesized causes, imaging modalities, and treatments.
- Main problem seems to come from the posterior wall of the inguinal canal.
- Term "sports hernia" is not accurate since there is no herniation of soft tissue, but this name has been used so widely by medical professionals and the media that is has been generally accepted by most.
- Also known as sportsman's hernia or Gilmore's groin.

Mechanism

- Weakness or injury to posterior wall of inguinal canal that may come from an inciting event causing injury to abdominal musculature or from chronic weakness of core musculature.
- Also some evidence now that FAI is associated with athletic pubalgia.

Presentation

- Typically unilateral burning or dull pain that is difficult to localize.
- Should indicate that the pain is above the inguinal ligament.
- Radiates to inner thigh and scrotum and even to contralateral side.
- Worse with activity and especially cutting or twisting, kicking, sprinting, or doing sit-ups.
- Pain free while inactive.

Physical Exam

- Palpation of inguinal crease and inguinal canal
- Hernia exam should be performed.
- Performing a sit-up with resistance should elicit pain (Figure 5.12).

Essential Diagnostics

- MRI and ultrasound are the diagnostic tests of choice, but there seems to be a dichotomy amongst the surgeons who specialize in these repairs.
- In the ED, ultrasound or CT may be useful to rule out an actual hernia if clinically indicated

- Due to location of pain, hip joint disorder should also be strongly considered and ruled out.

ED Treatment

- Splint: Not needed.
- Weight-bearing status: As tolerated
- Instructions to rest for at least seven to ten days and likely until seen by a sports medicine provider.
- NSAIDs are commonly prescribed for pain control.

Disposition

- Discharge
- Follow-up with sports medicine physician in one to two weeks
- Nonsurgical treatment typically consists of refraining from aggravating activity, physical therapy, and NSAIDs.
- If still concerned for athletic pubalgia, patient will likely be referred to a surgeon who specializes in athletic pubalgia.
- Surgical treatment may be done through an open procedure or laparoscopically.
- Return to activity must be determined by pain.

Complications

- Degree of pain often leads to cessation of sport.
- Chronic pain may lead to alterations in gait which may precipitate other injuries.

Pediatric Considerations

- Very little high-level evidence regarding athletic pubalgia in adults and even less in children.
- While adults typically have a high success rate for surgery, finding surgeon willing to perform the surgery on a pediatric patient may be challenging.

Pearls and Pitfalls

- ED workup should center on ruling out other causes of groin pain such as hip joint issue or a hernia.
- While still referred to as a "sports hernia," there is no true herniation of tissue involved in this disorder.

Hip

Femoral Neck Stress Fracture

General Description

- Stereotypical patient is one who recently started a new exercise program or began basic training for the military.
- Classified into two types
  - Tension type
  - Compression type
- Tension type located on superior aspect of femoral neck
  - More likely in older patients
  - Causes transverse fracture
  - High likelihood to displace
- Compression type located on inferior aspect of femoral neck
  - More likely in younger patients
  - More stable than tension type
  - Low likelihood to displace

Mechanism

- Repeated stress to femoral neck such as a sudden increase in physical activity.
- As with other stress injuries, may begin as stress reaction that will eventually result in stress fracture if the offending exercise is not stopped.

Presentation

- Pain localized to anterior hip or groin
- Deep ache that is relieved with cessation of activity.
- Difficulty walking without a limp.

Physical Exam

- Antalgic gait
- Painful and decreased internal rotation
- Unable to hop on one leg

Essential Diagnostics

- Initial hip radiographs may be negative but may rule out other fractures.
  - Bony changes such as radiolucent lines, periosteal bone formation, and sclerosis may not appear until two to four weeks after symptoms.
- AP pelvis radiograph useful for comparison of contralateral hip.

- MRI is imaging modality of choice but likely not necessary in the emergency department.
- SPECT may be positive as early as twenty-four to forty-eight hours after symptoms but positive predictive value is 80 percent.

ED Treatment

- Splint: Not needed.
- Weight-bearing status: Non-weight bearing
- Pain control
- If displaced, need orthopedic consult

Disposition

- Admit if displaced.
- Emergent orthopedic consult for ORIF if displaced.
- Tension type fractures should also get emergent orthopedic consult due to high likelihood of displacement.
- Compression type fractures may follow-up in one week with orthopedics or sports medicine physician.
    - Six to eight weeks for healing
    - Serial radiographs
    - May still need surgery for persistent pain or if displacement occurs.
- Return to work or sports will be determined by orthopedics or sports medicine physician.

Complications

- Displacement of tension type fractures if not treated soon enough.
- Even compression type fractures may lead to chronic pain.

Pediatric Considerations

- With open physes, a femoral neck stress fracture is extremely rare.

Pearls and Pitfalls

- High clinical suspicion of stress fracture should lead to non-weight bearing status and close follow-up.
- Any evidence of tension type fracture should prompt emergent orthopedic consult.
- Any displacement of femoral neck stress fracture should prompt emergent orthopedic consult for ORIF.

Femoroacetabular Impingement

General Description

- Relatively new diagnosis and corrective surgery but has shown promising results.
- Derangement in the bony structure of the hip joint leads to pain, labral injury, and early degenerative joint disease.
- If diagnosed and corrected early, goal is to prevent future complications and eventual hip replacement.
- As of yet, no reliable evidence for conservative treatment

Mechanism

- Hip joint composed of socket which is the acetabulum and ball which is the femoral head.
- The most common deformities
    - Loss of femoral head-neck offset (cam lesion).
    - Over-coverage by acetabulum (pincer lesion).
    - Combination of the two
- These bony abnormalities lead to frequent contact or impingement between the femoral neck and the rim of the acetabulum.
- This frequent contact leads to pain, labral tears, and early degenerative changes.

Presentation

- Pain localized to groin and anterior hip as well as posterior buttock at times.
- Many patients will cup the hand just superior to the greater trochanter to indicate both anterior and posterior pain.
- Frequently described as pinching or catching.
- Popping may occur which may be painful or painless.
- Exacerbated by flexing or internally rotating hip in actions such as getting into a car, sitting for a period of time, or walking up an incline or stairs.

Physical Exam

- Decrease in and painful with internal rotation
- *Flexion Adduction Internal Rotation Test* (FADDIR) (Figure 5.10)
- *Patrick test (FABER)* (Figure 5.9)
- Other testing to rule out other pathology should be used.

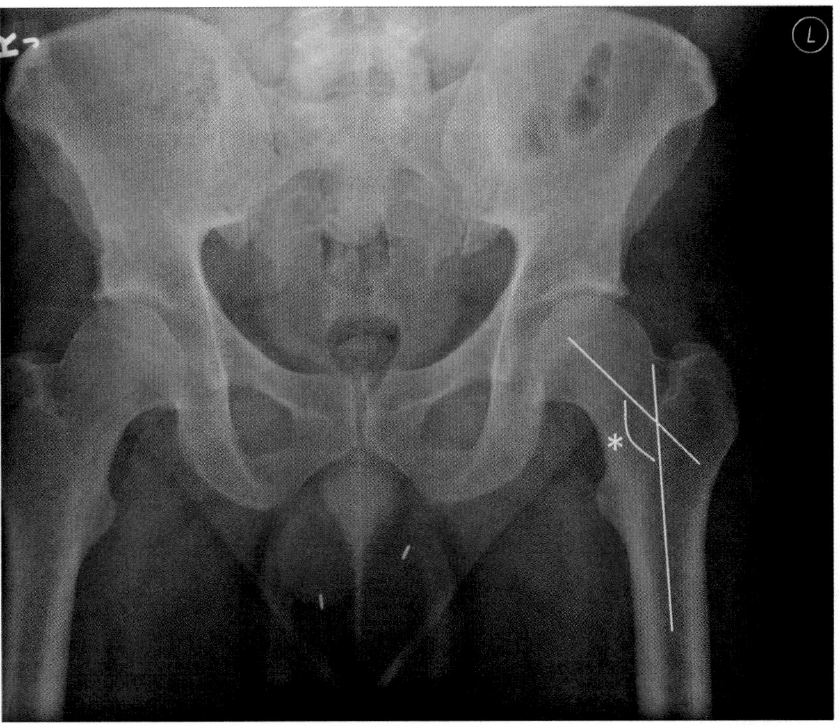

Figure 5.26. The neck-shaft angle (as signified by the asterisk) may be helpful in the diagnosis of femoroacetabular impingement. *Image courtesy of Thuan-Phuong Nguyen, West Virginia University.*

- *Straight leg raise* (lumbar radiculopathy) (Figure 5.8)
- *Ober's test* (IT band tightness) (Figure 5.13)
- *Thomas test* (tight iliopsoas musculature) (Figure 5.11)
- *Resisted sit-up* (athletic pubalgia) (Figure 5.12)

Essential Diagnostics

- Hip radiographs
  - Neck-shaft angle of the proximal femur of less than 120° or more than 135° may result in increased contact between femoral neck and acetabulum (Figure 5.26).
  - Offset femoral head noted with alpha angle on an AP radiograph, a modified Dunn radiograph, or a cross-table lateral radiograph. To calculate alpha angle, a circle is drawn to match the contour of the femoral head then a line is drawn from the center of the circle down the center of the femoral neck and another line from the center of the circle to the point where the femoral head exits the circle: greater than 55° between the lines is thought to be a cam lesion (Figure 5.27).
  - Overhanging superior acetabular edge measured by lateral center edge angle, the angle between vertical line through center of femoral head and line connecting center of femoral head and the edge of the acetabulum, with less than 25° being dysplasia and more than 40–45° being pincer impingement (Figure 5.28).
  - Crossover sign is another sign of a pincer lesion and is positive when the outline of the acetabulum makes a figure-of-eight (Figure 5.29).
- Other imaging such as ultrasound or MRI may be useful to rule out other pathology.

ED Treatment

- Splint: Not needed.
- Weight-bearing status: As tolerated
- Pain control typically attempted with NSAIDs

Disposition

- Discharge

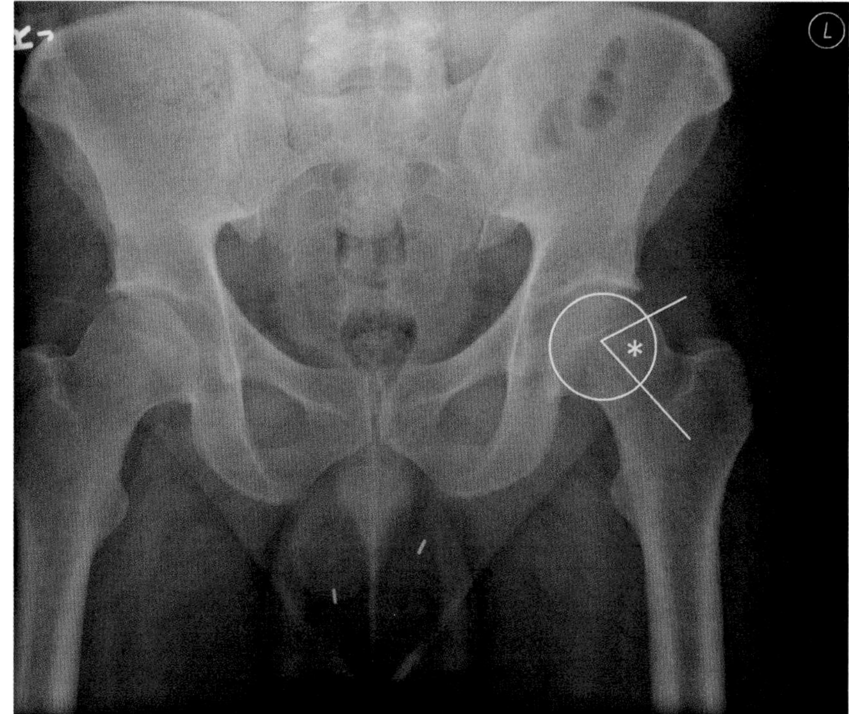

Figure 5.27. The alpha angle (as signified by the asterisk) may indicate an offset femoral head or cam lesion. *Image courtesy of Thuan-Phuong Nguyen, West Virginia University.*

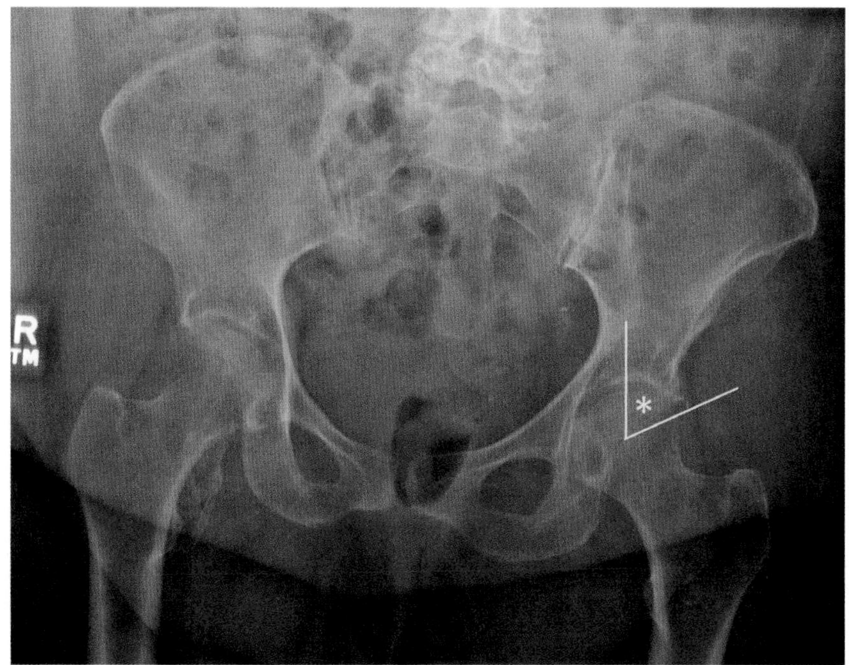

Figure 5.28. Lateral center edge angle (as signified by the asterisk) may assist with finding an overhanging superior acetabular edge or pincer lesion. *Image courtesy of Thuan-Phuong Nguyen, West Virginia University.*

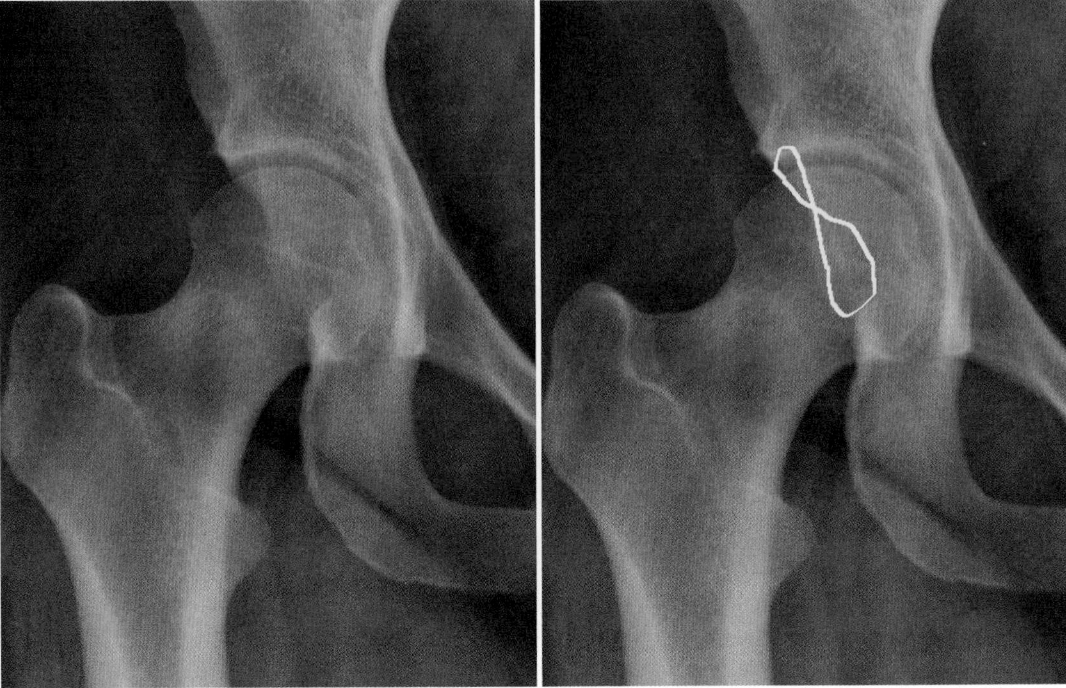

Figure 5.29. Crossover sign as shown in the second image is another sign of acetabular over-coverage or pincer lesion. *Image courtesy of Thuan-Phuong Nguyen, West Virginia University.*

- Consult orthopedics for severe pain with inability to ambulate.
- Follow-up as outpatient with orthopedic surgeon who specializes in hips and/or sports medicine.
  - Relatively small number of orthopedists who perform the surgery for FAI.
- Return to work or sports as tolerated.

Complications

- Left untreated, many patients develop labral tears or early degenerative joint disease which may be disabling.

Pediatric Considerations

- Increasingly recognized in pediatric patients as a cause of hip pain.
- May result from pediatric disorders such as Legg–Calve–Perthes disease or slipped capital femoral epiphysis.
- Early evidence suggests that arthroscopic hip surgery for FAI in pediatric patients has been reported as having good outcomes.

Pearls and Pitfalls

- Pain from FAI may present in several locations.
- FAI may progress to early degenerative joint disease.
- Only a small number of U.S. surgeons are doing these surgeries at this time so simple orthopedic referral may not suffice.

Snapping Hip

General Description

- Snapping or popping sensation that may or may not be audible.
- Typically occurs as tendons are pulled over bony prominences.
- May also occur with labral tears.
- May be accompanied by pain.

Mechanism

- Iliotibial band moving over greater trochanter is a common cause of snapping hip.
- Iliopsoas tendon moving over anterior inferior iliac spine, lesser trochanter, or iliopectineal ridge may also cause this disorder.
- Intra-articular causes such as labral tears that may flip over may be especially painful.

Presentation

- Often snapping hip syndromes are painless.

- Patient may display anxiety over frequent snapping.
- Iliotibial snapping will typically cause well-localized symptoms over the greater trochanter.
- Iliopsoas snapping may be difficult to localize and may present with inguinal crease or groin symptoms.
- Intra-articular snapping typically causes severe groin pain that may be disabling.

Physical Exam

- Most efficient is to ask the patient to recreate snapping.
- Iliotibial snapping may be recreated and palpated by having the patient internally and externally rotate the affected hip while standing.
- Iliopsoas snapping may be recreated and palpated by having the patient move the hip from a flexed position to a fully extended position which may be easiest to do when patient in lateral position.
- Intra-articular snapping and pain may cause limited internal rotation and an antalgic gait.

Essential Diagnostics

- Radiographs of the hip and pelvis will help rule out bony pathology and arthritic changes of hip.
- Radiographs are typically normal for snapping hip syndromes.
- Other imaging not needed in the emergency department in most cases.
- Outpatient MRI or MR arthrogram may be needed to detect labral tears.

ED Treatment

- Splint: Not needed.
- Weight-bearing status: As tolerated
- NSAIDs typically used for pain
- Instructions on activity modification and referral to physical therapy if patient particularly bothered by the symptoms

Disposition

- Discharge
- Follow-up with sports medicine physician in one to two weeks
- Return to work or sports as tolerated. If sports or work-specific activities aggravate symptoms, a period of rest or modification may be necessary.

Complications

- Untreated labral tears may cause continued irritation of the hip joint and early degenerative changes.
- In an attempt to prevent the snapping sensation, many patients alter gait or modify actions which puts them at risk for other injuries or overuse syndromes.

Pediatric Considerations

- Pediatric patients may be especially troubled by the snapping sensation and stop activities altogether without explanation.
- A careful exam may reveal the snapping hip.

Pearls and Pitfalls

- Several disorders may present with snapping hip.
- Treatment should focus on the source of the symptoms.
- Acetabular labral tears may need to be ruled out when snapping is especially painful or debilitating.

Acetabular Labrum Tear

General Description

- The acetabular labrum is a fibrocartilaginous ring that outlines the acetabulum.
- The labrum has several functions which include:
  - Increasing stability of hip
  - Distributing load on the acetabulum
  - Absorbing shock and trauma
  - Lubricating hip joint
- In patients with hip or groin pain, prevalence of labral tears has been reported as up to 55 percent.[4]
- Improved MRI techniques have led to increased recognition of tears.
- May be severely debilitating at times.
- Improved arthroscopic techniques have improved outcomes in these patients but there are relatively few orthopedic surgeons who are currently performing these surgeries.

Mechanism

- Five etiologies have been proposed at this time
  - Trauma
  - FAI
  - Hip hypermobility
  - Dysplasia
  - Degenerative joint disease
- Often associated with chondral abnormalities of the femoral head or acetabulum.
- In athletes, usually anterior/superior tears

Presentation

- Vast majority present with anterior hip or groin pain.
- Many will have pain for over two years before diagnosed with labral tear.
- May radiate to the knee.
- Many will include mechanical symptoms such as snapping, clicking, catching, giving way, or frank locking.
- Constant dull pain with intermittent episodes of sharp pain.
- Difficulty with using steps or walking long distance.

Physical Exam

- Extremely variable due to location of tear.
- Should ask patient how to recreate his or her symptoms.
- *Anterior impingement test* is most often positive
  - This test is performed by having the examiner flex the patient's hip to 90 degrees and then place the hip in 25 degrees of adduction.
  - The hip is then medially rotated to end range by the examiner.
  - The test is positive if anterior hip pain is produced.

Essential Diagnostics

- Hip radiographs may show evidence of degenerative changes or may be used to investigate other disorders such as FAI.
- It is unlikely that other testing will be necessary in the emergency department.
- Outpatient testing will likely include an MR arthrogram of the hip when there is concern for labral tear.
- Bone scan or SPECT has been proposed to look for characteristic bony changes that result from a labral tear but utility of this is still under debate.

ED Treatment

- Splint: Not needed.
- Weight-bearing status: As tolerated
- Pain control
- Some advocate intra-articular corticosteroid in the emergency department under ultrasound guidance but this is not a widely accepted practice.
  - In fact, many orthopedists strongly advocate against corticosteroid injections into the hip.

Disposition

- Discharge
- Consult orthopedics for severe, debilitating pain or inability to ambulate
- Follow-up with sports medicine physician in one to two weeks since this will likely be the fastest way to have the patient seen and worked up appropriately.
- Once there is MR arthrogram evidence of a labral tear, then the patient will be referred to an orthopedic surgeon who specializes in hip arthroscopy.
- Return to work or sports as tolerated, but this may take some time if pain is severe or if patient has a labor-intensive occupation.

Complications

- Untreated labral tears may lead to early onset degenerative joint disease.
- Severe pain with ambulation typically leads to antalgic gait and the cascade of other injuries caused by a gait disturbance.

Pediatric Considerations

- Labral tear in a pediatric patient will likely need aggressive treatment to prevent early degeneration and subsequent disability.
- While the number of surgeons who perform these procedures on adults is small, the number who perform them on pediatric patients is exponentially smaller.

Pearls and Pitfalls

- Clicking, snapping, or catching sensation in the groin or anterior hip should prompt a consideration of a labral tear.
- Initial trial of conservative therapy and relative rest may be appropriate.
- If symptoms persist, referral to an orthopedic surgeon is appropriate.
- There are a relatively small number of orthopedic surgeons who perform arthroscopic labral repairs so referral to a sports medicine physician will likely be the most expeditious way to get the patient appropriate follow-up and outpatient testing.
- Left untreated, a labral tear will lead to early degenerative changes and subsequent disability.

Slipped Capital Femoral Epiphysis (SCFE)

General Description

- There is a physis or growth plate near the midpoint of the femoral head.
- A SCFE is a displacement of the capital femoral epiphysis, which is the femoral head, in relation to the femoral neck.
- It is a Salter–Harris I fracture.
- Most common in boys between 13 and 15 years old and in girls between 11 and 13 years old.
- Known risk factors include.
  - Above 95th percentile for weight
  - Male
  - Athletic participation
  - Increased femoral retroversion
  - Hypothyroidism
  - Growth hormone deficiency
- Bilateral SCFE in 40–61 percent of cases[5-6]

Mechanism

- During the adolescent growth spurt, the orientation of the physis changes from horizontal to oblique which increases the potential stress on the physis.
- In children and adolescents, an open physis often is the weakest link in the skeletal chain.
- With repeated stress, there are microfractures in the physis and gradual slippage of the femoral head.
- Patients who are younger than 11 years or older than 16 years should have additional workup for endocrinologic or metabolic disorders.

Presentation

- Most will complain of pain in the anterior proximal thigh but about 23 percent have been found to have distal thigh pain.[7]
- Pain is worse with activity.
- Most describe a gradual progression of symptoms but it may have an acute onset after an injury.

Physical Exam

- Most sensitive and specific finding is a loss of internal rotation that is made worse with a flexed hip.
- Abduction and extension are also decreased.
- Shortening of affected leg by 1–3 cm.
- Will often walk with a limp with the affected leg in external rotation.

Essential Diagnostics

- AP and frog-lateral radiographs are often diagnostic as they will show the characteristic displacement.
- In the early stages of the disease, only a subtle irregularity or widening of the physis may be evident.
- Klein line on AP radiographs may be helpful in finding an abnormality.
  - This is drawn along the superior border of the femoral neck and should intersect the lateral capital femoral epiphysis (Figures 5.30 and 5.31).
- Lateral view often most sensitive for detecting the degree of displacement.
- Displacement classified with respect to angulation as mild (less than 30°), moderate (30–50°), or severe (greater than 50°).
- Outpatient MRI may be needed in early stages.

ED Treatment

- Splint: Not needed.
- Weight-bearing status: Non-weight bearing
- Pain control

Disposition

- Admission vs. discharge to be determined by degree of displacement or angulation in conjunction with pediatric orthopedic surgeon.

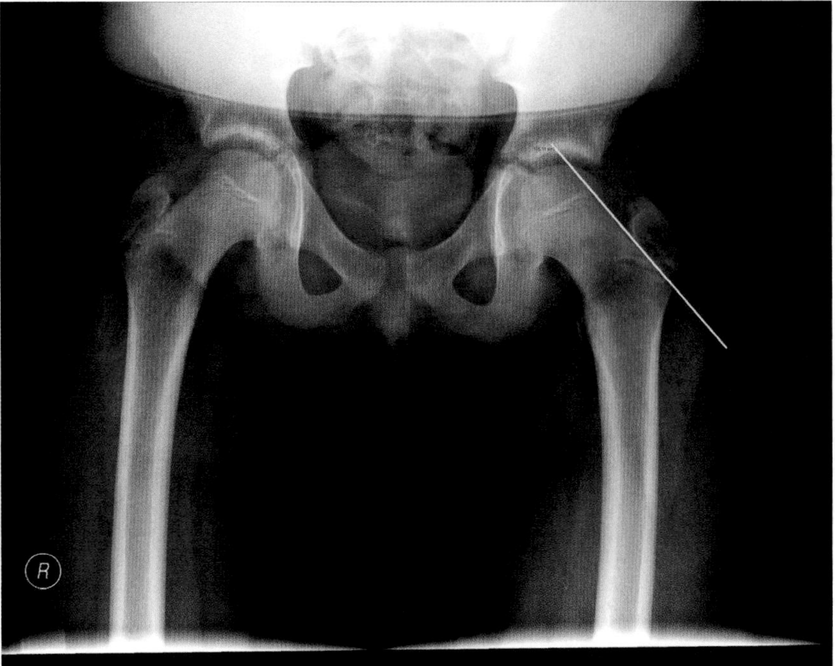

Figure 5.30. This is a normal pediatric hip with a normal Klein line. *Image courtesy of Thuan-Phuong Nguyen, West Virginia University.*

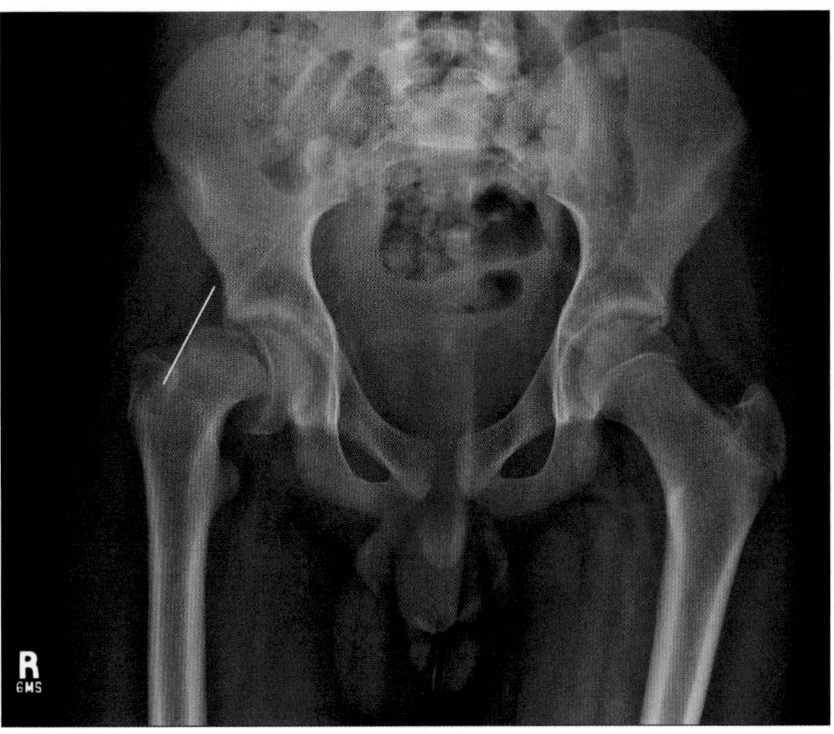

Figure 5.31. This is a pediatric hip with slipped capital femoral epiphysis and an abnormal Klein line. *Image courtesy of Mary Cannon, West Virginia University.*

- If discharged, follow-up with pediatric orthopedic surgeon will likely occur in next three to five days.
- Surgery for this typically involves one or possibly two screws to secure the femoral head from slipping further and has good outcomes.
- Patients will then be allowed toe-touch weight-bearing for the first six weeks.
- Return to sports and activities not permitted until physis closes, typically six to nine months.

Complications

- Most serious complication is osteonecrosis of the femoral head which is closely associated with the degree of stability.
    - In stable SCFE, only 5 percent develop osteonecrosis.
    - In unstable SCFE, up to 50 percent develop osteonecrosis.
- Gait disturbance may lead to degenerative changes in the hip or overuse injuries.
- The irregularity in the bony surface of the base of the femoral head may lead to impingement of the acetabular labrum and labral tears.

Pearls and Pitfalls

- Loss of internal rotation is most sensitive and specific exam finding and is made worse with hip in flexion.
- In early disease, radiographic changes may be very subtle or even absent, so close follow-up should be arranged.
- Due to high incidence of bilateral disease, some advocate prophylactic pinning of contralateral hip, but this is still debated.
- Worst complication is osteonecrosis of the femoral head and may occur in up to 50 percent of patients with an unstable SCFE.

Trochanteric Bursitis

General Description

- Greater trochanteric bursa lies between greater trochanter and iliotibial band
- Irritation of this bursa may be caused by several disorders and these should be investigated

Mechanism

- Bursa becomes irritated, inflamed, or infected and causes pain.
- Irritation and inflammation may be caused by local trauma, leg-length discrepancy, abnormal gait, inflammatory arthritis, intra-articular pathology, lumbar spinal disease, or hardware left in the hip.

Presentation

- Pain over greater trochanter.
- Pain may radiate distally or proximally.
- Pain worse when patient first rising from a seated position.
- Has night pain and unable to lay on affected side.
- Signs or symptoms of infection, if present, should be investigated further.

Physical Exam

- Point tenderness over greater trochanter.
- Pain worse with adduction of hip.

Essential Diagnostics

- Radiographs of the pelvis and hip

ED Treatment

- Splint: Not needed.
- Weight-bearing status: Full
- Pain control with NSAIDs
- Instruct the patient on activity modification
- Utility of corticosteroid injections is still debated by some
    - Despite this, an injection of lidocaine or bupivacaine alone into the trochanteric bursa may resolve the patient's pain and thus be diagnostic.

Disposition

- Discharge
- Follow-up with sports medicine physician in one to two weeks.
- Return to work or sports: As tolerated

Complications

- Left untreated, trochanteric bursitis will precipitate further injuries due to alteration in gait and other actions.
- In addition, cause of trochanteric bursitis should be investigated.

Pearls and Pitfalls

- Trochanteric bursitis is a common condition in which the affected area is point tender.
- Cause of trochanteric bursitis should be investigated.
- Carefully consider other diagnoses prior to reaching decision that patient has trochanteric bursitis.

Hip Fracture

General Description

- Classified by location of the fracture and may be intercapsular (femoral neck and head) or extracapsular (trochanteric, intertrochanteric, and subtrochanteric).
- Elderly are most susceptible due to underlying osteoporosis and increased susceptibility to falls.
  - Women more often affected than men due to increased incidence of osteoporosis.
  - Femoral neck and intertrochanteric fractures are most common.
  - Associated with high rates of morbidity and mortality.
- Trochanteric avulsion fractures are more common in the young, active population.

Mechanism

- Falls from standing are the most common causes of hip fractures in the elderly.
- Younger patients with femoral neck or intertrochanteric fractures are usually due to major trauma.
- Trochanteric avulsion fractures usually occur due to forceful muscular contraction of the gluteus medius or minimus.
  - May also be caused by direct trauma in the older population.

Presentation

- Sudden onset, severe pain is usually localized to the hip/groin
- Usually unable to bear weight
- Trochanteric avulsion fractures may present with referred pain in the knee or posterior thigh

Physical Exam

- Observe for deformity and position of extremity
  - Displaced intercapsular fractures may present with externally rotated, shortened leg.
  - Intercapsular fractures usually have no obvious bruising or swelling.
  - Extracapsular fractures often have significant swelling and ecchymoses.
- Palpate for tenderness.
- Assessment of hemodynamic status after an intertrochanteric or subtrochanteric fracture is essential because they can be associated with significant blood loss.
- Trochanteric avulsion fractures may have tenderness over the greater trochanter.
  - Pain may be exacerbated with hip abduction, flexion, and/or rotation.
- A complete neurovascular exam of the affected extremity is essential.

Essential Diagnostics

- Two view hip radiographs including AP and lateral views, as well as a pelvis radiograph to evaluate for occult pelvic fractures and to compare to uninvolved hip.
  - Evaluate integrity of cortex, trabecular pattern, and angle of the femoral neck.
    - Normal angle between femoral neck and shaft on AP radiograph is 45 degrees.
    - Normal angle between the medial femoral shaft and trabecular lines is 160 to 170 degrees.
    - Assess for any disruption in Shenton's line, an imaginary curvilinear line drawn along the superior border of the obturator foramen and the medial femoral neck.
- MRI is indicated if high suspicion for hip fracture but plain radiographs are unrevealing.

ED Treatment

- Adequate pain management is essential.
  - Narcotic pain medications are often required.
  - May also consider ultrasound guided femoral nerve block.
- Patient should be made non weight-bearing status.
- Skeletal traction is contra-indicated in patients with femoral neck fractures because it may further disrupt blood supply.

Disposition

- Most femoral neck and intertrochanteric fractures will require surgical management which may include internal fixation or hip arthroplasty.
  - Occasionally, non-operative treatment is preferable in debilitated patients and those with stable, impacted fractures.
- Trochanteric avulsion fractures are usually managed non-operatively as long as displacement is less than one centimeter.
  - Will need to be non-weight bearing for three to four weeks.
- Return to work or sports to be determined by extent of fractures.
  - Young, healthy patients with non-displaced trochanteric avulsion fractures may be able to return to sports within two to three months.

Complications

- Femoral neck fractures associated with higher risk of malunion or nonunion and avascular necrosis due to tenuous blood supply, however intertrochanteric fractures are also at risk.
- Infection
- Thromboembolism
- Pressure ulcers

Pearls and Pitfalls

- Make sure to assess the reason for the fall in elderly patients who have sustained a hip fracture, as well as concomitant injuries (e.g. intracranial or cervical spine injury).
  - Additional work-up may be necessary if due to such causes as syncope, stroke, GI bleed, and so forth.
- Consider type and crossmatch blood in elderly patients with intertrochanteric fracture and initial hemoglobin below 12g/dL.
- Consider pathologic fracture in evaluation of trochanteric avulsion fractures in the elderly.
- Negative plain films do not rule out a fracture.
  - Essential to perform further testing if clinical suspicion is high, especially if patient is unable to bear weight or has significant pain with weight-bearing.
- Disposition should be determined in consultation with Orthopedic Surgery.

Hip Dislocation

General Description

- May be anterior, posterior, or central
  - Posterior most common
- High rate of other associated injuries including fractures of the acetabulum and femoral head, as well as ipsilateral knee and sciatic nerve injuries.

Mechanism

- Usually due to high mechanism trauma
  - Posterior hip dislocation is often due to a dashboard injury with a direct force applied when hip is flexed and adducted.
  - Anterior hip dislocation often occurs after direct force applied when hip is abducted and externally rotated.

Presentation

- Usually present with significant pain, deformity, and inability to bear weight.

Physical Exam

- Assess for areas of tenderness and deformity of the affected extremity.
  - Posterior dislocations often present with a shortened, adducted and internally rotated extremity.
  - Anterior dislocations often present with an abducted and externally rotated hip.
- Limited range of motion
- Unable to bear weight
- Assess neurovascular status
  - Sciatic nerve injury occurs in approximately 10% of posterior hip dislocations.

Essential Diagnostics

- AP, lateral hip, and pelvis radiographs, as well as ipsilateral femur and knee.
  - Femoral head often appears smaller in posterior dislocations and larger in anterior dislocations due to placement of the cassett.
  - Judet view helpful to assess for acetabular fractures after a posterior hip dislocation.

- CT scan post-reduction after any traumatic hip dislocation is essential to evaluate for other associated femoral head fractures, acetabular fractures, or loose bodies.

ED Treatment

- Adequate analgesia is essential.
- Prompt closed reduction within six hours of injury.
  - Any delays in reduction correspond with increase risk of avascular necrosis.
  - Ensure adequate sedation and muscle relaxation prior to attempted reduction.
    - Procedural sedation is required.
  - Reduction techniques involve applying in-line traction with patient in supine position.
  - Consultation with orthopedics prior to reduction is required if there is an associated fracture.
- Limit number of reduction attempts in the ED and consult orthopedics early if unable to successfully reduce.

Disposition

- Most patients can be discharged home after reduction of simple dislocation.
  - Protected weight-bearing for four to six weeks.
- Orthopedics consult for any unsuccessful reduction or associated fractures.
  - Closed reduction under general anesthesia or open reduction for irreducible dislocations may be required.
  - ORIF is usually indicated for dislocations with associated fractures.
- Return to work or sports to be determined by extent of injury.
  - May return to full activity after simple dislocation after has regained full strength and function, usually in three to four months post-injury.

Complications

- Avascular necrosis
- Injury to the sciatic nerve
- Post-traumatic arthritis
- Recurrent dislocations

Pearls and Pitfalls

- Make sure to perform thorough primary and secondary survey as hip dislocations are often associated with concomitant injuries.
- Hip dislocations represent a true orthopedic emergency and need prompt reduction within six hours of injury to minimize further risk of avascular necrosis.

Transient Synovitis of the Hip

General Description

- Also known as coxalgia fugax and toxic synovitis
- Common source of limping for children from 2–7 years old
- Boys affected two to three times more often than girls.
- Self-limited condition that typically lasts four to six weeks.
- Should be a diagnosis of exclusion with a differential that includes septic arthritis, pelvic osteomyelitis, proximal femur osteomyelitis, Lyme disease, LPCD, inflammatory diseases, and traumatic injuries.

Mechanism

- Sterile hip joint effusion with unknown etiology
- Mild trauma may explain some cases.
- Many patients will have history of recent viral infection which may be upper respiratory or gastrointestinal.

Presentation

- Most common presentation is that parents noticed a limp that may or may not be painful.
- The limp may be intermittent and may get worse later in the day.
- If old enough, child may complain of pain anywhere in lower extremity although hip pain and knee pain are most common.
- May refuse to walk altogether.

Physical exam

- Noticeable limp
- General restriction of hip motion during gait.
- Range of motion testing may reveal decreased or painful abduction and internal rotation.
- Most are afebrile.

Essential Diagnostics

- A diagnosis of exclusion, the other more serious conditions will need further investigation.
- Radiographs of hip and other areas where patient is in pain.
  - AP and frog-lateral views needed.
- Due to concern for septic arthritis, patient workup should include a CBC with differential, ESR, and CRP.
- Other lab tests should be considered in appropriate patients such as Lyme titers, antistreptolysin-O (ASO), and rheumatologic tests but these will not provide results in a timely fashion in most emergency departments.
- An ultrasound of the hip may show a joint effusion which is not necessarily diagnostic, but an ultrasound-guided hip arthrocentesis may be performed at the same time and may be diagnostic.
  - When arthrocentesis is performed, fluid should be sent for cell count with differential, crystals, culture, Gram stain, protein, and glucose.

ED Treatment

- For mild symptoms, observation period may be okay.
- When there is concern for septic arthritis, antibiotics should be started once arthrocentesis has been performed or if the patient appears severely ill or septic.
- In Lyme endemic areas or with history consistent with Lyme disease, doxycycline is first-line treatment.
- Pain should be controlled.
- Splint: Not needed.
- Weight-bearing status: As tolerated.
- For those diagnosed with transient synovitis, most will be treated with activity restriction, NSAIDs, and possibly other analgesics.

Disposition

- Admit for IV antibiotics or possible washout when concerned for septic arthritis.
- If patient unable to ambulate, should be admitted even if septic arthritis ruled out.
- Mild symptoms may be discharged with close orthopedic follow-up.
- Indications to consult orthopedics include inability to ambulate, severe pain, or concern for septic arthritis.
- Follow-up should be in next two to three days when sending home with mild symptoms.
- Return to sports will be as tolerated.

Complications

- No significant complications since it is a self-limited condition.
- Legg–Calve–Perthes disease develops in 1–3 percent of patients with transient synovitis but there is no clear association between the two diseases.[8]
- Sequelae of septic arthritis may be severe and include early arthritis, need for hip replacement, severe disability, sepsis, and even death.

Pearls and Pitfalls

- Transient synovitis of the hip is a diagnosis of exclusion so great care should be taken in ruling out more severe diagnoses such as septic arthritis, and so forth.
- Workup will typically center around laboratory evaluation and ultrasound with arthrocentesis.
- Most common presentation is limp that may or may not be painful.
- Self-limited condition that will typically last four to six weeks.

Septic Arthritis of Hip

General Description

- Infection of hip joint may be a severely disabling condition.
- For a total of all joint infections, it has been estimated that about 20,000 occur in the United States each year.
  - The hip has been implicated in about 20 percent of these cases.
- Increasing numbers of prosthetic joints are causing a rapid increase in these numbers.
- Increasing use of immunosuppressants has also paralleled an increase in joint infections.

- Bacterial infections are often classified as gonococcal and nongonococcal.
  - *Neisseria gonorrhoeae* is still the most prevalent pathogen in younger sexually active patients.
  - *Staphylococcus aureus* infection has rapidly grown as a source of nongonococcal septic arthritis.

Mechanism

- Hematogenous spread is the most common mechanism, but bacteria may be introduced into the joint through direct inoculation and contiguous spread as well.
- Once bacteria enter the joint space and overwhelm the body's immune response, the bacteria and the immune response itself cause destruction of the synovium.

Presentation

- As with most processes that involve the hip joint, pain will most often be localized to the groin, but this should not be used to rule out septic arthritis.
- Acute onset of pain.
- Fever present in 40–60 percent of cases.
- Impaired range of motion.
- Limp or inability to ambulate altogether.
- Elicit history of possible sexually transmitted disease, immunosuppressants, diabetes, or rheumatoid arthritis.

Physical Exam

- Temperature should be checked for fever.
- All joints should be examined for possible polyarthritis.
- Inguinal crease tenderness may be present.
- Log roll of hip.
- Range of motion limited by pain.
- *FABER test* (Figure 5.9) will typically cause severe pain due to significant tension placed on synovium.
- Signs may be unreliable in patients who are immunocompromised, elderly, or intravenous drug abusers.

Essential Diagnostics

- Hip radiographs are first-line test as these will help rule out other causes as well.
- For laboratory evaluation, CBC with differential, ESR, and CRP should be ordered.
- Other lab tests should be considered in appropriate patients such as Lyme titers, ASO, and rheumatologic tests but these will not provide results in timely fashion in most emergency departments.
- An ultrasound of the hip may show a joint effusion which is not necessarily diagnostic, but an ultrasound-guided hip arthrocentesis may be performed at the same time and may be diagnostic.
  - When arthrocentesis is performed, fluid should be sent for cell count with differential, crystals, culture, Gram stain, protein, and glucose.
- Arthrocentesis under fluoroscopy necessary if no practitioner skilled in ultrasound-guided procedure.

ED Treatment

- Splint: Not needed.
- Weight-bearing status: Non-weight bearing in emergency department.
- Early antibiotics are recommended but may be delayed in stable patients if emergent washout in the operating room is planned.
  - Adult non-gonococcal: vancomycin 15–20 mg/kg IV PLUS one of cefotaxime 1 g IV, ceftriaxone 1 g IV, ciprofloxacin 400 mg IV, OR levofloxacin 750 mg IV.
  - Adult gonococcal: ceftriaxone 1 g IV OR ciprofloxacin 400 mg IV.
  - Pediatric: vancomycin 10 mg/kg IV PLUS one of cefotaxime 50 mg/kg IV OR Ceftriaxone 50 mg/kg IV.
  - Prosthesis Infection: rifampin 600 mg PO/IV PLUS one of vancomycin 15–20 mg/kg IV, ciprofloxacin 400 mg IV, OR levofloxacin 750 mg IV.
- Pain control.
- NPO for emergent washout.

Disposition

- Admit all patients with septic arthritis for either emergent washout or IV antibiotics with serial exams and observation.
- Orthopedic surgery should be consulted for all patients with septic arthritis.

- Return to work or sports determined by orthopedic surgery but typically four-to-six-week range barring any complications.

Complications

- Even a small delay in treatment may cause severe degeneration and destruction of the joint.

Pediatric Considerations

- Septic arthritis in an otherwise healthy child should prompt at least a consideration of further workup for other conditions such as rheumatoid arthritis, Lyme disease, or other immunosuppressive conditions if clinically indicated.
- Antibiotic choices are slightly different than for adults and are outlined above.

Pearls and Pitfalls

- Rare disorder but must be considered due to significant complications.
- Physical exam may be unreliable in patients who are immunosuppressed, elderly, or intravenous drug abusers.
- Blood tests may also be unreliable, and the diagnosis relies on an arthrocentesis that may be performed with ultrasound guidance or under fluoroscopy.
- Antibiotics should only be delayed in stable patients when emergent washout in the operating room is eminent.

Osteonecrosis of the Hip

General Description

- Also known as aseptic necrosis of the hip or avascular necrosis of the hip.
- Affects between 10,000–20,000 new patients each year.
- Greatest frequency in third to fifth decades of life.
- There are many disorders and offending agents that may precipitate osteonecrosis of the hip.
  - Trauma (especially hip dislocation or femoral neck fracture).
  - Corticosteroid use which is generally related to dose and duration but cases have been reported after only one or two uses.
  - Sickle cell disease.
  - Rheumatoid arthritis
  - Alcohol abuse
  - Systemic lupus erythematosus
  - Other less prevalent associated disorders such as Caisson disease (scuba diving), chronic pancreatitis, Crohn's disease, Gaucher disease, HIV, myeloproliferative disorders, radiation treatments, and smoking.

Mechanism

- Blood supply to femoral head is precarious.
- A disruption to blood supply to femoral head causes portions of bone to die which leads to weakening of bony architecture and subsequent collapse of femoral head.

Presentation

- Gradual onset of dull pain in groin, lateral hip, or buttock area.
- While bone is infarcting, pain is typically more severe then later becomes chronic pain that may be indistinguishable from osteoarthritis.
- May complain of limited range of motion.
- Limping or difficulty walking.
- Often is bilateral.

Physical Exam

- Pain with active *straight leg raise*
- Pain with range of motion and decreased range of motion particularly internal rotation
- Antalgic gait that may eventually transition to Trendelenburg gait.

Essential Diagnostics

- Hip radiographs with AP and frog-lateral views and AP pelvis radiograph should be initial test.
- Femoral head will eventually develop patchy lucency and sclerosis (Figure 5.32).
- Femoral head will become less spherical with time which leads to acetabulum degeneration (Figure 5.32).
- MRI may show abnormalities when radiographs have appeared normal.
- MRI in the emergency department should be reserved for most severe cases such as inability to ambulate due to pain or for high-risk patients with convincing story.

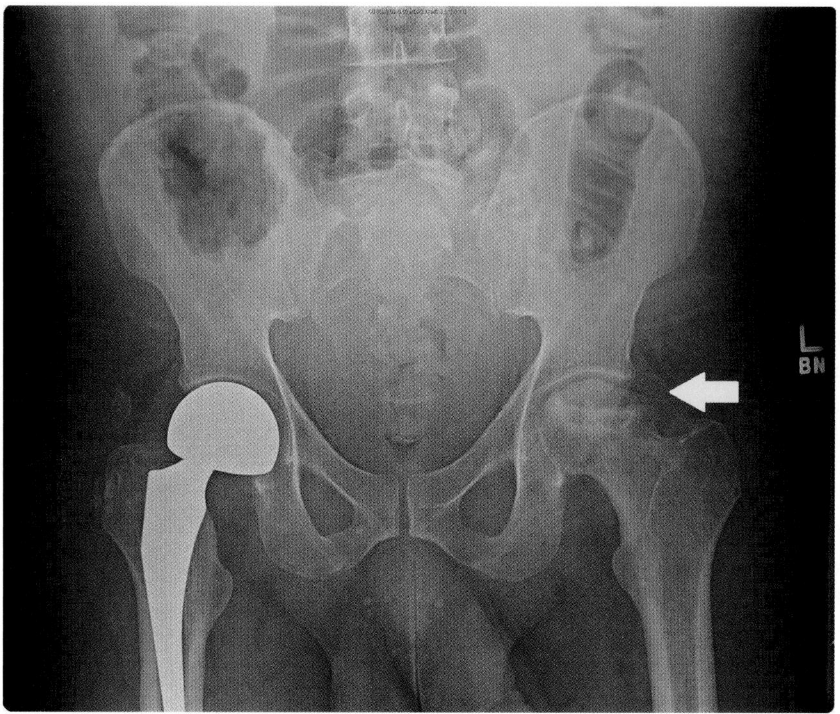

Figure 5.32. This radiograph shows osteonecrosis of the hip with patchy lucency and irregularity of the same of the femoral head. *Image courtesy of William Krantz, West Virginia University.*

- If pain and symptoms are bilateral, then bilateral imaging studies should be ordered.
- Once diagnosis is made, many orthopedic surgeons advocate MRI of unaffected hip so a diagnosis may be made early in subclinical disease and early surgical intervention may prevent further disease progress and eventual disability.
- Other testing may be useful to rule out other intra-articular disorders.

ED Treatment

- Splint: Not needed.
- Weight-bearing status: Non weight bearing
- Pain control
- If femoral head is showing collapse, patient will need arthroplasty, so coordination with orthopedics is important.

Disposition

- Most will be discharged unless symptoms are severe.
- Orthopedics should be consulted anytime diagnosis of osteonecrosis of the hip is made.
- Follow-up will happen at the direction of orthopedics but will likely happen within a few days for severe disease and one to two weeks for mild disease.
- Return to work or sports will be determined by the orthopedist but will likely be several weeks after arthroplasty.
- Lifelong activity modifications may be needed.

Complications

- If lesion is in weight-bearing portion, pain will typically increase until unbearable.
- Collapse of the femoral head leads to severe degenerative changes that may occur very quickly.

Pediatric Considerations

- LCPD is idiopathic osteonecrosis of the femoral head in children and typically affects boys between 4 and 8 years old (Figure 5.33).
- LCPD is very similar to the adult disease process but the healing process in pediatric bone may actually resolve this disorder without surgery.

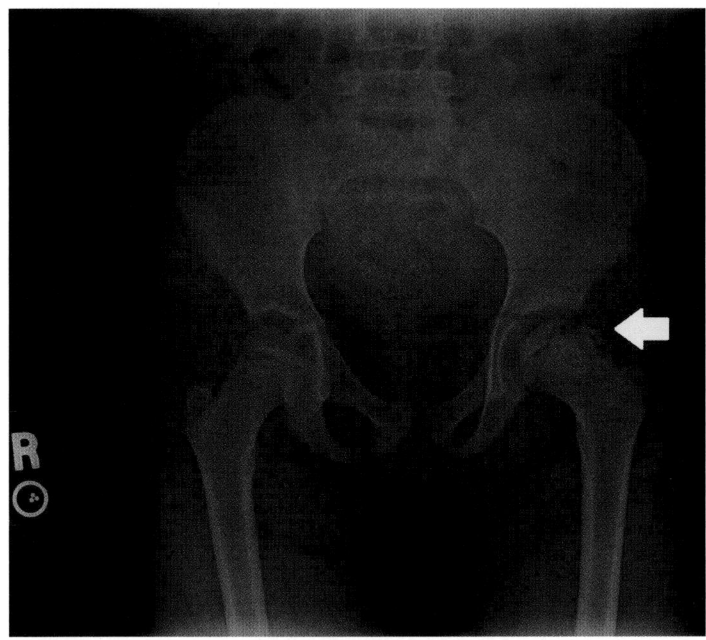

Figure 5.33. Legg-Calve-Perthes disease is a potentially debilitating disorder, but with proper conservative management, patients may do well. *Image courtesy of William Krantz, West Virginia University.*

- Activity restriction is the hallmark of treatment and is usually effective in those with mild to moderate disease.
- Severe disease may lead to an aspherical femoral head and subsequent early osteoarthritis for which arthroplasty is the typical treatment of choice once the symptoms are bad enough.

Pearls and Pitfalls

- Disease should be caught early for best outcomes.
- For high-risk patients with normal radiographs, strongly consider MRI in the emergency department due to significant complications that may result if left untreated.
- Mild to moderate disease may have strict activity restrictions but will likely need some type of surgery in adults and eventually arthroplasty.
- Children with LPCD may do well with activity restrictions alone.

Thigh

Meralgia Paresthetica

General Description

- Lateral femoral cutaneous nerve is a purely sensory nerve that supplies the lateral portion of the thigh down to just proximal to the knee.
- Nerve is most in jeopardy of compression just medial to the anterior superior iliac spine where it exits the pelvis.
- Historically, it was taught that the nerve actually passed lateral to the anterior superior iliac spine in 10 percent of the population, but a study of 68 hips in 50 cadavers by Hospodar in 1999 found no instances where the nerve passed laterally.[9]
- It divides into anterior and posterior branches.

Mechanism

- Mechanical compression of the lateral femoral cutaneous nerve due to obesity, tight-fitting clothing or straps around the waist such as belts or back pack straps, post-surgical scarring, or trauma.

Presentation

- Symptoms should cover the lateral aspect of the thigh down to the knee.
- Patients may describe frank numbness or decreased sensation but many describe pain and burning or dysesthesia.
- Runners may describe this as electric shock pain with every foot strike.
- No motor weakness with this disorder.

Physical Exam

- No motor weakness

- Symptoms should be localized to distribution of the nerve in lateral thigh down to knee.
- The most reproducible spot of decreased sensation is just above the knee on the lateral aspect of the leg.
- Many times, applying pressure from the anterior superior iliac spine medially from 0–5 cm (most commonly 1–1.5 cm) will find a spot that is tender and reproduces the symptoms.
- Pain may also be reproduced with hip extension.

Essential Diagnostics

- AP pelvis radiograph and AP/lateral hip radiographs will allow for exclusion of bony abnormality.
- Once a spot is found medial to anterior superior iliac spine that recreates the symptoms, a local injection of lidocaine here may prove diagnostic if it resolves pain or burning.
- CT pelvis with contrast would likely be the study of choice in the emergency department if intrapelvic mass is suspected.

ED Treatment

- Splint: Not needed.
- Weight-bearing status: As tolerated.
- Attempt to discover the offending source of compression and discuss alternatives.
- Neuropathic pain medications such as gabapentin or pregabalin may be useful for severe symptoms.

Disposition

- Discharge
- Indications to consult orthopedic surgery would include persistent severe symptoms despite prior treatment.
- May need general surgery, surgical oncology, or interventional radiology consultation if a mass is found in the pelvis.
- Follow-up with a sports medicine physician in one to two weeks.
- At follow-up patient may receive a corticosteroid injection, but this is usually reserved for circumstances where the patient may be followed up which is not typical in emergency department setting.
- Return to work or sports as tolerated; if uniform for work or sports or if the required actions of work or sports are thought to be the source of nerve compression, then significant modifications or a period of rest for several weeks may be necessary.

Complications

- Continued symptoms will persist if no treatment is pursued and symptoms may even continue with treatment.
- For severe and protracted cases for which all conservative measures have been exhausted, an orthopedic surgeon may attempt a surgical decompression of the nerve but this is very rare occurrence.

Pearls and Pitfalls

- There should be no motor component of this complaint so further investigation into lumbar disc disease should be undertaken if both motor and sensory components are present.
- If a tender spot is found medial to the anterior superior iliac spine which reproduces the symptoms, a local injection of lidocaine into this spot may prove diagnostic.
- Attempt to find the cause for nerve compression and treat this.

Iliotibial Band Syndrome

General Description

- Most common cause of lateral knee pain in athletes.
- Overuse injury common in runners and especially with downhill running.
- Also may commonly affect participants in cycling, volleyball, soccer, skiing, tennis, weight lifting, and aerobics.
- In U.S. Marine Corps recruits, ITBS incidence found to be up to 22 percent during basic training.[10]

Mechanism

- Typically results from irritation of bursa between iliotibial band and lateral femoral epicondyle.
- Posterior portion of iliotibial band contacts the lateral femoral epicondyle just after foot strike in the gait cycle at approximately 30° of knee flexion.

Presentation

- Gradual onset of lateral knee pain at first only present during activity but will increase in frequency until constant pain.
- Localized over lateral femoral epicondyle.
- Exacerbated by running downhill or climbing stairs.

Physical Exam

- During gait exam, the patient may keep knee extended to prevent sliding of iliotibial band.
- Tenderness where iliotibial band slides over lateral femoral epicondyle.
- *Ober's test* (Figure 5.13) may indicate iliotibial band tightness.
- Genu varum and hyperpronation of feet may predispose runners to iliotibial band syndrome so these should be looked for on exam.

Essential Diagnostics

- Knee radiographs are typically performed to investigate other causes of pain in this area.
- With pain at rest, the medical provider must include neoplasm, infection, or inflammatory arthropathy on differential and proceed with testing that is clinically necessary.

ED Treatment

- Splint: Not needed.
- Weight-bearing status: typically as tolerated, but once pain is constant or nearly constant, non-weight bearing on crutches should be recommended.
- Ice may be placed at the site.
- NSAIDs are typically used.

Disposition

- Discharge
- Orthopedic consultation should not be needed.
- Follow-up in one to two weeks with sports medicine physician.
- Return to work or sports as tolerated.
- Period of rest or avoidance of activity that aggravates pain such as downhill running.
- Should discuss stretching of iliotibial band.
    - Two such stretches shown in Figures 5.34 and 5.35
- Long-term treatment may include stretching, icing, and orthotic devices.

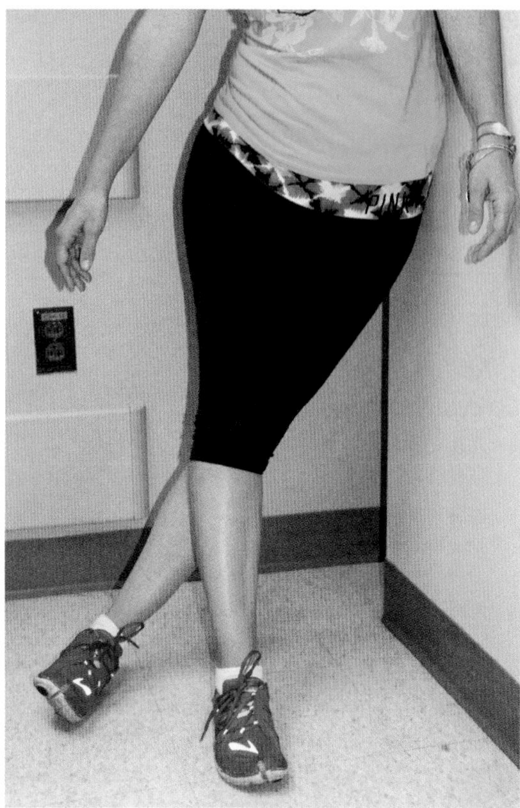

Figure 5.34. In this iliotibial band stretch, the affected leg is placed behind while leaning toward the wall.

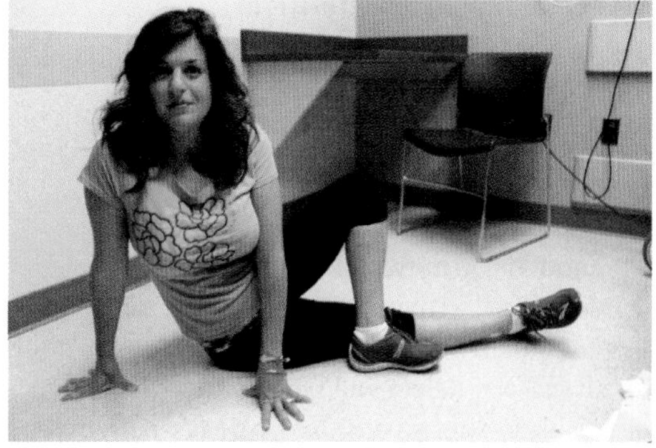

Figure 5.35. In this iliotibial band stretch, the affected leg is extended on the ground while placing the weight on the lateral aspect of the hip and getting the torso as vertical as possible.

Complications

- Left untreated and with continued activity, pain will become constant and may radiate to hip, knee, and lower leg.
- Differential should include meniscus tear, popliteus tendinosis, patellofemoral pain syndrome, and discoid lateral meniscus.

Pediatric Considerations

- For pediatric patients, careful consideration of other diagnoses is imperative.

Pearls and Pitfalls

- Rest from offending activity and stretching of iliotibial band are mainstays of treatment.
- Remember to consider other, more serious, diagnoses in the differential.

Quadriceps Hernia

General Description

- This is a muscle hernia through a defect in the overlying fascia.
- Many times a traumatic cause is found such as a collision during an athletic event or a strain of the muscle.
- Others are thought to be caused by overuse injuries.
- Many have no identifiable cause.
- Have also been called fascial herniation or pseudotumor.
- Aside from causing pain, many patients find this cosmetically unappealing and may be very anxious that it is a cancerous tumor.
- Most cases of muscle herniation occur in the anterior tibialis but rectus femoris is also a common muscle herniation.
  - Other quadriceps muscle herniations have been reported as well.

Mechanism

- Once a defect in the fascia becomes large enough for muscle to protrude through, continued activity will enlarge the defect.
- Eventually, the pressure the muscle exerts on the fascial defect will be overcome by resistance to expansion of the fascial defect.
- At that point, expansion will stop.
- If relatively small defect with large volume of muscle that has herniated, blood supply to the muscle may be restricted or even cut off completely.

Presentation

- Most patients will complain of a mass over the anterior quadriceps which gets larger during muscle contraction.
- Many are asymptomatic.
- Those that are painful may limit sport participation.
- Pain may be localized to the mass or may be more vague and diffuse in the muscle.

Physical Exam

- Typically, an ovoid mass is palpated that may or may not be tender.
- Mass will enlarge and become firm with quadriceps contraction.
- Mass should not be movable like lipomas.

Essential Diagnostics

- Ultrasound in the emergency department may be useful to identify muscle tissue in the mass
- This is largely a clinical diagnosis.
- If concern for muscle infarction, CK levels should be checked.

ED Treatment

- Splint: Not needed.
- Weight-bearing status: As tolerated
- As with other hernias, if patient is in pain and hernia is firm, attempt at reduction should be made.
  - Pain control will likely be necessary for this.

Disposition

- Admit if concerned for muscle infarction; others discharged.
- Consult orthopedics when concerned for muscle infarction to assess need for emergent fasciotomy.
- Follow-up with sports medicine physician in one to two weeks.
- Most treatment plans begin with activity modification, a compressive device, physical therapy, and NSAIDs.
- There are very little published data on conservative management.
- Recent published study looking at fasciotomy in muscle herniations is promising.[11]
- Return to work or sports could be immediate when not painful, but may need period of rest and avoidance of exercise if herniation is symptomatic.

Complications

- Large herniation with poor blood supply may cause muscle infarction.

- Will be considered by most to be cosmetically unappealing.

Pearls and Pitfalls

- Imaging may be helpful but this is largely a clinical diagnosis.
- If there is concern for muscle infarction, emergent consult to orthopedics for possible fasciotomy is necessary.

Hamstring and Quadriceps Strain or Tear

General Description

- Muscle injuries lie on a continuum upon which normal muscle is on one end and a full tear is on the other.
- Muscle strains are thought to be microtears.
- Muscle injuries are the hallmark of the "weekend warrior" and may be significantly debilitating.
- Hamstring injuries are very common in high school and college-age athletes, but proximal hamstring avulsions occur most often in the 30s and 40s.
- Quadriceps injuries are less common than hamstring injuries in young athletes but may be very common in the "weekend warrior" population.
  - Full quadriceps tears most commonly occur in the 50s and 60s and are likely associated with decreased vasculature.

Mechanism

- In strains, a sudden contraction overcomes the strength of the muscle fibers and microtearing results.
- In tears, a sudden contraction overcomes the strength of the musculotendinous junction, where most muscle tears occur.
  - The "weekend warrior" has not done enough training to strengthen the musculotendinous junction but still attempts to exert maximal force.

Presentation

- Increased risk is associated with diabetes, renal failure, corticosteroid injections, hyperthyroidism, and gout.
- For tears or avulsions, instantaneous onset of severe pain with painful ambulation and movement of hip and knee.
- For strains, may still have instantaneous onset but may also have delayed onset (i.e., when waking up the morning after hard workout).
- Localized to area of injury.

Physical Exam

- Localized tenderness at site of injury
  - Quadriceps strain typically at midpoint of thigh to distal.
  - Quadriceps rupture typically at distal musculotendinous junction.
  - Hamstring strain typically at midpoint to proximal.
  - Hamstring rupture typically at proximal insertion.
- Weakness corresponding to muscle.
- For quadriceps rupture, decreased strength in extensor mechanism of knee may present with inability to lift a straight leg off the exam table when laying supine.
- Pain with passive stretch of corresponding muscle.

Essential Diagnostics

- Plain radiographs are needed to rule out bony avulsion.
- Bedside ultrasound may be useful to get real-time dynamic imaging of the muscles in action (Figures 5.36 and 5.37).
- MRI may be utilized but likely as outpatient.

ED Treatment

- Splint: Not usually needed.
  - Knee immobilizer recommended for complete quadriceps tear.
- Weight-bearing status: Full tears will likely need crutches and non-weight bearing but others may be as tolerated.
- Pain control
- Ice to the painful area
- Patients should be instructed to not stretch the muscle at this time.
  - For some reason, most patients with hamstring and quadriceps strains feel the need to stretch the muscle, but this will only increase the microtearing in the acute setting.

Disposition

- Discharge is likely.
- Orthopedics should be consulted for complete tears.
- A complete tear of a hamstring or quadriceps will likely need an early (first seven days) surgical intervention to regain prior strength and function.
- Follow-up of tears will be coordinated by the orthopedic surgeon but should occur in one to two days.
  - Follow-up of strains may occur with a sports medicine physician in the next one to two weeks.
- With a complete tear, patient should be instructed that muscle needs full rest until seen by orthopedics.
- With a strain, patient will need at least three to seven days of rest with a gradual progression in activity after that.
- Return to work or sports as tolerated with strains and only after cleared by orthopedist for a complete tear.

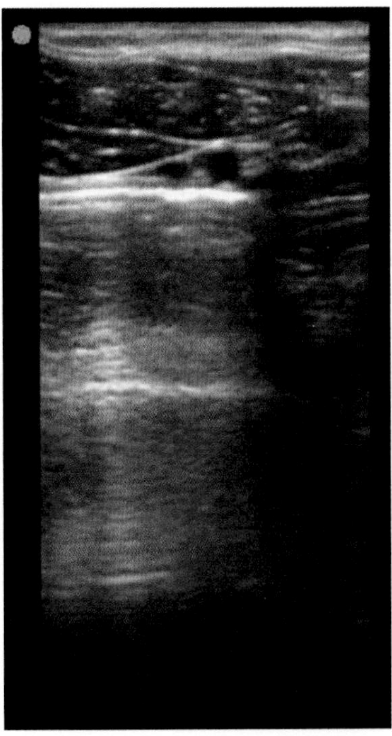

Figures 5.36. These ultrasound images show a normal muscle (Figure 5.36) and a partial muscle tear (Figure 5.37). Notice the orderly, homogeneous pattern of the normal muscle in contrast to the disorderly, heterogeneous pattern of the torn muscle. *Images courtesy of Joseph Minardi, West Virginia University.*

Complications

- A full tear that is not treated with early surgery will likely scar down and limit future strength, function, and flexibility.
- Surgery attempted after first seven days may have difficulty getting muscle back out to length and may still have associated disability.
- Many strains lead to chronic pain and recurrent strains if not permitted adequate rest and given proper rehabilitation.

Pediatric Considerations

- Due to the weakness of the physis, pediatric patients will often suffer an avulsion fracture when adult patients tear or strain a muscle so be diligent when examining radiographs in pediatric patients.

Pearls and Pitfalls

- Ultrasound or MRI are useful for diagnosing a complete tear.
- Early operative intervention is key to full recovery after a full tear of the hamstring or quadriceps.
- Closely examine radiographs to rule out avulsion fractures especially in pediatric patients.

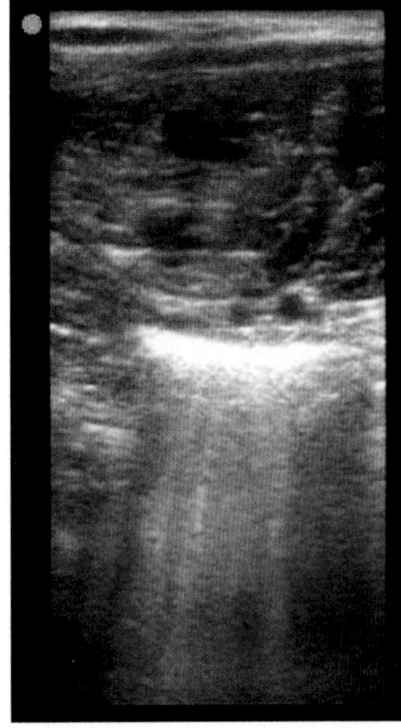

Figures 5.37.

- For hamstring and quadriceps strains in the acute setting
  - No stretching
  - Ice 15–20 minutes at a time at least four times per day
  - Rest for at least three to seven days and longer if continued severe pain
  - Progress back to full activity very slowly
  - Will benefit from physical therapy to prevent recurrent strains

Table 5.5 Indications for Orthopedic Surgery Consultation in the Emergency Department

Pelvic fracture
Hip fracture
Hip dislocation
Ischial tuberosity avulsion fracture
Femoral neck stress fracture
Slipped capital femoral epiphysis
Transient synovitis of the hip
Septic arthritis
Osteonecrosis of the hip
Hamstring full tear
Quadriceps full tear

Recommended Reading

A. Bedi, B. Kelly. Femoroacetabular impingement. *J Bone Joint Surg Am.* 2013; **95**(1): 82–92.

J. J. Minardi, O. M. Lander. Septic hip arthritis: Diagnosis and arthrocentesis using bedside ultrasound. *J Emerg Med.* 2012; **43**(2): 316–8.

A. Brown, S. Abrahams, D. Remedios, et al.. Sports hernia: A clinical update. *Br J Gen Pract.* 2013; **63**(608): e235–7.

T. A. Miller, K. P. White, D. C. Ross. The diagnosis and management of Piriformis Syndrome: Myths and facts. *Can J Neurol Sci.* 2012; **39**(5): 577–83.

M. M. Groh, J. Herrera. A comprehensive review of hip labral tears. *Curr Rev Musculoskelet Med.* 2009; **2**(2): 105–17.

References

1. Christmas C, Crespo CJ, Franckowiak SC, et al.. How common is hip pain among older adults? Results from the Third National Health and Nutrition Examination Survey. *J Fam Pract.* 2002; **51**(4): 345–8.
2. Dawson J, Linsell L, Zondervan K, et al.. Epidemiology of hip and knee pain and its impact on overall health status in older adults. *Rheumatology (Oxford).* 2004; **43**(4): 497–504.
3. Cecchi F, Mannoni A, Molino-Lova R, et al.. Epidemiology of hip and knee pain in a community based sample of Italian persons aged 65 and older. *Osteoarthritis Cartilage.* 2008; **16**(9): 1039–46.
4. Groh M, Herrera J. A comprehensive review of hip labral tears. *Curr Rev Musculoskelet Med.* 2009; **2**(2): 105–117.
5. Riad J, Bajelidze G, Gabos PG. Bilateral slipped capital femoral epiphysis: Predictive factors for contralateral slip. *J Pediatr Orthop.* 2007; **27**(4): 411–4.
6. Hagglund G, Hansson LI, Ordeberg G, Sandstrom S. Bilaterality in slipped upper femoral epiphysis. *J Bone Joint Surg Br.* 1988; **70**(2): 179–81.
7. Matava MJ, Patton CM, Luhmann S. Knee pain as the initial symptom of slipped capital femoral epiphysis: An analysis of initial presentation and treatment. *J Pediatr Orthop.* 1999; **19**(4): 455–60.
8. Mukamel M, Litmanovitch M, Yosipovich Z. Legg-Calve-Perthes disease following transient synovitis. How often? *Clin Pediatr (Phila).* 1985; **24**(11): 629–31.
9. Hospodar PP, Ashman ES, Traub JA. Anatomic study of the lateral femoral cutaneous nerve with respect to the ilioinguinal surgical dissection. *J Orthop Trauma.* 1999; **12**(1): 17–9.
10. Linenger JM, West LA. Epidemiology of soft-tissue/musculoskeletal injury among U.S. Marine recruits undergoing basic training. *Mil Med.* 1992; **157**(9): 491–3.
11. Kramer DE, Pace JL, Jarrett DY, et al.. Diagnosis and management of symptomatic muscle herniation of the extremities: A retrospective review. *Am J Sports Med.* 2013; **41**(9): 2174–80.

Chapter 6

Knee

Allison Lane

Background/Epidemiology

- There are more than 1 million Emergency Department (ED) visits per year for knee pain.
- Increasing number of patients presenting with knee pain due to increased activity levels and rising obesity.
- Female athlete has a higher incidence of injury rate than the male athlete.
- Given the large number of patients who present to the ED for knee pain, a clinical decision rule called the Ottawa Knee Rules has been developed to help identify patients with knee trauma that require radiographic imaging, in an attempt to reduce unnecessary radiographs.
  - This decision rule has a high sensitivity for clinically significant fractures and good inter-observer agreement.
  - Indications for x-rays in the ED based on the Ottawa Knee Rules:
    - Age 55 or older
    - Fibular head tenderness
    - Isolated patellar tenderness (no other bony tenderness)
    - Inability to flex knee to 90°
    - Inability to bear weight
      - Unable to take four steps (two steps on each leg), regardless of limping, at time of injury and at presentation

Anatomical Considerations/ Pathophysiology

- Knee is the largest joint in the body (Figures 6.1 and 6.2).
- Three articulations: patellofemoral, medial tibiofemoral, lateral tibiofemoral
- Static stabilizers: bones, menisci, ligaments, capsule, articular cartilage
- Anterior cruciate ligament (ACL) prevents anterior tibial translation
- Posterior cruciate ligament (PCL) prevents posterior tibial translation
- Medial collateral ligament (MCL) prevents excessive valgus force
- Lateral collateral ligament (LCL) prevents excessive varus force
- Medial and lateral menisci stabilize against rotational forces
- Muscle/tendon knee stabilizers: vastus medialis, vastus intermedius, vastus lateralis, rectus femoris, biceps femoris, semitendinosus, semimembranosus, (ITB), sartorius, gracilis, popliteus, gastrocnemius
- Major nerve structures: tibial nerve and common peroneal nerve branch from sciatic nerve in proximal popliteal fossa
- Major vascular structures: popliteal artery and vein run, and are tethered, in the posterior fossa
- Acute vs. chronic injury
- Extrinsic vs. intrinsic factors leading to injury
  - Extrinsic: improper shoes, hard or uneven training surface, new or increased training regimen
  - Intrinsic: ligamentous laxity, decreased muscle flexibility, muscle weakness, atypical foot alignment
- Pay special attention to the pediatric population, as there may be injury to the growth plate

Focused History and Physical Exam

- A focused history in the ED should include:
  - Injury/trauma: mechanism, pain location, time course, weight-bearing status, presence of mechanical symptoms (locking/catching), instability or giving

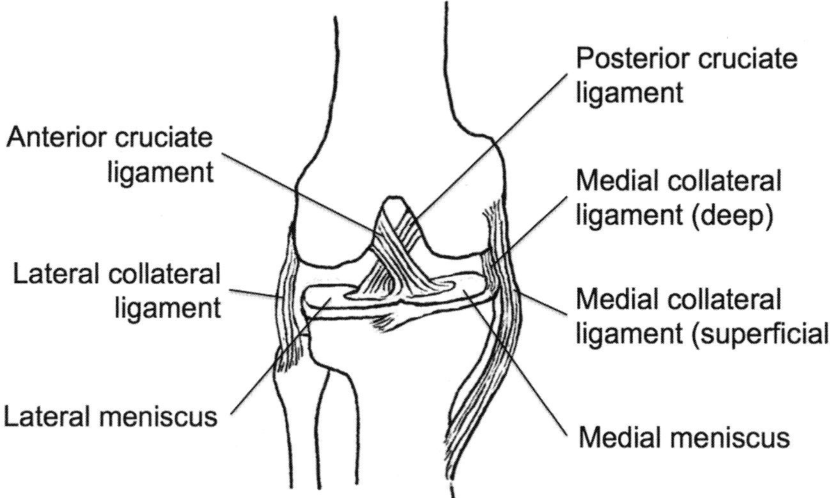

Figure 6.1. Frontal view of knee. Illustration by Yvonne Chow.

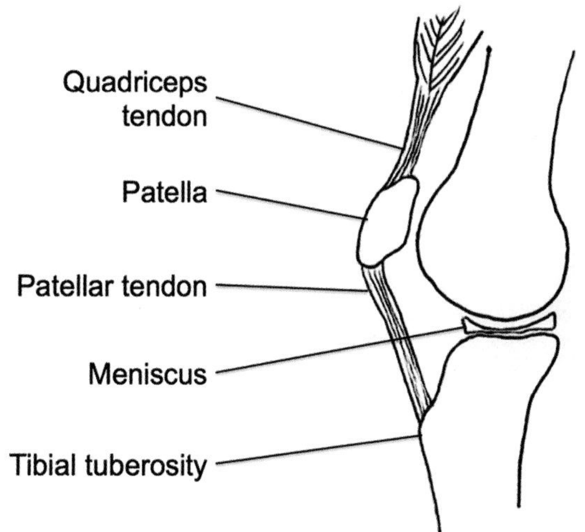

Figure 6.2. Lateral view of knee. Illustration by Yvonne Chow.

way, swelling or ecchymosis, paresthesias or weakness.

- Prior treatment: medications, physical therapy/rehab ilitation, RICE (rest, ice, compression, elevation).
- Prior history: prior injury, surgery, medical history, work history, sports history, family history.

- A focused physical exam in the ED should include:
  - Inspection: gait, alignment, skin, muscular symmetry, soft tissue swelling, effusion, ecchymosis.
  - Palpation: assess for point tenderness, effusion and increased skin warmth.
    - Make sure to palpate the medial and lateral femoral condyles and tibial plateaus, quadriceps and inferior patellar tendons, tibial tuberosity, patella, medial and lateral collateral ligaments, and medial and lateral joint lines.
    - Palpation of joint lines is best performed with the knee in slight flexion.
    - An effusion may be detected with ballottement or by sweeping the joint space.
      - Ballottement is performed by applying downward pressure on the patella towards the foot with one hand and then applying pressure on the superior pole of the patella with the other hand.
        - The test is positive if there is a sensation of bogginess felt while applying pressure on the patella.
      - Sweeping the joint space is performed by sweeping either the medial or lateral joint space and looking for a fluid wave, or bulge, on the other side.
- Range of motion: active and passive range of motion, evaluation for crepitus, patellar tracking
  - Normal flexion: 130–150°
  - Normal extension: 0–10°
- Special testing: bony, muscular, ligament, meniscus
  - ACL

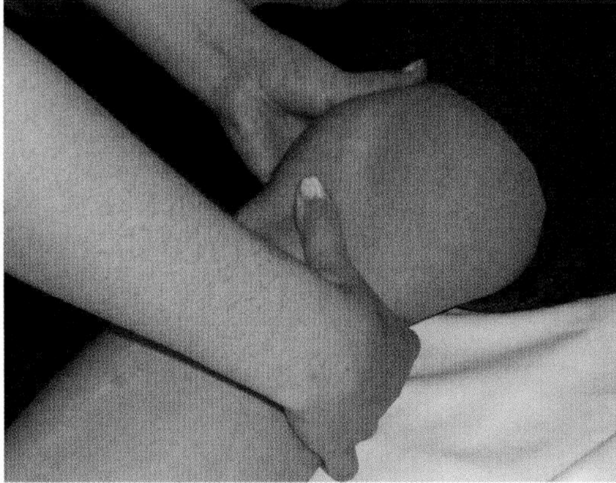

Figure 6.3. Lachman test.

- *Lachman test* (most sensitive) (Figure 6.3)
  - May be difficult to perform in the acute setting, and is operator dependent.
  - Patient supine, knee flexed 20–30°, stabilize distal femur with one hand, apply anterior force to proximal tibia with other hand.
  - The test is positive if there is subluxation of tibia anteriorly with no firm endpoint.
- *Pivot shift test* (highest positive predictive value, but only in a patient without guarding)
  - Patient supine, knee fully extended, internally rotate foot and tibia, apply mild valgus stress while flexing knee.
  - The test is positive if the tibia subluxates anteriorly at around 30° of knee flexion.

- *Anterior drawer test* (Figure 6.4)
  - Patient supine, knee flexed to 90°, stabilize foot in neutral position on the table, apply anterior force to the proximal tibia with thumbs placed along the joint line on either side of the patellar tendon.
  - The test is positive if there is subluxation of tibia anteriorly.

- PCL
  - *Posterior drawer test* (Figure 6.4)
    - Patient supine, knee flexed to 90°, foot stabilized on the table, thumbs placed along the joint line on either side of the patellar tendon, posterior force applied to the proximal tibia.

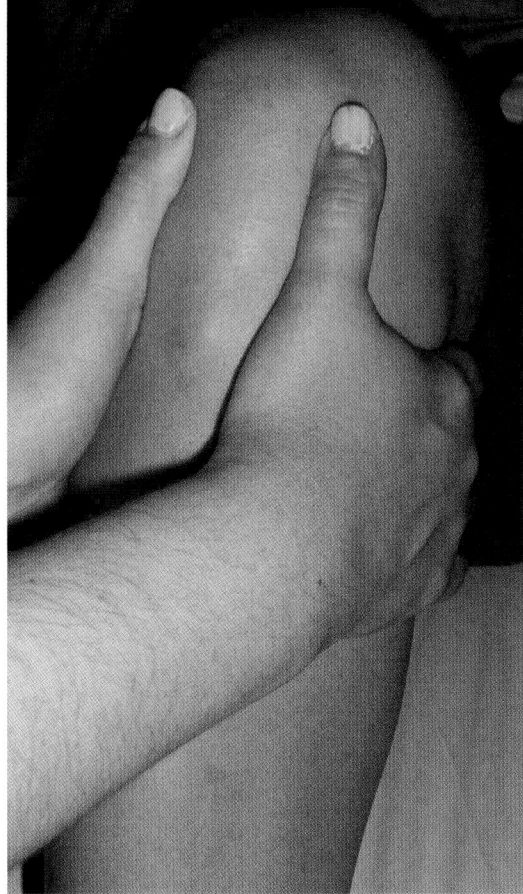

Figure 6.4. Correct positioning of hands to perform anterior and posterior drawer tests.

    - The test is positive if there is posterior subluxation of the tibia.
  - *Posterior sag test*
    - Patient supine, knees and hips flexed to 90°
    - The test is positive if there is a sagging or translation of tibia posteriorly.
  - *Dial test*
    - Assesses for both injury to the posterolateral corner structure (PLC) and PCL.
    - Patient supine, foot/tibia over side of table, femur stabilized on table, passive rotation of the tibia laterally at both 30 and 90°, compare to opposite side.
    - Look for asymmetry compared to uninjured leg at both 30 and 90°:

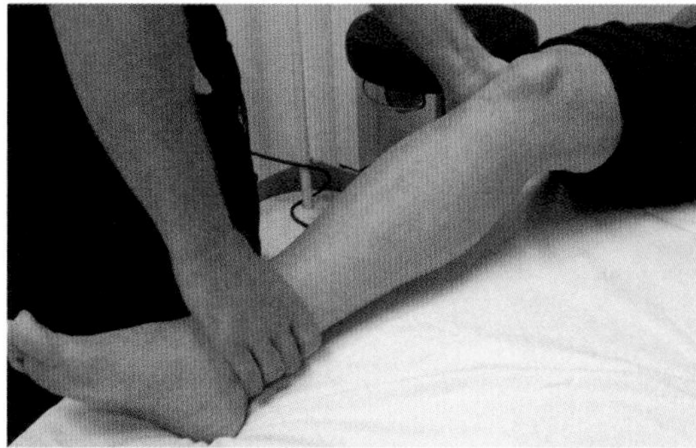

Figure 6.5. Valgus stress test.

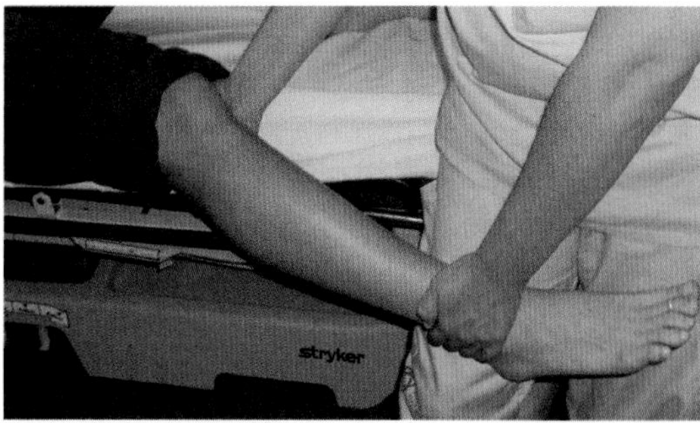

Figure 6.6. Varus stress test.

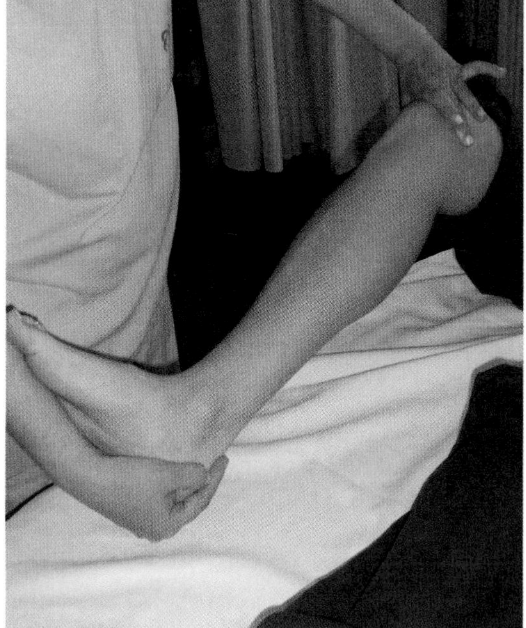

Figure 6.7. McMurray test for medial meniscus.

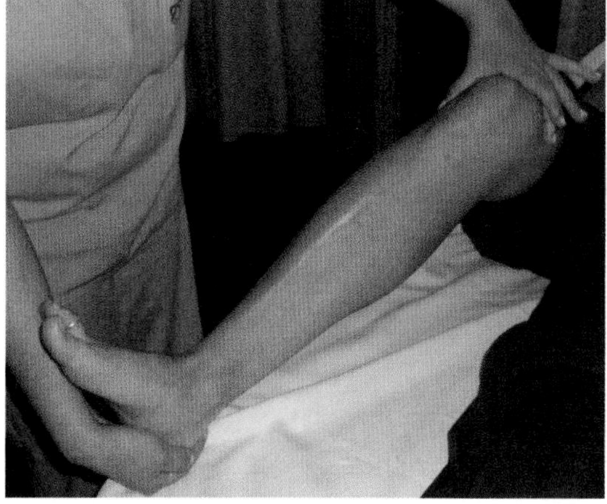

Figure 6.8. McMurray test for lateral meniscus.

    - More rotation at 30° indicates PLCS injury
    - More rotation at 90° indicates PCL injury
    - Asymmetry compared to uninjured leg at both 30 and 90° indicates both PLCS and PCL injury.

- MCL
  - *Valgus stress test* (Figure 6.5):
    - Apply valgus pressure to knee while stabilizing the ankle
    - Test with knee in 0 and 30° flexion and compare to opposite side, knee in 30° of flexion isolates superficial MCL.
    - Test is positive if there is pain and/or opening of the medial joint space.
- LCL
  - *Varus stress test* (Figure 6.6)
    - Apply varus pressure to knee while stabilizing the ankle.
    - Test with knee in 0 and 30° flexion, and compare to opposite side, knee in 30° of flexion isolates LCL.
    - Test is positive if there is pain and/or opening of the lateral joint space.
- PLCS
  - *Dial test*: see in the earlier section under PCL injury
- Menisci
  - *McMurray test* (Figures 6.7 and 6.8)
    - Patient supine, one hand holding patient's heel, other hand on the patient's joint line, maximally flex

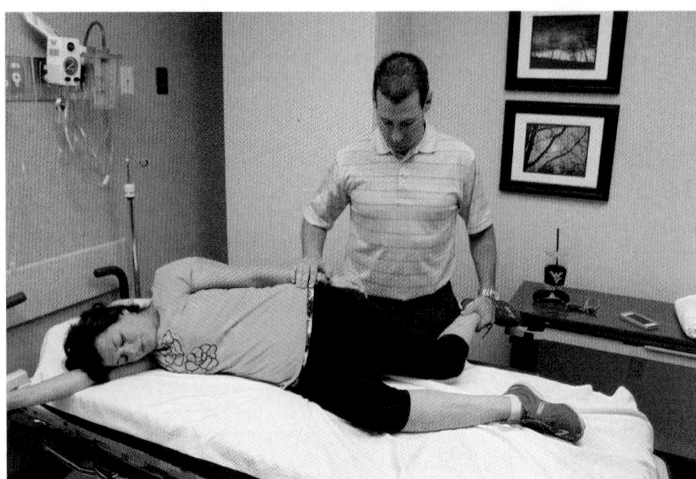

Figure 6.9. Ober's test.

knee, apply external tibial rotation (medial meniscus) or internal tibial rotation (lateral meniscus), and bring knee into full extension while maintaining rotation.
    - The test is positive if there is a painful pop/click over the appropriate joint line.
  - *Apley compression test*
    - Patient prone, knee flexed to 90°, apply downward axial load to tibia with internal (lateral meniscus) or external (medial meniscus) rotation.
    - The test is positive if there is a painful pop/click over the affected joint line.
- Patellofemoral pain syndrome
  - *Grind test*
    - Retropatellar pain with compression of the articular patellofemoral surfaces during quadriceps contraction.
    - Retropatellar pain with half or full-squat
- ITB friction syndrome
  - *Ober's test* (Figure 6.9)
    - This test is used to evaluate for ITB tightness.
    - Patient lying on side with symptomatic side up, knee resting on the exam table is flexed 45°, pelvis is at 90° to exam table and stabilized with examiner's hand, other arm supports the affected knee and then brings hip from flexion/abduction into extension/adduction, allow hip to passively adduct.

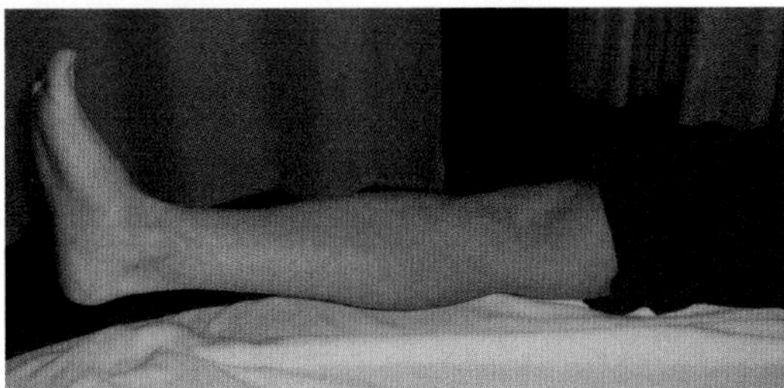

Figure 6.10. Test for integrity of extensor mechanism.

    - The test is positive if the leg does not adduct past parallel.
  - *Noble compression test*
    - Hip and knee passively flexed to 90°, apply pressure with thumb over ITB proximal to lateral femoral condyle, patient actively extends hip and knee
    - The test is positive if there is pain over distal ITB (just proximal to lateral femoral condyle) at 30° of extension.
  - Extensor mechanism (Figure 6.10)
    - Used to evaluate the integrity of the entire extensor mechanism of the knee including quadriceps, quadriceps tendon, and patellar tendon.
    - While keeping the leg extended at knee, the patient attempts to actively raise their straight leg off the exam table.
    - Inability to actively raise a straightened leg off the exam table is an indication that there has been a disruption of the extensor mechanism.

- *Patellar apprehension test* (Figure 6.11)
  - Used to assess for instability of patella after a patellar dislocation.
  - While the patient is supine, the examiner places lateral pressure on the patella while flexing the knee; test is positive if the patient contracts quadriceps, resists further attempts at manipulation of the knee, and has the same sensation of patellar instability as at the initial dislocation.
- Neurovascular exam: sensation, strength, reflexes (patellar, Achilles), pulses (popliteal, dorsalis pedis, posterior tibialis), and capillary refill
  - Nerve distribution:
    - Common peroneal nerve
      - Motor innervation for ankle dorsiflexion and great toe extension, sensation to web space between first and second toes and lateral leg
    - Saphenous nerve
      - Sensation to anteromedial aspect of the leg and foot
    - Tibial nerve
      - Sensation to posterolateral leg, lateral foot, sole of foot, and motor innervation to posterior compartment of the leg including plantarflexion, toe flexion, and weak inversion
- Skin exam
  - Check for color, warmth, erythema, or ecchymosis

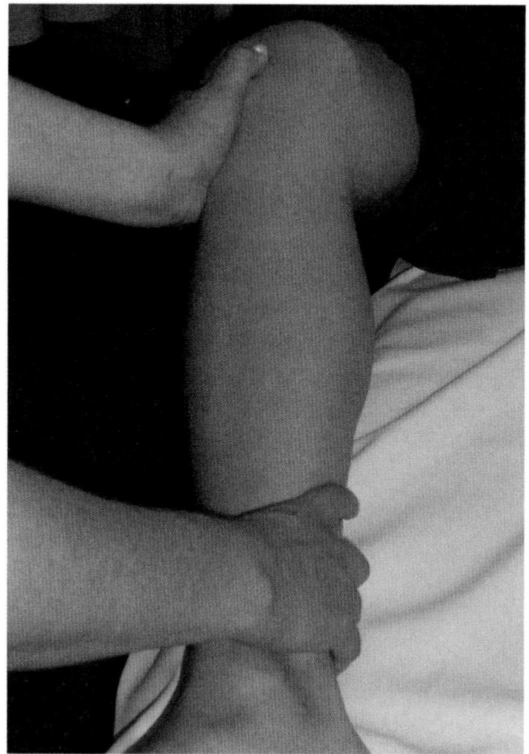

Figure 6.11. Patellar apprehension test.

Differential Diagnosis – Emergent and Common Diagnoses

Patellar Fracture

General Description

- Patella is the largest sesamoid bone.
- Patella increases leverage and efficiency of the quadriceps muscle.
- Typically triangular, apex pointing distally
- Rectus femoris and vastus muscles insert on proximal pole.
- Patellar ligament attaches to distal pole of patella, inserts on tibial tuberosity.
- Quadriceps tendon passes over patella, joins patellar ligament distally.
- Fracture classified by fracture pattern or location.
  - Location: lower, middle, or upper pole
  - Pattern: transverse, stellate or comminuted, vertical, and osteochondral

Table 6.1. Emergent and Common Diagnoses in the Emergency Department

Emergent Diagnoses	Common Diagnoses
Patellar fracture	ACL injury
Patellar dislocation	MCL injury
Extensor mechanism disruption	Meniscus injury
Proximal tibiofibular joint dislocation	Patellar tendinopathy
Total knee dislocation	Patellofemoral pain syndrome
Tibial plateau fracture	Popliteal cyst
Pre-patellar septic bursitis	Osteoarthritis
Septic arthritis	
Pediatric physis injury	

    - Transverse most common, stellate next common
    - Transverse typically lower third of patella
    - Vertical typically along the margins of the patella
    - Osteochondral fracture involving medial patellar facet may occur after patellar dislocation or subluxation.
- May be displaced or nondisplaced.
- Normal variants that may be mistaken for a fracture
  - Bipartite patella
    - Persistence of an accessory ossification center that fails to fuse in childhood
    - May involve inferior, lateral, or superolateral (most common) margin
    - Usually asymptomatic and able to differentiate from patellar fracture by history and physical exam
    - This is best seen on AP view
      - Has well-defined zone of separation
      - View of opposite knee usually confirms this diagnosis, as bipartite patella may be bilateral
  - Fabella
    - Small sesamoid bone in the tendons posterior to knee joint
    - Best seen on lateral view

Mechanism

- May be caused by direct or indirect forces
  - Direct forces include fall onto anterior knee or striking knee on dashboard.
    - Typical fracture pattern is stellate and nondisplaced
  - Indirect forces include forceful quadriceps muscle contraction usually in an attempt to prevent a fall.
    - This force may exceed the intrinsic strength of the patella leading to fracture.
    - With repeated quadriceps contraction there is tearing of the medial and lateral retinacula resulting in displacement.
    - Typical fracture pattern is transverse and displaced.

Presentation

- Pain and swelling over anterior knee after injury
- Inability to fully extend the knee

Physical Exam

- Tenderness and soft tissue swelling over patella
- Effusion likely
- Displaced fracture may have palpable defect or separation if swelling not excessive
- Evaluate for disruption of the extensor mechanism (Figure 6.10)

Essential Diagnostics

- Obtain an x-ray of the knee including AP, lateral, oblique, and sunrise views
  - Lateral view is most useful in delineating fracture lines and determining displacement, especially for transverse fractures
  - Separation of more than 3 mm between fragments or articular step-off more than 2 mm constitutes a displaced fracture
  - Marginal vertical fractures best seen on sunrise views

ED Treatment

- Ice, compression, elevation to decrease swelling
- Nondisplaced fractures with intact extensor mechanism may be placed in a knee immobilizer in full extension and allowed to weight bear as tolerated.
- Orthopedic surgery consult indicated for displaced, open, or severely comminuted fractures, or any patella fracture with a disrupted extensor mechanism.

Disposition

- Nondisplaced patellar fractures with extensor mechanism intact may be discharged.
  - Patient should be instructed to follow-up with sports medicine or orthopedic surgery within five to seven days.
- Return to work
  - May return as tolerated based upon requirements.

  - Sedentary jobs: may return after a few days of rest, ice, compression, elevation, though consider waiting until after first follow-up appointment (five to seven days).
  - Jobs requiring knee flexion: even climbing stairs, should not return until cast or brace is discontinued and range of motion has progressed to allow for ability to perform these activities with reasonable comfort, which is typically six to eight weeks.
- Return to sport
  - May begin activities requiring little knee flexion soon after immobilization.
  - Begin straight leg raises, and ankle range of motion while in immobilizer.
  - No clearance for return until fracture has healed, typically six to eight weeks, with no pain and normal strength and range of motion.
- Displaced, severely comminuted, or open patellar fractures should be admitted for surgical repair by orthopedic surgery.

Complications

- Infection
- Loss of reduction or failure of internal fixation
- Avascular necrosis
- Delayed union, nonunion, malunion
- Chondromalacia
- Osteoarthritis
- Stiffness and weakness
- Extensor mechanism disruption

Pediatric Considerations

- Patella ossifies in early childhood, first visible on radiographs between ages 3 and 6.
  - Up to six ossification centers, correlate with clinical exam for tenderness and obtain comparison view of normal knee.
- Unlike adults, knee effusions are rarely due to ligamentous injury.
  - Patellar dislocation or fracture is much more likely.
- MRI or arthroscopy may be required for adequate evaluation because fracture may primarily involve cartilage.
- Most patellar fractures in children are osteochondral or avulsion injuries.
- Osteochondral fractures usually result from patellar dislocations, occurring in about 10 percent of dislocations.
- Patellar sleeve fractures
  - Usually results from high-impact jumping activity.
  - Type of osteochondral avulsion fracture of the patella.
  - Patellar avulsion fracture, which includes a large amount of articular cartilage and retinaculum.
  - Will often see a high-riding patella on lateral knee x-ray.
- Orthopedic consult is indicated for children with patella sleeve fractures, displaced avulsion fractures, or avulsion fractures complicated by inability to fully extend the knee.
- Obtain MRI in a child if there is concern for disruption of the extensor mechanism.

Pearls and Pitfalls

- Always make sure to check integrity of the extensor mechanism.
- Beware of what appear to be small patella avulsion fractures in pediatric patients because they often represent a much larger injury.

Patellar Dislocation

General Description

- Typically underlying patellofemoral malalignment.
  - Factors that increase risk of subluxation or dislocation include shallow femoral groove, hypoplasia of lateral femoral condyle, small or high-riding patella, genu valgum, external tibial torsion, atrophy of vastus medialis muscle.
- Nearly all occur laterally

Mechanism

- Several mechanisms may result in patellar dislocation:
  - External pivotal motion on partially flexed knee followed by a forceful contraction of the quadriceps that pulls the patella laterally.

- Sudden cutting motion or sudden contraction of quadriceps during deceleration.
- Direct blow to medial patella forcing it laterally.
- Spontaneous reduction, knee went out of place and slipped back after extension of the knee.

Presentation

- Acute knee pain and swelling after injury.
- Patient will often report that they felt or heard "a pop."
- Patient may not present with an obvious deformity if the patella has spontaneously reduced prior to ED presentation.

Physical Exam

- If there is an obvious deformity, the patella is typically laterally displaced.
- Patient will often have an effusion.
- Tenderness over medial retinaculum and lateral femoral condyle.
- Positive *apprehension test* (Figure 6.11).
- Assess integrity of extensor mechanism (Figure 6.10).

Essential Diagnostics

- Knee x-rays should include AP, lateral, oblique, and sunrise views.
- Pre- and post-reduction x-rays to rule out accompanying fracture, even if spontaneous reduction.
    - Pay particular attention to the medial edge of the patella to evaluate for osteochondral fracture.

ED Treatment

- Any patient with a laterally displaced patella will need reduction.
    - Patient should be placed in either a supine or seated position.
    - Hip is flexed to decrease tension on the quadriceps.
    - Gradually extend the knee while gently pushing patella medially.
    - The same technique is used for a medially displaced patella, except apply an anterolateral force to the patella.
- Ice, compression, elevation to decrease swelling.
- Place patient in a knee immobilizer to limit knee flexion.
- May weight bear as tolerated.
- Crutches as needed for ambulation.

Disposition

- Most patellar dislocations may be discharged as long as they are successfully reduced and there is no associated fracture.
- Follow-up may be with either sports medicine or orthopedic surgery within seven days.
    - Initial patella dislocations are usually managed conservatively with bracing and functional strengthening and conditioning.
- Recurrent dislocations may need operative stabilization of patella.
- Return to work or school based on job requirements, as the patient is able.
- Rehabilitation
    - Early isometric quadriceps exercises to maintain strength.
    - Early range of motion exercises when pain and swelling decreased (usually seven to ten days).
    - Resistance exercises of quadriceps once full range of motion is achieved.
- Return to sport after full, pain-free range of motion, full strength, and sport-specific agility progression program.

Complications

- Recurrent dislocation
- Degenerative arthritis
- Osteochondral fracture
- Osteoarthritis

Pediatric Considerations

- Unlike adults, knee effusions are rarely due to ligamentous injury.
    - Patellar dislocation or fracture is much more likely.
- Recommend orthopedic surgery consultation if there is an associated osteochondral fracture.
- Obtain MRI if x-rays are normal but child is unable to perform a straight leg raise.

Pearls and Pitfalls

- Lateral patella dislocation is most common.

- Consider this diagnosis in any patient with suggestive history even if the patella is not displaced on exam as the patella may have spontaneously reduced prior to presentation.
- Reduction is generally safe and simple.
- Obtain x-rays to look for osteochondral fractures.
- Check integrity of extensor mechanism

Disruption of the Extensor Mechanism

General Description

- Disruption of the extensor mechanism of the knee includes quadriceps tendon rupture, patellar tendon rupture, tibial tubercle avulsion fracture.
- Quadriceps tendon rupture typically occurs in patients greater than 40 years old at bone-tendon junction, and is more common than patellar tendon rupture.
- Patellar tendon rupture typically occurs in patients less than 40 years old, and is most common at inferior pole of patella.
- Tibial tubercle avulsion fractures occur most commonly in pediatric patients.
- Tendon rupture may be partial or complete.
- Risk factors include: systemic inflammatory disease, chronic renal disease, diabetes, tendinopathy, corticosteroid injection, anabolic steroids, chronic degeneration, history of prior ACL repair using patellar tendon autograft.

Mechanism

- Several mechanisms may lead to disruption of the extensor mechanism:
    - Sudden, forceful contraction of quadriceps during vertical or horizontal deceleration, that is, jumping sports.
    - Direct trauma to anterior knee, especially in younger patients.
    - Patellar tendon rupture usually occurs due to a tensile overload of the extensor mechanism.
        - Most occur with knee in flexed position, greater than 60°.
        - Increased risk if history of patellar tendon allograft for repair of prior ACL injury.
    - Quadriceps tendon rupture usually occurs due to an eccentric contraction of the quadriceps muscle.
        - Most often occurs with the foot planted and the knee slightly bent.

Presentation

- A “pop” may have been heard during injury.
- Difficulty weight-bearing
- Patellar tendon rupture: infrapatellar pain
- Quadriceps tendon rupture: suprapatellar pain

Physical Exam

- Effusion
- Tenderness over injured tendon
- May be able to palpate defect.
    - A gap may be present below inferior pole of patella in patellar tendon disruption.
    - A gap may be present superior to patella in quadriceps tendon rupture.
- Loss of extension
    - A partial tendon injury does not extend into retinaculum, and patient may be able to extend against gravity.
        - May, however, still have an extensor lag.
    - A full-thickness tendon injury will result in the patient being unable to perform an active straight leg raise or maintain a passively extended knee (Figure 6.10).

Essential Diagnostics

- X-ray views should include AP, lateral, oblique, and sunrise views.
    - The AP and lateral views are the best views to assess patella height and position, as well as possible associated fracture pattern.
        - The Insall–Salvati ratio may be used to assess patellar height.
            - This is the ratio of length of patella to length of patellar tendon.
            - Measured on lateral x-ray with knee flexed 30°.
                - Normal ratio is 1:1
                - Consider patella alta, which may be an indication of patellar tendon rupture, if ratio is less than 0.8.
                - Consider patella baja, which may be an indication of quadriceps tendon rupture, if ratio is greater than 1.2.
    - The sunrise view may be used to further delineate fracture displacement and osteochondral defects.
- Ultrasound may be used to look for tendon continuity.

ED Treatment

- Knee should be placed in a knee immobilizer in extension.
- Consult orthopedic surgery for tibial tubercle avulsion fractures or complete tendon ruptures.
  - Complete tendon ruptures need urgent repair or reconstruction and are most successful if performed within fourteen days from initial injury.
- Partial tendon ruptures with intact extensor mechanism may be placed in a knee immobilizer in full extension, allowed to weight bear as tolerated, and may begin early range of motion.

Disposition

- Patients with complete tendon ruptures will likely require admission or urgent orthopedic surgery follow-up for surgical repair or reconstruction.
- Patients with partial tendon ruptures may be discharged home.
  - Patients should follow-up with sports medicine or orthopedics within seven days for repeat evaluation.
- Return to work or sports depends on degree of tear and operative management
  - Patients may return to sport after partial tears when they are pain free and have regained full range of motion and normal strength.
  - Patients with full tears who require operative treatment may generally return to sport in nine to twelve months after repair and completion of a rehabilitation program.

Complications

- Re-rupture
- Persistent quadriceps atrophy and weakness
- Loss of motion/stiffness
- Functional impairment

Pediatric Considerations

- It is important to evaluate pediatric patients for tibial tubercle avulsion fracture if they present with a disruption in their extensor mechanism.
  - This is an avulsion fracture of tibial tuberosity, Salter–Harris type III of proximal tibial physis.
  - May present with either complete or partial disruption of the extensor mechanism.
  - Best seen on lateral view with patella alta depending on displacement of tuberosity.
  - Consider in adolescents.
  - Often occurs during jumping.
  - May be confused with Osgood–Schlatter disease, which has more insidious onset.
  - Compartment syndrome may be a complication.
  - Orthopedic surgery should be consulted in all cases as surgical repair may be required.

Pearls and Pitfalls

- Always evaluate the integrity of the extensor mechanism after acute knee injuries.
- When there is a deficit in the extensor mechanism, be sure to consider quadriceps tendon ruptures, especially in patients greater than 40 years old, patellar tendon ruptures in patients less than 40 years old, and tibial tubercle avulsion injury in adolescents.

ACL Injury

General Description

- Origin at posteromedial aspect of intercondylar notch of lateral femoral condyle.
- Insertion in front of intercondylar eminence of tibia and medial to anterior horn of lateral meniscus.
- Functions as the primary restraint of anterior translation of tibia on femur.
- Secondary restraint to internal rotation of the tibia when knee is in full extension.
- Associated with meniscal injury, lateral meniscus tear more common with ACL injury.
- The classic unhappy triad consists of ACL tear and medial meniscus and MCL injury.

Mechanism

- Usually low-energy, noncontact injury that occurs with deceleration, hyperextension, or rotational force at the knee.

Presentation

- Patient may have noticed a "pop."
- May have been unable to bear weight initially.
- Swelling usually occurs within hours.
- Often complain of a sensation of giving way or instability.

Physical Exam

- Effusion usually present
  - Often presents with large effusion, but on occasion may have little to no effusion, especially in younger patients.
- Guards or limits active extension of knee to avoid activation of the quadriceps muscle which may cause pain and/or symptoms of instability.
- *Lachman* (Figure 6.3), *anterior drawer* (Figure 6.4), and *pivot shift tests* are often positive.
  - These tests may be falsely negative in patients with significant pain and guarding after acute injury.

Essential Diagnostics

- Knee x-rays should include AP, oblique, and lateral views to exclude underlying bony injury.
  - Usually only show indirect evidence of ACL tear, but often normal.
    - Effusion may be visible.
    - May have bony avulsion of anterior tibial intercondylar eminence.
    - May have a Segond fracture, which is an avulsion fracture of lateral aspect of tibial condyle and pathognomonic for ACL injury.
- MRI often used to confirm ACL injury, and look for associated injuries such as meniscal tear or osteochondral lesions.
  - This is not needed emergently in the ED and may be performed as an outpatient.

ED Treatment

- Ice, compression, elevation to decrease swelling.
- Activity modification, rest
- Crutches if needed for ambulation, weight bear as tolerated.
- Knee immobilizer only if instability symptoms for short period of time (i.e., seven to ten days).
  - Prolonged immobilization may complicate rehabilitation.

Disposition

- Almost all ACL injuries may be discharged from the ED.
- Emergent orthopedic consult is not indicated.
- Patients may follow-up as an outpatient with orthopedic surgery or sports medicine.
  - Reconstruction is indicated for most, but usually delayed three to six weeks post injury.
- Patients may return to work or school as tolerated based on job requirements.
- Patients may return to play after reconstruction following normalization of range of motion and strength and progression of sport-specific activities without pain or instability, usually after six to nine months.

Complications

- Chronic instability, especially if not surgically repaired
- Multiligamentous injury
- Meniscal injury
- Loss of motion/muscle weakness
- Osteoarthritis

Pediatric Considerations

- Strongly consider surgery for ACL tear, as activity limitation not realistic in children.
- Consider tibial spine fracture in late childhood to mid-adolescence.
  - Consider with mechanism that would cause ACL injury in adults.
  - Usually associated with bicycling after a foot gets caught in spokes of the wheel.
  - May also occur after hyperextension of knee during a fall.
  - Nondisplaced fracture in long-leg cast for five to six weeks, with knee in 5–10° of flexion.
  - Consult orthopedics if there is a displaced fracture.

Pearls and Pitfalls

- *Lachman*, *anterior drawer*, and *pivot shift tests* are used to diagnose ACL tears, however may be falsely negative acutely and are operator dependent.
- Knee immobilizers are only indicated for patients with symptoms of instability and should only be used for a short period of time (seven to ten days).
- Often associated with other injuries, such as meniscal tears.

PCL Injury

General description

- Origin at anterolateral aspect of medial femoral condyle.
- Inserts on posterior tibia, below the articular surface.
- It functions as the primary restraint of posterior translation of tibia and secondary restraint of external rotation of tibia.
- May be associated with other injuries
  - Consider PLC when associated injuries occur, that is, common peroneal nerve or vascular injury.

Mechanism

- Several mechanisms may lead to injury to the PCL
  - Hyperextension, hyperflexion with plantar-flexed ankle, or rotational stress to knee.
  - Posteriorly directed force to anterior proximal tibia with flexed knee after direct blow, that is, car dashboard or contact sports.

Presentation

- Posterior knee pain
- May have knee instability with ambulation

Physical Exam

- Effusion
- Tenderness in popliteal fossa
- Hyperextension of the knee compared to opposite side
- Positive *posterior drawer test* (Figure 6.4)
  - Grade I (partial) injury: 1- to 5-mm posterior tibial translation, tibia anterior to femoral condyles.
  - Grade II (complete isolated) injury: 6- to 10-mm posterior tibial translation, anterior tibia flush with femoral condyles.
  - Grade III (PCL and capsuloligamentous) injury: greater than 10-mm translation, tibial plateau displaced posterior to the condyles, often associated ACL and/or PLCS (see later) injury.
- Positive *posterior sag test*
- Also important to assess integrity of PLC with *dial test*.

Essential Diagnostics

- X-rays should include AP, oblique, and lateral views
  - May see avulsion fractures with acute injuries, that is, bony avulsion from proximal tibia.
- Lateral stress view may be obtained:
  - Asymmetric posterior tibial displacement indicates PCL injury.
  - Difference greater than 12 mm suggests combined PCL and PLC injury.
- MRI is often used to confirm PCL injury and evaluate for other associated injuries.
  - Usually not needed emergently in the ED and may be obtained as an outpatient.

ED Treatment

- Ice, compression, and elevation to decrease swelling.
- Activity modification, rest
- Crutches to assist in ambulation, weight bear as tolerated.
- Grade III injuries: knee immobilization in extension for two to four weeks.
- Grade I and II injuries: hinged knee brace with early quadriceps strengthening.

Disposition

- Almost all patients with PCL injuries may be discharged safely from the ED.
- Orthopedic consult is not needed emergently in the ED.
- Patients should follow-up with sports medicine or orthopedics in seven days.
  - Isolated PCL injuries are usually treated conservatively with a rehabilitation program.
  - Combined ligamentous injuries and grade II or III injury with bony avulsion may require surgical repair/reconstruction.
  - Surgical repair/reconstruction may be needed for chronic PCL injury with continued functional instability despite rehabilitation.
- Patients may return to work or school as tolerated based on job requirements.
- Patients may return to play after rehabilitation program, with ability to perform sports-

specific drills without pain or instability, generally two to four weeks for grade I and II injuries.

Complications

- PLC injuries
- Multiligamentous injury
- Popliteal artery injury
- Chronic pain/osteoarthritis

Pediatric Considerations

- Rare, usually treated conservatively

Pearls and Pitfalls

- Perform *posterior drawer* and *posterior sag tests* for diagnosis.
- Consider associated PLC injury in suspected PCL injuries.

MCL Injury

General Description

- Primary and secondary valgus stabilizer of the knee.
- Originates from medial femoral epicondyle anterior to adductor tubercle.
- Inserts on anteromedial tibia below the joint line.
- Most commonly injured knee ligament.
- Composed of superficial and deep layers.
  - Deep layer has fibers that attach to the medial meniscus.

Mechanism

- Valgus force on partially flexed knee.
- External rotational force on tibia relative to the femur.

Presentation

- Acute medial knee pain
- May have noticed an associated "pop" to medial side of knee.
- Unlikely to have large knee effusion or instability with isolated MCL injury.

Physical Exam

- Medial knee soft tissue swelling
- Possible small effusion
- Medial joint line and MCL tenderness
- Positive *valgus stress test* (Figure 6.5)
  - Laxity with knee in full extension (0°) suggests associated injury to ACL, posterior oblique ligament, posteromedial capsule.
  - Grade I sprain (stretch injury): pain along MCL during valgus testing at 30°, with minimal laxity (0- to 5-mm opening).
  - Grade II sprain (partial tear): laxity with 5- to 10-mm joint space opening, firm endpoint present, with valgus testing at 30°.
  - Grade III sprain (complete tear): gross laxity (greater than 10-mm opening) with soft endpoint or no endpoint, with valgus testing at 30°.
- Assess integrity of saphenous nerve
  - Injury may cause numbness to infrapatellar region that is worse with flexion of the knee or with compression.

Essential Diagnostics

- X-rays of the knee including AP, oblique, and lateral views to exclude other associated bony injuries.
  - X-ray may show avulsion fracture of medial femoral condyle.
    - Pellegrini–Stieda lesion is a calcification from prior injury at the medial femoral condyle.
- MRI may be obtained on nonemergent basis as an outpatient to further characterize MCL or associated injury.
  - Grade I tears show edema around the ligament.
  - Grade II tears show displacement of ligament fibers.
  - Grade III tears show complete loss of continuity of ligament.

ED Treatment

- Ice, compression, elevation to decrease swelling.
- Activity modification, rest
- Crutches if needed for ambulation, weight bear as tolerated.
- Stabilizing brace for stage II and III sprains to assist with sensation of instability and during rehabilitation.

Disposition

- Patients may be discharged from the ED and do not require emergent orthopedic consult.
- Follow-up with sports medicine or orthopedics in seven days.
- Most injuries are managed conservatively with a rehabilitation program.
- Surgical repair considered acutely if multiligamentous injury, displaced distal avulsion fractures, entrapment of torn end of medial compartment.
- Surgical repair considered sub-acutely if continued instability with conservative management.
- May return to work or school as tolerated based on job requirements.
- May return to sport after functional training program, full range of motion and strength, sport-specific drills, with minimal or no pain and without instability.
  - Grade I sprain: immediate range of motion exercises, quadriceps and hamstring training, return to play in five to seven days.
  - Grade II sprain: one week of rest before range of motion and strengthening, return to play in two to four weeks.
  - Grade III sprain: one week of rest before range of motion and strengthening, return to play in four to eight weeks.

Complications

- Multiligamentous injuries
- Meniscal injury
- Loss of motion/stiffness
- Saphenous nerve injury
- Continued laxity, especially with distal MCL injuries

Pediatric Considerations

- Consider obtaining valgus stress views on x-ray to help detect physeal injury.

Pearls and Pitfalls

- Perform *valgus stress test* to assess integrity of MCL.
- Check for associated saphenous nerve injury.

LCL and PLC Injury

General description

- LCL is the primary restraint to varus stress at 5 and 25° of knee flexion.
- LCL is taut at full extension and lax after 30° flexion.
- Originates on lateral femoral condyle
- Inserts onto anterolateral fibular head
- Isolated injury to LCL uncommon
  - Typically associated with PLC injury
- PLC components resist varus stresses, external tibial rotation, and less so, posterior tibial translation.
- PLC has three layers
  - First layer includes ITB and biceps femoris tendon.
    - Common peroneal nerve lays between layers I and II
  - Second layer includes patellar retinaculum and lateral patellofemoral ligament.
  - Third layer includes LCL (superficial), popliteus muscle and tendon, popliteofibular ligament, arcuate ligament, lateral capsular fibers.

Mechanism

- Often results from excessive varus stress, hyperextension, and/or external tibial rotation.

Presentation

- Acute onset of lateral knee pain after injury
- Feeling of instability with knee in full extension, may have buckling into hyperextension.
- Difficulty going up and down stairs
- Difficulty with cutting and pivoting

Physical Exam

- Pain and soft tissue swelling to the lateral knee, anywhere along lateral femoral condyle to fibular head
- *Varus stress test* positive (Figure 6.6)
  - Grade I sprain (minimal): mild lateral knee pain but minimal laxity (0- to 5-mm opening) with varus stressing in 30° flexion

- Grade II sprain (partial): 5- to 10-mm joint space opening, firm endpoint, with varus stressing at 30°
- Grade III sprain (complete): greater than 10-mm opening, soft endpoint, with varus stressing at 30°, associated with other PLC or cruciate ligament injuries
- Laxity, joint opening in full extension (at 0°) suggests combined LCL and/or ACL/PCL injury

- Further evaluate for PLC injury with the *dial test*
- Neurological exam to evaluate common peroneal nerve injury in LCL/PLCS injuries
- Injury to peroneal nerve may result in numbness/tingling to lateral leg and weakness with ankle dorsiflexion

Essential Diagnostics

- Knee x-rays should include AP, oblique, and lateral views.
- MRI may be obtained nonemergently as an outpatient to further characterize injury severity and location.

ED Treatment

- Ice, compression, elevation to reduce swelling
- Crutches if needed for ambulation, weight bear as tolerated.
- Stabilizing brace for stage II and III sprains to assist with stability and during rehabilitation.

Disposition

- Patients with LCL and/or PLC injuries may be discharged home and do not require orthopedic consult while in the ED.
- Patients may follow-up with sports medicine or orthopedics as an outpatient.
  - Some PLC injuries may require early surgical repair or reconstruction.
- May return to work or school as tolerated based on job requirements.
- May return to play after functional training program, full range of motion and strength, sport-specific drills, with minimal or no pain and without instability.

Complications

- Associated PLC injury
- Peroneal nerve injury
- Multiligamentous injuries
- Stiffness
- Persistent laxity

Pediatric Considerations

- Consider obtaining stress views on x-ray to help detect physeal injury.

Pearls and Pitfalls

- Perform *varus stress test* to assess LCL injuries
- Perform the *dial test* to assess for associated PLC injury.
- Always perform a thorough neurovascular exam with particular attention to the integrity of the peroneal nerve.

Meniscus Injury

General Description

- Fibrocartilaginous discs that help with load transmission between femoral and tibial condyles.
- Include medial and lateral menisci.
- Injuries may be acute or degenerative.
  - Degenerative meniscal tears are common in patients with underlying osteoarthritis and result from a decrease in meniscal elasticity.
- Patients age less than 30 typically sustain acute, traumatic tears located in the periphery.
- Patients age greater than 30 typically have degenerative tears, which are usually located in the posterior horn of medial meniscus.
- Medial meniscus tears more common than lateral.
- Lateral tear associated with acute ACL injury.

Mechanism

- Acute tears are usually traumatic and result from a twisting injury or direct blow.
- Degenerative tears may occur due to minor trauma or may develop insidiously.

Presentation

- Acute tears
  - Acute pain to medial or lateral joint line after an injury, may have heard a "pop."
  - May describe locking, popping, or clicking
  - May have swelling.
- Degenerative tears

- Insidious onset of pain
- Typically no mechanical symptoms (locking, catching)
- May have swelling with activity

Physical Exam

- Acute tears:
  - May have effusion
  - May be unable to passively extend the knee if large, displaced flap
  - Joint line tenderness is best palpated with knee bent to 90°
  - *McMurray test* is often positive (Figures 6.7 and 6.8)
  - *Apley compression test* is often positive
- Degenerative tears:
  - Typically normal range of motion
  - May have effusion
  - Tenderness over respective joint line
  - *McMurray* and *Apley compression tests* may cause pain, though typically no pop/click
  - Common with underlying osteoarthritis

Essential Diagnostics

- Knee x-rays should include AP, oblique, and lateral views
  - Generally normal in young patients with acute injury
  - Evaluate for fracture or osteochondral loose body
  - Obtain weight-bearing films if concern for degenerative meniscal tear
  - May have joint space narrowing and osteoarthritis.
- MRI may be obtained nonemergently as an outpatient for evaluation of an acute meniscal tear to further characterize injury.

ED Treatment

- Acute tears
  - Ice, compression, elevation to decrease swelling
  - Activity modification, rest
  - Crutches as needed for ambulation, weight bear as tolerated
- Degenerative tears
  - Activity modification, ice, compression, elevation
  - Pain management with nonsteroidal anti-inflammatories if no medical contraindications

Disposition

- Patients with meniscal injuries may be discharged from the ED and do not require an orthopedic consult emergently
- Patients may follow-up as an outpatient with sports medicine or orthopedics.
  - Surgical repair more common in younger population.
  - Management of degenerative tears is usually conservative (including corticosteroid injection and physical therapy) and aimed at pain control and treatment of underlying condition, that is, osteoarthritis.
- May return to work or school as able based on job requirements.
- May return to play after full, painless range of motion, full strength, and ability to perform sport-specific drills.

Complications

- Instability
- Osteoarthritis
- Pain
- Persistent mechanical symptoms such as locking, popping, and catching

Pediatric Considerations

- Children have a better blood supply to the meniscus and may be able to heal some tears.
- If operative management, consider surgical repair, and avoid meniscectomy if possible, as osteoarthritis may develop at a younger age.

Pearls and Pitfalls

- Physical exam findings include joint line tenderness, positive *McMurray* and *Apley compression tests.*
- Medial meniscus tears are more common than lateral tears.
- Consider operative repair with tear in younger patients, and rehabilitation with strengthening and conditioning exercises in older patients with degenerative tears.

Proximal Tibiofibular Joint Dislocation

General description

- Majority are anterolateral.
- Posteromedial also seen in athletes
- Superior more commonly associated with displaced tibia fractures or congenital knee dislocation.

Mechanism

- Anterolateral: fall on flexed, adducted leg with inverted ankle.
- Posteromedial: direct trauma to flexed knee

Presentation

- Lateral knee pain
- Instability

Physical Exam

- Fibular head prominent, tender, excessively mobile
- Assess integrity of common peroneal nerve, especially with posterior dislocations

Essential Diagnostics

- Knee x-rays should include AP, oblique, and lateral of both knees.
  - Best seen on AP view with evidence of laterally displaced fibular head and widening of proximal interosseous space compared to opposite leg.

ED Treatment

- Closed reduction for acute dislocation
  - Flex knee to 80–110° and place pressure over fibular head opposite to direction of dislocation.
  - Immobilization in extension

Disposition

- Most patients may be discharged from the hospital.
- Orthopedics should be consulted in the ED if there is an associated open fracture, hip dislocation, fracture of the knee or ankle, or common peroneal nerve injury.
- Patients should follow-up with sports medicine or orthopedics as an outpatient in approximately seven days.
- May return to work or school as able based on job requirements.
- May return to sport after pain is resolved and after regaining normal strength and range of motion.
  - Early rehabilitation program is usually recommended

Complications

- Common peroneal nerve injury
- Osteoarthritis, rare
- Recurrent dislocations/chronic subluxation

Pediatric Considerations

- Children may have idiopathic subluxation of the proximal fibula, which is self-limited, and symptoms decrease once the patient reaches skeletal maturity.

Pearls and Pitfalls

- Make sure to evaluate for associated peroneal nerve injury.
- Majority of dislocations are anterolateral.

Knee Dislocation

General description

- Multiligamentous and soft tissue injury
- Classification is positional or anatomical
  - Positional: position of tibia relative to femur
    - Anterior, posterior, medial, lateral, rotary
    - More than 50 percent anterior or posterior, anterior greater than posterior
  - Anatomical: based on ligamentous, bony, arterial, nerve injury
- Anterior dislocation results in PCL and ACL + MCL or LCL disruption with possible popliteal artery injury.
- Posterior dislocation results in ACL and PCL disruption with possible extensor mechanism disruption and possible popliteal artery injury.
- Lateral dislocation results in ACL and PLC disruption and has the highest rate of peroneal nerve injury.
- Medial dislocation results in PLC and PCL disruption.
- Rotary usually results in posterolateral dislocation and is usually irreducible.

Mechanism

- Anterior dislocation: hyperextension usually greater than 30°
- Posterior dislocation: axial load on flexed knee forcing tibia posteriorly, that is, dashboard
- Lateral/medial dislocation: varus/valgus force
- Rotary dislocation: combination of forces, usually posterolateral dislocation
- High velocity vs. low velocity
  - Low-velocity, that is, sport injuries are typically associated with less neurovascular damage and soft tissue injury

Presentation

- Pain, deformity, and instability after acute injury
  - Rarely these may reduce prior to ED presentation and do not have an obvious deformity on presentation
- Often hear/feel a "pop"

Physical Exam

- Deformity, if not spontaneously reduced
- Diffuse tenderness
- Limited ROM
- Consider spontaneously reduced knee dislocation if evidence of LCL disruption with peroneal nerve palsy or if three or more torn ligaments
- Thoroughly assess peroneal and tibial nerves
- Thoroughly assess for vascular injury and compare to opposite side
  - Hard signs: absence of pulses, expanding/pulsatile hematoma, thrill/bruit, pulsatile hemorrhage
- Avoid strength testing, initially, given the amount of soft tissue and ligamentous injury
- Perform x-rays prior to assessment of ligaments

Essential Diagnostics

- Knee x-rays should include AP, oblique, and lateral views.
  - May be normal if spontaneous reduction
  - Commonly associated with fractures
- Perform ankle brachial index (ABI)
- Perform vascular studies on all knee dislocations (even if normal ABI): arteriography, duplex ultrasonography, CT angiography based on vascular surgery or orthopedic surgery recommendations.

ED Treatment

- Emergent orthopedic surgery consultation
- Emergent vascular surgery consultation if signs of vascular injury
- Reduction
  - Immediate reduction using longitudinal traction if vascular compromise
  - Except if there is a contraindication to closed reduction
    - "Dimple sign" occurs when the medial femoral condyle buttonholes through the anteromedial capsule.
      - This indicates a posterolateral dislocation and risk of skin necrosis
- Splint in 20° flexion once reduced

Disposition

- Admit for serial perfusion checks, regardless of imaging, if immediate revascularization not required.
- Orthopedics should be consulted for all knee dislocations.
- Vascular surgery should be consulted anytime there is evidence of acute vascular injury.
- Immediate surgical revascularization for hard signs of vascular damage or ABI less than 0.9.
- Surgical orthopedic treatment generally required, though may be one to three weeks post injury.
- Conservative treatment with immobilization only for older or sedentary individuals with relatively stable knee.
- Usually long and difficult rehabilitation
- Low-velocity injuries generally have a better prognosis than high-velocity injuries.
- Return to sport is at least nine to twelve months after injury, and likely not with ability to perform at pre-injury level.

Complications

- Frequent complications, rarely will knee return to pre-injury state.
- Vascular injury, due to tethering at popliteal fossa
  - Anterior dislocation: popliteal artery injury, intimal tear more common
  - Posterior dislocation: popliteal artery injury, highest rate of complete tear.

- Nerve injury: peroneal and tibial
  - Lateral dislocation: highest rate of peroneal nerve injury
- Inability to reduce dislocation
  - Posterolateral dislocation: often requires operative reduction
  - Dimple sign, associated with skin necrosis, do not attempt to reduce
- Compartment syndrome frequent, requiring fasciotomy
- Persistent instability
- Post-traumatic arthritis
- Loss of motion

Pediatric Considerations

- Extremely rare in pediatrics, though high morbidity if unrecognized
- Consider associated distal femur physeal fracture
- Consider associated proximal tibial physis, tibial spine, tibial tubercle fracture

Pearls and Pitfalls

- Severe ligamentous and soft tissue injury
- Vascular injury common, all patients need vascular studies
- Nerve injury common
- Consider spontaneously reduced knee dislocation if evidence of LCL disruption with peroneal nerve palsy or if three or more ligaments disrupted
- Consult both orthopedic surgery and vascular surgery immediately

Tibial Plateau Fracture

General description

- Medial and lateral tibial plateaus are the articular surfaces for the tibial condyles
- Separated by the intercondylar eminence (ACL attachment)
  - Intercondylar eminence fracture associated with ACL injury
- Covered by meniscus
- Medial plateau and condyle are larger and stronger.
- Lateral plateau and condyle are smaller and weaker.
- Lateral plateau fractures are more common.
- Consider neurovascular injury, ligamentous injury, and compartment syndrome with high-energy mechanisms.
- Frequently associated with soft tissue injury (ligamentous).
- Split fracture in younger patients due to dense cancellous bone.
- Split or depressed fracture in older patients due to osteoporotic bone.

Mechanism

- Lateral tibial plateau fractures usually occur from medially directed force (valgus), that is, pedestrian hit by car with bumper hitting outside of leg.
- Medial tibial plateau fracture requires more force, varus.
- Consider tibial plateau fracture in elderly osteoporotic patients with twisting mechanism.
- Proximal tibia fracture from axial compression, that is, fall from height.
- Femoral condyle hits the tibial plateau, resulting in depressed or split fracture.

Presentation

- Painful, swollen knee
- Unable to bear weight

Physical Exam

- Proximal tibia tenderness
- Usually has associated large effusion
- Limited flexion and extension
- Assess distal pulses
- Assess peroneal nerve
- Assess for compartment syndrome, especially if tibial plateau fracture extends to tibial shaft
- Medial or lateral tibial plateau fracture: assess for ACL injury.
- Lateral plateau tibial fracture: assess for MCL and lateral meniscus injury
- Medial plateau tibial fracture: assess for LCL and medial meniscus injury

Essential Diagnostics

- Knee x-rays should include AP, lateral, internal and external oblique views.
  - AP view does not demonstrate normal plateau slope (anterosuperior to posteroinferior), so fracture findings may

be subtle and likely cannot characterize extent of depression.
  - AP view may show area of increased bone density correlating to fracture depression
  - Obtain tunnel (notch) view if suspecting intercondylar eminence fracture.
- CT scan is indicated to better assess extent of articular involvement and degree of fracture depression.
  - Also consider CT scan if initial x-rays are negative but there is a high degree of suspicion for fracture.

ED Treatment

- Place in long-leg compressive dressing from metatarsals to thigh.
- Immobilize knee with knee immobilizer or long-leg posterior splint.
  - Knee should be maintained in full extension and ankle at 90°.
- Non-weight-bearing for four to six weeks, until radiographic evidence of healing.
- Ice, elevation.

Disposition

- Admit if concern for vascular injury or compartment syndrome.
- Consult orthopedic surgery for most tibial plateau fractures including those associated with vascular injury, compartment syndrome, or displaced or depressed fracture.
- If nondisplaced tibial plateau fracture with no evidence of neurovascular injury or compartment syndrome, may discharge home with close outpatient orthopedic follow-up in two to three days.
- Return to work or school based on job requirements and access to transportation, as patient is unable to bear weight for at least four to six weeks.
  - May return to work at sedentary jobs likely once knee flexion increased and patient starts partial weight-bearing.
  - May return to work with jobs requiring standing/walking gradually once radiographic evidence of solid union and toleration of full weight-bearing.
- May begin non-weight-bearing exercise like swimming or bicycling once full weight-bearing tolerated.
- Twelve to twenty weeks for full healing and restoration of function.

Complications

- Vascular injury
- Nerve injury
- Compartment syndrome
- Loss of knee motion
- Osteoarthritis

Pediatric Considerations

- Longitudinal growth of tibia occurs at proximal tibia physis
  - Consider physis fracture for mechanisms that would cause tibial plateau fracture or knee dislocation in adults.
  - Complications include popliteal artery injury.
    - If concern, consider arteriogram
- Fracture of proximal metaphysis of tibia associated with chance of future deformity.
- Orthopedic consult for proximal tibia fractures.

Pearls and Pitfalls

- Immobilize knee in extension and make patient non-weight-bearing.
- Assess for vascular and nerve injury
- Maintain high degree of suspicion if patient presents with effusion and inability to bear weight, even if no evidence of fracture on x-rays.
  - Take extra caution with elderly patients because seemingly minor injury mechanisms may still result in tibial plateau fractures.

Patellar Tendinopathy (jumper's knee)

General Description

- Typically a chronic overuse injury in a skeletally mature patient.
- Most commonly affects the patellar tendon at the attachment to the inferior patellar pole.
- May also be at the attachment of the patellar tendon to the anterior tuberosity of the tibia, or the quadriceps tendon to the superior patellar pole.
- Not due to tendon inflammation (tendinitis), but rather tendon degeneration.

- Associated with decreased quadriceps and hamstring flexibility.

Mechanism

- Repetitive stress on patellar or quadriceps tendon.
  - Common in jumping sports

Presentation

- Insidious onset of anterior knee pain
- Generally pain is infrapatellar, but may also be suprapatellar
- Usually worsened with activity, and may become constant if activity continued.

Physical Exam

- Effusion rare
- Tenderness over patellar tendon, generally inferior pole of patella, though may be over superior patellar pole or tibial tuberosity
- Pain worse with resisted knee extension
- Normal range of motion, though likely hamstring and quadriceps muscle tightness

Essential Diagnostics

- Not necessary, as diagnosis is clinical, though may want to rule out other causes of symptoms.
- Knee x-ray may possibly show radiolucency at involved inferior patellar pole, or elongation of involved pole.
- Ultrasound may show thickening and hypoechogenicity of tendon fibers and peritendinous neovascularization.
  - Not necessary in the ED and may be performed as an outpatient

ED Treatment

- Conservative treatment, healing may be slow, four to six months
- Normal weight-bearing
- Activity modification, decrease activity that increases patellofemoral pressure, that is, jumping and squatting
- Ice massage
- Rehabilitation includes working on flexibility of quadriceps, hamstrings, and calves, as well as strengthening of quadriceps and core muscles
- May try patella tendon strap
- NSAIDs as needed

Disposition

- May be discharged home and does not require orthopedics consult in the ED unless there is a complete patellar tendon rupture.
- Follow-up with sports medicine or primary care physician in seven to ten days.
- May return to sport once full strength, range of motion, and able to perform sport-specific activity without pain.

Complications

- Persistent pain
- Weakness
- Complete tendon rupture

Pediatric Considerations

- Sinding–Larsen–Johansson disease is a traction apophysitis of the inferior pole of the patella
  - Usually an overuse injury that may occur during periods of rapid growth
  - Workup and treatment is similar to that of patellar tendinopathy

Pearls and Pitfalls

- Conservative treatment is the mainstay of therapy.
- Corticosteroid injection into the tendon is contraindicated as it increases the risk of complete tendon rupture.
- Knee immobilization is contraindicated, as it will increase stiffness of joint and muscles
- Complete tendon rupture requires surgical repair.

Popliteal Cyst (Baker's cyst)

General Description

- Most common synovial cyst
- Due to fluid distention of gastrocnemius-semimembranosus bursa, which communicates with knee joint, or herniation of synovial membrane through the joint capsule typically associated with osteoarthritis.

Mechanism

- Cyst communicates with joint space.
- Effusion and fibrin are pumped from joint into cyst, which enlarges, exerts mass effect, and prevents return of fluid to joint space.

- Effusion may be reabsorbed, though fibrin is usually left in the space.
- May leak and/or rupture.

Presentation

- Aching posterior knee pain
- Feeling of fullness in posterior fossa
- May fluctuate in size given communication with the joint
- May restrict range of motion based on size
- May also present with swelling of lower extremity if it has ruptured or is leaking

Physical Exam

- May note a cystic mass in medial side of popliteal fossa.
- Evaluate for pulsatility, consider popliteal artery aneurysm
- May be tender.
- May have decreased range of motion due to size of cyst.
- Cyst may transilluminate.
- May have joint effusion.
- May have lower extremity swelling if cyst is leaking or has ruptured.

Essential Diagnostics

- Not necessary, but may want to look for underlying osteoarthritis or rule out other causes of posterior knee pain, such as other benign cysts, cystic tumors, solid mass, popliteal artery aneurysm/pseudoaneurysm, or deep vein thrombosis.
  - X-ray of the knee may be performed to look for underlying osteoarthritis and degenerative joint disease.
    - AP bilateral standing film helpful to assess for joint space narrowing.
  - Ultrasound may show cystic structure with communication in to the joint space, and is useful to help rule out deep venous thrombosis, especially if there is lower extremity edema or pain.
  - MRI is not usually indicated in the ED, but may be used to rule out other causes of symptoms.
    - Cyst is best seen with intermediate signal on T1 and high signal on T2 images.
    - Cyst may be seen medial to the lateral head of the gastrocnemius and in the axial plane should see fluid-filled neck of cyst connecting to cyst in the joint space.

ED Treatment

- Activity modification
- Ice, compression, elevation to decrease swelling.
- Nonsteroidal anti-inflammatories as needed.
- Aspiration not recommended because the fluid is too viscous for drainage, there is a high rate of recurrence, and there are important surrounding neurovascular structures.
- Treatment is usually aimed at other underlying conditions, such as osteoarthritis.

Disposition

- May be discharged from the ED and does not require orthopedic surgery consult from the ED.
- May refer to sports medicine, primary care or orthopedics for further outpatient management.
  - Most treatment is conservative.
  - In rare cases cyst excision is performed if conservative therapy fails after several months and symptoms are severe.
- May return to work, school, and sport as able.

Complications

- Persistent pain, swelling
- Cyst may drain or rupture and cause pain and diffuse calf swelling

Pediatric Considerations

- Common in children
- However, typically cyst does not communicate with the joint as it does in adults.
- Intra-articular pathology is rare
- Majority with spontaneous resolution
- Diagnostics are indicated to rule out other diagnoses.

Pearls and Pitfalls

- Associated with effusion, meniscus tear, degenerative arthropathy
- Aspiration not recommended
- Cyst removal is not first-line therapy.

- Treatment is usually conservative with rest, ice, compression, and elevation.
  - Aimed at treatment of underlying condition which is usually osteoarthritis.

Prepatellar Bursitis

General Description

- Inflammation and increase of fluid within the prepatellar bursa
- Prepatellar bursa is superficial, has a thin synovial lining, and normally does not communicate with the joint space

Mechanism

- Overuse, recurrent minor trauma (i.e., excessive kneeling in certain professions or sports)
- Trauma to the knee (i.e., fall)
- May also be insidious

Presentation

- Knee pain and swelling of the prepatellar bursa
- Pain worse with walking, improved with rest
- Unable to kneel on the knee
- Occasionally may drain spontaneously

Physical Exam

- Erythema
- Fluctuant edema over the lower pole of the patella
- Tenderness of the patella
- Decreased flexion due to pain
- Intra-articular knee effusion is rare

Essential Diagnostics

- X-rays are only necessary to rule out other causes, though may show soft tissue swelling

ED Treatment

- Normal weight-bearing
- Activity modification, rest, ice, elevation, and compression
- If there is concern for septic bursitis (i.e., warmth, overlying erythema, fever) consider:
  - Aspiration of fluid for analysis
  - Antibiotics to cover skin flora

Disposition

- Most may be discharged from the ED and does not require emergent orthopedic consultation.
  - Uncomplicated septic bursitis may be discharged on antibiotics and given one- to two-day follow-up with sports medicine or orthopedics.
    - Orthopedic consult is needed for incision and drainage of septic prepatellar bursitis if no improvement after thirty-six to forty-eight hours of treatment.
    - Orthopedic referral for consideration of chronic or recurrent prepatellar bursitis.
  - Severe septic bursitis, if there is a concern for concomitant septic arthritis, and/or patients with underlying co-morbidities need orthopedic consult and need to be admitted for IV antibiotics.
- Return to work, school, or sport as able based upon requirements.
  - May need initial modifications if job includes kneeling.
- Knee pads if job/sport requires kneeling
- Consider physical therapy for range of motion and hamstring/quadriceps flexibility.

Complications

- Septic prepatellar bursitis
- Recurrent or chronic bursitis
- Septic arthritis

Pediatric Considerations

- If prepatellar bursitis is present in a pediatric patient, it is most likely septic, especially in an immunocompromised patient.

Pearls and Pitfalls

- Prepatellar bursitis without evidence of infection may be managed conservatively with rest, ice, elevation, and compression.
- Always consider septic bursitis and septic arthritis in differential diagnosis.

Osgood–Schlatter Disease

General description

- Apophysitis of the tibial tubercle

- Repetitive microfractures at tendon insertion site, cartilaginous portion.
- Most commonly occurs in pre-adolescence, and may occur during rapid growth spurt.

Mechanism

- Repetitive quadriceps contraction affecting patellar tendon at the insertion on the tibial tubercle, which is skeletally immature.

Presentation

- Pain and swelling of the tibial tubercle
- Typically insidious onset, or history of pain even before an inciting event
- Able to ambulate
- Pain often worsened with running/jumping activities, squatting, and going up and down stairs
- Pain improved with rest

Physical Exam

- No effusion
- Point tenderness at tibial tubercle, may be enlarged
- Full range of motion of knee
- Normal knee extension without limitations, but may have pain with resisted knee extension
- No evidence of knee instability
- Normal hip and ankle exam

Essential Diagnostics

- Imaging not necessary, as diagnosis is clinical, however may want to rule out other causes.
- AP and lateral knee x-rays may be obtained.
  - Imaging generally normal, especially if child in pre-ossification phase
  - X-ray evidence of Osgood–Schlatter disease is best seen on lateral view with knee in 10–20° internal rotation.
    - Acutely, may show soft tissue edema proximal to the tibial tuberosity.
    - More severe cases may show irregular ossification center at proximal tibial tuberosity, calcification or thickening in patellar tendon, superficial ossicle in the patellar tendon.
    - In advanced stages may also show heterotopic ossification at the tibial tubercle.

ED Treatment

- Normal weight-bearing
- Activity modification (especially running, jumping, squatting), ice, rest, compression
- Protective padding if needed
- Analgesics and nonsteroidal anti-inflammatories as needed

Disposition

- May be safely discharged home and does not require orthopedic consultation in the ED.
- Follow-up with sports medicine or primary care physician in seven to ten days.
  - May consider resection by orthopedics if continued problems after patient reaches skeletal maturity.
- Quadriceps and hamstring stretching/strengthening is recommended once acute pain has resolved
- Return to sport as tolerated, but usually need an initial period of rest

Complications

- Pain on kneeling even as an adult
- May continue to have bony prominence at the anterior knee
- Less likely, but may have continued pain requiring excision

Pediatric Considerations

- If there is an acute onset of pain, consider avulsion of the tibial tubercle

Pearls and Pitfalls

- Consider avulsion of tibial tubercle with acute onset of pain in a pediatric patient
- Most important treatment is activity modification and strengthening and conditioning knee rehabilitation program.

Patellofemoral Pain Syndrome (Runner's knee)

General Description

- Most common overuse injury of the knee
- More common in adolescents, young adults, and females
- Chondromalacia patella is thought to be a result of long term patellofemoral syndrome, leading to softening and degeneration of the cartilage behind the patella.

Mechanism

- Likely multifactorial
- Patella normally glides in the trochlear groove on the femur, creating a fulcrum for the quadriceps.
- Anatomical alignment issues and quadriceps muscle weakness may cause improper tracking of the patella in the groove.
- There may be an imbalance of the quadriceps muscle group, with the lateral over-powering the medial, pulling the patella out of the normal groove.
- Malalignment of the foot, leg, or pelvis may cause an abnormal pull of the muscles on the patella and create poor tracking on the femur.
- Actual source of pain is unclear as there is no innervation of the articular cartilage.
  - May be due to force transmission to underlying bone.
  - May be from nociceptive stimulation of adjacent structures (i.e., peripatellar retinaculum, extensor mechanism).

Presentation

- Insidious onset of anterior knee pain
- Pain may be described as under or around the patella.
- May be unilateral or bilateral.
- May have history of increased eccentric loading of the quadriceps (i.e., running).
- Pain worse with loading of the patellofemoral joint (i.e., stairs, squatting, running down hill)
- Positive theater sign: pain when standing from prolonged period of sitting.
- Cracking or popping, especially after prolonged periods of sitting, may decrease pain.
- May be sensation of giving way due to pain.

Physical Exam

- Inspection
  - Assess for intrinsic biomechanical factors that may predispose to the condition.
    - Excessive varus or valgus deformity, femoral anteversion, external tibial torsion, patellar malposition, excessive lateral insertion of patellar tendon (increased quadriceps angle), pes cavus or planus, increased Q-angle.
  - J-tracking may be present: excessive lateral tracking of the patella when passively extending the knee (resembles upside-down "J").
  - Effusion unlikely, although may have trace.
- Palpation
  - May have tenderness to palpation of the femoral condyles and patellar facets.
- Range of motion
  - Usually normal
- Special tests
  - May have positive *Clarke sign* or *grind test*: retropatellar pain with compression of the articular patellofemoral surfaces during quadriceps contraction.
  - May have pain with half or full squats
  - Assess for functional factors that may contribute to the condition.
    - This may include tightness of the hamstrings, ITB (positive *Ober's test*), or rectus femoris, as well as atrophy of the vastus medialis and/or a tight lateral retinaculum

Essential Diagnostics

- Knee x-rays may be obtained to rule out other underlying etiologies of pain
  - Sunrise or merchant views may show abnormalities of patellar alignment within the trochlear groove.
  - Sunrise view also shows underside of the patella, looking for cartilage softening and defects.

ED Treatment

- Acetaminophen or nonsteroidal anti-inflammatories for pain control
- Relative rest, avoid activities that exacerbate symptoms
- Ice massage, rest with elevation, and compression as needed

Disposition

- These patients may be safely discharged from the ED with outpatient sports medicine or primary care follow-up.
  - Consider referral to orthopedics if failure of conservative management after one year
- May return to work and sport as able.

- Rehabilitation
  - Exercises to strengthen core muscles and vastus medialis muscle.
  - Stretching of hip flexors, ITB, calf, and hamstrings.
- Consider patellar support or patellar tracking brace to decrease patellar mobility.
- Ice massage, especially after activity
- Slow, gradual, progressive return to activity
- Evaluation of footwear

Complications

- Chondromalacia patella

Pediatric Considerations

- Common in adolescence
- Consider osteochondritis dessicans, a disorder in which there is damage to the articular cartilage and subchondral bone.
  - This causes deprivation of blood supply to subchondral bone and may lead to avascular necrosis.

Pearls and Pitfalls

- Usually presents with anterior knee pain with descending steps or hills, or with prolonged sitting.
- Diagnosis may be made based on history and physical exam.
- Majority of people respond to conservative therapy with a temporary avoidance of exacerbating activities and rehabilitation.
- Consider chondromalacia patella in those with chronic patellofemoral pain syndrome.

Lliotibial Band Friction Syndrome

General Description

- ITB helps to abduct the leg and stabilize the pelvis in single-leg stance.
- Originates from the lateral iliac crest and inserts on the lateral aspect of the tibial tubercle.
- ITB syndrome is considered an overuse or overload syndrome.

Mechanism

- Repetitive overload of ITB distal fibers at insertion on the tibial tubercle (Gerdy tubercle) or excessive friction from the ITB over the lateral femoral epicondyle.
- Repetitive shifting of ITB over lateral femoral condyle with flexion and extension leads to irritation and inflammation
- Risk factors include ITB tightness, pes cavus, gluteal/hip abductor weakness, and/or sudden increased training intensity

Presentation

- Insidious onset of pain to posterolateral knee, generally over lateral femoral condyle
- Worse with running on hills or banked surfaces (uphill leg)
- Most common in runners, cyclists, sports with repetitive knee flexion and extension
- Usually relieved with rest

Physical Exam

- May have swelling over ITB.
- May have underlying foot or knee malalignment, which are risk factors.
- Tenderness along distal ITB, worst over lateral femoral condyle
- May have reduced hip/knee range.
- Weakness with hip abduction
- Pain with single leg squat
- Positive *Ober's test* (Figure 6.9)
- Positive *Noble compression test*

Essential Diagnostics

- None needed unless diagnosis is unclear and need to rule out other underlying etiologies.
  - Diagnosis usually based on history and physical exam

ED Treatment

- Ice massage
- Oral analgesics
- Relative rest

Disposition

- Patients may be discharged from the ED and do not require orthopedic consultation.
- May-follow up with sports medicine or primary care physician.
- Return to work and sport as able, as long as does not exacerbate symptoms.
- Training modifications recommended.
  - Change shoes every 300–500 miles
  - Avoid sudden increase in training

- Rehabilitation
  - Aggressive ITB stretching
  - Strengthening of core, gluteal, hip abductor, and knee musculature
  - Gradual return to full activity as long as symptoms have resolved
  - Consider corticosteroid injection if conservative treatment fails
    - However use caution as it may increase risk of ITB rupture

Complications

- Trochanteric bursitis
- Lateral synovial recess cyst or bursitis

Pediatric Considerations

- Similar to adults

Pearls and Pitfalls

- Consider ITB friction syndrome as a cause of lateral knee pain
- Conservative management is the mainstay of therapy

Osteoarthritis

General Description

- Most common type of joint disease
- Classified as a non-inflammatory arthritis, however there is evidence that inflammation does occur in this disease via cytokines and metalloproteinases released into the joint.
- Degenerative disease causing progressive loss of articular cartilage, synovial fluid, underlying bone, overlying joint capsule, and other joint tissues.
- Greater loss of joint space in areas with highest load, generally medial femorotibial compartment.
  - Lateral femorotibial compartment and patellofemoral compartment may also be affected.
- May be symptomatic or asymptomatic.
- Risk factors include age, female sex, African American ethnicity, obesity, trauma, manual labor, and muscle weakness.

Mechanism

- Progressive degenerative cascade involving the articular cartilage, synovium, and bone.
- Subchondral bone attempts to remodel once there is cartilage breakdown, which may produce fibrocartilage in areas of denuded bone, and bone cysts in late stages with lytic lesion and sclerotic edges.

Presentation

- Usually insidious onset over years or decades.
- Pain, often worse in the morning and with extensive use.
- Initially, pain may be relieved with rest, but as the disease progresses may become constant
- Swelling
- Stiffness during rest
- Decreased range of motion and crepitus
- Feeling of instability

Physical Exam

- Effusion
- Crepitus
- Diffuse tenderness, especially over joint lines
- Decreased range of motion, especially at extremes of flexion and extension
- Special tests may be positive for meniscus or ligament abnormality, which is likely degenerative in nature.
- Malalignment may be present, especially in advanced disease.
  - Collapse of medial compartment may lead to varus deformity.
  - Collapse of lateral compartment may lead to valgus deformity.

Essential Diagnostics

- Knee x-rays should include bilateral weight-bearing views, lateral and sunrise.
  - Help detect joint space narrowing, osteophytes, eburnation of bone, subchondral sclerosis or cysts.

ED Treatment

- Relative rest, avoidance of activities that exacerbate symptoms, especially during pain exacerbations.
- Ice, compression, and elevation for pain and swelling
- May recommend oral or topical nonsteroidal anti-inflammatories (if no contraindications), other analgesics, such as acetaminophen, or topical capsaicin.

Disposition

- Patients may be safely discharged from the ED and do not require orthopedic consultation.
- May follow-up with sports medicine or primary care physician for nonoperative treatment.
- Rehabilitation program for knee strengthening and conditioning.
  - Most improvement with combination of supervised and home exercise program
- Bracing with varus/valgus unloading brace may be helpful in unicompartmental disease
- Corticosteroid joint injection
- Viscosupplementation
- Orthopedic surgery referral for those who have failed conservative management to consider surgical management including:
  - Arthroscopic debridement for symptomatic degenerative meniscal tears
  - Joint replacement for advanced symptomatic disease
- May return to work or sport as able

Complications

- Continued joint degeneration
- Muscle atrophy
- Chronic pain
- Malalignment or deformity

Pediatric Considerations

- Inflammatory arthritis, rather than primary osteoarthritis is more likely in the pediatric population
  - Osteoarthritis is unusual in pediatric population

Pearls and Pitfalls

- Bilateral weight-bearing x-rays are recommended to fully assess extent of joint space narrowing and degenerative joint disease.
- The goal of treatment is to alleviate pain and improve functional status with a combination of non-pharmacologic and pharmacologic treatments.
- If patient presents to the ED for a painful flare of their osteoarthritis, be sure to also rule out underlying fracture, such as tibial plateau fracture, or septic arthritis.

Septic Arthritis

General Description

- Joint inflammation due to bacterial or fungal infection
- Knee joint is most commonly affected.
- May causes irreversible cartilage destruction and joint damage.
- Increased risk in older, male patients, but also consider in IV drug users, immunocompromised patients, those with prior knee surgeries/prosthesis, those with history of crystal arthropathies, and younger sexually active patients.

Mechanism

- Bacterial seeding of joint, which may occur due to:
  - Bacteremia
  - Direct inoculation from trauma or surgery
  - Contiguous spread from adjacent osteomyelitis
- Common pathogens include:
  - *Staphyloccus aureus* (most common) and epidermidis
  - *Neisseria gonorrhoeae* (most common in healthy sexually active adolescents and young adults)
  - *Streptococcus*
  - *Salmonella* (associated with sickle cell disease)
  - *Pseudomonas aeruginosa* (associated with IV drug abuse)
  - *Pasteurella multocida* (associated with dog or cat bites)
  - *Eikenella corrodens* (associated with human bites)
  - Consider fungal and Candida infection in immunocompromised hosts

Presentation

- Pain
- Swelling
- Erythema
- Warmth
- Fever
- Inability to bear weight

Physical Exam

- Erythema, warmth, effusion
- Diffuse tenderness
- Pain with both active and passive range of motion

Essential Diagnostics

- Knee x-rays may show effusion and help to rule out osteomyelitis.
- Labs, serum
  - Leukocytosis with left shift
  - CRP (most helpful)
    - Rises within hours of infection
    - Normalizes within one week of treatment
  - ESR
    - Rises within two days of infection, and three to five days after treatment
    - Normalizes in three to four weeks
- Joint fluid aspirate (gold standard for diagnosis)
  - Cell count with differential, Gram stain, culture, glucose, and crystal analysis
  - Cloudy or purulent-appearing fluid
  - WBC count more than 50,000 diagnostic, though lower counts may still be consistent with infection
    - WBC count more than 1,100 in prosthetic joint considered septic
  - Organism identified only one-third of the time on Gram stain.
  - Glucose less than 60 percent of serum level suggestive of septic joint.

ED Treatment

- Combined medical and surgical approach recommended
  - Consult orthopedics emergently as a septic joint is a surgical emergency needing operative joint irrigation and drainage, or repeated closed needle aspirations.
  - Initiate intravenous antibiotic therapy in consultation with orthopedic surgery after knee aspiration is performed, and should consider age and risk factors when choosing antibiotics.
    - Young and healthy patients have increased risk of *Staphylococcus aureus and Neisseria gonorrhoeae* causing septic arthritis.
    - Immunocompromised patients have increased risk of *Staphylococcus aureus and Pseudomonas aeruginosa* causing septic arthritis.
- Consult orthopedics for arthrocentesis if prosthetic joint infection suspected.

Disposition

- All patients with suspected prosthetic and diagnosed native joint septic arthritis need emergent orthopedic consult in the ED with admission for intravenous antibiotics, and definitive management by orthopedic surgery.
- Return to work or sports will be determined by orthopedics but generally not until infection improved, pain free, and completion of a progressive rehabilitation program.

Complications

- Cartilage destruction
- Bony destruction
- Functional loss of joint
- Secondary infection
- Osteomyelitis
- Sepsis

Pediatric Considerations

- Consider septic arthritis in children with an atraumatic limp.
- Always consider knee pathology even if child describes hip pain.

Pearls and Pitfalls

- Always consider septic arthritis in a warm, swollen, erythematous, painful knee with painful passive range of motion.
- *Staphylococcus aureus* is the most common pathogen.
- Consider septic arthritis in a patient that has painful passive range of motion.
- Orthopedic consult immediately for arthrocentesis if suspected septic joint with prosthetic.
- Initiate intravenous antibiotic therapy in consultation with orthopedics as patient may be taken to the OR prior to beginning antibiotics.

Table 6.2 Key Diagnosis, History, Physical Exam Findings, and Treatment

Diagnosis	History	Physical Exam Findings	Treatment
Patellar fracture	Direct trauma or forceful quadriceps contraction Anterior knee pain	Patellar tenderness and swelling	Knee immobilizer in extension *WBAT **RICE
Patellar dislocation	Direct blow or quadriceps contraction Anterior pain Possible deformity	Laterally displaced patella, usually	Reduction Knee immobilizer in extension WBAT RICE
Disruption of the extensor mechanism	Direct trauma or forceful quadriceps contraction	Unable to actively raise the leg with knee in full extension	Complete: Orthopedic consult Partial: knee immobilization in extension with progressive WBAT
Anterior cruciate ligament injury	Noncontact direction change while running, hyperflexion or hyperextension Acute swelling Giving way	Effusion Positive Lachman, pivot shift, anterior drawer tests	RICE WBAT Outpatient orthopedic follow-up
Posterior cruciate ligament injury	Posteriorly directed trauma to flexed anterior tibia, hyperflexion with plantar-flexed ankle, hyperextension Posterior pain	Popliteal fossa tenderness Positive posterior drawer and sag tests	Grade I/II: hinged brace Grade III: knee immobilizer in extension WBAT RICE Outpatient orthopedic follow-up
Medial collateral ligament injury	Valgus force on partially flexed knee Medial pain	Tenderness along MCL Positive valgus stress test	RICE WBAT Grade II/III: stabilizing brace Grade III: outpatient orthopedic follow-up
Lateral collateral ligament injury	Varus force, hyperextension, external tibial rotation Lateral pain	Tenderness along LCL Positive varus stress test	RICE WBAT Grade II/III: stabilizing brace Grade III: outpatient orthopedic follow-up
Posterolateral corner injury	Varus force, hyperextension, external tibial rotation Posterolateral pain	Posterolateral joint line tenderness Positive dial test	RICE WBAT Stabilizing brace Outpatient orthopedic follow-up
Meniscus injury	Twisting or hyperflexion Medial/lateral pain Locking, clicking	Joint line tenderness Positive McMurray, Apley compression tests	RICE WBAT Outpatient orthopedic follow-up for young patients and/or mechanical symptoms
Proximal tibiofibular joint dislocation	Direct trauma or fall Lateral pain Instability	Tender and mobile fibular head	Reduction Immobilization in extension

Table 6.2 *(cont.)*

Diagnosis	History	Physical Exam Findings	Treatment
Knee dislocation	Hyperextension, axial load on flexed knee, varus/valgus force Pain, deformity, instability	Deformity if not reduced Possible peroneal nerve palsy Possible vascular injury	Immediate orthopedics and vascular consult Reduction Splint 20° flexion Admit
Tibial plateau fracture	Valgus force or axial compression Unable to bear weight	Tenderness proximal tibia Limited range of motion Inability to bear weight	Long-leg compression dressing Immobilizer in extension Non-weight-bearing
Patellar tendinopathy	Repetitive stress on patellar/quad tendon Jumping sports Insidious onset	Tenderness over tendon Pain with resisted knee extension	RICE Activity modification Normal weight-bearing
Popliteal cyst	Posterior pain/swelling History of osteoarthritis	Effusion Posterior tenderness Mass medial side popliteal fossa Transillumination	RICE Normal weight-bearing
Prepatellar bursitis	Repetitive kneeling or trauma Anterior pain and swelling	Fluctuant edema over patella Tenderness of patella	Normal weight-bearing RICE Activity modification Knee pads
Osgood–Schlatter disease	Pain/swelling tibial tubercle Insidious onset Pre-adolescence Able to ambulate Worse with running/jumping	Tibial tubercle tenderness Full ROM, though pain with resisted extension	Normal weight-bearing Activity modification Padding if needed
Patellofemoral pain syndrome	Anterior knee pain Insidious onset Eccentric loading of the quadriceps (i.e., running) Worse with loading of the patellofemoral joint (i.e., stairs, squatting, running downhill) Positive theater sign	Positive Clarke sign or grind test	RICE Normal weight-bearing Pain control Strengthen core muscles and vastus medialis obliques Stretching of hip flexors, iliotibial band, calf, and hamstrings
Iliotibial band friction syndrome	Posterolateral pain Insidious onset Runners, cyclists, sports with repetitive knee flexion and extension Relieved with rest	Distal ITB tenderness: lateral femoral condyle Pain with single leg squat Positive Ober's test Positive Noble compression test	RICE Pain control ITB stretching Strengthening of core, gluteal, hip abductor, knee musculature Gradual return to activity once pain is improved

Table 6.2 *(cont.)*

Diagnosis	History	Physical Exam Findings	Treatment
Osteoarthritis	Insidious onset over years or decades Worse in the morning and with extensive use Swelling and stiffness Decreased range of motion and crepitus Feeling of instability	Effusion Malalignment in advanced disease Diffuse tenderness, especially over joint lines Crepitus Decreased range of motion Positive tests for meniscus or ligament injury	RICE Oral or topical nonsteroidal anti-inflammatories Other analgesics, i.e., acetaminophen Topical capsaicin Rehabilitation recommendations
Septic arthritis	Pain Swelling Warmth Fever Inability to bear weight	Erythema Warmth Effusion Diffuse tenderness Pain with passive range of motion	Arthrocentesis If prosthetic joint consult orthopedics for arthrocentesis Initiate intravenous antibiotic therapy

*RICE-Rest, ice, compression, elevation
**WBAT-Weight-bearing as tolerated

Table 6.3 Indications for Orthopedic Surgery Consultation in the Emergency Department

Injury	Indication for Consult
Patellar fracture	Displaced, comminuted, open fracture Disruption of extensor mechanism
Patellar dislocation	Inability to maintain patellar position Osteochondral fracture Disruption of extensor mechanism
Disruption of extensor mechanism	Complete rupture
Ligamentous injury	Multiligamentous injury Associated displaced bony avulsion Nerve injury Vascular injury
Proximal tibiofibular joint dislocation	Associated fracture Nerve injury
Total knee dislocation	*ALL knee dislocations Also consult vascular surgery
Tibial plateau fracture	Displaced or depressed fracture Compartment syndrome Vascular injury Nerve injury
Patellar tendon rupture	Complete rupture

Table 6.3 *(cont.)*

Injury	Indication for Consult
Prepatellar septic bursitis	Complicated septic bursitis
Pediatrics	Any physis injury
Septic arthritis	Concern for septic arthritis in prosthetic joint After arthrocentesis performed in native septic joint

Recommended Reading

Seidenberg P, Beutler A. The Sports Medicine Resource Manual. 2008.

Eiff M, Hatch R, Calmbach W. Fracture Management for Primary Care, 2nd Ed., 2003.

Harris J, Harris W, Novelline R. The Radiology of Emergency Medicine, 3rd Ed., 1993.

Chapter 7

Lower Leg and Ankle

Christopher A. Gee

LOWER LEG (TIBIA/FIBULA)

Background/ Epidemiology

- The lower leg is commonly injured in active people.
- Impact-related activities create repetitive low levels of trauma that build over time resulting in a variety of injuries.
- A review of 100 US high schools reported that over the course of one year there were over 800,000 lower extremity injuries reported.[1]
  - The most common sport involved was soccer, but injuries also occur commonly in basketball, football, and track (running/jogging).
- Emergency physicians (EP) must be aware of some basic principles of injury to the lower leg to effectively examine and assess for pathology.

Anatomic Considerations/ Pathophysiology

- The anatomy of the lower leg is comprised of the larger anteromedial tibia that bears the majority of the body's weight and the laterally positioned fibula, which contributes mostly to leg stability and rotational strength.
  - Proximally, the tibia interfaces with the femur to create the knee joint, while the fibula connects laterally to the proximal tibia.
    - The proximal tibiofibular joint has very little motion, but is important in the distribution of rotational forces from the ankle to the leg.[2]
    - Rarely, this joint may be symptomatic from increased motion leading to instability or cystic structure formation.
  - The interosseus membrane (Figure 7.1) is a thick fibrous connection between the tibia and fibula that effectively creates a ring structure of the lower leg.
  - Fascial layers divide the musculature of the leg into four distinct compartments.
    - Anterior, lateral, superficial posterior, deep posterior (Figure 7.2)
- The causes of pain in the lower leg may be from a wide variety of sources. Most commonly the following processes are involved:
  - Bone stress: May be due to acute traumatic injuries resulting in acute fractures or chronic injuries from repeated low level impacts causing stress reactions or fractures.
  - Inflammation: Often due to muscle units pulling on the periosteum of the lower leg; this leads to focal pain, especially with repeated activities
  - Elevated compartment pressures: Muscle action during athletic or work activities requires increased blood flow, which increases the pressures within facial compartments of the lower leg; these pressures may increase to the point of causing injurious compression of vascular, neurologic, and muscular structures.
  - Nerve entrapment: Scar tissue or other structures may impinge nerves traversing the lower leg leading to distal leg/ foot pain or weakness.

Focused History and Physical Exam

- A thorough history will include focused questions on the onset, timing, character of pain, injury mechanism, exacerbating/ relieving factors and history of prior injuries.
- A recent traumatic event with sufficient forces involved increases the possibility of acute fracture or muscle tears, while a more insidious onset and development of

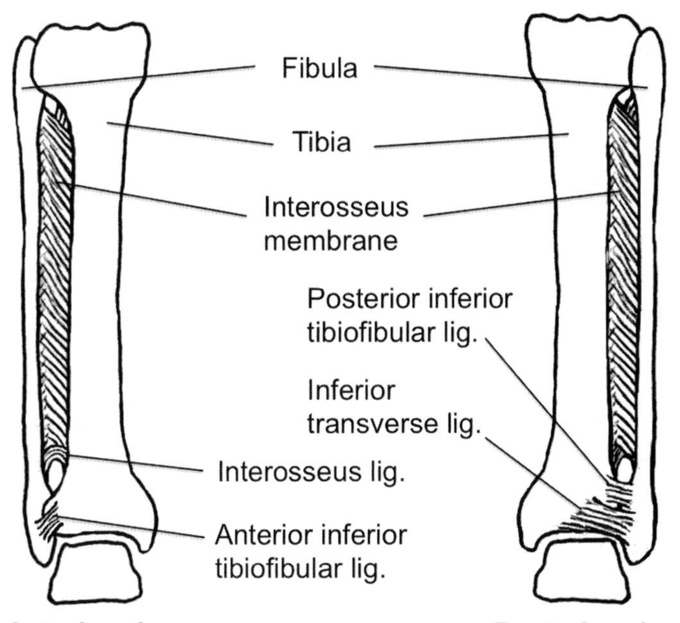

Figure 7.1. Interosseus membrane and syndesmosis of the lower leg. Illustration by Yvonne Chow.

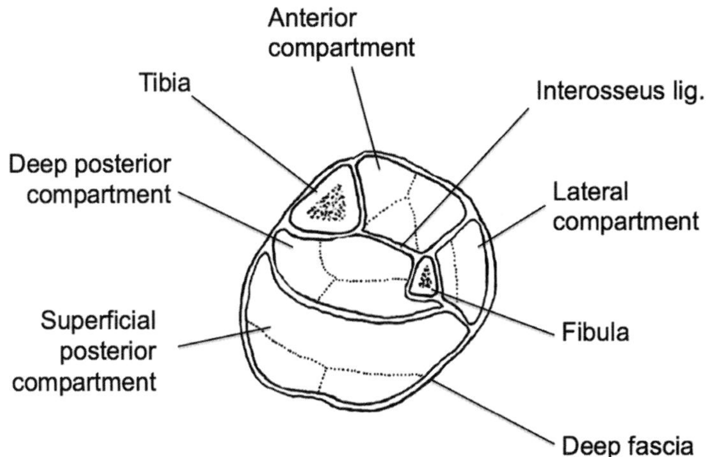

Figure 7.2. Fascial compartments of the lower leg. Illustration by Yvonne Chow.

pain may involve stress injuries, nerve or vessel entrapment, or inflammatory conditions.

- Other contributing factors may include training regimens, dietary restrictions, and comorbid conditions.

- A broad review of systems may be helpful in identifying potentially associated symptoms.
  - At times a musculoskeletal complaint or a limitation of athletic performance may be due to a systemic metabolic condition leading to early limitation of activities or other painful conditions (i.e., pulmonary disease may limit aerobic performance).
- Examining the lower leg in a systematic fashion will ensure a thorough exam to provide evidence of injury or disease

Inspection

- Look for any asymmetric swelling, ecchymosis, deformity, soft tissue swelling, or discoloration.
- Since the leg is involved in locomotion, it is imperative to evaluate the leg at rest and during standing and walking.

- Evidence of varus or valgus alignment from the knee down may indicate knee pathology or the propensity for such pathology.
- Observe any evidence of tibial torsion (in-toeing or out-toeing) or pes planus (flat feet). These conditions contribute to alterations in gait that may cause injury.
- Observe the patient's gait; watching for asymmetry between legs or potential weaknesses of certain muscle groups.

Palpation

- Because the entire lower leg is connected in a ring-like structure, the entire tibia and fibula should be palpated, in addition to the area of identified pain.
- The anterior tibial shaft is very shallow beneath the skin and stress injuries, and fractures or inflammation may be focally tender to palpation.
- The full length of the fibula should be palpated for any focal or diffuse tenderness as well as any areas of step-off or mass.
- The gastrocnemius, soleus, and plantaris muscle bellies, musculotendinous junctions, and Achilles tendon should be palpated for tenderness, swelling, gaping, or nodularity. These muscle groups should be assessed for overall bulk and tone.
- Finally, the four major compartments of the leg should be palpated for tightness, firmness, or pain. Rarely, a mass may be felt consistent with muscle hernia through a fascial defect.

Range of motion (ROM)

- While the leg does not have any testable motions outside of the knee or ankle joints, the muscles that cause the joint motion are attached to particular points on the leg.
  - While observing active motion of the knee and particularly the ankle, the examiner may watch for muscle action, bulk, and symmetry during particular motions.
  - This may provide clues to muscular involvement leading to weakness or other pathology.

Special tests

- Due to the stability of the lower leg, there are not many specialized tests; however, it is important to differentiate between a bony injury and soft tissue inflammation.
  - When there is concern for a stress injury, placing a vibrating tuning fork or ultrasound on the site of pain may elicit pain over a stress fracture.
    - A positive test is indicated by an increase in pain.
    - A recent systematic review found that while some studies reported relatively acceptable test performance characteristics of tuning fork and ultrasound tests, overall these tests didn't perform well enough to be used alone without confirmatory imaging.[3]
  - The *single leg hop test* is another useful test for stress fractures.
    - The patient is asked to hop on the affected leg; a positive test occurs when the patient has extreme pain and cannot hop more than once or twice.
    - Generally, patients with medial tibial stress syndrome (MTSS) can hop up to ten times.

Neurovascular exam

- Sensory dermatomes of the L4-S1 nerve roots are located in the lower leg.
  - The L4 dermatome is on the medial aspect of the leg.
  - The L5 dermatome is on the proximal lateral leg.
  - The S1 dermatome is located on the distal posterior calf, heel, and lateral malleolus.
  - Vascular structures traversing the lower leg are important to assess, but are most easily assessed at the knee or ankle.
    - The easiest way to assess circulation is to palpate the dorsalis pedis pulse.
  - Overall leg perfusion should be generally assessed, as well as evaluating for swelling or edema that may indicate other pathology, like thrombotic disease.

Differential Diagnosis-Emergent and Common Diagnoses

General

- A list of differential diagnoses for leg pain includes the common issues of shin splints (medial tibial stress syndrome), acute fractures, arthritis, cysts, stress fractures, proximal and midshaft fibular fractures, and the less common but important diagnoses of CECS nerve entrapments, and gastrocnemius musculotendinous tears.

Shin Splints

Background

- The term shin splints is commonly used in active runners and may, at times, be a vague "catch-all" term for any lower leg pain.
- MTSS is a more specific term for this condition.
- It is most common in runners, but may occur in other athletes.

Table 7.1 Emergent and Common Diagnoses in the Emergency Department

	Emergent Diagnoses	Common Diagnoses
Leg	Open fractures	Shin splints
	Fractures with neurovascular compromise	Arthritis
	Acute compartment syndrome	Stress fractures
	Displaced fractures	Chronic exertional compartment syndrome
		Nerve entrapments
		Gastrocnemius strains/tears
Ankle	Ankle dislocation	Ankle instability
	Displaced fractures	Ankle sprain
	Open fractures	Tendinopathy
		Osteochondral lesions
		Arthritis

Mechanism

- MTSS is caused by excessive pull of lower leg muscles on the periosteal lining of the tibia.
- These muscles generally include the tibialis posterior, soleus, and flexor digitorum longus.
- The excess traction causes a periosteal reaction along the tibial shaft that may be diffusely tender to palpation.
- Excessive foot pronation (flat feet), training errors, and inadequate shoe support may contribute to the development of this condition.

Presentation

- Patients will present with a gradual onset of pain that will be worse in the morning and after exercise.
- Symptoms will often improve with rest, adequate warmup before exercise, and stretching.

Physical Exam

- The patient will complain of diffuse pain along the medial tibial border.
- The area will be diffusely tender to palpation; occasionally mild swelling may be visible in the area.
- Any focal tenderness along the tibial shaft should cause the examiner to consider a diagnosis of stress fracture.

Essential Diagnostics

- Radiographs of the tibia and fibula are not mandatory, but may be useful to rule out fracture or stress reaction.

ED Treatment

- ED treatment consists of pain control, thorough evaluation for other conditions (i.e., fractures), and reassurance.
- Often times, symptoms may be improved with altering training regimens (introducing cross training, changing running surface), improving shoe type, or using shoe arch supports.
- Symptomatic treatments that may be helpful are focal ice massage and nonsteroidal antiinflammatory drug (NSAID) creams.
- These are particularly useful just after activity.
- In recalcitrant cases there may be more severe gait abnormalities and referral for a formal gait analysis may guide treatment, especially with custom orthotics.

- Severe cases may benefit from foot/ankle bracing to limit motion and allow any inflammatory processes to heal.

Disposition

- Patients may be discharged home with primary care or sports medicine follow-up.
- Patients may need referral for physical therapy to work on stretching, soft tissue treatments, and foot/ankle strengthening.
- Athletes may continue activities as tolerated by pain, but need to modify their activities to prevent progression to stress fracture.

Complications

- Continued pain may force the athlete to modify or stop their activities.
- Persistent symptoms raise the concern for the development of a stress fracture.

Pediatric Considerations

- This condition may be common in children, especially those just starting to run or those running intermittently (i.e., physical education classes).
- Usually, an evaluation to rule out other pathology as well as reassurance and conservative treatments are adequate to return patient to activity.

Pearls and Pitfalls

- Whenever the diagnosis of MTSS is considered, other diagnoses like stress fractures, muscle imbalance, neuropathies, or CECS should be considered.
- Often times these diagnoses have other historical or physical exam findings that point toward the alternate diagnosis, but they should be adequately evaluated for and ruled out, especially in MTSS cases that are not improving.

Stress Fracture

Background

- Stress fractures in the tibia (and slightly less in the fibula) are a feared complication of running and impact activities.
- Stress fractures occur as a result of multiple repetitive smaller forces directed at the bone resulting in a stress injury or fracture.
  - Stress injury refers to the early signs and symptoms prior to the development of a discrete fracture line.
- A fracture line in the anterior tibial cortex is referred to as "the dreaded black line" because it is often difficult to heal and requires significant change in activities for the patient.
- Stress fractures may occur anywhere in the body, but most concerning in a running population are those in the hip, tibia, navicular, and metatarsals.

Mechanism

- Bone metabolic processes include the continual reshaping of bony structures to adapt to ongoing forces applied to the bone.
- When a bone is placed under repetitive stresses that exceed its capacity to withstand such stress, it begins a process of remodeling.
- This initiates with resorption of bony material along the site of stress.
- This weakens the area and results in eventual fracture of the cortex.
- Finally bone is laid down around the fracture area, starting directly below the periosteum.
- This causes the periosteum to elevate directly over the fracture area. This may be seen on x-rays as a hazy heaped-up line running parallel to the cortex.
- This is referred to as a periosteal reaction and is indicative of a stress fracture.

Presentation

- Stress fractures occur in patients who have experienced a relative increase in impact activities over a period of time sufficient to induce bony changes.
- Often the patient may remain asymptomatic for a period of time, and only after one to two months of sustained activity does the patient begin to manifest symptoms.
- Patients will complain of gradual development of pain over focal area of bone.
- As time progresses, the pain will worsen with activity and eventually become symptomatic during routine walking.
- The stress injury may also produce a deep achy pain at night.
- Other important considerations are overall patient health, gender, diet, calcium intake, and age.

- With female patients in particular, identification of an eating disorder and a lack of regular menses may indicate conditions of increased risk for potential stress fractures.

Physical Exam

- Patients will have a focal area of pain directly over the bone, usually the tibia.
    - This is in contradistinction to MTSS, which will generally have a diffuse area of tenderness.
- As time goes on and a bony callous grows, an area of swelling and bony growth may occasionally be palpated.
- Other tests which may be performed include:
    - Placing a vibrating tuning fork, or active ultrasound probe, directly on the painful area
    - *Single leg hop test*
        - This is performed by having the patient hop on the affected leg while evaluating for reproduction of their pain.

Essential Diagnostics

- A standard two view x-ray of the tibia and fibula should be obtained any time the diagnosis of stress fracture is considered.
    - These should be evaluated for evidence of a periosteal reaction, callous development, or frank fracture.
    - In some cases, a bone scan or MRI may be needed to determine the presence of a stress injury or fracture.
        - These studies are generally not necessary while the patient is in the ED.

ED Treatment

- When a stress fracture is suspected, the patient should be placed into a fracture walker boot, even if initial x-rays are negative.
    - This will cushion the leg and prevent ongoing trauma.
    - The patient may be weight-bearing as tolerated.
    - On occasion, patients may be symptomatic enough, or the fracture may be tenuous enough (i.e., anterior tibia), that the patient should be made non-weight bearing.
    - Patients should be advised to avoid further impact activities.
- Patients should also be advised regarding adequate calcium, vitamin D, and protein intake.
- In addition, any other ongoing comorbid conditions (i.e., female athlete triad) should be identified and adequately managed.

Disposition

- Patients should be advised to follow-up with orthopedics or sports medicine within one week from ED discharge.
    - Patients will need ongoing care and repeat imaging to ensure healing over time.
- After a period of immobilization, progressive weight-bearing and return to activities may be incorporated, provided the patient is pain free with walking and other activities.

Complications

- Once a stress injury progresses to a stress fracture the major concern becomes adequately stabilizing the area and removing the stress to ensure appropriate healing.
- Stress fractures of the anterior tibial cortex are particularly concerning due to their risk of progressing to complete fractures.
    - They are also at risk for delayed healing and nonunion.
    - In these cases, the patient may need surgery to stabilize the area.

Pediatric Considerations

- Due to active bone growth and turnover, children could be considered to be at an increased risk of stress injury.
- However, stress fractures tend to be fairly uncommon in children.

Pearls and Pitfalls

- Given the high morbidity of displaced fractures and the often vague presentation, the risk of missing this diagnosis is substantial
- X-rays findings may be very subtle and easily missed
- Serial imaging and a low threshold for removing patients from activities or even making them non-weight bearing should be considered if there is a high index of suspicion
    - It may take ten to fourteen days for a fracture line to manifest itself on x-rays.

Proximal and Midshaft Fibular Fractures

Background

- Isolated fibular proximal and midshaft fibular fractures are rare.
  - By definition, there are no other associated bony or ligamentous injuries.
- The fibula typically bears only about 5–15 percent of the body's total weight and may sometimes be overlooked as a site of injury.
- However, its integrity is important to the stability of the lower leg and serves as a critical source of attachment of muscles and ligamentous structures.

Mechanism

- Fibular fractures may occur by direct or indirect measures.
  - A direct blow to the lateral leg may fracture the proximal or midshaft of the fibula.
  - An indirect twisting force to the foot or leg may cause a spiral fracture, which may be unstable.
    - This force may also cause disruption of the ankle ligaments, the tibiofibular syndesmosis, or a fracture of the medial malleolus.
      - This type of fracture is called a Maisonneuve fracture.
- Although much less common, stress injuries may occur in the fibula in runners or individuals who sustain a significant amount of repetitive impact force to leg.

Presentation

- Patients may present with localized pain in the lateral leg with a history of a direct blow.
- They may be able to weight bear with minimal or no pain.

Physical Exam

- It is always important to palpate the entire length of the fibula, including the proximal fibular head, in any injury to the leg.
- Patients may have tenderness over the site of fracture, swelling, and ecchymosis and have variable degrees of difficulty walking after acute injuries.
- More chronic injuries may be subtle and only have symptoms during exercise, so any exacerbating symptoms should be asked about.
- It is important to also evaluate the ankle for any signs of injury and exclude an unstable Maisonneuve injury.
  - The integrity of the medial and lateral ankle, as well as the tibiofibular syndesmosis, should be evaluated with the *compression* and *dorsiflexion eversion tests* (Figures 7.3 and 7.4). See ankle section for descriptions of tests.
- It is also important to pay particular attention to the integrity of the peroneal nerve.

Essential Diagnostics

- Two-view x-rays of the tibia and fibula should be obtained to fully evaluate for fracture.
  - Ankle and/or knee x-rays may also be needed, depending on the clinical suspicion of concomitant injury.

ED Treatment

- Patients should have the affected leg elevated, iced, and splinted in a position of comfort until definitive x-rays are obtained.

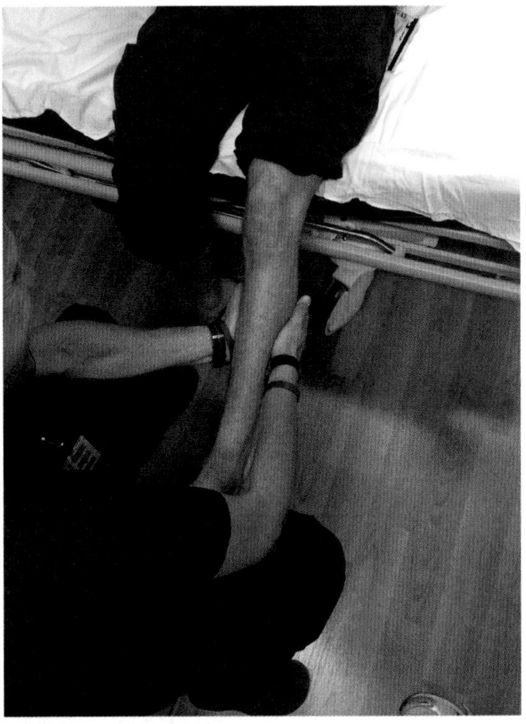

Figure 7.3. Compression test.

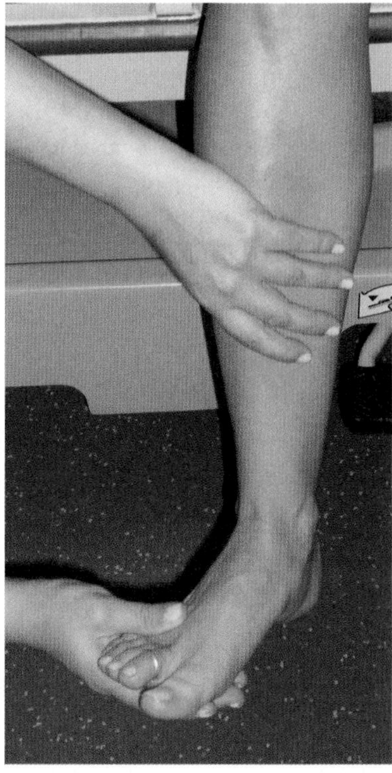

Figure 7.4. Dorsiflexion eversion test.

- Once a fibular fracture is determined, the stability of the ankle should be evaluated.
  - Stable, isolated proximal or midshaft fibula shaft fractures may be treated based upon patient's symptoms:
    - If there is no or minimal pain with ambulation, a simple compression dressing may be used.
    - If there is difficulty with ambulation, then a splint, cast, or walking boot may be used.
    - Rest, ice, elevation, and weight-bearing as tolerated may be recommended.
  - Unstable Maisonneuve fractures should be splinted with a posterior splint with the ankle at 90° and the patient made non-weight bearing.

Disposition

- Most isolated proximal and midshaft fibula fractures may be referred for outpatient management.
  - Stable, isolated fractures may be followed up by sports medicine or primary care physicians.
    - Patients may begin to return to play with a rehabilitation program once they are symptom free, usually after four to six weeks. Return to contact activities usually takes longer due to increased risk of re-fracture.
  - Unstable Maisonneuve injuries need close follow-up within two to three days with orthopedic surgery.
- Open fractures or grossly displaced fractures that are unable to be reduced in the ED need emergent orthopedic consultation.

Complications

- Painful nonunion or malunion are possible, but given the small amount of weight-bearing by the fibula, this is usually not a major problem.
- Instability of the ankle from a Maisonneuve-type injury may lead to foot and ankle dysfunction and posttraumatic arthritis.
- Neurovascular injury may occur.

Pediatric Considerations

- Children are not at any special risk for these types of injury.
- Similar patterns of injury as adults should be considered.

Pearls and Pitfalls

- The major issue to consider with proximal or midshaft fibular fractures are associated ligamentous ankle injuries resulting in Maisonneuve injuries.
  - These are unstable and easy to miss if the provider only evaluates the ankle and/or leg in isolation.
  - Consideration should be given to obtaining leg or knee films in these situations.
- Pay particular attention to the integrity of the peroneal nerve.

Chronic Exertional Compartment Syndrome

Background

- Chronic exertional compartment syndrome (CECS) is an entity not much different from acute compartment syndrome during its acute phase, but quickly resolves once activities stop.
- CECS is due to acute swelling of muscles during exercise within defined fascial compartments

that leads to tissue compression causing pain, numbness, or weakness.

- Usually, the pain causes the patient to stop the activity and the symptoms resolve spontaneously (typically within 30 minutes).
- The compartments most commonly affected in the lower leg are the anterior and lateral compartments, although any of the four compartments may be involved (Figure 7.2).

Mechanism

- Exercise induces increased blood flow to active muscles, which effectively swell within the enclosed fascial compartments.
- As the pressure increases, muscular pain increases.
- Eventually, pressures may become high enough to compress vascular and neurologic structures, which further exacerbates pain and leads to other symptoms like pallor, coolness, loss of pulse, or neuropathies.
- The fascial compartments are likely abnormally stiff or noncompliant in these patients, thus not allowing for adequate expansion during exercise.

Presentation

- Symptoms will usually develop after a particular period of continuous exertion.
- This period may be variable, depending on the patient and the severity of disease.
- Most commonly described is an achy constant pain in the affected compartment that slowly develops as the patient exercises.
- The pain usually gets intense enough that the patient will have to stop exercising.
- With rest, the pain gradually improves but may take over 30 minutes to resolve.
- The patient's symptoms may be variable, depending on the structure(s) compressed.
- Patients may simply have pain from muscle compression, but also temporary paresthesias and weakness during the acute phase of the disease.

Physical Exam

- While the patient is at rest, he/she will have a normal physical exam.
- However, during exertion the muscles of the affected compartment may become visibly enlarged, and the compartment will become tense and firm to palpation.
- Occasionally, muscle herniations and swelling may be seen.
- One way to provoke this is to have the patient lay supine and actively dorsiflex and plantarflex the ankles against resistance. Reproduction of pain, swelling, or paresthesias is considered a positive test.
  - Absences of pulses should prompt investigation for arterial insufficiency.

Essential Diagnostics

- Most commonly this is initially a clinical diagnosis that is based upon a typical history and exam features.
  - Other etiologies such as MTSS and stress fracture should also be evaluated.
  - Imaging diagnostics like x-ray or MRI should be considered to evaluate for other causes of pain (fractures or soft tissue masses causing external compression).
- No workup is indicated in the ED if CECS is suspected, as long as there is not concern for acute compartment syndrome or fracture.
- In the clinic setting, compartment pressures of the anterior, lateral, and sometimes posterior superficial compartments should be obtained.
  - This is usually done in a clinical setting where the patient may run or exercise enough to bring on symptoms.
  - The patient usually runs at least 5 minutes into the "pain zone," and then the compartment pressures are tested in the standard fashion.
  - Typically compartment pressures are obtained at rest prior to exercise, at 1 minute post exercise, and again at 5 minutes post exercise.

ED Treatment

- These patients will not routinely present to the ED, however, they may present while in the acute phase of the disease.
  - In these cases they may be treated conservatively with ice, compression, and anti-inflammatories.
- If there is concern for acute compartment syndrome, they should be treated with imaging, pain control, compartment pressure testing, and orthopedic consultation for possible fasciotomy.

Disposition

- Patients with CECS may be sent home with follow-up with orthopedics or sports medicine.
- A period of rest and a reduced exercise program should be advised.
  - Patients should avoid exercises that provoke symptoms as there is a small risk of causing acute compartment syndrome.
- Physical therapy may be beneficial to work on soft tissue mobilization and stretching/ strengthening of the affected compartments.
- Any biomechanical problems (e.g., pes planus) should be corrected in an attempt to offload the overstressed muscles and improve symptoms.
- Once conservative therapies fail, fasciotomy or fasciectomy may be considered to alleviate symptoms.

Complications

- Severe, untreated CECS could potentially progress to full-blown acute compartment syndrome with the ensuing complications of muscle necrosis, nerve damage, contractures, or even loss of limb.

Pediatric Considerations

- This condition is uncommon in children, but not impossible.
- Other conditions like fractures, tumors, or metabolic disorders should be considered.

Pearls and Pitfalls

- As with acute compartment syndrome, CECS is a difficult diagnosis to make and takes a thorough history and an astute physical exam.
- It is typically a diagnosis that takes several encounters to make and confirm.
- Unfortunately, it is a difficult entity to treat and may often cause patients to alter their exercise or work patterns due to pain and other debilitating symptoms.
- Once acute compartment syndrome and fracture has been ruled out, patients may be referred to sports medicine or orthopedics for further evaluation and workup.

Nerve Entrapment

General Description

- As nerves traverse the lower leg, they may become entrapped at a number of different sites from a variety of conditions.
- Typically this is a condition that occurs with the slow growth of masses or scar tissue.
- However, casts and other compressive braces may cause focal impingement that may cause the patient to be symptomatic.
- The location and extent of entrapment will determine the extent of symptoms.

Mechanism

- Prior trauma, surgery, tight-fitting casts, braces, contusions, or arthritis may cause the development of scar tissue, cysts, masses, or osteophytes that effectively entrap nerves.
- Symptoms usually develop over time, as the structure is progressively impinged.

Presentation

- Patients generally complain of insidious onset of burning pain or paresthesias in a particular dermatome that maps to the affected nerve.
- They may also present with weakness of the innervated muscles or subtle muscle atrophy.

Physical Exam

- A key to diagnosis is to determine the specific area involved to further assist in the identification of the particular nerve that is entrapped.
- The common peroneal nerve may become entrapped at the fibular head causing neuropathic pain on the anterolateral aspect of the leg that extends into the foot.
  - They may also have a foot drop and recurrent ankle injuries.
  - The distal branches of the common peroneal nerve may also be entrapped and symptomatic.
- The sural and saphenous nerves may also become entrapped and cause pain.
- Any overlying restricting devices should be removed and the area of complaint fully examined for scars, masses, or deformities that may cause pressure or stretching of nerves.
- A *Tinel's sign* may be performed at the presumed site of impingement.

- A recurrent tapping on the nerve will cause a distinct shooting pain into the affected area that will reproduce the patient's symptoms.

Essential Diagnostics

- Imaging is important to rule out bony or soft tissue structures that are compressing the nerve.
- This may begin with x-rays but an MRI scan may be needed to fully assess for soft tissue masses.
- Nerve conduction studies may be useful in determining the location and severity of nerve entrapments.

ED Treatment

- The EP should evaluate for acute causes of compression, such as fractures, masses, or cysts, utilizing the physical exam and standard x-rays.
  - In most cases, more advanced imaging may be done as an outpatient.
- Generally, conservative treatment is all that is needed in the ED.
- Patients should be advised to rest, remove any compressive devices, use NSAIDs for pain and avoid activities that exacerbate symptoms.

Disposition

- Patients will need further imaging and possible nerve conduction studies and should be referred to sports medicine or orthopedics for further workup.

Complications

- Progressive weakness, paresthesias, and loss of function are the most common outcomes in untreated disease.

Pediatric Considerations

- There are no specific pediatric considerations.

Pearls and Pitfalls

- Don't forget other causes of neuropathy, like diabetes or multiple sclerosis.
- In addition, it is important to rule out a more proximal cause of symptoms such as impingement from the low back or spine.
- A broad differential diagnosis should always be considered and evaluated with a thorough history and physical exam.
- The diagnosis of nerve entrapment is often a difficult one to make and it may be missed on the first encounter.

Gastrocnemius Musculotendinous Tears

General Description

- Acute strains and tears of the gastrocnemius musculotendinous complex usually occur on the medial aspect.
- Patient are often over 30 years of age.

Mechanism

- A strong force is applied across the calf musculature, as often occurs in running up a hill, playing tennis, or jumping.

Presentation

- Patients feel an acute tearing or stabbing sensation in the posterior mid calf.
- They may complain of weakness after the injury and will have moderate swelling and ecchymosis of the area.
- Occasionally, they may hear a distinct popping sound at the time of injury.

Physical Exam

- The musculotendinous junction at the posterior distal aspect of the gastrocnemius is often focally tender, swollen, and ecchymotic.
- It is important to rule out other conditions, particularly an Achilles tendon rupture or deep vein thrombosis.

Essential Diagnostics

- Radiographs may be useful to evaluate for associated fracture, and bedside ultrasound may be utilized to demonstrate focal edema and disruption of the muscle tendon complex.
- If the diagnosis of Achilles tendon rupture is being considered, a formal ultrasound may confirm the integrity of the tendon.
- An MRI may also demonstrate Achilles rupture, or other pathologies.

ED Treatment

- Patients should be provided with pain control, compression, crutches, and possibly a fracture boot for a short period of time.
- The boot will limit plantarflexion and effectively offload the gastrocnemius muscle.
- Ice, elevation, and activity restrictions are important treatments as well.

- The patient should be instructed to begin gentle ankle range of motion exercises once pain is controlled to the point of relative comfort.

Disposition

- Patients will need referrals to sports medicine and physical therapy for ongoing treatment.
- Soft tissue therapies and eccentric exercises (loadbearing while lengthening the muscle) are effective in improving symptoms and strengthening the musculotendinous junction.

Complications

- Patients will often have a prolonged period of time before returning to full activity.
- Given the immobility and swelling over the leg, the patient will be at risk for developing DVTs.
- This should be discussed with the patient, and if any concerning symptoms develop they should seek care right away.

Pediatric Considerations

- This condition is more common in adults, especially over 30 years old.
- Certain genetic connective tissue disorders may make this more common in young patients.

Pearls and Pitfalls

- The biggest pitfall with this condition is not considering Achilles tendon rupture.
  - While almost all gastrocnemius muscle tears will heal with time and conservative treatment, Achilles tendon tears require much more intense evaluation and treatment.
  - If there is any concern that the Achilles tendon may be ruptured, the patient should be splinted in plantarflexion, made non-weight bearing, and have close follow-up for additional imaging arranged.
  - Failure to do so could change a nonoperative case into an operative one.

ANKLE

Background/Epidemiology

- The ankle is a very commonly injured joint and patients will commonly present with ankle-related pain to the ED.
- Ankle injuries, particularly sprains, are common. The vast majority of patients with ankle injuries likely do not seek medical treatment initially and may only present once symptoms are not improving with conservative treatment.
- Severe ankle injuries or recurrent untreated injuries may predispose patients to recurrent injuries from relatively minor traumas.
- The Ottawa Ankle Rules are useful for eliminating unnecessary radiographs.[7] An x-ray is only required if:
  - There is bony tenderness to palpation along the distal 6 cm posterior edge of the medial malleolus.
  - There is bony tenderness along the distal 6 cm posterior edge of the lateral malleolus.
  - The patient is unable to bear weight both immediately or for four steps in the emergency department.
- A systematic review and meta-analysis found that ankle sprains occur more commonly in females than in males (13.6 vs. 6.94 per 1000 exposures), in children compared to adolescents (2.85 vs. 1.94 per 1000 exposures), and in adolescents compared to adults (1.94 vs. 0.72 per 1000 exposures).[5]

Anatomic Considerations/ Pathophysiology

- The ankle joint is formed from the ends of the distal tibia, fibula, and the superior aspect of the talus.
- This joint allows forward flexion, called dorsiflexion, and extension, referred to as plantarflexion.
- Other motions occur just below the ankle joint proper at the talocalcaneal joint, referred to as the subtalar joint.
- The subtalar joint allows for inversion and eversion of the foot relative to the leg.
- A combination of inversion, plantarflexion, and foot adduction create foot supination, while eversion, dorsiflexion, and abduction create foot pronation.
- Patients may have a degree of baseline pronation or supination while standing or running that will cause compression of the

foot and ankle joints or overload certain musculotendinous units.

- Often times, a basic biomechanical analysis may determine the root cause of the patient's pain and simple adjustments of stance and gait may markedly improve symptoms.

- The ankle joint is held together with several ligaments that provide important stability to the joint while allowing for motion that provides for ambulation.
  - Laterally, the ankle is supported most anteriorly by the anterior talofibular ligament (ATFL), posteriorly by the posterior talofibular ligament (PTFL), and by the calcaneofibular ligament (CFL) in between (Figure 7.5).
    - The ATFL crosses from the anterior distal tip of fibula, called the lateral malleolus, to the anterior lateral aspect of the talus.
    - The PTFL crosses horizontally from the posterior lip of the lateral malleolus to the posterior talus.
    - The CFL runs nearly vertically from the distal tip of the lateral malleolus to a projection on the lateral aspect of the calcaneus.
    - These ligaments prevent excessive inversion of the ankle.
    - In addition, the distal extension of the tibia known as the medial malleolus also prevents inversion; however, it is relatively short compared to the lateral malleolus and therefore allows more inversion than eversion injuries.
- The medial ankle is supported by the broad, strong deltoid ligament (Figure 7.6).
  - While this is often considered as one single ligament it is actually composed of four distinct ligaments: the anterior tibiotalar, tibiocalcaneal, posterior tibiotalar, and tibionavicular ligaments.
  - The strength of the deltoid is further buttressed by the longer lateral malleolus, making eversion-type ankle sprains much less common.
- The ankle joint is further supported by ligaments and a fibrous syndesmosis (Figure 7.1) that spans the distance between the distal tibia and fibula.
  - The anterior inferior tibiofibular ligament and the posterior inferior tibiofibular ligament are structures that support the ring of the lower leg and prevent separation of the tibia and fibula.
  - A force sufficient to disrupt the ankle ligaments and force the tibia and fibula apart may sprain these ligaments and the interosseus membrane that runs the length of the two bones.
  - This is what is often referred to as a "high ankle sprain."

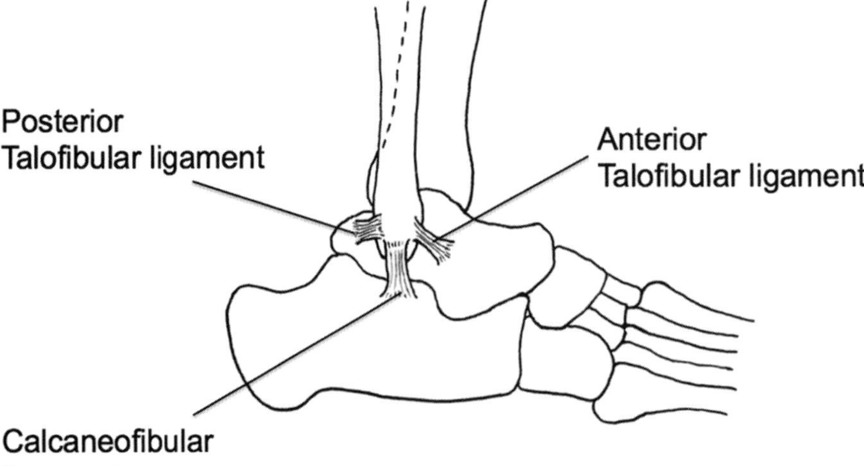

Figure 7.5. Lateral ankle ligaments. Illustration by Yvonne Chow.

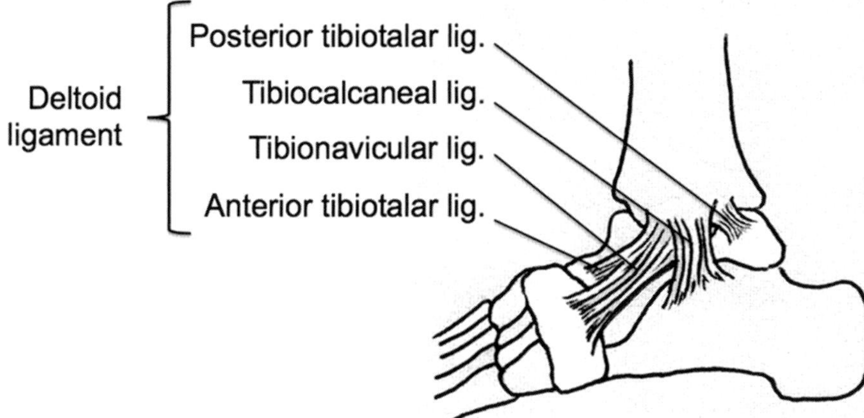

Figure 7.6. Deltoid ligament. Illustration by Yvonne Chow.

- Ligamentous injuries may be graded in a simple fashion.
  - Grade 1 refers to stretching of the ligament without tearing.
  - Grade 2 involves partial tearing but with some fibers still intact.
  - Grade 3 occurs with a total disruption of the ligament.
- When the ankle moves quickly into an inverted position that initiates an ankle injury, the first ligament to come under stress is the ATFL.
  - This will begin stretching and eventually fail.
  - As the force is continued, the CFL gets overwhelmed and tears.
  - Finally, with continued force, the PTFL will fail.
  - This sequence is frequently followed with lateral ankle injuries.
- Eversion ankle injuries are less common, but when they occur they cause injury to the deltoid ligament on the medial ankle.
  - The deltoid may become disrupted at several locations, but one particular concern is that the force will cross through the joint and extend into the tibiofibular syndesmosis more proximally through the interosseus membrane (Figure 7.1).
  - These injuries may be unstable.
- The edema and ecchymosis from ankle sprains may be quite impressive and may cause significant pain. Patients should not only be reassured but also encouraged to take measures to decrease swelling (i.e., elevation, compression, rest, and ice).

Focused History and Physical Exam

History

- Acutely, patients will often present with significant pain, swelling, and limited ambulation.
- They often report a history of trauma in which the ankle "gave way" during walking or running. Loud pops or cracks may occur with ankle ligament rupture as well as fractures.
- Frequent giving-way episodes may be indicative of instability.
- Occasionally, the history is more gradual in nature.
- Patients may complain of grinding, popping, or catching sensations within the joint.
- They may notice consistent swelling without significant trauma. This may be associated with a dull chronic achy pain in the ankle.
- Previous surgeries or trauma may lead to significant degeneration of joint surfaces, evidenced by arthritic changes on imaging or limited ROM on exam.

Physical Exam

- Inspection
  - The ankle should be visualized without any clothing on and in positions of rest and standing (if possible).
  - The alignment of the foot relative to the leg should be evaluated, because not only may

acute changes in position indicate fracture or dislocation but may also be evidence for underlying structural abnormalities that may cause overuse injuries.
- A patient's stance and gait may be helpful in identifying biomechanical issues that may cause injury.
- The examiner should look for areas of focal and diffuse swelling as well as ecchymosis that may point toward the ultimate diagnosis.

Palpation

- When examining the ankle it is often easiest to have the patient seated on the edge of the bed with the leg hanging down (if possible).
- This allows for access to the areas that need to be palpated and for testing of motion and strength.
- The examiner should first palpate along the anterior aspect of the ankle joint, looking for swelling, fullness, bony abnormalities, or tenderness.
- This palpation may then be carried along the medial and lateral malleoli to assess for areas of tenderness and swelling.
- Areas away from ligamentous attachments (i.e., the posterior lip of lateral malleolus) should be assessed for bony tenderness.
  - This is because, regardless of the degree of sprained ligament, focal bony tenderness may indicate potential fracture.
- Make sure to palpate along the distal aspect of the tibiofibular syndesmosis (along the tibiofibular junction, just superior to ankle joint proper).
  - The anterior aspect of the distal syndesmosis may be an area of focal pain after severe ankle injuries that sprain or stretch the syndesmotic fibers.

ROM

- The cardinal motions to be tested in the ankle are: dorsiflexion, plantarflexion, eversion, and inversion.
- The typical ranges for each motion are:
  - 0–20° for dorsiflexion
  - 0–50° for plantarflexion
  - 0–25° for eversion
  - 0–35° for inversion
- Passive ROM should be assessed if there are limitations with active range of motion.

Special Tests

- The *anterior drawer test* (Figure 7.7) is useful in testing the stability of the ATFL.
  - The ankle is tested in a small amount of plantarflexion, approximately 20°.
  - The examiner cups the heel in one hand and stabilizes the lower leg with the other.
  - The hand cupping the heel is then pulled forward and the degree of anterior translation of the foot relative to the tibia is assessed.
  - It is important to assess for side-to-side differences because of possible chronic laxity that may cause the exam to be positive.
  - This exam will often be very painful in an acute injury and the patient may not be able to cooperate well. (The patient may counter the exam with muscle resistance causing a falsely negative exam.)
- *Compression test* (Figure 7.3)
  - This test is used to test for high ankle sprain or injury to the syndesmosis.

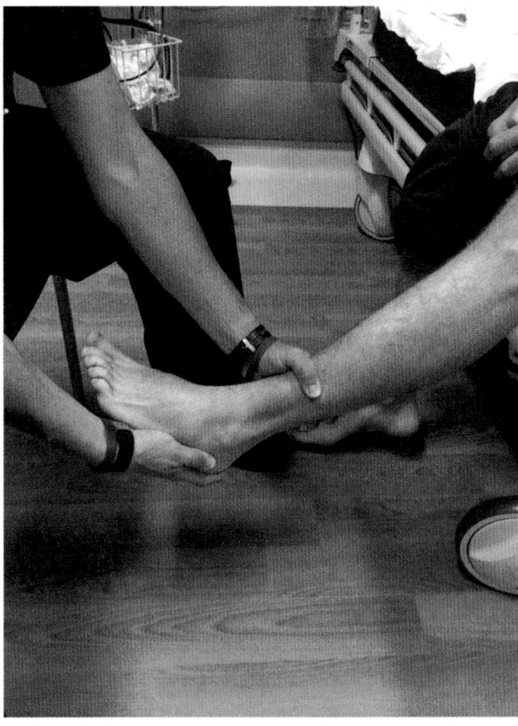

Figure 7.7. Anterior drawer test.

- This test is performed by the examiner compressing the proximal tibia and fibula and assessing for pain anteriorly over the syndesmosis or for any instability.

- *Dorsiflexion eversion test* (Figure 7.4)
  - This test is also used to test the integrity of the syndesmosis.
  - With the patient sitting on the exam table, the examiner passively dorsiflexes and everts the foot while stabilizing the proximal calf with the other hand.
  - This test is positive if it causes pain or instability over the syndesmosis.

Neurovascular Exam

- Posterior to the medial malleolus is the posterior tibial artery.
  - This pulse should be evaluated during an ankle examination.
- Any areas of paresthesia should be noted.
- Some muscle power may be tested with the patient seated.
  - The examiner holds the patient's lower leg and asks the patient to resist eversion, inversion, and dorsiflexion.
  - Subtle changes may be assessed from side to side.
  - However, a patient may often generate much more power for plantarflexion since this is used routinely in locomotion.
  - Therefore, subtle differences may be missed if the patient's strength is tested while seated.
- The patient should be asked to stand and walk on the toes to test plantarflexion (or heels to test dorsiflexion).
- Standing behind the patient may be helpful in assessing calf muscle symmetry and bulk.
- Finally, the ankle jerk reflex and the presence/absence of clonus should be evaluated while examining the ankle.

Differential Diagnosis

- The differential diagnosis of ankle pain and injury should include medial ankle sprains, lateral ankle sprains, ankle instability, posterior tibial tendinopathy, peroneal tendinopathy, osteochondral lesions, ankle fractures (medial, lateral, or posterior malleoli), ankle dislocations, and arthritis (not covered in this chapter).

Medial Ankle Sprains

Background

- The ankle is a commonly injured joint, but only 20 percent of ankle injuries are medial in nature.
  - This is usually due to the fact that the medial ligament complex (deltoid) is much larger and stronger than the lateral side, and the lateral malleolus is longer than the medial.
  - This provides additional support against lateral movement of the foot into an everted position.
- General principles of treatment for ankle sprains do not necessarily vary from medial to lateral; however, there are special types of injuries that may occur with a medial ankle sprain that need to be considered, such as high ankle sprains and Maisonneuve fractures.
- High-risk activities for medial ankle sprains include basketball, football, volleyball, and long jumping.

Mechanism

- As the patient is ambulating, a force is directed to the foot that pushes it into an everted position.
- The posterior tibialis muscle ideally resists this motion, but if it occurs too quickly the deltoid ligament acts as the major restraint to forceful eversion.
- The forces typically pass across the deltoid ligament from an anterior to posterior position, progressing from spraining or pulling the ligaments to fully tearing the ligament.
- While the lateral malleolus may act as a secondary buttress to ankle eversion, a significant enough force may disrupt the deltoid ligament and fracture part of the lateral malleolus or sprain part of the tibiofibular syndesmosis.
- A particularly unique injury that may occur with this injury pattern is a Maisonneuve fracture.
  - This usually occurs with a medial ankle sprain (or fracture) and results due to an extension of force superiorly up the tibiofibular syndesmosis.
  - As this force propagates up the syndesmosis, it may break out by fracturing through the more proximal aspect of the fibula.

- This fracture tends to be inherently unstable and often needs surgical repair.

Presentation

- Patients will present after an acute eversion injury and complain of pain, moderate swelling, and ecchymosis.
- While the pain may be focused on the medial side, swelling and mild tenderness may diffuse.
- Patients may have a difficult time walking.
- More subacute injuries may present with tingling in the toes or foot from nerve stretching or irritation from blood or swelling.
- Patients may report hearing or feeling a loud pop or crack as ligaments gave way.

Physical Exam

- The examiner should start by palpating along the anterior joint line and then progress medially and laterally along the ligamentous restraints.
- Patients will be very tender over areas of ligamentous disruption, but any area of bony tenderness that does not have a nearby ligament attachment should increase the suspicion of fracture.
- An *anterior drawer test* (Figure 7.7) should be performed to assess for gross instability.
  - This will likely be painful regardless of the injury pattern.
- It is important to palpate along the shaft of the fibula when suspecting medial ankle injuries.
  - Any focal bony tenderness (even as far away as the fibular head) should cause the EP to evaluate for fibular fracture.
- High ankle sprain, or injury to the syndesmosis, should always be evaluated.
  - Compression of the leg (Figure 7.3) may be helpful in identifying syndesmotic injury.
  - Passive dorsiflexion with eversion may also cause pain or instability over the syndesmosis (Figure 7.4).
- Neurovascular integrity should be assessed.

Essential Diagnostics

- X-rays may be useful in distinguishing fracture from sprain.
- Algorithms, such as the Ottowa ankle rules, have been designed to indicate when to obtain x-rays.
  - If the clinical suspicion is high x-rays should be obtained regardless of these rules.
- Both the AP and mortise views should be examined closely for both evidence of fracture and instability.
  - The mortise view is a view of the talar dome inserting between the medial and lateral malleoli.
  - Special attention should be paid to evaluating the medial clear space (between the talus and medial malleolus).
    - This should be less than 4 mm.
  - The tibiofibular clear space between the tibia and fibula should also be evaluated.
    - This should be less than 5-6 mm.
  - Furthermore, stress views may be helpful in investigating the integrity of the mortise.
- The provider should consider obtaining tibia/fibula films if any more proximal bony tenderness is present.
- Occasionally, MRI may be useful in assessing for further soft tissue injury, but is rarely needed in the ED.
- Bedside ultrasound may be utilized to assess the integrity of ligaments and other structures.

ED Treatment

- Acute treatment of medial ankle sprains involves a "PRICE" protocol (Protection, Rest, Ice, Compression, Elevation).
- Patients should be provided with some sort brace for protection and compression.
- Weight-bearing devices like a walking boot or compressive cast are ideal, but occasionally patients may need a non-weight bearing period.
  - Removable walking boots are often well tolerated.
- Ice and elevation may be very helpful during the acute phase.
- Patients should be advised to attempt to keep the extremity elevated on a pillow, ideally above the level of the heart.

- Ice should be applied for 20 minutes three to four times a day.
  - Patients should be cautioned about placing ice directly on the skin, especially if there are any comorbid neuropathies or vascular insufficiency.
- Anti-inflammatories may be useful for pain control.
- Phase 1 of treatment (one to two weeks) focuses on ice, elevation, and improving swelling.
  - Patients may be advised in the ED to begin gentle ROM exercises (i.e., spelling the alphabet with toes, moving from full dorsiflexion to plantarflexion) as soon as pain allows.
- Phase 2 (two to four weeks) focuses on beginning to regain full ROM and weight-bearing.
- Phase 3 (four to six weeks) begins to incorporate more aggressive strengthening and rehabilitation exercises.
  - There is evidence that a program of proprioception exercises is effective at reducing the rate of recurrent ankle sprains in active patients.[6]

Disposition

- Patients should be referred to primary care or a sports medicine physician to ensure that proper rehabilitation is obtained.
- Patients may return to play when pain and swelling have resolved and they have regained near normal strength and ROM
  - They often benefit from a functional ankle brace when returning to play.
  - It often takes four to eight weeks for full return to sports after an ankle sprain.
- Any evidence of fibular fracture above the level of the mortise (i.e., Maisonneuve fracture) should be discussed with orthopedics for further management, as these are often inherently unstable.

Complications

- Once an ankle is injured, the inherent proprioception feedback from foot to brain becomes disrupted.
- This unfortunately leads to an increased risk of further injury.
- Exacerbating this concern is the fact that ligaments may not heal normally (especially if torn significantly).
- Without close follow-up and rehabilitation these patients often go on to have recurrent ankle injuries and gross instability.

Pediatric Considerations

- Children frequently have ankle sprains and should generally be treated the same as adults.
- However, the one salient difference in a growing child is the presence of open physeal plates, which places them at risk for Salter–Harris-type fractures.
- This is due to the fact that the ligamentous structures tend to be stronger than the physeal plates, and forces directed at the ankle may disrupt the physis prior to tearing the ligaments.
- When examining a child, a provider should closely assess for any focal growth plate tenderness and subsequently image and protect as needed.

Pearls and Pitfalls

- Referrals for physical therapy may be very helpful to fully return patients to prior levels of activity.
- In addition, ongoing use of an ankle brace when going back to sports may prevent further injury.
- When the deltoid ligament is injured, always assess for injury to the syndesmosis and Maisonneuve fracture.

Lateral Ankle Sprains

Background

- Lateral ankle sprains are very common and routinely affect both the athletic and non-athletic population.
- While ankle sprains in general are fairly common, nearly 80 percent of them are lateral in nature, making this the much more common injury.
- They are also seen in many different settings, from the primary care physician's office to the ED.
- Ankle sprains may occur during many different types of athletic events, including basketball, soccer, volleyball, and tennis.

- In some types of sports, they become so common that most athletes have "turned" their ankles many times.
- They may also occur during simple activities of daily living, such as with simple walking on uneven ground.
- Unfortunately, these common injuries are not always properly assessed or treated with the appropriate rehabilitation therapies.
- This potentially leads to chronic pain or instability that may worsen over time and lead to further injury.

Mechanism

- Lateral ankle sprains occur when the foot lands on an uneven surface and inverts at the ankle.
- Rapid proprioceptive messages are sent back to the nervous system about the potentially abnormal motion in the ankle.
- Ideally, the peroneal muscles will react to the ground reaction forces and provide a stabilizing force before the ankle is inverted to the critical point at which the ligaments and capsule are sprained or torn.
- During an acute injury, the ground reaction forces overwhelm the intrinsic stability of the ankle and force the foot into an inverted position.
- The ligaments of the lateral ankle are engaged in a predictably sequential pattern.
  - First the ATFL is engaged and recruited to resist the excessive motion.
  - If the force is exceeds the limits of the ATFL's tensile strength, then the ligament will be pulled, stretched, and then torn in a progressive fashion.
  - The CFL is the next ligament to be engaged and potentially torn, followed by the PTFL.
- A posterior rotational force could potentially reverse this order, and sprain the PTFL first.
- However, the CFL is rarely injured in isolation.
- When the forces on the ankle are directed superiorly toward the distal tibiofibular joint, the fibers of the anterior inferior tibiofibular ligament and tibiofibular syndesmosis may be sprained or torn.
- The force will continue vertically up the syndesmosis causing what is referred to as a "high ankle sprain."
- Due to the relative strength of the syndesmosis, the amount of force required to cause a high ankle sprain is quite high.
- In addition, the soft tissue damage is relatively large; therefore, this injury tends to take a prolonged time to heal.

Presentation

- Patients will usually present after an acute inversion injury complaining of lateral-sided ankle pain with a moderate degree of swelling and early ecchymosis.
- Depending on the overall stability of the ankle, the inversion injury that caused them to present may be relatively minor if the ankle is unstable.
- Patients may have difficulty walking
- They may report a history of turning the ankle inward and hearing or feeling a series of "pops," usually related to the ligaments giving way.

Physical Exam

- An acutely injured ankle will often have moderately diffuse swelling and ecchymosis, not just isolated to the lateral side.
- The examiner should take a consistent approach to examining the ankle.
- This usually involves starting over the anterior joint line and progressing medially and laterally over the restraining ligaments.
- These areas will often be swollen and focally tender to palpation.
- The space between the distal tibia and fibula should be palpated to evaluate for any tenderness of the distal syndesmosis.
- *Compression test* of the tibia and fibula (Figure 7.3) and *passive dorsiflexion with eversion test* (Figure 7.4) should be performed to test the integrity of the syndesmosis.
- An *anterior drawer test* (Figure 7.7) should be performed on these patients, but the examiner should be aware that this will invariably cause acute pain.
  - The real diagnostic value of the test is in estimation of relative anterior translation of the foot relative to the distal tibia.
  - This may be performed on a delayed basis after the acute swelling as decreased.
- Active ROM should be tested including inversion.

- Particularly important is to test for peroneal tendon subluxation.
  - This may be done with passive circumduction of the ankle while feeling for subluxation of the tendons over the posterior lip of the lateral malleolus.
  - Peroneal tendon and muscle function should be grossly assessed as well.
- Neurovascular exam should be performed.

Essential Diagnostics

- X-rays may be useful in assessing for fractures.
  - Decision algorithms such as the Ottowa ankle rules may be used to guide the decision of whether or not to image.
  - The ankle mortise view should be examined particularly closely for any evidence of instability.
    - For further details, please see medial ankle sprain.

ED Treatment

- Acute treatment of lateral ankle sprains involves a PRICE protocol (Protection, Rest, Ice, Compression, Elevation).
- Patients should be provided with some sort brace for protection and compression.
- Weight-bearing devices like a walking boot or compressive cast are ideal, but occasionally patients may need a non-weight bearing period.
- Ice and elevation may be very helpful during the acute phase.
  - Patients should be advised to attempt to keep the extremity elevated on a pillow, ideally above the level of the heart.
  - Ice should be applied for 20 minutes three to four times a day.
  - Patients should be cautioned about placing ice directly on the skin, especially if there are any comorbid neuropathies or vascular insufficiency.
- NSAIDs may be useful for pain control.
- Phase 1 of treatment (one to two weeks) focuses on ice, elevation, and improving swelling.
  - Patients may be advised in the ED to begin gentle ROM exercises (i.e., spelling the alphabet with toes, moving from full dorsiflexion to plantarflexion) as soon as pain allows.
- Phase 2 (two to four weeks) focuses on beginning to regain full ROM and weight-bearing. Phase 3 (four to six weeks) begins to incorporate more aggressive strengthening and rehabilitation exercises.
  - There is evidence that a program of proprioception exercises is effective at reducing the rate of recurrent ankle sprains in active patients.[6]
- Patients may return to play when pain and swelling have subsided and they have regained near normal strength and ROM
  - They may benefit from using a functional ankle brace upon returning to sports.

Disposition

- Patients should be referred to a primary care or sports medicine physician to ensure proper rehabilitation is obtained.
- Once an ankle is injured, the inherent proprioception feedback from foot to brain becomes disrupted.
- This unfortunately leads to an increased risk of further injury.
- Exacerbating this concern is the fact that ligaments may not heal normally (especially if they are torn significantly).
- Without close follow-up and rehabilitation these patients often go on to have recurrent ankle injuries and gross instability.

Pediatric Considerations

- Children frequently have ankle sprains and should generally be treated the same as adults.
- However, the one salient difference in a growing child is the presence of open physeal plates, which places them at risk for Salter–Harris-type fractures.
- This is due to the fact that the ligamentous structures tend to be stronger than the physeal plates and forces directed at the ankle may disrupt the physis prior to tearing the ligaments.
- When examining a child, a provider should closely assess for any focal growth plate tenderness and subsequently image and protect as needed.

Pearls and Pitfalls

- Referrals for physical therapy may be very helpful in fully returning patients to prior levels of activity.
- In addition, ongoing use of an ankle brace when going back to sports may prevent further injury.
- Always assess for injury to the syndesmosis and Maisonneuve fracture.

Ankle Instability

Background

- Repeated injuries to the ankle will progressively stretch and disrupt the ligaments until they are no longer able to support the joint.
- This may occur with a single injury or, more often, with repeated injuries.
- A good history and physical exam often points to chronic instability, and aggressive rehabilitation may prevent further injury.
- Occasionally, these patients have ankle injuries that are unstable enough to need surgery to repair ligaments and tighten the joint capsule.

Mechanism

- Whenever an ankle sprain occurs, the affected ligaments are stretched and potentially torn.
- This microscopic injury may progressively weaken the ligaments, or recurrent injuries may cause the ligaments to progressively stretch.
- In some patients, frank tears of the ligaments prevent further healing and the ligaments do not heal at all.

Presentation

- Patients present with recurrent ankle sprains that become progressively easier to induce with relatively minor trauma.
- Often they present with a recent acute ankle sprain in the setting of recurrent injuries.
- Many patients have a history of a severe ankle injury in the past, and, as time passes, more minor trauma causes recurrent sprains.
- Things as simple as uneven ground may cause a significant ankle sprain. Patients may also complain of popping or grinding in the ankle.

Physical Exam

- A thorough exam of the ankle is important, particularly palpating the joint margins and medial/lateral ligamentous restraints.
- Any bony tenderness should be noted, as should any knee or foot pathology that may potentially predispose the patient to recurrent ankle injuries.
- The most important test for ankle instability is an *anterior drawer test* (Figure 7.7), which will demonstrate gross instability in the affected ankle.
- Occasionally, patients have instability bilaterally, but still the relative amount of anterior translation will be grossly obvious.

Essential Diagnostics

- X-rays are useful in evaluating for other conditions, such as fractures, but usually an MRI is necessary to determine the nature of the soft tissue injury and to confirm the diagnosis.
- MRI is not usually indicated in the ED and may be performed as an outpatient.

ED Treatment

- Since these patients often present at the time of an acute exacerbation, they should be treated as for any acute ankle sprain (as noted earlier in lateral and medial ankle sprain sections).

Disposition

- These patients need to follow-up with a sports medicine or orthopedic physician.
- Patients need a referral for formal physical therapy to work on strengthening and proprioception-type rehabilitation programs.
  - If they fail these regimens, they may need surgery.
- Patients may return to play when pain has subsided and they have near normal strength and ROM
  - They should wear a functional brace for an indefinite amount of time when returning to sports.

Complications

- The complications of ankle instability include recurrent ankle sprains, arthritis, fractures, dislocations, and disruption of joint cartilage possibly leading to loose bodies or osteochondral lesions.

Pediatric Considerations

- Children do have repeated ankle sprains and often ongoing growth spurts may cause relatively increased joint mobility.

- It is important to ensure appropriate conservative treatment and rehabilitation for these patients since allowing repeated injury may lead to long-term complications.

Pearls and Pitfalls

- This diagnosis is a complication of repeated ankle injuries and may be avoided with proper acute treatment.
- Anytime a patient reports a history of frequent ankle injuries, this diagnosis should be considered and appropriate treatment/ follow-up arranged.
- Further injury and joint damage may be avoided with early, aggressive treatment.

Posterior Tibial Tendinopathy

Background

- The posterior tibial tendon is one of the main supporting structures of the medial ankle and arch.
- It originates on the posterior aspect of the tibia, fibula, and interosseous membrane.
- It then travels distally along the posterior medial malleolus and turns around the distal malleolus to insert on the bases of the second through fourth metatarsals, the second through third cuneiforms, and the cuboid.
- The action of this muscle helps support the medial arch of the foot.
- The area of the tendon that wraps around the medial malleolus is particularly at risk of injury because of its limited blood supply. This watershed zone creates an area that is difficult to heal.
- Overuse or acute injury (i.e., ankle sprain) may cause inflammation of the tendon leading to pain along the tendon or even dysfunction that allows the arch of the foot to flatten.

Mechanism

- Medial ankle sprains, obesity, diabetes, hypertension, or overuse may cause the tendon to become inflamed and lead to dysfunction.
- Overuse injuries may occur especially in runners who wear worn-out running shoes or who have flat feet causing strain on the posterior tibial tendon.

Presentation

- Patients complain of pain along the medial side of the foot and ankle and may occasionally have an unsteady gait.
- They may notice swelling along the medial aspect of the ankle, particularly along the posterior distal medial malleolus.

Physical Exam

- Patients have tenderness and swelling along the course of the posterior tibial tendon.
- They may have weakness and/or pain inverting the foot, and commonly have difficulty standing on the toes of the affected side.
- In advanced cases with tendon dysfunction the medial arch is decreased or completely flattened.
  - The heel shows increased valgus from behind and the forefoot is abducted revealing the "too many toes sign."
    - This sign is seen when the forefoot abducts laterally and more than the two most lateral toes are viewed from the back when the patient is standing facing away from the examiner.
    - Eventually, the lateral foot will abut against the distal fibula, causing impingement and lateral pain.

Essential Diagnostics

- Basic radiographs are important to evaluate for fracture or congenital fusion of the foot bones that may cause ankle dysfunction.
- Ultrasound and MRI are adjunctive imaging modalities in the outpatient setting but are rarely indicated in the ED.
  - Ultrasound may be useful in evaluating the integrity of the tendon and surrounding edema.
  - MRI may be needed to identify tendon rupture or inflammation.

ED Treatment

- Acute treatment should include basic imaging to evaluate for fracture.
- Patients may be placed in a cam fracture boot or air cast to support and limit motion of the posterior tibial tendon.

- NSAIDs, focal icing, and rest are all key components of acute therapy.
- A medial arch support will also help improve alignment of the foot until the tendon heals.

Disposition

- Patients should be referred to sports medicine or primary care for follow-up.
    - Occasionally, in severe cases of tendinopathy, casting for four weeks may be indicated to resolve inflammation.
- After a period of relative rest and improvement in acute symptoms, physical therapy is often helpful for working on strengthening programs to improve posterior tibial function.
- Patients may return to play once pain has resolved and they have regained normal strength and ROM
    - Some may benefit from arch supports.

Complications

- The most problematic complication is tendon rupture and loss of the medial arch.
    - Acutely, the tendon may be repaired and the arch restored.
    - In cases of prolonged tendon dysfunction, the foot may become arthritic and have limited flexibility.
        - This makes primary tendon repair very difficult and may require an ankle fusion to remedy the problem.

Pediatric Considerations

- Young athletes are at risk for this condition, especially if involved in extensive running sports.
- The provider should always consider other entities, such as growth plate injuries or congenital foot fusions.
- Often a break in sporting activities with improved shoe wear, arch supports, and therapy to strengthen the posterior tibial tendon may be helpful.

Pearls and Pitfalls

- Posterior tibial tendinopathy and dysfunction lie along a spectrum of disease, with the former being much easier to treat.
    - Once the patient begins to have tendon dysfunction, bracing or even surgery may be indicated.
- Posterior tibial tendinopathy should be considered in the differential diagnosis of medial ankle pain.

Peroneal Tendinopathy

Background

- Symptoms of peroneal tendinopathy include pain and swelling along the course of the peroneal tendons just posterior and distal to the lateral malleolus.
- The peroneal muscles (peroneus longus and peroneus brevis) originate from the lateral surface of the fibula and the intermuscular septa of the lower leg.
    - They run together around the posterior lateral malleolus then divide with the brevis, attaching on the base of the fifth metatarsal and the longus coursing under the foot to attach on the base of the first metatarsal.

Mechanism

- Runners who run along slopes which cause excess eversion of the foot are more susceptible to peroneal tendinopathy.
- Also, overpronation of the foot causes the tendon to run against the malleolus and inflames the tissue.
- Tight calf muscles will effectively increase the tension in the peroneal tendons and cause more friction between the tendons and the bone.
- Overuse often plays a factor, especially in basketball players, runners, or dancers.

Presentation

- Patients present with pain and swelling along the course of the peroneal muscles or near the attachment of the peroneus brevis tendon at the base of the fifth metatarsal.
- This may have occurred over time with overuse, or may have occurred with an acute injury (i.e., lateral ankle sprain).
- The pain is often worse during activity and improves with rest.

Physical Exam

- Patients often have tenderness to palpation along the peroneal tendons.
- There may also be focal swelling in this area.
- Resisted eversion and passive inversion causes pain over the course of the peroneal tendons.

Essential Diagnostics

- X-rays of the ankle are helpful to evaluate for bony deformity, avulsion, or fracture.
- Ultrasound and MRI may be used to diagnose the peroneal tendon tears or edema consistent with tendinopathy, but are rarely indicated in the ED.

ED Treatment

- The mainstay of treatment is rest, since many of these injuries are due to overuse.
- Focal ice massage and NSAIDs may be helpful in alleviating pain.
- A cam fracture boot or air cast may be helpful in offloading the affected tendons and providing rest.

Disposition

- Once other acute injuries have been ruled out, patients may be sent home to follow-up with their primary care doctor or a sports medicine specialist.
- Patients may return to sport once they are pain free and have regained full strength and ROM
  - Some may benefit from the addition of orthotics.

Complications

- Untreated cases may go on to develop chronic symptoms and limit an individual's ability to participate in running types of activities.
- In some patients, the fascia restraining the peroneal tendons from moving over the lateral malleolus may be become disrupted.
  - This allows the tendons to sublux over the posterior aspect of the lateral malleolus.
  - Patients present with popping in the lateral ankle, and this may be visualized or palpated when the patient circumducts or flexes the ankle.
  - This often requires a surgical repair.

Pediatric Considerations

- Young athletes may be at risk for this, especially if involved in extensive running sports.
- The provider should always consider other entities such as growth plate injuries or congenital foot fusions.
- Often a break in sporting activities with improved shoe wear, arch supports, and therapy to strengthen the peroneal tendons may be helpful.

Pearls and Pitfalls

- Patients with lateral ankle sprains may develop a component of peroneal tendinopathy, either from the initial injury or from compensated ambulation.
- Occasionally an x-ray shows a small avulsion off the proximal fifth metatarsal at the attachment of the peroneus brevis tendon.
- Peroneal tendinopathy is treated similarly to other lateral ankle sprains with rest, ice, bracing, and ROM exercises.

Osteochondral Lesions

Background

- At times, injuries to the ankle joint may introduce a shear or impaction force onto the hyaline cartilage that lines the ends of the tibia or talus.
- When this occurs, a piece of cartilage or cartilage-bone complex may be disrupted off the end of the bone.
  - This may still be partly attached or loose in the joint.
- Osteochondritis dissecans (OCD) is a condition of idiopathic subchondral avascularity that may predispose patients to developing osteochondral lesions.
- These lesions then fissure and potentially collapse.
- This disrupts the joint surface and leads to free bodies, early arthritis, and progressive joint destruction.

Mechanism

- In OCD, the relative avascularity of the underlying cartilage matrix allows the cartilage to be lifted away from the joint with less traumatic force than when cartilage is healthy.

- These lesions may then delaminate the ends of the bone and lead to joint destruction.
- They may be loose or lay within a crater on the end of the bone.

Presentation

- Patients will present with recurrent pain, swelling, and complaints of popping or catching sensations.
- There may have been a single previous injury or a history of recurrent episodes of turning the ankle.

Physical Exam

- The ankle is usually diffusely swollen and often exhibits a limited passive and active ROM
- There may be a recurrent popping or catching with circumduction of the ankle.
- Depending on the location of the lesion, there may be focal joint line tenderness to palpation (most commonly along the anterior joint).
- Generally, the ligaments and musculotendinous units that surround the ankle are stable on exam.

Essential Diagnostics

- The first step in diagnosing an osteochondral lesion is to obtain an x-ray.
- Early on in the course of disease, there may not be any discrete changes seen on x-rays.
- However, mortise views of the ankle may show a scooped-out lucency along the talar dome or tibial plafond that may appear small and wafer-like acutely or deep and cup-shaped in OCD disease.
- CT may be helpful in distinguishing the extent of bony involvement of the lesion, and MRI may further characterize the cartilaginous involvement.
    - Particularly helpful with MRI is to see fluid tracking between the lesion and the remaining talar dome, indicating a loose body.
- CT scan and MRI should usually be obtained as an outpatient and rarely need to be performed emergently, unless other diagnoses need to be ruled out.

ED Treatment

- When an osteochondral lesion is seen or suspected, the ankle should be immobilized and the patient should be made non-weight bearing until follow-up for further imaging.
- Symptoms of pain should be addressed and rest, ice, and elevation recommended.

Disposition

- Patients need follow-up with a sports medicine physician or orthopedist to determine the need for surgical intervention.
- Younger patients may be able to heal the lesion, and a trial of conservative therapy may be indicated for a lesion that is not totally loose yet.
- Subacute or chronic OCD lesions may also be treated initially with conservative therapy.
- Patients may return to play when pain has subsided and they regain normal strength and ROM

Complications

- Osteochondral lesions may become loose and move around the joint further disrupting existing cartilage.
- This may lead to early osteoarthritis and more cartilage damage.

Pediatric Considerations

- Children who are not yet fully skeletally mature will have a better chance of healing an osteochondral lesion back down to the existing joint surface.
- With age and skeletal maturity, the likelihood of spontaneous healing of these lesions decreases.

Pearls and Pitfalls

- An osteochondral lesion may occasionally be misdiagnosed as an ankle sprain.
- The examiner should be careful to examine the ligamentous restraints of the ankle for tenderness, swelling, or instability.
- If none of these exist but the patient still has ankle joint swelling and pain, the possibility of an osteochondral lesion must be considered.
- Close follow-up must be ensured to prevent further joint damage.

Ankle Fractures

Background

- Ankle fractures may involve various combinations of the medial, lateral, and posterior malleoli.
- Stable injury patterns tend to involve just one malleolus, while two or more fractured malleoli (bimalleolar or trimalleolar fractures) are considered unstable.
  - Fractures of the medial malleolus and injury to the deltoid ligament also increase the risk for unstable injuries.
- Stable injuries may often be treated nonoperatively with casting, while unstable injuries frequently need surgery to ensure stability of the joint and to prevent subsequent posttraumatic arthritis.
- The Weber grading system is used to classify lateral malleoli fractures.
  - Type A fractures occur below the level of the ankle joint.
    - The deltoid and tibiofibular syndesmosis are usually intact.
    - This pattern is typically stable because enough of the mortise joint of the ankle is intact to provide stability to the talotibial joint.
  - Type B fractures occur at the level of the ankle joint.
    - The tibiofibular syndesmosis is mostly intact and provides some additional support to the joint.
    - This fracture pattern tends to be unstable approximately 50 percent of the time.
      - This depends on the integrity of the medial deltoid ligaments.
  - Type C fractures occur above the level of the ankle joint.
    - These are known to be inherently unstable due to the loss of the mortise of the ankle.
    - In addition, the involvement of the tibiofibular syndesmosis further destabilizes the joint and potentially allows the talus to push between the tibia and fibula with weight-bearing.

Mechanism

- Patients usually present with acute pain and inability to ambulate after trauma.
- Even minor trauma (tripping off a curb) may cause an ankle fracture.
- Usually there is some element of rotational force involved that exceeds the torsional strength of the malleoli and results in a fracture.

Presentation

- Patients present with ankle pain and swelling and typically an inability to bear weight.

Physical Exam

- Pain is often very focal along the lateral or posterior edges of the malleoli (where ligaments do not attach).
- Any motion of the joint will cause significant pain and there may be ecchymosis and significant swelling.
- In cases where fractures are suspected, radiographs should be obtained prior to ligamentous stressing due to the potential for displacement of fracture fragments.

Essential Diagnostics

- The clinician should use a clinical decision rule like the Ottawa ankle rules to determine the need for radiographs.
- If radiographs are obtained, three views of the ankle including the AP, mortise, and lateral should be obtained.
  - Also consider foot x-rays in the appropriate clinical setting.

ED Treatment

- The patient should have the ankle elevated, iced, and splinted in a position of comfort, with pain medication provided as needed.
- Small distal avulsion fractures of any malleoli may usually be treated as ankle sprains, with protection with a fracture boot, icing/elevation, and weight-bearing as tolerated.

- Larger malleolar fractures may lead to more instability and require manipulation, splinting, or even surgery.
    - Any malignment of the ankle joint should be reduced into anatomical alignment in the ED.
    - These fractures should be immobilized in a posterior short leg stirrup splint.

Disposition

- Most patients may be discharged from the ED.
    - Patients with small, stable avulsion fractures may be weight-bearing as tolerated and follow-up with a primary care physician or sports medicine specialist.
        - Patients may return to play once they no longer have pain and have full ROM usually in six to eight weeks, depending on the sport.
    - Larger fractures with concerns for the stability of the ankle joint should be made non-weight bearing and should follow-up with either a sports medicine specialist or an orthopedic surgeon.
        - Return to play decisions are made based upon the stability of the injury and evidence of healing. If no surgery is required, patients may usually return to play once there is both clinical and radiographic evidence of healing and they have regained full strength and ROM. This may take twelve weeks or longer.
- Orthopedic surgery should be consulted any time there is an open fracture, neurovascular injury, or the fracture is unable to be reduced into anatomical alignment.

Complications

- Ankle fractures may cause posttraumatic arthritis and, depending on the injury to the supporting ligaments, may lead to chronic instability if not treated appropriately.

Pediatric Considerations

- Open physeal plates in children are weaker than ligaments.
    - It is more likely for a child with an open growth plate to have sustained a Salter–Harris fracture than a ligament sprain.
    - The clinician should have a strong suspicion for involvement of the growth plates if the patient has tenderness in these areas.
    - If there is any concern for an injury to an open growth plate, a splint should be placed and the child should be made non-weight bearing and have close outpatient follow-up with orthopedics or sports medicine.

Pearls and Pitfalls

- Maintain a high degree of suspicion for concomitant ligamentous disruption in conjunction with malleolar fractures because they may lead to significant instability, chronic pain, and posttraumatic arthritis in the ankle.

Ankle Dislocations

Background

- Isolated ankle dislocations without fracture are relatively uncommon.
- Typically, the foot sustains a significant force that causes the talus to slip out from below the tibial plafond. This often will fracture the medial, lateral, or posterior malleolus.
- Due to the traction on neurovascular structures, quick reduction is a priority.

Mechanism

- A dislocation begins with an axially loaded foot with a force that eventually overwhelms the restraining ligaments and capsule and allows the talus to escape anteriorly or posteriorly from under the talus.
- Typical mechanisms include motor vehicle accidents, falls, and high-speed or contact sports.

Presentation

- Patients will present with an obviously deformed ankle that may be open or closed.
- They may complain of neurologic symptoms of numbness or tingling due to nerve stretch.

Physical Exam

- The foot is displaced either anteriorly or posteriorly and may be turned to the side if one of the malleoli is fractured.
- A quick neurovascular exam should be performed, checking sensation, motion, and pulse.
  - It is important to reduce the dislocation quickly, so a focused exam should be performed.
- Skin integrity should be evaluated since occasionally these are open dislocations.

Essential Diagnostics

- Radiographs of the ankle are important to evaluate for acute fracture.
  - Do not delay ankle reduction to obtain x-rays if there is any evidence of neurovascular compromise.

ED Treatment

- After analgesia or sedation has been administered, a rapid reduction should be performed.
- The patient's knee and hip should be bent.
  - To reduce a posterior ankle dislocation, apply constant axial traction to the foot while an assistant places posterior force on the distal tibia proximal to the injury and anterior force over the heel of the foot.
  - To reduce an anterior ankle dislocation, apply constant axial traction to the foot while an assistant places anterior force on the distal tibia proximal to the injury and posterior force over the foot distal to the injury.
- The neurovascular status should once again be checked and documented.
  - The ankle should be splinted in neutral position with a well-molded posterior short leg stirrup splint, with the leg elevated.
  - The patient may then be sent for post-reduction x-rays.

Disposition

- Consultation with orthopedic surgery is recommended for all ankle dislocations to ensure timely definitive management of the injury.
- Almost all ankle dislocations need surgical stabilization.
  - If adequate alignment is achieved in the ED, patients may often be made non-weight bearing and have close follow-up with orthopedic surgery as an outpatient.
  - This decision should be made in consultation with an orthopedic surgeon.
- Open fractures, persistent neurovascular injury after reduction, or dislocations that are unable to be adequately reduced need to go the operating room urgently.

Complications

- Neurovascular injury is the most concerning complication and should be closely evaluated and documented.
- Even without a fracture, significant ligamentous injuries may occur and lead to ongoing ankle instability.
- Additional concerns include cartilage disruption with the initial dislocation or reduction that may lead to osteochondral defects.

Pediatric Considerations

- Close evaluation of any existing physes should be ensured, given that these areas are often weaker than ligamentous structures.
- A force strong enough to cause a dislocation may easily disrupt growth plates, so anatomic alignment and joint protection with close follow-up should be arranged.

Pearls and Pitfalls

- Do not wait to obtain radiographs prior to reduction of an ankle dislocation if there is any evidence of neurovascular injury.
- Even if the patient does not have a neurovascular injury on presentation, rapid reduction of this injury is essential.
- Patients often have severe pain and anxiety prior to reduction, but, with analgesia or sedation, a quick reduction may greatly ease the patient's discomfort.

Table 7.2 Key Diagnosis, History, Physical Exam Findings, and Treatment

Diagnosis	History	Physical Exam Findings	Treatment
Lower Leg			
Shin splints	Diffuse shin pain, worse in the morning and after exercise	Diffuse pain and tenderness along medial tibial border	*RICE Activity modification
Stress fracture	Progressive shin pain over a specific area, may be worse at night	Focal area of tenderness and reproduction of pain with single leg hop test	RICE May be *WBAT No impact activities until symptoms resolve
Proximal and midshaft fibula fractures	Usually direct blow or twisting injury	Localized pain, swelling, and tenderness over site of fracture	RICE If stable fracture, may be WBAT and splint only as needed for comfort If unstable, splint with posterior short leg stirrup splint and arrange close orthopedic follow-up
Chronic exertional compartment syndrome	Pain and swelling in either (or both) the anterior and lateral lower leg with exertion that resolves with rest, may have associated paresthesias with exertion	During exertion may have swelling or muscle herniation from anterior or lateral lower leg compartment, may also have decreased sensation and/or weakness	Avoid provocative activities Refer to orthopedic surgery or sports medicine for further workup, which may include compartment pressure testing
Nerve entrapment	Entrapment of nerves due to a variety of compressive forces	Pain and/or weakness in area of nerve injury	RICE Anti-inflammatories Removal of any compressive devices Follow-up with orthopedics or sports medicine as outpatient, may need nerve conduction studies
Gastrocnemius sprain/tear	Acute tearing sensation in posterior calf with associated swelling	Swelling, ecchymosis, and tenderness of posterior distal aspect of calf at musculotendinous junction	RICE WBAT Activity modification
Ankle			
Ankle sprain	Usually inversion or eversion injury	Swelling and tenderness over medial and/or lateral ankle Rule out high ankle sprain with squeeze and dorsiflexion/eversion tests	RICE WBAT Anti-inflammatories May need immobilization in walking boot due to pain or concern for high ankle sprain Activity modification Progressive range of motion as tolerated after initial period of rest
Ankle instability	Recurrent ankle sprains	Swelling and tenderness over medial or lateral ankle, positive anterior drawer test	WBAT RICE Activity modification Physical therapy Functional brace when return to sports

Table 7.2 *(cont.)*

Diagnosis	History	Physical Exam Findings	Treatment
Posterior tibial tendinopathy	Pain and swelling along medial ankle and foot	Tenderness and sometimes swelling over medial ankle and foot, pain and/or weakness with inversion	RICE Activity modification Anti-inflammatories Walking boot
Peroneal tendinopathy	Pain and swelling over lateral ankle, may notice a clicking or catching sensation	Pain and sometimes swelling over peroneal tendons, pain with eversion	RICE Activity modification Anti-inflammatories
Osteochondral lesions	Recurrent pain or swelling in ankle joint, may be acute or chronic injury	Swelling with decreased *ROM	RICE Activity modification Anti-inflammatories WBAT
Ankle fractures	Usually similar to ankle sprains and due to inversion or eversion injury	Pain and swelling along affected area	RICE Stable fractures may be treated with CAM boot, WBAT Potentially unstable fractures should be placed in a posterior short leg stirrup splint and referred for close outpatient orthopedic follow-up Fractures which cannot be reduced in the ED need emergent orthopedic surgery consultation
Ankle dislocations	Typically due to high-energy mechanism, such as *MVA, which causes axial loading of foot	Severe pain, swelling, ecchymosis, and deformity, high risk for neurovascular compromise	Urgent reduction and placement of posterior short leg stirrup splint RICE If adequate reduction, may have close outpatient follow-up with orthopedic surgery If inadequate reduction, need emergent orthopedic surgery consultation

*RICE = Rest, ice, compression, and elevation
*WBAT = Weight-bearing as tolerated
*ROM = Range of motion
*MVA = Motor vehicle accident

Table 7.3 Indications for Orthopedic Surgery Consultation in the Emergency Department

Any unstable fractures, e.g., Maisonneuve injury
Acute compartment syndrome
Open fractures
Any fracture or dislocation associated with neurovascular injury
Any fracture or dislocation which is not able to be reduced in the emergency department

Recommended Reading/ References

1. J. A. Rechel, E. E. Yard, R. D. Comstock. An epidemiologic comparison of high school sports injuries sustained in practice and competition. *J Athl Train.* 2008 Apr–Jun; **43** (2): 197–204.
2. M. Milankov, V. Kecojević, N. Gvozdenović, et al. Dislocation of the proximal tibiofibular joint. *Med Pregl.* 2013 Sep–Oct; **66** (9–10): 387–91.
3. A. G. Schneiders, S. J. Sullivan, P. A. Hendrick, et al.. The ability of clinical tests to diagnose stress fractures: a systematic review and meta-analysis. *J Orthop Sports Phys Ther.* 2012 Sep; **42** (9): 760–71.
4. A. Soroceanu, F. Sidhwa, S. Aarabi, et al.. Surgical versus nonsurgical treatment of acute Achilles tendon rupture: a meta-analysis of randomized trials. *J Bone Joint Surg Am.* 2012 Dec 5; **94** (23): 2136–43.
5. C. Doherty, E. Delahunt, B. Caulfield, et al.. The incidence and prevalence of ankle sprain injury: a systematic review and meta-analysis of prospective epidemiological studies. *Sports Med.* 2014 Jan; **44** (1): 123–40.
6. G. S. Schiftan, L. A. Ross, A. J. Hahne. The effectiveness of proprioception training in preventing ankle sprains in sporting populations: a systematic review and meta-analysis. *J Sci Med Sport.* 2014 Apr 26; **14**: 74–77.
7. I. G. Steill, R. D. Greenberg, R. D. McKnight, et a.l. A study to develop clinical decision rules for the use of radiography in acute ankle injuries. *Ann Emerg Med.* 1992 Apr; **21** (4): 384–90.

Chapter 8 Foot

Brenden J. Balcik, Aaron J. Monseau, and William Krantz

Background / Epidemiology

- Patients with foot injuries commonly present to the emergency department (ED).
- As participation in athletic activities increases, so do the frequency of these injuries.
- The emergency physician is often the first provider to care for these patients and should be able to recognize, manage and treat both emergent and nonemergent conditions involving the foot.

Anatomical Considerations

- The foot contains 28 bones and 57 articulations, which allows for a wide range of motion (ROM), including plantar flexion, dorsiflexion, inversion, eversion, supination and pronation.[1] (Figures 8.1, 8.2 A–E).
- The foot is composed 2 arches: longitudinal (midfoot) and transverse (forefoot).
- The foot's anatomical divisions include the hindfoot, midfoot, and forefoot (Figure 8.3).
  - The hindfoot is made up of the calcaneus and talus, with its distal border marked by the Chopart joint.
  - The midfoot is comprised of the navicular, the cuboid, and the three cuneiform bones, with its proximal border marked by the Chopart joint and the distal border marked by the Lisfranc joint.
    - The midfoot is also composed of two columns, medial and lateral. The medial column is comprised of the navicular, cuneiforms, and the first three tarsometatarsal joints. The lateral column is made up of the cuboid and the fourth and fifth tarsometatarsal joints.
    - The midfoot is the least mobile portion of the foot.
  - The forefoot is made up of the metatarsals and phalanges, with the proximal border marked by the Lisfranc joint.

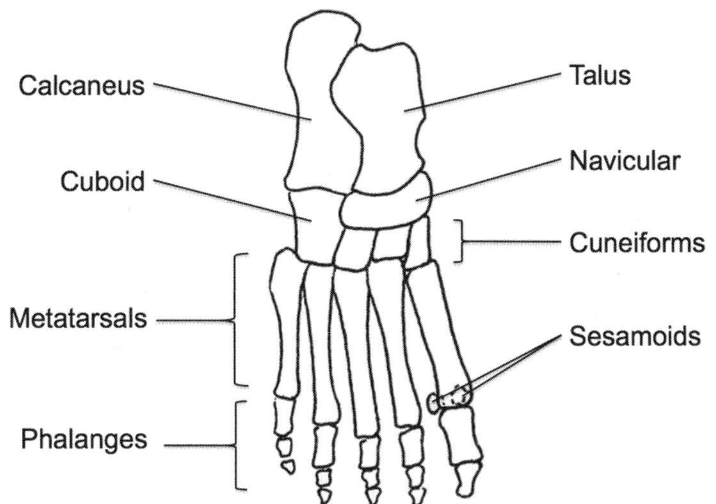

Figure 8.1. Bony anatomy of the foot. Illustration by Yvonne Chow.

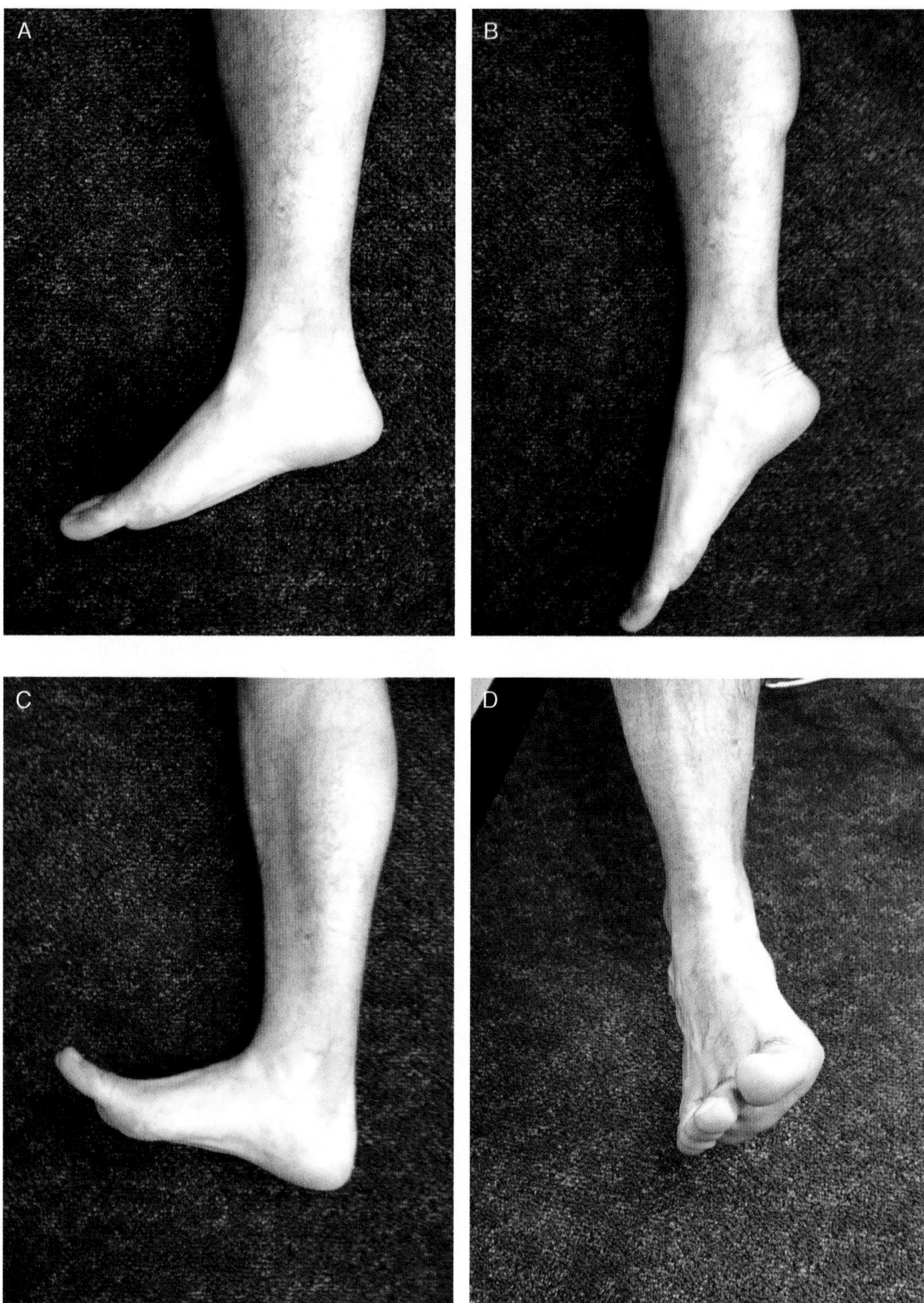

Figure 8.2. Range of motion of the foot.

A) Neutral
B) Plantarflexion
C) Dorsiflexion
D) Inversion
E) Eversion

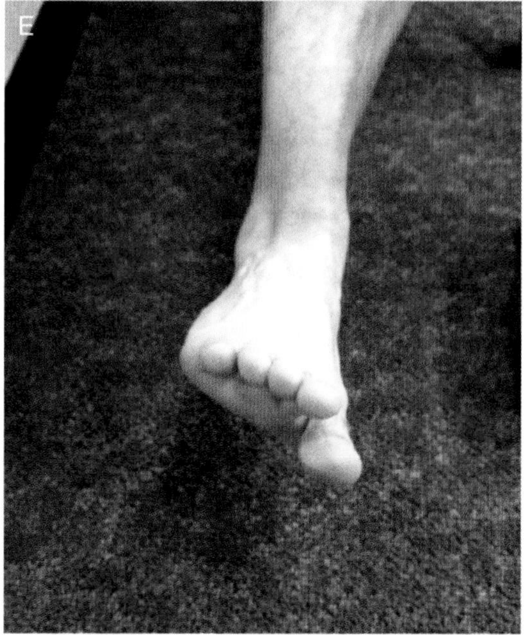

Figure 8.2. *(cont.)*

- Vascular supply.
  - The popliteal artery gives rise to several branches.
    - The anterior tibial artery gives rise to the dorsalis pedis which supplies the dorsum of foot.
    - The posterior tibial and peroneal arteries supply the sole of foot.
- Nerve supply.
  - The foot is supplied by the tibial, deep fibular, superficial fibular, sural, and saphenous nerves, which originate from the sciatic and femoral nerves.
    - All five of these nerves contribute to the cutaneous (sensory) innervation of the foot (Figures 8.4 and 8.5).
    - The tibial nerve and its branches, the medial plantar nerve and the lateral plantar nerve, innervate all intrinsic muscles of the foot except for the extensor digitorum brevis, which is innervated by the deep fibular nerve.
      - The medial plantar nerve is the major sensory nerve in the sole of the foot.

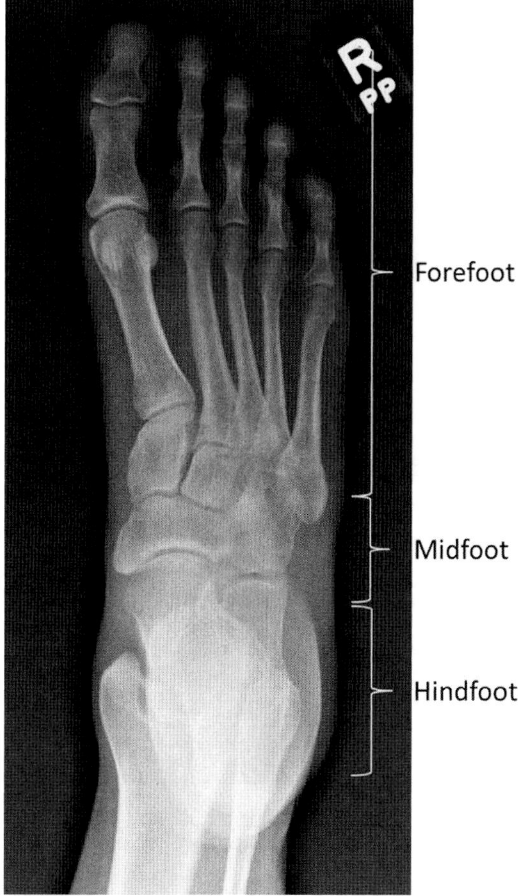

Figure 8.3. Normal radiograph depicting the divisions of the foot: hindfoot, midfoot, and forefoot.

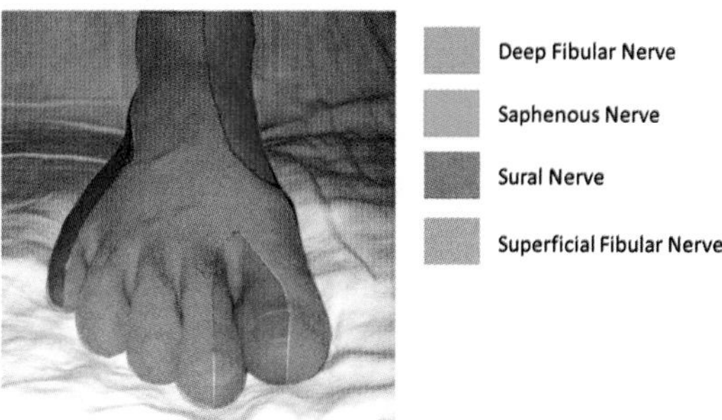

Figure 8.4. Sensory distribution of the dorsal surface of the foot.

      - The lateral plantar nerve is an important contributor to motor function as it innervates intrinsic muscles in the sole of the foot.
    - The deep fibular nerve often contributes to the innervation of the

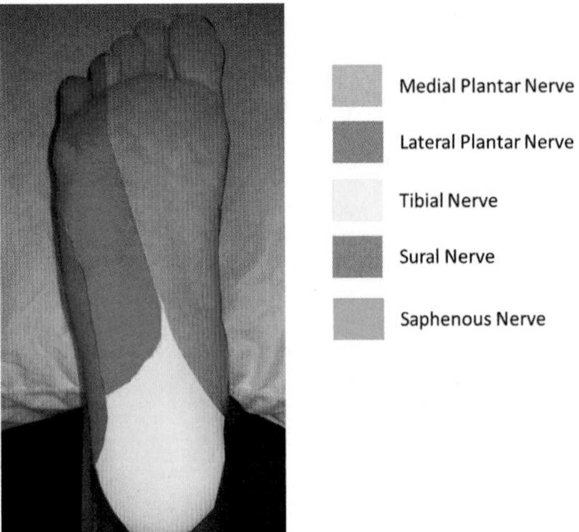

Figure 8.5. Sensory distribution of the plantar surface of the foot.

first and second dorsal interossei and provides sensory innervation for the web space between the first and second toes.
  - The superficial fibular nerve provides sensory innervation for the dorsal aspect of the foot.
  - The sural nerve serves as cutaneous innervation for the lateral surface of the foot and the dorsolateral surface of the fifth toe.
  - The saphenous nerve provides sensory innervation for the medial surface of the foot.

Pathophysiology

- Injuries to the foot involve three basic mechanisms.[2]
  - Indirect trauma includes twisting forces, axial loading, or other extremes of movement.
  - Direct trauma may involve direct impact, crush injuries, falls from height, or motor vehicle collisions (MVC).
  - Overuse may also cause injury.

Focused History

- Points of emphasis in the history of foot injury should include:[3]
  - The mechanism of injury, including the type of force and direction.
  - The location of the pain and time to onset of swelling or bruising.
  - The consistency and character of the pain since the injury.
  - The ability to bear weight, if any.
  - The presence of prior injuries or surgeries which may predispose the foot to specific injuries.
  - The treatments, if any, that were used following the injury.
  - The presence of associated or distracting injuries that may make evaluation of the injury difficult.

Focused Physical Exam

Inspection

- The injured foot should be compared to the noninjured foot and any asymmetry should be noted.
- All aspects of the foot should be examined, including anterior, posterior, medial, lateral, and plantar surfaces.
- Special attention should be made to note any deformity, swelling, or discoloration.
- The arch should be evaluated for pes planus (flat foot) and pes cavus (high arch).

Palpation

- The area of palpation should include the injured area but should also extend beyond area of pain.
- Areas of focus should include the base of the fifth metatarsal, the base of the second metatarsal, and the navicular.
- Specific tendons should be evaluated for tendonitis.
  - The peroneal tendons should be palpated posterior to the lateral malleolus.
  - The posterior tibial tendon should be palpated posterior and distal to the medial malleolus.
  - The Achilles tendon should be palpated along the length of the tendon and at the insertion on the calcaneus.

Range of motion

- Active ROM should be assessed first, followed by passive ROM if there are any abnormalities in active ROM.

- It is important to evaluate the noninjured side as well, and to assess for symmetry of movements.
- Included in the assessment is examination of the joint proximal and distal to the injured joint.
- Individual joints of the foot should be evaluated independently.
  - Dorsiflexion should reach 20°.
  - Plantar flexion should reach 50°.
  - Inversion at the subtalar joint should reach 40°.
  - Eversion at the subtalar joint should reach 20°.
  - Forefoot abduction and adduction should reach 5°.
  - The first metatarsalphalangeal (MTP) joint should be able to flex (plantarflex) to 70° and extend (dorsiflex) to 45°.
  - The lesser MTP joints should reach 40° in both flexion and extension.

Special Tests

- The *Thompson test* is used to evaluate for Achilles tendon rupture.
  - The patient lies prone with the ankle and foot hanging off the edge of the bed. The calf is squeezed and the foot is observed for plantarflexion.
    - An intact tendon will transmit the force to the foot, resulting in plantarflexion.
    - A ruptured tendon will not transmit the force, and the foot will not plantarflex when the calf is squeezed.
- A variant of the *Thompson test*, called the *knee flexion test*, places the patient prone with the knee flexed to 90° (Figure 8.6).
  - As above, the calf is squeezed and the foot is observed for plantarflexion.
  - In addition, the foot may be observed to fall into neutral or dorsiflexion if a rupture is present.
- *Tinel's sign* is used to evaluate for tarsal tunnel syndrome.
  - Percussion of the posterior tibialis nerve as it courses through the tarsal tunnel (inferior to the medial malleolus) will cause pain to radiate to the medial and lateral plantar surfaces of the foot.

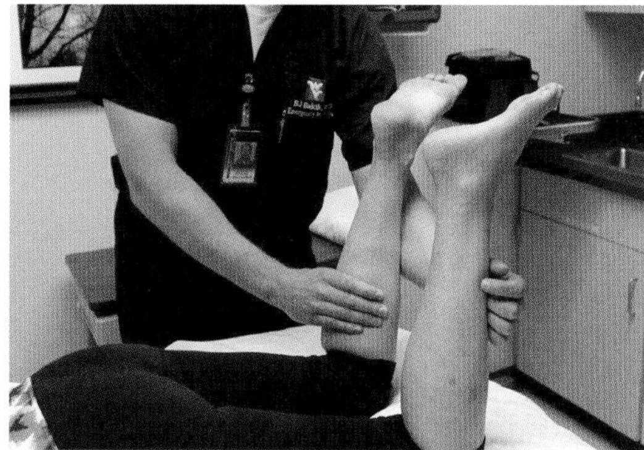

Figure 8.6. The knee flexion variant of the Thompson test.

- *Morton's test* is used in detection of interdigital neuromas.
  - A compressive force is applied to the first and fifth metatarsal heads (squeezed together), causing pain to the affected area.
  - An audible or palpable click called *Mulder's sign* may be elicited.

Neurovascular Exam

- Strength should be assessed and compared to the noninjured side.
  - Resisted plantarflexion, dorsiflexion, inversion, and eversion should all be included.
- Posterior tibialis and dorsal pedis pulses should be palpated and compared to the noninjured side.
- Capillary refill of all toes should be assessed.
- Sensation of the foot should be tested and should include all surfaces of the foot[4]
- Gait should be assessed if the patient is able to ambulate.

Differential Diagnosis – Emergent and Common Diagnoses

Fractures

Calcaneus Fractures

Epidemiology

- Fractures of the calcaneus account for 2 percent of all fractures.
- The calcaneus is the most frequently fractured tarsal bone and accounts for 60 percent of all tarsal fractures.

Table 8.1 Emergent and Common Diagnoses in the Emergency Department

Emergent Diagnoses	Common Diagnoses
Any open fracture	Uncomplicated fractures
Any injury with neurovascular compromise	Stress fractures
Certain variants of calcaneus, talus, navicular, and Lisfranc fractures.	Phalangeal fractures
Any subluxation	Sprains/strains
Any dislocation	Achilles tendinopathy
Compartment syndrome (acute)	Plantar fasciitis
	Bursitis
	Morton's neuroma

- A total of 90 percent of these fractures occur in men 21 to 45 years old, the majority of which are industrial workers.[1,2,3,5,6]

Anatomic Considerations

- The anterior portion of the calcaneus is the body.
- The posterior portion of the calcaneus is the tuberosity.
- The principal articulation is with the talus, forming the subtalar joint.
- Calcaneus fractures may be intra- or extra-articular. Approximately 75 percent of calcaneus fractures are intra-articular, and of these 75 percent are depressed.[1]

Mechanism

- Axial loading.
  - Falls from height drive the talus down into calcaneus and cause most intra-articular fractures.
- Generally falls of greater than 8 feet are required unless osteoporosis is present.
  - Motor vehicle accidents (MVAs) account for the remainder of these fractures, in which the accelerator or brake pedal impacts the plantar surface of the foot.
  - Twisting of the foot is the cause of most extra-articular fractures.
- Tuberosity fractures in diabetics typically occur via avulsion by the Achilles tendon.

Presentation

- The patient will present with moderate to severe heel pain after a mechanism as described earlier.

Physical Exam

- The foot will appear swollen with ecchymosis extending to the arch of the foot.
- There may be widening and shortening of heel, with tenderness to palpation.
- Fracture blisters may be present if presentation is delayed, as these develop within twenty-four to forty-eight hours.
- It is important to assess for compartment syndrome as this occurs in 10 percent of calcaneus fractures.

Essential diagnostics

- Radiography (X-ray): anteroposterior (AP), lateral, and Harris axial views along with a full ankle series are required (Figures 8.7 and 8.8).
  - X-ray should be reviewed and Bohler's angle should be assessed.
    - Bohler's angle is composed of a line drawn from the highest point of the anterior process of the calcaneus to the highest point of the posterior facet and a line drawn tangential from the posterior facet to the superior edge of the tuberosity.
    - Normal angle is between 20 and 40° (Figure 8.9).
    - Any angle less than this indicates collapse of the posterior facet. However, this angle may be normal in the presence of fracture, and therefore this measurement cannot be used to exclude fracture. The most important function of this measurement is for prognosis, as fractures with a decreased Bohler's angle have worse outcomes. If the diagnosis is in question, a comparison X-ray of the opposite foot may be useful.
  - The Gissane angle may also be used to assess for fractures of the calcaneus. It is

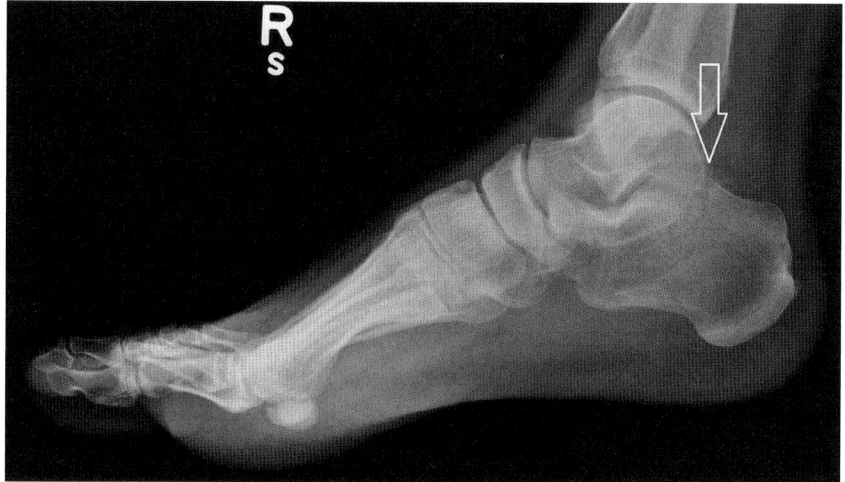

Figure 8.7. Calcaneus fracture. Lateral view.

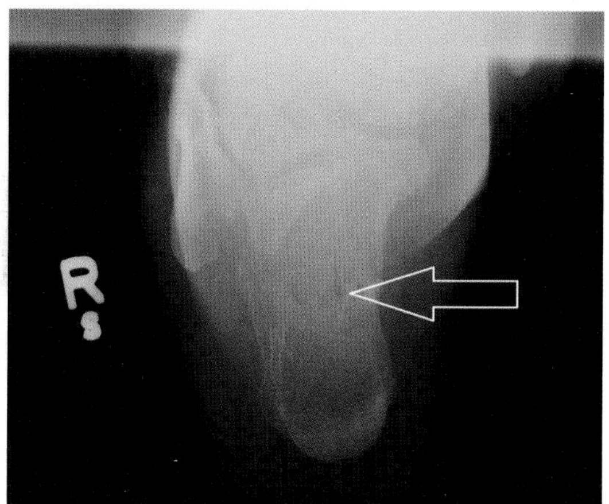

Figure 8.8. Calcaneus fracture. Harris view.

formed by the downard and upward slopes of the superior surface of the calcaneus. It is best evaluated on the lateral view.

- Normal angle is between 105 and 135°.
- An increase in this angle indicates collapse of the posterior facet.[2]

- CT is useful in determining the extent of the fracture and for preoperative planning.

ED Treatment

- Open fractures of any kind require immediate orthopedic consultation in the ED.
- Calcaneal body fractures.
  - These require immobilization with a bulky, well-padded posterior splint. As with all splints, adequate padding will help to prevent fracture blisters and skin injury. Often a stirrup slab is used to increase stability and immobilization.
  - The patient should be kept on strict non-weight bearing status (NWBS). Crutches, with instructions on their use, should be provided.
  - Ice and elevation are recommended to prevent or minimize swelling.
  - Adequate analgesia should be provided.

Disposition

- Most patients may be discharged safely from the ED. However, if there is significant swelling and there is concern for the development of compartment syndrome, the patient should be admitted to the hospital.
- For intra-articular fractures of the calcaneal body, orthopedic referral should be made and the patient should be seen within twenty-four hours.
  - Definitive management depends on the degree of displacement. Nondisplaced fractures may be managed nonoperatively with NWBS for six to eight weeks. This may be followed with a gradual increase in activity. Management of displaced fractures varies from conservative (nonoperative) to surgical repair. Thus urgent orthopedic consult is recommended.

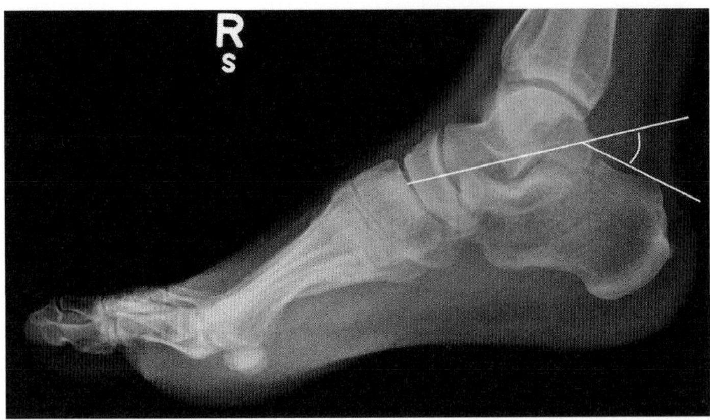

Figure 8.9. Lateral radiograph depicting Bohler's angle. Note that despite the fractured calcaneus Bohler's angle is within normal range.

- For all other extra-articular fractures, orthopedic or sports medicine referral should be made and the patient should be seen within two weeks.
  - Nondisplaced fractures are managed with NWBS for four to six weeks with gradual return to activity.
  - Displaced fractures may be managed nonoperatively or with surgical repair, so early orthopedic consult is recommended.

Complications

- Posttraumatic arthritis is the most frequent complication. Typically, patients will present with stiffness and chronic pain.
- Compartment syndrome may occur in 10 percent of calcaneus fractures.
- Wound dehiscence, if surgical intervention required.
- Calcaneal osteomyelitis
- Increased heel width.
- Loss of subtalar motion.
- Peroneal tendonitis
- Sural nerve injury.

Pediatric Considerations

- Calcaneus fractures in children rarely occur and typically involve children older than 9 years old.
- Most occur secondary to a fall or jump from heights similar to those of adults; however, the mechanism requires less energy than adults.
- Initial injury is missed in 45–55 percent of pediatric cases.
- Nonoperative management is recommended for extra-articular fractures and intra-articular fractures with less than 4-mm displacement. Children are typically made non-weight bearing for six weeks.
- Operative management is recommended for displaced intra-articular fractures[2].

Pearls and Pitfalls

- More than 50 percent of calcaneus fractures are associated with additional injuries.
- A total of 26 percent of calcaneus fractures are associated with additional lower extremity injuries.
- Calcaneus fractures are bilateral in 7 percent of cases.
- Compression fractures of the thoracolumbar spine occur in 10 percent of cases.
- Compartment syndrome develops in 10 percent of calcaneus fractures.
- Bohler's angle may be used to assess for subtle fractures.
- Intra-articular fractures typically carry a worse prognosis than extra-articular fractures.[1,2,3,5,6]

Talus Fractures

Epidemiology

- Fracture of the talus is the second most common tarsal fracture.
- The incidence ranges from 0.1–0.85 percent of all fractures and 5–7 percent foot injuries.
- The most common talus fractures involve the neck of the talus. Of these, 14–26 percent have associated medial malleolus fractures.

- Fractures of the lateral process of the talus account for 2.3 percent of all snowboarding injuries and 15 percent of all ankle injuries.
- Fractures of the talar head are rare, accounting for only 3–5 percent of all talus fractures.[1,2,3,6]

Anatomic Considerations

- The talus is divided into three segments, the head, neck, and body.
- Fractures of the talus are divided into major fractures, those involving the head, neck, or central portion of the body, and minor fractures, those that do not involve the central portion of the bone.
  - Minor fractures include the posterior process, lateral process, and osteochondral talar dome fractures.
- A total of 60 percent of the surface of the talus is covered by articular cartilage.
- There are no tendinous muscle insertions and the bone itself is held in place by ligaments.
- Vascular supply does not penetrate cartilage but is delivered by surrounding ligaments. This predisposes the talus to avascular necrosis, especially in the cases of proximal talus fractures.

Mechanism

- Talar head fractures are typically the result of direct impact such as a fall from height onto a dorsiflexed foot.
- Talar neck fractures are also typically the result of falls from heights onto a dorsiflexed foot or following an MVA with the foot in a dorsiflexed position.
- Talar body fractures are the result of acute hyperextension of the foot.
- Lateral process fractures are the result of axial loading, dorsiflexion, eversion, and external rotation. Typically these are seen after falls, MVAs, or snowboarding injuries.
  - Fractures of the lateral process are often termed "snowboarder's ankle."
- Posterior process fractures are often the result of extreme plantarflexion.

Presentation

- Patients typically present with ankle pain after mechanisms as described earlier.

Physical Exam

- Generally edema, ecchymosis, and tenderness are present.
- ROM is typically limited by pain.
- Palpation may elicit crepitus.
- Specific aspects of the physical exam may provide clues to determine what portions of the talus may be involved.
  - Talar head fractures are associated with tenderness concentrated over the talar head and talonavicular joint. Typically ankle motion is normal, but inverting the foot exacerbates pain over the talonavicular joint.
  - Talar neck fractures present with the foot in hyperextension if an associated dislocation is present.
  - Lateral process fractures cause pain and swelling over the lateral malleolus with point tenderness anteroinferior to the lateral malleolus.
  - Posterior process fractures present with posterolateral tenderness and edema. Pain is exacerbated by plantarflexion. Dorsiflexion of the great toe may exacerbate pain as the flexor hallucis longus tendon slides along the bone.

Essential Diagnostics

- X-ray: Full evaluation requires multiple views of the foot and ankle. Views of the ankle should include AP, mortise, and lateral views while AP, lateral, and oblique views of the foot should be obtained (Figure 8.10).
  - Talar neck fractures are best seen on lateral views.
  - The Canale view provides optimum evaluation of the talar neck, but due to the manipulation of the foot and ankle required to obtain the view may be difficult to obtain in the acute setting.
- CT may be necessary as some fractures may not be adequately visualized using only X-ray.
- CT may help further characterize the fracture pattern and assess any articular involvement.

ED Treatment

- Open fractures of any kind require immediate orthopedic consultation in the ED.

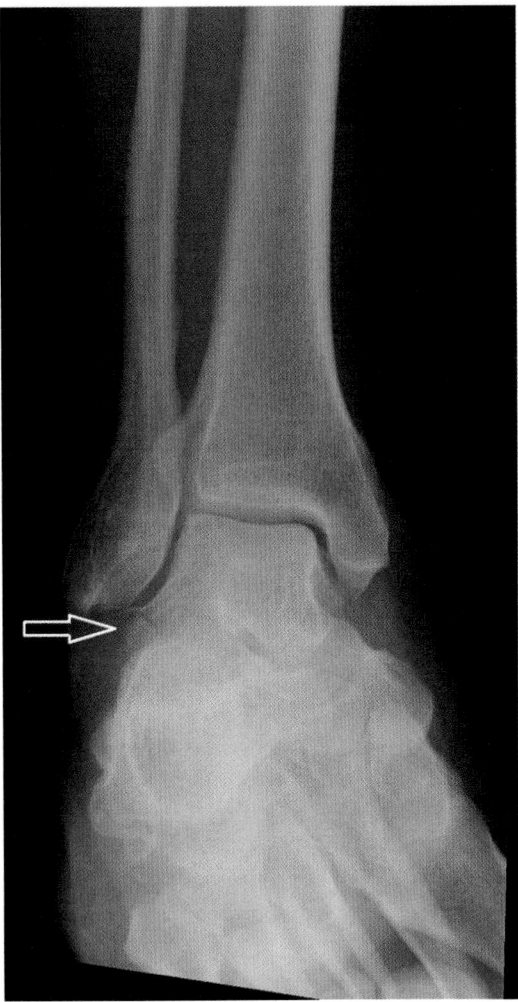

Figure 8.10. Lateral process fracture of the talus.

- Talus fractures require immobilization with a bulky, well-padded posterior splint. A stirrup slab may be placed to increase stability.
- The patient should be kept on strict NWBS. Crutches, with instructions on their use, should be provided.
- Ice and elevation are recommended to prevent or minimize swelling.
- Adequate analgesia should be provided.

Disposition

- Most talus fractures may be safely discharged home, with the exception of open fractures and those with neurovascular compromise. These injuries require orthopedic consultation in the ED.
- Major fractures of the talus require immediate orthopedic referral, with follow-up within twenty-four hours.
- Minor fractures of the talus require early orthopedic or sports medicine referral, with follow-up within two weeks.
  - The posterior splint for lateral process fractures should maintain the ankle in a neutral position while the splint for a posterior process fracture should maintain the foot in 15° of plantarflexion.
- Return to activity largely depends on the approach to treatment.
  - Talar head fractures are treated in a non-weight bearing cast for six to eight weeks. However, open reduction with internal fixation (ORIF) is recommended if there is instability of the talonavicular joint, there is an articular step-off, or if the fracture involves more than 50 percent of the articular surface.
  - Talar neck fractures are definitively managed with a short-leg non-walking cast for six weeks followed by three weeks of partial weight-bearing. Displaced fractures require surgical intervention and anatomic reduction.
  - Talar body fractures that are nondisplaced are treated definitively with a short-leg non-walking cast for six to eight weeks. Displaced or comminuted fractures require surgical intervention for anatomic reduction.
  - Lateral process fractures are typically managed nonoperatively with immobilization in a non-weight bearing short-leg cast for four weeks and an additional two weeks of partial weight-bearing. ORIF is indicated for large fragments or for more than 2-mm of displacement.
  - Posterior process fractures are managed similarly to lateral process fractures. ORIF is indicated for large fragments or fractures with a large degree of displacement.

Complications

- Talar head fractures may lead to talonavicular osteoarthritis or chondromalacia.
- Talar neck fractures may lead to peroneal tendon dislocations, avascular necrosis, or delayed union.

- Displaced or comminuted talar body fractures may lead to avascular necrosis.
- Lateral process fractures may lead to malunion or nonunion.
- Avascular necrosis may develop in any case of fracture dislocation.

Pediatric Considerations

- Fractures of the talus are extremely rare in children and the talar neck is most often involved.
- These fractures are typically managed in a long-leg cast with non-weight bearing for six to eight weeks followed by progressive weight-bearing for an additional two-three weeks.
- Operative management is indicated if there is more than 5-mm displacement or more than 5° malalignment of fracture fragments on AP radiograph.[2]

Pearls and Pitfalls

- Talar fractures, especially to of the neck, are predisposed to avascular necrosis, so diagnosis, management, and appropriate referral are essential to preventing this complication.[1,2,3,6]

Navicular Fractures

Epidemiology

- The navicular bone is the most commonly fractured bone of the midfoot.[1]

Anatomic Considerations

- Fractures are classified as dorsal avulsion (most common), tuberosity fractures, body fractures, or compression fractures.
    - Body and compression fractures are the rarest of these types.

Mechanism

- Typically these fractures are the result of a direct blow or axial loading. In the case of axial loading, the force may be directly along the long axis of the foot or in an oblique orientation.
    - Dorsal avulsion fractures often have a component of foot inversion while tuberosity fractures often follow an acute eversion force.
    - Navicular stress fractures may occur as a result of overuse, most commonly in sports which require explosive movements and sudden changes in direction (e.g., soccer, basketball, high jumpers).

Presentation

- Patients present with pain and swelling over the dorsal medial aspect of the foot.

Physical Exam

- Dorsal navicular fractures have tenderness to palpation over the dorsal medical aspect of the foot.
- Tuberosity fractures have tenderness to palpation distal to the medial malleolus. In the case of this fracture, eversion of the foot elicits pain.
- It is important to palpate all bony structures of the foot and ankle as navicular fractures often involve concomitant injuries.

Essential Diagnostics

- X-ray: AP, lateral, medial oblique, and lateral oblique views often demonstrate these injuries.
    - If possible, these should be done with patient weight-bearing.
    - Comparison views of the unaffected foot may be required.
- Subtle, nondisplaced fractures may not be visualized with X-ray, so CT may be required if suspicion is high.

ED Treatment

- Navicular fractures require immobilization with a bulky, well-padded posterior splint.
- The patient should be kept on NWBS. Crutches, with instructions on their use, should be provided.
- Ice and elevation are recommended to prevent or minimize swelling.
- Adequate analgesia should be provided.

Disposition

- Most navicular fractures may be safely discharged to home, with the exception of open fractures and those with neurovascular compromise. These injuries require orthopedic consultation in the ED.
- Displaced fractures of the navicular require immediate orthopedic referral, with follow-up within twenty-four hours.
- Nondisplaced fractures of the navicular require early orthopedic or sports medicine referral, with follow-up within two weeks.

  - These fractures require repeat X-ray in ten to fourteen days.
  - If joint instability or associated injuries are seen on the follow-up X-ray, then surgical intervention is often required.
- Nonoperative management involves a short-leg cast with gradual weight-bearing over the course of six to eight weeks.
- Operative management requires a patient to be non-weight bearing in a short-leg cast for a period of twelve weeks from the time of surgical intervention.

Complications

- Avascular necrosis may develop after body fractures.
- Nonunion is often seen with tuberosity fractures.
- Arthritis
- Loss of normal foot alignment.
- Late instability of the foot.

Pearls and Pitfalls

- It is important to adequately evaluate all associated and surrounding structures when navicular fractures are found as there is a high rate of associated injury.
  - Dorsal avulsion fractures are often seen with associated lateral malleolar ligament injuries.
  - Tuberosity fractures are often seen with associated fractures of the cuboid.

Cuboid Fractures

Epidemiology

- Injury to the cuboid may be isolated but is often seen with associated injuries of surrounding midfoot structures.[1,2,3]

Anatomic Considerations

- The cuboid articulates with the calcaneus, navicular, and lateral cuneiform as well as the fourth and fifth metatarsals.

Mechanism

- Indirect trauma accounts for the majority of cuboid fractures. This involves a torsional stress or plantarflexion with abduction of the foot.
- Direct trauma may also cause a cuboid fracture and this typically involves a crush injury with a force applied to the dorsolateral aspect of the foot.[2]

Presentation

- Patients present with pain and swelling following a traumatic mechanism as described earlier.

Physical Exam

- There is swelling and tenderness to palpation of the dorsolateral aspect of the foot.
- Motion of the midfoot exacerbates the pain.
- All bony structures should be palpated to detect any associated injuries.[1,3]

Essential Diagnostics

- X-ray: AP, lateral, and oblique views may demonstrate these injuries.
  - If possible, xrays should be performed with patient weight-bearing.
  - Comparison views of the unaffected foot may be required.
- CT imaging may be required to further assess the extent of the fracture and any instability.

ED Treatment

- Cuboid fractures require immobilization with a bulky, well-padded posterior splint.
- The patient should be kept on strict NWBS. Crutches, with instructions on their use, should be provided.
- Ice and elevation are recommended to prevent or minimize swelling.
- Adequate analgesia should be provided.

Disposition

- Most cuboid fractures may be safely discharged to home, with the exception of open fractures and those with neurovascular compromise. These injuries require orthopedic consultation in the ED.
- Cuboid fractures require early orthopedic or sports medicine referral with follow-up within two weeks.
- Displaced or severely comminuted fractures or those fractures with more than 2-mm

joint surface disruption will require ORIF; however, these do not require immediate (i.e., twenty-four hours) orthopedic follow-up.
- Nondisplaced fractures managed nonoperatively should be treated with a short-leg cast for six to eight weeks. During this time patients are NWBS. Patients are then able to begin a gradual return to activity.

Complications
- Nonunion may occur in fractures with significant displacement or inadequate immobilization.
- Osteonecrosis may be seen following severely displaced or comminuted fractures.
- Posttraumatic osteoarthritis
- Foot instability

Pearls and Pitfalls
- Cuboid fractures are often associated with other soft tissue injuries.
- In the case of a fracture to the distal portion of the cuboid, a tarsometatarsal dislocation should be assumed present until proven otherwise.
- Cuboid fractures are often seen with concomitant calcaneus and metatarsal fractures.[1,2,3]

Cuneiform Fractures
Epidemiology
- Isolated injuries to the cuneiforms are very rare. Most often they coexist with other injuries.

Anatomic Considerations
- The cuneiforms articulate with the navicular, metatarsals, and the cuboid (lateral cuneiform).

Mechanism
- Often occur after axial loading.

Presentation
- Patients present with pain and swelling over the involved area.

Physical Exam
- There is localized tenderness to palpation over the cuneiform region.
- If the patient is able to bear weight, pain is elicited in the midfoot.
- Motion of the midfoot exacerbates the pain.

Essential Diagnostics
- X-ray: AP, lateral, and oblique may demonstrate these injuries.
  - If possible, these should be done with patient weight-bearing.
- CT imaging may be required to further assess the extent of the fracture and any instability.

ED Treatment
- Cuneiform fractures require immobilization with a bulky, well-padded posterior splint.
- The patient should be kept on strict NWBS. Crutches, with instructions on their use, should be provided.
- Ice and elevation are recommended to prevent or minimize swelling.
- Adequate analgesia should be provided.

Disposition
- Most cuneiform fractures may be safely discharged home, with the exception of open fractures and those with neurovascular compromise. These injuries require orthopedic consultation in the ED.
- Cuneiform fractures require early orthopedic or sports medicine referral with follow-up within two weeks.
  - Fractures of the medial cuneiform may require surgical intervention.
- Nondisplaced fractures managed nonoperatively should be treated with a short-leg cast for six to eight weeks. During this time patients are on NWBS. Patients are then able to begin a gradual return to activity.

Complications
- Similar to those seen with cuboid fractures.

Pearls and Pitfalls
- As with cuboid fractures, associated injuries are common, so it is imperative to adequately assess for these injuries.[1,2,3]

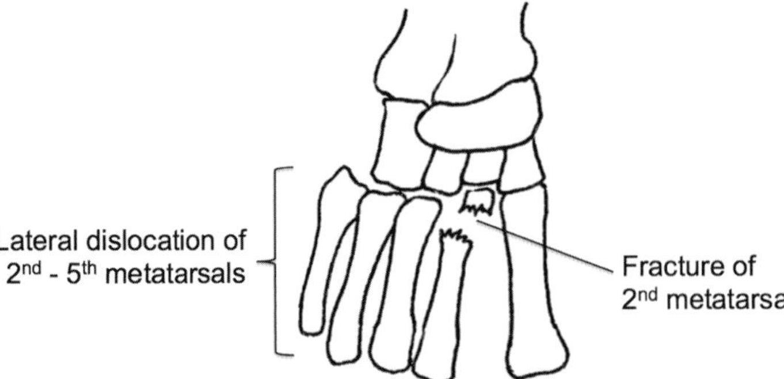

Figure 8.11. Lisfranc fracture-dislocation. Illustration by Yvonne Chow.

Lisfranc Fracture-Dislocation

Epidemiology

- Lisfranc injuries involve a spectrum of injuries from stable sprains to unstable fracture-dislocations.
- The unstable fracture-dislocation (Figure 8.11) is rare and accounts for only 0.2 percent of all fractures.
- Approximately 20 percent of these injuries are missed initially.
- These are becoming increasingly more common as the result of sports injuries, specifically soccer and football[1,2,3,6,7].

Anatomic Considerations

- The Lisfranc joint marks the articulation between the midfoot and forefoot (Figure 8.12).
- The cuneiforms articulate with the first three metatarsals while the cuboid aligns with the fourth and fifth metatarsals.
  - The articulation between the second metatarsal and the middle cuneiform is recessed, providing additional stability.
- In addition to the bony articulations, inherent to this joint's stability are the multiple ligamentous connections.
  - Tarsometatarsal ligaments connect the metatarsal bones to bones of the midfoot.
  - Transverse intertarsal ligaments connect the metatarsals, with the exception of the first and second metatarsals, which do not have ligamentous connection.
  - The intertarsal ligaments have a weaker dorsal component, making dorsal dislocations more likely.
  - The Lisfranc ligament extends obliquely from the plantar surface of the medial cuneiform to the plantar surface of the base of the second metatarsal, providing the primary stabilizing force of this joint (Figure 8.12).

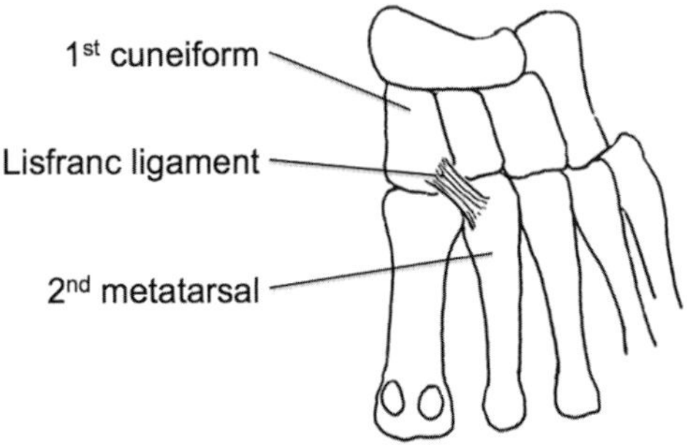

Figure 8.12. Normal Lisfranc joint and ligament. Illustration by Yvonne Chow.

- The dorsalis pedis artery dives between the first and second metatarsals, placing it at risk for compromise during injury.

Mechanism

- MVAs, falls, and athletics (football, soccer, and equestrian) account for the majority of these injuries, with MVCs accounting for 45 percent. [1,6]
- High-energy mechanisms (MVAs) lead to the more severe fracture-dislocations, while lower-energy mechanisms typically cause ligamentous injuries.
- Direct blows to the dorsum of the foot may cause significant soft tissue injury.
- Indirect trauma involves an axial load or a rotational force applied to a plantarflexed foot.

Presentation

- Depending on the extent of the injury, the patient may present ambulatory with minimal pain and swelling, or be unable to bear weight with significant pain and extreme swelling.

Physical Exam

- The foot may have gross deformity or may appear relatively normal, depending on the injury.
- Edema and ecchymosis to the dorsum and/or plantar surface[1,7] of the midfoot may be present.
- There will likely be tenderness to palpation over the area of the Lisfranc joint.
- Passive plantar and dorsiflexion of the foot may elicit pain, and this should heighten suspicion of injury and prompt further evaluation.
- Passive abduction and pronation of the forefoot with the hindfoot held fixed may exacerbate pain and is suggestive of injury.
- Passive movement of the metatarsal heads may produce pain at the tarsometatarsal joint.
- Passive dorsiflexion of the toes may elicit pain, suggesting the possibility of associated compartment syndrome.
- Although rare, vascular injury may occur, so pulses should be assessed.

Essential Diagnostics

- X-ray: AP, lateral, and oblique views are required (Figures 8.13A–D).
  - If possible, these should be done with patient weight-bearing.
  - Comparison views of the unaffected foot may be required.
  - The AP view allows for evaluation of the alignment of the first and second metatarsals and cuneiforms.
  - The distance between the bases of the first and second metatarsals should be on more than 2 mm, and any distance greater than this is a sign of unstable injury.
  - The lateral view allows for visualization of any dislocation in the plantar or dorsal directions.
  - The oblique view allows for evaluation of the alignment of the third and fourth metatarsals with the cuboid and lateral cuneiform.
  - An avulsion fracture of the second metatarsal or medial cuneiform, known as the fleck sign, is present in 90 percent of cases and may be the only radiographic indicator of injury.[1]
- CT imaging is ideal (although not necessarily required in the ED) and may be indicated where there is high clinical suspicion and when patients are unable to tolerate weight-bearing views.

ED Treatment

- Open fractures of any kind require immediate orthopedic consultation in the ED.
- Management of Lisfranc injuries depends on the severity of the injury, with displaced fracture dislocations (>2 mm) requiring orthopedic consultation in the ED.
- Nondisplaced injuries require immobilization with a bulky, well-padded posterior splint.
- The patient should be kept on strict NWBS. Crutches, with instructions on their use, should be provided.
- Ice and elevation are recommended to prevent or minimize swelling.
- Adequate analgesia should be provided.

Disposition

- Patients presenting with displaced or unstable injuries require an orthopedic consult in the ED and likely admission for ORIF.
  - Following operative repair, the patient is non-weight bearing in a short-leg cast for six to eight weeks.
  - Progressive weight-bearing is allowed at that time.
- Injuries with concern for the development of compartment syndrome should be admitted to the hospital.
- Nondisplaced injuries may be safely discharged to home with strict NWBS and orthopedic or sports medicine follow-up within two weeks.
  - Nonoperative management typically involves a short-leg cast for six weeks (NWBS) with repeat weight-bearing X-ray at four to six weeks.
  - Progressive return to activity may begin at that time.

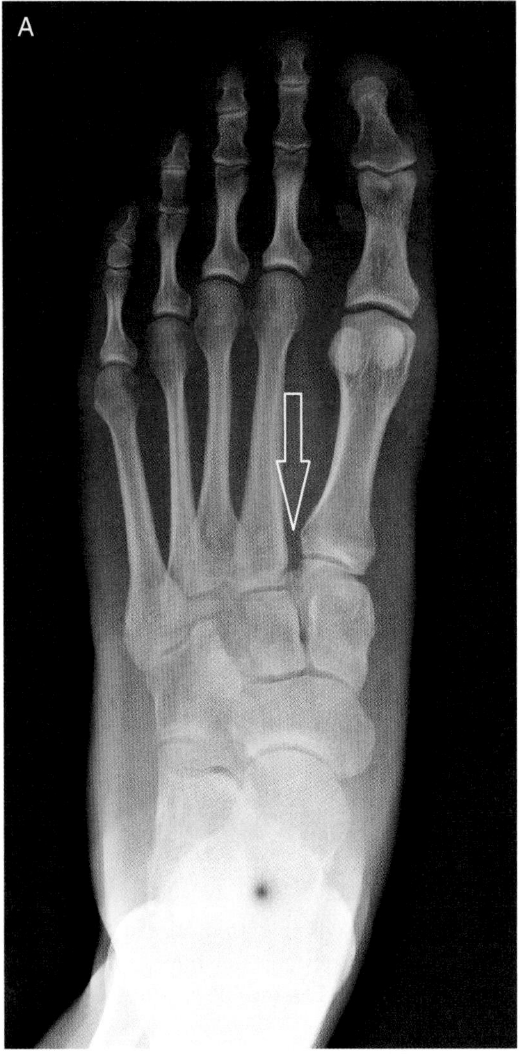

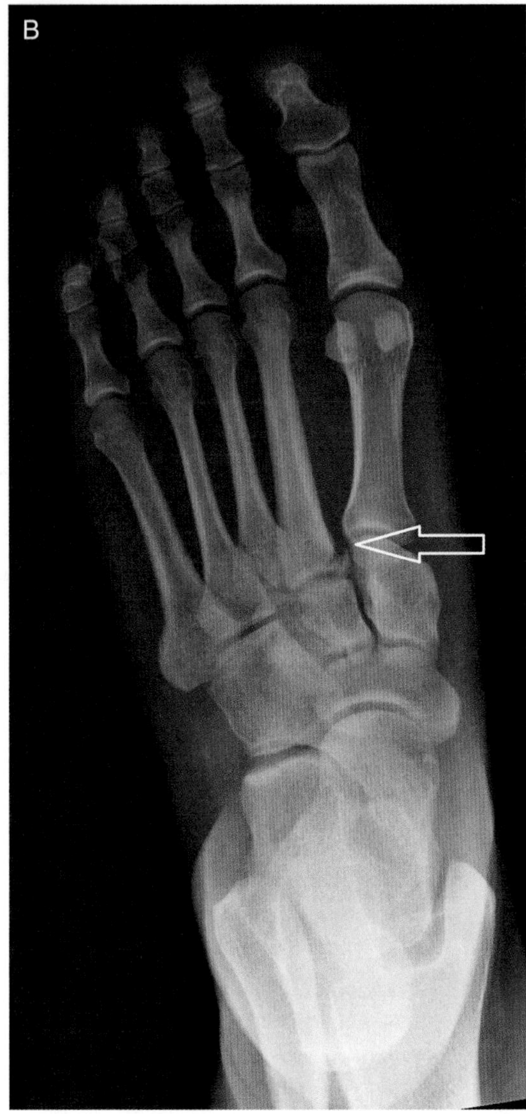

Figures 8.13A–D. Lisfranc fracture-dislocations
A) Subtle widening of the space between the first and second metatarsals
B) Fracture at the base of the second metatarsal
C) Lateral view with fleck sign
D) Severe Lisfranc fracture-dislocation

Complications

- Posttraumatic arthritis occurs in most cases.
- Compartment syndrome
- Chronic pain

Pediatric Considerations

- Lisfranc injuries are uncommon in children and when they occur are seen in children more than 10 years old.
- Displaced dislocations typically respond well to closed reduction.
- Surgical management is indicated when closed reduction is unsuccessful.[2]

Pearls and Pitfalls

- Due to the high risk of chronic pain and functional disability, any foot with pain and swelling after trauma should be suspected of having a Lisfranc injury.
- A fracture at the base of the second metatarsal suggests a Lisfranc fracture-dislocation until proven otherwise.

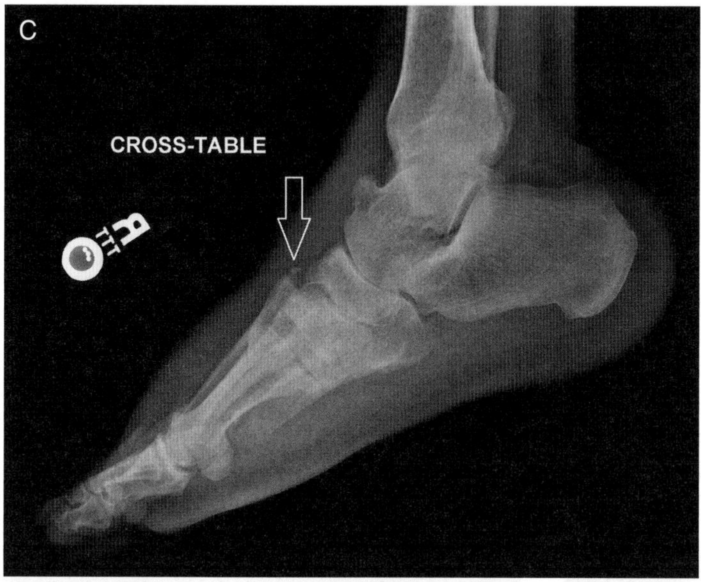

Figures 8.13A–D. *(cont.)*

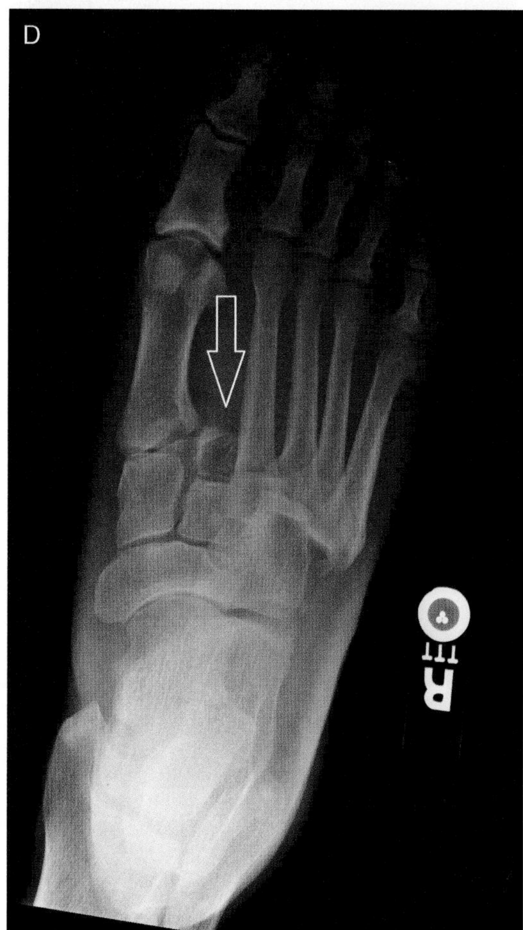

Figures 8.13A–D. *(cont.)*

- Plantar ecchymosis is pathognomonic for Lisfranc injury.[2]
- Delays in diagnosis may result in long-term pain and disability.[1,2,3,6,7,8]

First metatarsal Fractures

General Description

- The first metatarsal is larger and stronger than the second to fifth metatarsals and is less frequently fractured.

Anatomic Considerations

- A lack of interconnecting ligaments allows the first metatarsal independent movement.
- Displaced fractures disrupt the major weight-bearing complex of the foot.

Mechanism

- The majority of injuries are the result of direct trauma, specifically crush injuries.
- Indirect trauma in the form of a twisting mechanism in which torque is applied to the foot with the toes in a fixed position may also cause these fractures.

Presentation

- Patients present with pain and swelling over the dorsal and medial aspects of the foot.

Physical Exam

- There may be edema and tenderness to palpation over the fracture site.
- Axial compression longitudinally along the length of the metatarsal elicits pain.
- Presence of the dorsalis pedis pulse should be confirmed to rule out vascular compromise.

Essential Diagnostics

- X-ray: AP, lateral, and oblique views are adequate to identify these fractures (Figures 8.14A–B).
- Stress or weight-bearing views, while not necessary in ED, may be required to determine stability and ultimately surgical intervention.

ED Treatment

- First metatarsal fractures require immobilization with a bulky, well-padded posterior splint, ensuring metatarsals are in neutral position.
- The patient should be kept on NWBS. Crutches, with instructions on their use, should be provided.
- Ice and elevation are recommended to prevent or minimize swelling.
- Adequate analgesia should be provided.

Disposition

- Most first metatarsal fractures may be safely discharged to home with orthopedic or

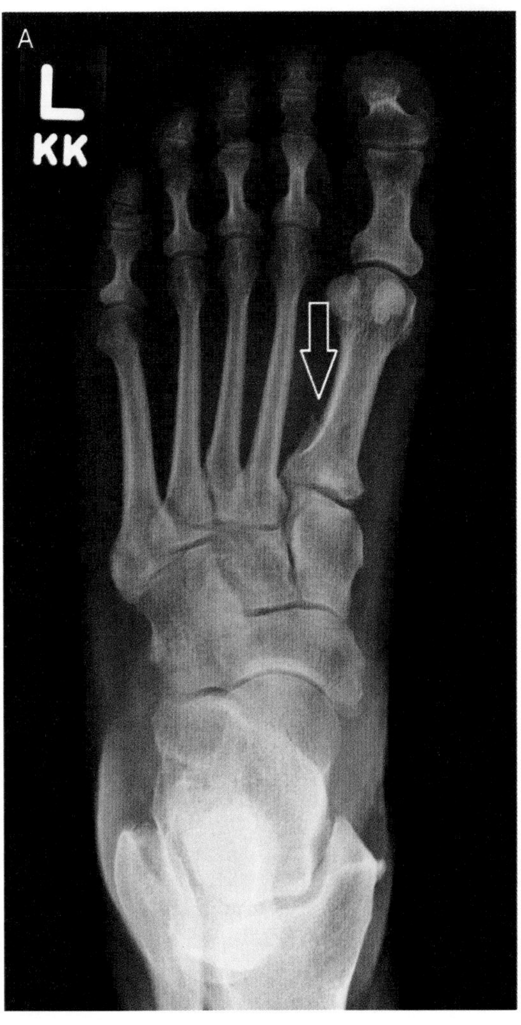

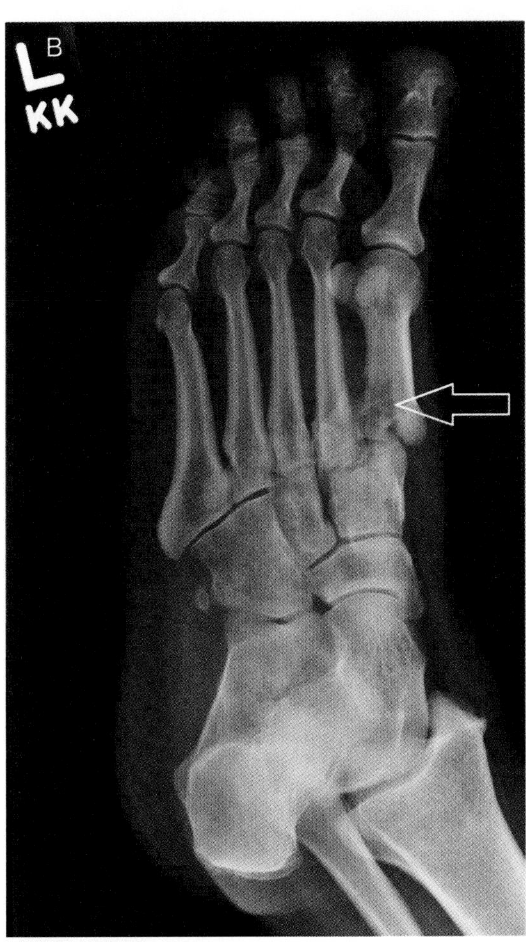

Figures 8.14A–B. Fracture of the base of the first metatarsal
A) AP view
B) Oblique view

sports medicine referral and follow-up within one week.

- Nonoperative management involves NWBS in a short-leg cast for four to six weeks with gradual return to activity once stability is confirmed with stress view X-ray.
- Indications for surgical repair (at follow-up) include displaced neck fractures and severely comminuted fractures.

Complications

- Nonunion
- Malunion
- Degenerative arthritis may develop in the case of an intra-articular fracture.

Pediatric Considerations

- Metatarsal fractures are common in children and account for 60 percent of pediatric foot fractures.
- Also termed "bunk bed fracture" as it may occur after a child jumps from a bunk bed and lands on a plantarflexed foot.

Pearls and Pitfalls

- First metatarsal fractures may be seen with associated fractures of the other metatarsals.
- It is important to consider compartment syndrome when significant soft tissue swelling is present.[1,2,3]

Second to Fourth (midshaft) Metatarsal Fractures

General description

- More common injuries than first metatarsal fractures.

Anatomic considerations

- Displaced fractures disrupt the major weight-bearing complex of the foot.
- These metatarsals are interlocked with several ligamentous attachments which work to provide stability to the complex.

Mechanism

- As with fractures of the first metatarsal, the majority of injuries are the result of direct trauma, especially crush injuries.
- Indirect trauma in the form of a twisting mechanism in which torque is applied to the foot with the toes in a fixed position may also cause these fractures.

Presentation

- Patients present with pain and swelling over the dorsal aspect of the foot.

Physical Exam

- There may be edema and tenderness to palpation over the fracture site.
- Axial compression longitudinally along the length of the metatarsal elicits pain.

Essential Diagnostics

- X-ray: AP, lateral, and oblique views are adequate to identify these fractures.

ED Treatment

- Any open fracture requires orthopedic consultation in the ED.
- Midshaft metatarsal fractures, if nondisplaced, may be placed in a hard-sole shoe with instructions for the patient to weight bear as tolerated.
- Fractures which are displaced (>3 mm) or angulated (>10°) require closed reduction in the ED.
  - Once adequate reduction is achieved the foot should be immobilized in a bulky, well-padded posterior splint, ensuring metatarsals are in neutral position.
  - The patient should be kept on strict NWBS. Crutches, with instructions on their use, should be provided.
  - Ice and elevation are recommended to prevent or minimize swelling.
  - Adequate analgesia should be provided.

Disposition

- Most midshaft metatarsal fractures may be safely discharged to home with orthopedic or sports medicine referral and follow-up within one week.
  - Nonoperative management involves weight-bearing as tolerated in a hard-sole shoe.
  - Indications for surgical repair (at follow-up) include those fractures which were

displaced or angulated at initial presentation or those that continue to be unstable or were inadequately reduced.

Complications

- Nonunion
- Malunion
- Degenerative arthritis may develop in the case of an intra-articular fracture.

Pediatric Considerations

- Metatarsal fractures are common in children and account for 60 percent of pediatric foot fractures.

Pearls and Pitfalls

- These are often seen with concomitant phalanx fractures.
- A Lisfranc injury should be suspected if the base of the second metatarsal is involved.[1,2]

Proximal Fifth Metatarsal Fractures

General Description

- Most common site of midfoot fractures.[6]
- Classified based on zone of the injury.
  - Zone 1: Tuberosity avulsion fractures or pseudo-Jones fractures, which account for 90 percent of proximal fifth metatarsal fractures.
  - Zone 2: Metaphyseal-diaphyseal junction fractures or Jones fractures, which account for 4 percent of proximal fifth metatarsal fractures.
  - Zone 3: Diaphyseal stress fractures, which account for 3 percent of proximal fifth metatarsal fractures[2].

Anatomic Considerations

- Tuberosity avulsion fractures occur proximal to the articulation of the fourth and fifth metatarsals and are due to tension from the peroneus brevis tendon.
- Jones fractures occur distal to the tuberosity and may disrupt blood supply to the distal portion of the proximal fragment.
- Diaphyseal stress fractures are distal to the proximal ligaments and extend 1.5 cm into the diaphysis.

Mechanism

- Tuberosity avulsion fractures occur after inversion of the foot while the ankle is plantarflexed.
- Jones fractures are due to a medially directed force on a plantarflexed foot but may also be seen after forceful adduction or inversion of the forefoot as commonly seen in football or basketball.

Presentation

- Acute onset of pain with difficulty bearing weight, with the exception of diaphyseal stress fractures, which typically have a prodrome of symptoms prior to fracture.

Physical Exam

- There may be minimal swelling and ecchymosis after acute injury.
- There is tenderness over the base of the fifth metatarsal.
- Passive inversion elicits pain.
- Resisted eversion elicits pain.

Essential Diagnostics

- X-ray: AP, lateral, and oblique views are usually adequate to identify these fractures (Figures 8.15A–B).
  - Tuberosity avulsion fractures are transverse or oblique and are typically extra-articular but may extend to the articulation of the fifth metatarsal and the cuboid.
- High-performance athletes may require CT for more detailed imaging of the injury.

ED Treatment

- Nondisplaced tuberosity avulsion fractures require a hard-sole shoe with instructions to weight bear as tolerated.
- Tuberosity avulsion fractures with more than 2-mm displacement, more than 30 percent involvement of the articular surface of the cubometatarsal joint, or significant step-off require immobilization with a bulky, well-padded posterior splint.
  - The patient should be kept on strict NWBS. Crutches, with instructions on their use, should be provided.

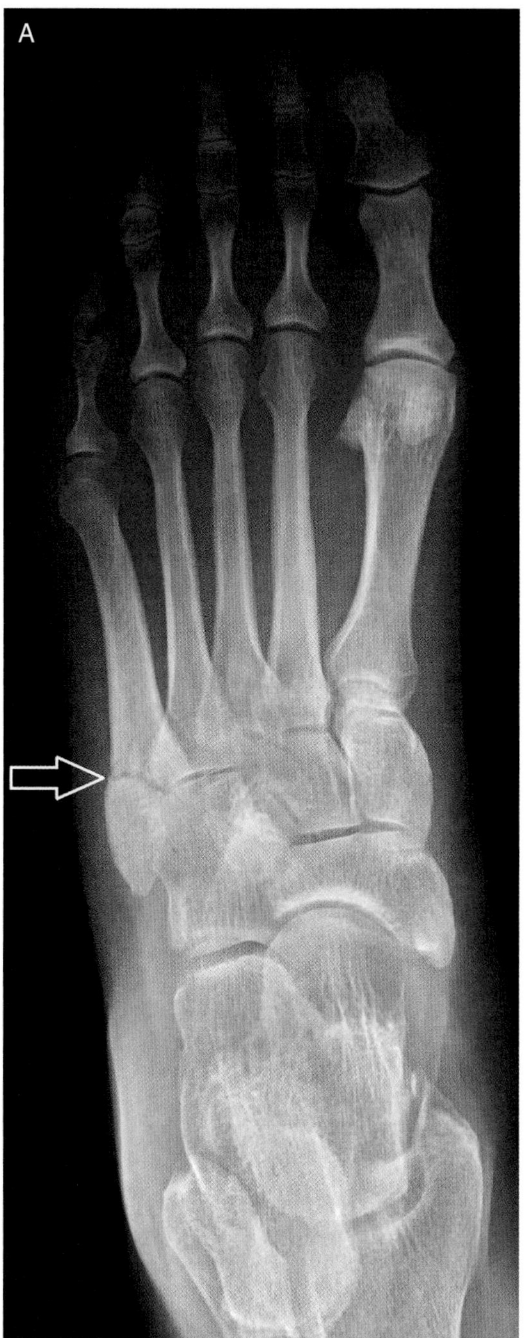

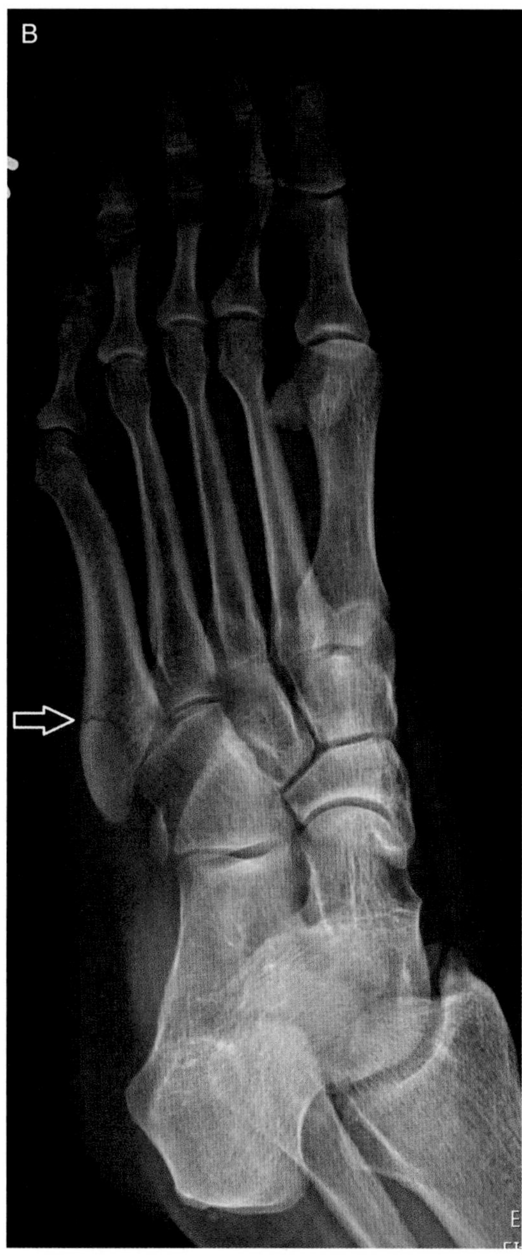

Figures 8.15A–B. Avulsion fracture of the proximal fifth metatarsal
A) AP view
B) Oblique view

  - Ice and elevation are recommended to prevent or minimize swelling.
  - Adequate analgesia should be provided.
- Jones fractures require immobilization with a bulky, well-padded posterior splint.
  - The patient should be kept on strict NWBS. Crutches, with instructions on their use, should be provided.
  - Ice and elevation are recommended to prevent or minimize swelling.

  - Adequate analgesia should be provided.
- Diaphyseal stress fractures require immobilization with a bulky, well-padded posterior splint.
  - The patient should be kept on strict NWBS. Crutches, with instructions on their use, should be provided.
  - Ice and elevation are recommended to prevent or minimize swelling.
  - Adequate analgesia should be provided.

Disposition

- Most fractures of the proximal fifth metatarsal may be discharged safely to home.
- Patients should have an orthopedic or sports medicine referral and follow-up within one week.
  - Tuberosity avulsion fractures should weight bear as tolerated for four to six weeks.
  - Jones fractures should remain NWBS for six to eight weeks.
  - Diaphyseal stress fractures should remain non-weight bearing for six to ten weeks.

Complications

- There is a high incidence of nonunion with Jones fractures and diaphyseal stress fractures.
  - For Jones fractures some advocate for early surgical intervention, especially in athletes.
  - Diaphyseal stress fractures are less likely to heal than Jones fractures and often require surgical intervention despite a long period of immobilization.

Pediatric Considerations

- Minimally displaced fractures may present with minimal swelling and tenderness.
- Avulsion fractures at the base of the fifth metatarsal should be treated with a short-leg walking cast for three to six weeks, until there is evidence of union.
- Fractures at the metaphyseal-diaphyseal junction have a higher rate of nonunion and require NWBS in a short-leg cast for six weeks.

Pearls and Pitfalls

- These fractures may present with concomitant phalanx fractures.
- Management of each type of proximal fifth metatarsal fracture differs, so knowing the type of fracture greatly improves the success of treatment.[1,2,3,6]

Phalangeal Fractures

Epidemiology

- Most common fractures of the forefoot.
- The most frequently injured is the first phalanx of the great toe.[1,2]

Anatomic Considerations

- The first and fifth phalanges are the most vulnerable due to their medial and lateral positions on the forefoot.

Mechanism

- The majority of phalanx fractures are due to a direct blow, such as when a heavy object is dropped on the foot, producing a transverse or comminuted fracture.
- An axial force or "stubbing the toe" with a varus or valgus component produces spiral or oblique fractures.

Presentation

- Patients present with pain, swelling, and ecchymosis to the injured area.

Physical Exam

- There is variable deformity to the phalanx depending on the degree of injury.
- Subungual hematoma may be present if the injury occurred more than twelve hours prior to presentation.
- Point tenderness is present over the phalanx.

Essential Diagnostics

- X-ray: AP, lateral, and oblique views are adequate to identify these fractures.

ED Treatment

- Open fractures require orthopedic consult in the ED.
- Nondisplaced fractures of all phalanges may be buddy taped, placed in a hard-sole shoe and instructed to weight bear as tolerated.
- Displaced fractures or those with gross deformity should be reduced in the ED, placed in a hard-sole shoe and instructed to weight bear as tolerated.

- Fractures of the first phalanx which are comminuted or which involve more than 25 percent of the joint surface should be placed in a posterior splint for added stability.

Disposition

- Phalanx fractures may be safely discharged home.
- Fractures of the first phalanx which are comminuted or involve more than 25 percent of the joint surface should have orthopedic or sports medicine referral with follow-up in one to two weeks.
  - Surgical intervention may be required for unstable or incongruous fractures.
- Patients may weight bear as tolerated and may progressively return to activity in two to three weeks.

Complications

- Nonunion rarely occurs.
- Posttraumatic osteoarthritis may develop after intra-articular fractures.

Pediatric Considerations

- Nonoperative management is indicated unless there is severe articular incongruity or there is an unstable displaced fracture of the first proximal phalanx.
- Children may be treated in a hard-sole shoe for two to four weeks (until pain free) and then should be held out of kicking or running sports for an additional two to three weeks.

Pearls and Pitfalls

- When buddy taping toes, it is important to place gauze between the affected toes to prevent skin maceration and breakdown.[1,2,3]

Sesamoid Fractures

General Description/Epidemiology

- Difficult diagnosis to make.
- Up to 30 percent of population may have bipartite sesamoids, and 85 percent have them bilaterally.
- Fractures usually involve the tibial sesamoid.
- May be acute or chronic.
- Fracture is usually transverse or comminuted.

Anatomic Considerations

- The sesamoid bones are two small bones located just proximal to the volar aspect of the first metatarsal head.
- They function to cushion the first metatarsal head.
- The tibial sesamoid receives the majority of the weight transmitted from the first metatarsal.

Mechanism

- Typically caused by either a direct blow or hard landing.
- May also be caused by overuse.

Presentation

- Pain with ambulation, especially with push-off.

Physical Exam

- There is often swelling, focal point tenderness, and decreased ROM at the metatarsophalangeal (MTP) joint.
- May have decreased strength with plantarflexion and dorsiflexion.

Essential Diagnostics

- Foot x-rays including AP, lateral, and oblique views as well as a sesamoid view.
- Bipartite sesamoid may mimic a fracture.
- If continued clinical concern, may consider obtaining x-rays of contralateral side or obtaining a bone scan, however rarely do these studies need to be obtained in the ED.

ED Treatment

- Place in short-leg posterior splint or boot with toe plate.
- May be weight-bearing as tolerated.

Disposition

- May be discharged home from the ED.
- Follow-up with sports medicine or orthopedic surgery.
- Will likely need to be placed in a short-leg walking cast or walking boot with toe plate for six weeks, followed by hard-sole shoe for an additional four to six weeks.

Complications

- Chronic pain

- May need surgical excision if fracture fragments are displaced or treatment is delayed.

Pearls and Pitfalls

- Need to have a high index of suspicion in order to recognize this injury.
- Make sure to obtain sesamoid views if this diagnosis is considered.

Stress Fractures

General Description/Epidemiology

- Stress fractures are common injuries, especially in runners or those engaging in repetitive impact activities.

Anatomic Considerations

- Commonly involved bones of the foot include the calcaneus, navicular, talus, bases of the second and proximal fifth metatarsals, and shafts of the metatarsals.[8]
- These may be categorized as low-risk or high-risk injuries, based on healing potential.[9]
  - Low-risk injuries include stress fractures to metatarsal shafts, commonly referred to as "march fractures."
  - High-risk injuries include stress fractures of the navicular body, talar neck, and bases of the second metatarsal and proximal fifth metatarsal.
  - The dorsal mid-portion of the navicular body has limited blood supply and predisposes this area to stress fractures.

Mechanism

- Typically caused by overuse or chronic repetitive forces.

Presentation

- Patients typically present with localized pain.
- Insidious onset
- Often complain of pain early in the course of activity.

Physical Exam

- There is often focal point tenderness.

Essential Diagnostics

- This is often a clinical diagnosis.
- X-ray: These are often negative as they have a low sensitivity during the first two to three weeks.
- Often advanced imaging in the form of CT, MRI, or bone scans are needed to identify these fractures, however these do not need to be done in the ED.

ED Treatment

- Low-risk stress fractures do not need specific treatment in the ED.
- High-risk stress fractures should be immobilized in a well-padded posterior splint and placed on NWBS.

Disposition

- Stress fractures may be safely discharged to home.
- Low-risk stress fractures require activity modification with relative rest.
  - These fractures do not necessarily need orthopedic referral or follow-up unless the symptoms persist despite rest and activity modification.
  - Once patients are asymptomatic they may slowly return to activity.
  - A total healing time of four to eight weeks should be expected.
- High-risk stress fractures should be referred to orthopedics or sports medicine with follow-up in one to two weeks.
  - Navicular stress fractures often require immobilization with NWBS and gradual return to activity at that time.
  - Stress fractures at the base of the second metatarsal should be immobilized and non-weight bearing for a total of six weeks, with gradual return to activity.
  - Stress fractures of the proximal fifth metatarsal often require immobilization for six to ten weeks.
  - Surgical fixation should be considered for these high-risk injuries, especially in athletes or those fractures showing signs of nonunion.

Complications

- Talar neck stress fractures, if they are allowed to progress to complete fractures, may lead to avascular necrosis.
- Chronic pain

Pearls and Pitfalls

- Stress fractures, especially early in their course, may not be visible on X-ray, therefore diagnosis often depends on history, physical exam, and clinical suspicion.[1,2,3,8,9]

Dislocations

Subtalar Dislocation

Epidemiology

- This type of dislocation is rare and accounts for 1–2 percent of all dislocations.[1]
- Also called a peritalar dislocation.
- Most commonly occurs in young men.

Anatomic Considerations

- Subtalar dislocations involve the simultaneous dislocations of the talus from the calcaneus and the navicular bones.
- May be classified as medial, which is more common, accounting for 80–85 percent, or lateral.[1,2]

Mechanism

- These may be the result of low-energy (i.e., stepping off a curb) or high-energy mechanisms (i.e., MVAs or falls from height).
- Medial dislocations occur after inversion of a plantar flexed foot.
- Lateral dislocations occur after eversion of a plantarflexed foot.
    - These typically require a high-energy mechanism.

Presentation

- Patients present with gross deformity of the foot after a mechanism described earlier.

Physical Exam

- There is gross deformity.
- There may be tenting of the skin.
- A neurovascular exam should be completed to assess for any neurovascular compromise.

Essential Diagnostics

- X-ray: AP, lateral, and oblique views are typically adequate in showing this dislocation.
    - Careful review of the X-ray should be undertaken to assess for any associated fractures (malleolus, talus, tarsals) as these may occur in up to two-thirds of cases.

ED Treatment

- This is considered an orthopedic emergency so prompt recognition of the injury is imperative.
- An open dislocation requires orthopedic consultation in the ED.
- For closed dislocations, reduction should be performed once the patient has received adequate analgesia.
    - To perform the reduction, the knee should be flexed to 90° to relax the gastrocnemius, with a second clinician prepared to hold the knee in this position for countertraction.
    - Longitudinal traction should be applied to the foot and the injury should be "recreated" to disengage the calcaneus.
    - Once the calcaneus is disengaged the deformity should be reversed, often with a palpable and sometimes audible clunk.
- Post-reduction X-ray should be obtained to assess adequacy of reduction.
- CT imaging may be required to evaluate for any associated fractures or the presence of talocalcaneal subluxation.
- Following adequate reduction the foot should be immobilized in a well-padded posterior splint.
- The patient should be made NWBS and crutches with instructions on their use should be provided.

Disposition

- If adequately reduced, subtalar dislocations may be safely discharged to home with orthopedic referral and instructions to follow-up in one week.
    - These patients will remain in a short-leg cast with NWBS for four to six weeks, with gradual return to activity at that time.
- If reduction is not possible in the ED, then orthopedic consultation should be obtained and the injury may need to undergo open reduction.

Complications

- Posttraumatic arthritis
- Ischemic skin
- Avascular necrosis of the talus

Pearls and Pitfalls

- It is imperative to recognize this injury immediately so that reduction may be performed as soon as possible to prevent any neurovascular compromise.[1,2]

Toe Dislocations

General Description/Epidemiology

- These are rare dislocations, but when they occur they typically occur in the dorsal direction.[1]

Mechanism

- Dislocations of the first MTP joint typically occur after extreme dorsiflexion or hyperextension of the toe.
- Dislocations of the second to fifth MTPs may occur after hyperextension or low-energy stubbing mechanisms.

Presentation

- The patient presents with difficulty walking as well as pain and swelling of the injured toe.

Physical Exam

- There is swelling to the affected toe.
- There may be a dorsal prominence if swelling is not severe.
- Passive ROM produces pain.

Essential Diagnostics

- X-ray: AP, lateral, and oblique views are typically adequate in demonstrating this injury.

ED Treatment

- Open dislocations require orthopedic consultation in the ED.
- Closed dislocations should undergo reduction in the ED by simultaneously hyperextending the toe and applying longitudinal traction.
- If adequate reduction is obtained, the toe should be buddy taped and then placed in a hard-sole shoe with instructions to weight bear as tolerated.
- If unable to achieve adequate reduction, an orthopedic consultation should be made and the patient should undergo open reduction.

Disposition

- If adequately reduced, toe dislocations may be safely discharged home with orthopedic or sports medicine referral and instructions to follow-up in one week.
  - These patients should remain in the hard-sole shoe for four weeks.
- If reduction is not possible in the ED, then orthopedic consultation should be obtained and the injury may need to undergo open reduction.

Complications

- Arthritis

Pearls and Pitfalls

- It is important to review the X-ray for associated injuries, as subtle fractures may occur with these injuries.[1,2]

Soft Tissue Injuries

Achilles Tendon Rupture

Epidemiology

- Achilles tendon rupture is a common injury, occurring in 18 of 100,000 persons per year.
- Seen in both recreational and serious athletes, typically in males 30–50 years old.
- Approximately 75 percent of ruptures occur during sporting activity.
- Approximately one-third of patients have symptoms prior to rupture.
- Diagnosis of Achilles tendon rupture is missed in approximately 25 percent of cases.
- Risk factors include episodic athletic participation (“weekend warrior”), chronic steroid use, or quinolone use.[1,3,6,7]

Anatomic Considerations

- The Achilles tendon is the largest tendon in the body.
- The tendon is the confluence of the gastrocnemius and soleus muscles and spans a distance of 15 cm to where it inserts on the calcaneus.

- It lacks a true synovial sheath but instead has a paratenon with visceral and parietal layers.
- Most ruptures occur 2–6 cm above the calcaneus where the tendon is the narrowest and the blood supply the weakest.

Mechanism

- Rupture often occurs when eccentric force is suddenly applied to a dorsiflexed foot.
- Other mechanisms include forceful dorsiflexion while the ankle is relaxed or direct trauma to a taut tendon.
- During sports activities, this typically occurs while accelerating, decelerating, or jumping.

Presentation

- At the time of injury, the patient may report a loud pop or snap and the sensation of being kicked or struck in the back of the leg.
- The patient reports acute onset of pain, difficulty with ambulation, and inability to stand on the toes.
- The pain often subsides by the time the patient is evaluated in the ED.
- Patients may report previous episodes of "tendinitis."

Physical Exam

- There may be swelling and ecchymosis present in the area.
- There may be a palpable defect present 2–6 cm above the calcaneus, however this may be obscured if significant swelling is present.
- The patient may still be able to plantarflex the foot as accessory ankle flexors (posterior tibialis, flexor hallucis longus, and flexor digitorum longus) are still intact, but significant weakness should be evident when compared to the uninjured side.
- The *Thompson test* is positive, meaning squeezing the calf does not cause plantarflexion.

Essential Diagnostics

- X-ray: There is no role for X-ray in the diagnosis of Achilles tendon rupture.
  - Plain films should be obtained only if there is concern for associated fracture or other injury.
- Ultrasound may be used to confirm the diagnosis, but is highly operator dependent.
- MRI may be obtained to fully characterize the tear (i.e., partial vs. complete), however this is not necessary in the ED.

ED Treatment

- These injuries should be immobilized in a well-padded posterior splint with the ankle in a slightly plantarflexed position.
- These patients should be non-weight bearing and should be given crutches and instructed on their use.
- Adequate analgesia should be provided.

Disposition

- Achilles tendon ruptures may be safely discharged to home with orthopedic or sports medicine referral and follow-up within one week but ideally in two days.
- Definitive management is controversial, with some authors advocating surgical management, citing decreased rates of recurrent rupture, while others advocate conservative treatment, citing lack of risk of postsurgical complications, such as infection.
  - The trend in young athletes is to undergo surgical repair, as this allows faster return to activity.
- Patients typically regain full function.

Complications

- Recurrent rupture.
- Postsurgical complications including wound dehiscence, infection, or nerve injury.

Pearls and Pitfalls

- Recognition of the injury is important as they are missed in 25 percent of cases.[6]

Achilles Tendinopathy

General Description

- Achilles tendinopathy is pain due to inflammation of the Achilles tendon.
- This condition is also known as Achilles tendonitis, tenosynovitis, peritendonitis, paratendonitis, and tendinosis.
- It is common in distance runners (present in approximately 10 percent) and ballet dancers.[1,9]

Mechanism

- This condition is most often secondary to acute overexertion, acute change in activity, or chronic overuse.

Presentation

- Patients often present with pain and swelling of insidious onset.

Physical Exam

- There is swelling around the tendon with tenderness to palpation over the area 2–6 cm proximal to the insertion on the calcaneus.
- Crepitus may be felt with passive ROM of the foot.
- Passive dorsiflexion exacerbates the pain.

Essential Diagnostics

- Achilles tendinopathy is usually a clinical diagnosis.
- There is no role for diagnostic imaging in the ED unless concomitant injury is suspected.

ED Treatment

- There is no specific treatment indicated in the ED.

Disposition

- These patients may be safely discharged home.
- Conservative management is indicated.
  - Patients should be instructed to increase activity as pain allows.
  - They may place a heal cup or pad in the shoe to elevate the heel.
  - Achilles complex stretches should be prescribed.
  - Ice should be applied to the area following activity.
  - Nonsteroidal anti-inflammatories may be used.
- Orthopedic referral for operative intervention should be made for those patients who do not respond to a six-month trial of conservative management.

Complications

- Repeated episodes may predispose to Achilles tendon rupture.

Pearls and Pitfalls

- It is important to prevent recurrent flare-ups as recurrent episodes place patients at higher risk for rupture.[1,8,9]

Sprain of First MTP Joint (Turf Toe)

General description/epidemiology

- Sprains of the first MTP joint are common, especially in athletic activities.
- Incidence has risen due to artificial playing surfaces and more flexible shoes, permitting greater flexibility at these joints, hence the moniker "turf toe."[2]
- Represents a range of injuries of the plantar plate and joint capsule.
- Injury is graded by severity, with grade 1 injuries usually due to a minor stretch or tearing injury, grade 2 injuries due to partial tear of the capsuloligamentous complex, and grade 3 injuries due to a complete tear.

Mechanism

- This occurs when the first toe is hyperextended while the foot is in plantarflexion.

Presentation

- Patients present with pain and swelling of the toe.

Physical Exam

- Tenderness on plantar side of the joint.
- Pain with passive ROM.
- May have a limp.

Essential Diagnostics

- Diagnosis is typically made from history and physical exam.
- If there is concern for fracture, AP, lateral, and oblique X-ray views should be obtained. These may show a capsular avulsion, the hallmark of this injury.

ED Treatment

- For grade 1 and 2 injuries, no specific treatment in the ED is needed, but the patient may be placed in a hard-sole shoe with buddy taping of the toe for additional comfort or support.
- The patient may weight bear as tolerated.
- For grade 3 injuries, the patient should be given crutches and made non-weight bearing.

Disposition

- Patients presenting with sprains of the first MTP joint may be safely discharged to home.

- In grade 1 and 2 injuries, symptoms typically improve in two to three weeks and patients may gradually return to activity at that time.
- Grade 3 injuries may require longer treatment, up to six weeks.
- If returning to sports a reinforced shoe may be of benefit for additional support.

Complications

- Arthritis.[1,2,3]
- Persistent pain and joint stiffness.

Pearls and Pitfalls

- This is a common injury, especially in football players.
- While most of these injuries heal well within two to three weeks, Grade 3 injuries may take longer to heal and require an initial period of non-weight bearing.

Compartment Syndrome of the Foot

General Description

- Compartment syndrome occurs when there are elevated tissue pressures within a fascial compartment leading to vascular compromise resulting in pain due to ischemia.[3]
- Compartment syndrome of the foot may be challenging for the ED physician to diagnose as the presentation may be subtle.
- Many cases are acute secondary to traumatic injury, but compartment syndrome may also be chronic, termed chronic exertional compartment syndrome (CECS).
- CECS has been reported in as many as 33 percent of runners with leg pain.[9]

Anatomic Considerations

- There are nine compartments in the foot, all of which are susceptible to compartment syndrome.
- The medial, central, and lateral compartments run the entire length of the plantar surface.
- The four interosseous compartments lie dorsally between the metatarsals.
- The calcaneal compartment is deep to the central compartment in the heel region.
- The adductor compartment is in the deep plantar aspect of the forefoot.

Mechanism

- Acute compartment syndrome is typically caused by a high-energy mechanism which results in multiple fractures, such as a crush injury, but may also be associated with burns.
- CECS is due to overuse, as seen with running or cycling.[9]

Presentation

- Patients with acute compartment syndrome present with pain and swelling after injury.
  - Pain is typically out of proportion to the degree of injury.
  - The patient may complain of paresthesias in advanced cases.
- Patients with CECS complain of pain in a well-defined area during activity that resolves with rest.

Physical Exam

- After an acute injury, the foot is swollen, possibly tense, without well-defined tenderness to palpation.
- Passive dorsiflexion of the toes elicits pain in 86 percent of patients.
- Advanced cases may have neurovascular compromise such as decreased sensation, diminished pulses, or delayed capillary refill, so neurovascular exam should be completed and documented.
- CECS will often have a normal physical exam, so may require an exercise challenge to elicit symptoms.

Essential Diagnostics

- Measurement of intracompartmental pressure confirms the diagnosis.
  - A difference of less than 30 mmHg between the diastolic blood pressure and the compartment pressure is an indication for fasciotomy.

ED Treatment

- Acute compartment syndrome of the foot is an orthopedic emergency; consultation in the ED is indicated and emergent fasciotomy should be performed.
  - Permanent damage may result with more than eight hours of ischemia.
  - Neurologic deficits may occur early on, as nerves begin to lose conduction

capacity within two hours of onset of elevated pressures.

- While awaiting surgical intervention, any restrictive casts, splints, or dressing should be removed and the affected foot should be placed at the level of the heart.
- Adequate analgesia should be provided.
- There is no specific treatment for CECS in the ED.

Disposition

- Patients with acute compartment syndrome should be admitted to the hospital for serial compartment checks or fasciotomy, if indicated.
- Patients with CECS may be safely discharged to home with instructions to avoid activity until they are able to follow-up with an orthopedist or sports medicine physician in one to two weeks.
  - Conservative management includes reduction/cessation of activity, NSAIDs, stretching, and specialized orthotics.
  - If conservative management fails, surgical intervention is indicated.

Complications

- Neurologic deficits
- Muscle necrosis
- Ischemic contractures

Pearls and Pitfalls

- Prognosis of compartment syndrome is dependent on rapid diagnosis and treatment.
- Pain out of proportion to injury is a key diagnostic indicator in compartment syndrome.[1,3,9]

Plantar Fasciitis

Epidemiology

- Most common cause of plantar heel pain, affecting one to two million people in the United States each year.
- The peak incidence is between 40 and 60 years of age.[1,9,10]

Anatomic Considerations

- The plantar fascia functions to anchor the plantar skin to the bone.

Mechanism

- Plantar fasciitis was initially thought to be an inflammatory process but now is thought to be a degenerative process secondary to repetitive microtrauma.[9]
- It is commonly seen in patients who experience excessive standing, walking, or running, are obese. or wear poorly cushioned footwear.

Presentation

- Patients present with gradual onset of heel pain.
- The pain is typically worse after waking up in the morning or after activity.
- Patients may report worsening pain while walking barefoot, upstairs, or on their toes.

Physical Exam

- It is uncommon to have any signs of trauma such as ecchymosis or swelling on inspection of the foot.
- There is tenderness to palpation at the anteromedial aspect of the calcaneus (the origin of the plantar fascia) although there may be tenderness anywhere along the length of the fascia.
- Passive dorsiflexion elicits pain.

Essential Diagnostics

- Imaging is not indicated in the ED unless another diagnosis is being considered.
- If obtained, X-ray may show a heel spur at the plantar aspect of the calcaneus.

ED Treatment

- There is no specific treatment indicated in the ED.

Disposition

- Patients with plantar fasciitis may be safely discharged home.
- Approximately 90 percent of cases respond to conservative treatment.[9]
  - Short-term management includes rest, ice, NSAIDs, massage, and heel/arch support.
  - Patients should be instructed to avoid barefoot walking and replace worn footwear.

- Patients should be referred to an orthopedist, sports medicine physician, podiatrist, or primary care physician and have follow-up in two to four weeks.
  - At the time of follow-up, additional intervention such as stretching and strengthening exercises may be employed.
  - Additionally, corticosteroid injections may be considered if symptoms are not improving as expected.
- Return to activity is dependent on improvement of symptoms.
  - Pain may persist for up to six to twelve months despite therapeutic intervention.

Pearls and Pitfalls

- Early treatment, within six weeks of symptom onset, will speed recovery.[1,9,10]

Nerve Entrapment Syndromes

Tarsal Tunnel Syndrome

General Description

- Tarsal tunnel syndrome is a condition characterized by foot and heal pain caused by compression of the posterior tibial nerve.
- This is commonly seen in athletes engaged in activities which place stress on the tibiotalar joint.

Anatomic Considerations

- The tarsal tunnel is on the medial aspect of the foot, posterior to the medial malleolus.
- The tunnel is formed by the talus, calcaneus, tibialis posterior, flexor hallucis longus, and flexor digitorum longus on the plantar surface, while the flexor retinaculum composes the dorsal surface.
- The tarsal tunnel includes nerves, arteries and tendons, including the posterior tibial nerve, which provides sensation to the bottom of the foot.

Mechanism

- Compression may be both intrinsic (edema, osteophytes, fibrosis) or extrinsic (running with hyperpronation, restrictive footwear).

Presentation

- Patients present with foot pain of insidious onset.
- It is often described as burning pain and is localized to the medial malleolus, with radiation to the toes, heel and sole.
- Patient typically report increased pain with activity which is relieved by rest.
- Patients may also report paresthesias.

Physical Exam

- Pain is exacerbated by simultaneous dorsiflexion and eversion of the ankle.
- Advanced cases may have weak toe flexion.
- A positive *Tinel's sign* is present when percussion inferior to the medial malleolus causes pain to radiate to the medial or lateral plantar surfaces of the foot.

Essential Diagnostics

- Diagnosis is typically made clinically.

ED Treatment

- There is no specific treatment indicated in the ED.

Disposition

- Patients diagnosed with tarsal tunnel syndrome may be safely discharged to home.
- Patients should be instructed to use ice and NSAIDs and to avoid exacerbating activities.
- Patients should be referred to orthopedics or a sports medicine provider for follow-up in two to three weeks, especially if symptoms have not improved with conservative management, as surgical release of the flexor retinaculum may be required.

Pearls and Pitfalls

- Tarsal tunnel syndrome may be mistaken for plantar fasciitis or Achilles tendinitis so it is important differentiate between these entities, as surgical intervention may be required for tarsal tunnel syndrome.[1,3]

Deep Peroneal Nerve Entrapment

General Description

- Deep peroneal nerve entrapment or “ski boot compression syndrome” is a condition characterized by pain to the dorsum of the foot.

Anatomic Considerations

- The deep peroneal nerve courses beneath the inferior extensor retinaculum and may become entrapped or compressed, causing pain or paresthesia to the dorsum of the foot or the web space between the first and second toes.

Mechanism

- Recurrent ankle sprains, repetitive trauma, edema, or tight-fitting outerwear such as ski boots may cause symptoms.

Presentation

- Patients present with dorsal and medial foot pain which is exacerbated by activity and relieved by rest.
- They may complain of hypoesthesia of the first and second web space.

Physical Exam

- Severe pain is elicited by palpation of the dorsum of the foot.
- Dorsiflexion and plantarflexion produce pain.
- There is diminished or absent sensation between the first and second web spaces.
- In more advanced cases, toe extension may be limited secondary to extensor muscle wasting.

Essential Diagnostics

- This is a clinical diagnosis.

ED Treatment

- There is no specific treatment required in the ED.

Disposition

- Patients diagnosed with deep peroneal nerve entrapment may be safely discharged to home.
- Patients should be instructed to use ice and NSAIDs and to avoid exacerbating activities.
- Pain typically resolves in thirty-six to forty-eight hours, however return of sensation may be delayed up to four weeks.
- Patients should be referred to orthopedics or a sports medicine provider for follow-up in four weeks, especially if symptoms have not improved with conservative management, as neurolysis may be required.

Complications

- Chronic pain
- Muscle atrophy

Pearls and Pitfalls

- History and physical exam are keys to the diagnosis.[1,3]

Plantar Interdigital Neuroma (Morton's Neuroma)

General Description

- Morton's neuroma is a condition characterized by pain on the plantar aspect of the foot near the metatarsal heads.
- This commonly affects middle-aged women[1].

Anatomic Considerations

- A neuroma is a fusiform swelling of a nerve, in this case the interdigital nerve, causing an entrapment neuropathy.
- The neuroma may be found in any interspace but most commonly occurs in the third interspace.

Mechanism

- Pain is due to local irritation of the nerve, commonly due to tight-fitting shoes.

Presentation

- Patients present with burning pain to the plantar surface of the foot which radiates to the toes.
- The pain is worse with walking or standing and typically relieved with rest and removal of shoes.

Physical Exam

- The foot should appear normal to inspection.
- Palpation of the affected (usually third) interspace produces pain, and often a discrete mass may be felt.
- *Morton's test* is positive, yielding *Mulder's sign.*[1,4]
  - Audible, painful click of the neuroma as it subluxes out from between the metatarsal heads after application of a compressive force to forefoot.

Essential Diagnostics

- This is a clinical diagnosis.

ED Treatment

- There is no specific treatment indicated in the ED.

Disposition

- Patients diagnosed with Morton's neuroma may be safely discharged to home.
- Initial management consists of conservative treatment, including shoes with a wide toe box and support to offload pressure from the metatarsal heads.
- The patient should be referred to orthopedics or sports medicine should conservative management not improve symptoms, as steroid injections may be beneficial.
- Surgical intervention may be indicated for refractory cases.

Pearls and Pitfalls

- The key to diagnosis and treatment is recognition through history and physical exam.[1,3,4]

Bursitis

General Description

- Bursitis is an inflammatory condition involving the bursa.
- In the foot, the retrocalcaneal and forefoot bursas are most commonly affected.

Mechanism

- This is typically due to pressure or repetitive use or trauma.

Presentation

- Patients present with pain to the involved area.

Physical Exam

- There may erythema and edema overlying the area.
- There is tenderness to palpation over the site.

Essential Diagnostics

- This is a clinical diagnosis unless septic bursitis is suspected, in which case fluid aspiration needs to be performed, with the fluid sent for analysis.

ED Treatment

- There is no specific treatment indicated in the ED for nonseptic bursitis.
- The patient may weight bear as tolerated.

Disposition

- Patients with nonseptic bursitis may be safely discharged to home.
- Management includes relative rest with avoidance of precipitating activity, ice, equipment modification, padding to the affected area, and NSAIDs.

Pearls and Pitfalls

- If there is concern for septic bursitis then the bursa should be aspirated and the patient should be treated accordingly; otherwise, conservative management is typically successful,[1,3]

Pediatric Considerations

Sever's Disease (Calcaneal Apophysitis)

General Description

- Traction apophysitis at the Achilles insertion on the calcaneus in skeletally immature patients.
- Usually presents during a period of rapid growth.

Mechanism

- This is typically due to overuse, or occasionally trauma.

Presentation

- Patients present with aching heel pain.

Physical Exam

- Tenderness of posterior heel.
- Commonly have decreased dorsiflexion.
- Tight heel cord.

Essential Diagnostics

- Radiographs including AP, lateral, and oblique views may be obtained to rule out other underlying diagnoses such as stress fracture or osteomyelitis.
- May show evidence of fragmentation of the apophysis.
  - These findings, however, are not necessarily pathologic and may be present on contralateral side.

ED Treatment

- There is no specific treatment indicated in the ED.

Disposition

- Patients with Sever's disease may be safely discharged to home.
- Management includes rest, ice, stretching of heel cord, heel cups, and NSAIDs.
- Patients may return to sports as tolerated, usually two to four weeks after initiation of treatment.

Pearls and Pitfalls

- Most cases of Sever's disease are benign and self-limiting.
- Make sure to consider other diagnoses such as stress fractures, bone cysts, or osteomyelitis in the appropriate clinical setting.

Table 8.2 Key Diagnoses, History, Physical Exam Findings, and Treatment

Diagnosis	History	Physical Exam Findings	Treatment
Calcaneus fracture	Fall from height or *MVA with axial loading injury	Severe swelling, ecchymosis and limited range of motion	Bulky posterior splint *NWB Close outpatient Orthopedic surgery follow-up
Talus fracture	Direct impact on a dorsiflexed foot, such as MVA or fall from a height	Severe swelling, ecchymosis and limited range of motion	Posterior splint NWB Close outpatient Orthopedic surgery follow-up
Navicular fracture	Direct impact or axial loading	Pain and swelling on dorsomedial aspect of foot	Bulky posterior splint NWB Close outpatient Orthopedic surgery follow-up
Cuboid fracture	Indirect impact with torsional stress or direct impact with crush injury	Pain and swelling on dorsolateral aspect of foot, exacerbation of pain with any midfoot motion	Bulky posterior splint NWB Outpatient sports medicine or Orthopedic surgery follow-up
Cuneiform fracture	Axial loading	Pain and swelling over cuneiforms, exacerbation of pain with any midfoot motion	Bulky posterior splint NWB Outpatient sports medicine or Orthopedic surgery follow-up
Lisfranc fracture-dislocation	Axial-load to a plantar-flexed foot such as during MVA or with a direct blow	Pain, swelling, and ecchymosis over lisfranc joint on either/or dorsum or plantar aspect of foot, pain with passive range of motion of toes or metatarsals	Bulky posterior splint NWB Outpatient sports medicine or Orthopedic surgery follow-up
1st Metatarsal fracture	Direct blow or twisting mechanism	Pain and swelling over dorsal, medial aspect of foot, pain with axial loading	Bulky posterior splint NWB Outpatient sports medicine or Orthopedic surgery follow-up
2nd-4th Metatarsal fractures	Direct trauma or twisting mechanism	Pain and swelling along dorsum of foot, pain with axial loading	Non-displaced, midshaft fractures can be placed in hard-sole shoe and *RICE, *WBAT Displaced or angulated fractures need to be reduced and placed in posterior splint and NWB Fractures at base of metatarsals associated with Lisfranc injuries

Table 8.2 (cont.)

Diagnosis	History	Physical Exam Findings	Treatment
5th Proximal metatarsal fracture	Eversion or inversion injury	Pain and swelling at proximal 5th metatarsal, pain with passive inversion and resisted eversion	If avulsion fracture, may be placed in CAM walking boot and WBAT, RICE More proximal fractures, ie Jones fracture at diaphyseal-metaphyseal junction, need to be placed in posterior splint and made non-weight bearing
Phalangeal fracture	Direct blow or axial load, ie "stubbing"	Pain, swelling and ecchymosis over injured area	2nd-5th phalangeal non-displaced fractures can be buddy-taped and placed in hard sole shoe, WBAT Displaced fractures need to be reduced and placed in hard-sole shoe 1st phalangeal fracture needs to be placed in posterior splint and made non-weight bearing
Sesamoid fracture	Direct blow or hard landing Pain with ambulation and push-off	Tenderness , swelling and decreased range of motion at 1st MTP	Short-leg posterior splint or walking boot Weight-bearing as tolerated Follow-up sports medicine or Orthopedic surgery
Stress fracture	Overuse injury	Focal point tenderness over area of injury	Low risk stress fractures need activity modification, RICE, and weight-bear as tolerated High risk stress fractures need to be placed in posterior splint and made non-weight bearing with close sports medicine or Orthopedic surgery follow-up
Subtalar dislocation	Usually due to high force mechanism after inversion or eversion on plantarflexed foot	Swelling Obvious deformity	Reduction Well-padded posterior splint NWB Outpatient Orthopedic surgery follow-up if adequate reduction and neurovascularly intact
Toe dislocation	1st MTP-extreme dorsiflexion or hyperextension 2nd-5th MTP-hyperextension, usually low energy	Swelling, pain, and possible deformity	Reduction Buddy-tape Hard-sole shoe WBAT Orthopedic or sports medicine follow-up
Achilles Tendon Rupture	Loud pop or snap in posterior ankle, difficulty walking	Swelling, pain Palpable defect in Achilles tendon Positive Thompson test	Posterior splint in plantarflexion NWB Outpatient Orthopedic surgery follow-up

Table 8.2 *(cont.)*

Diagnosis	History	Physical Exam Findings	Treatment
Achilles Tendinopathy	Insidious onset of pain and swelling in posterior heel	Tenderness and sometimes swelling of Achilles tendon Passive dorsiflexion exacerbates pain	RICE Anti-inflammatories WBAT Activity modification Physical therapy
Sprain of 1st metatarsal joint (Turf toe)	Hyperextension of toe while foot is plantarflexed	Swelling Tenderness on plantar side of the joint Pain with passive range of motion May have a limp	Buddy-tape and hard-sole shoe WBAT (non-weight bearing if grade III injury) Activity modification with gradual return as symptoms allow
Compartment syndrome	High energy mechanism after multiple fractures, crush injury or burn	Swelling Tense compartments Pain with passive range of motion of toes Occasional neurovascular compromise	Measure compartment pressures Emergent Orthopedic surgery consult Elevate and remove any constrictive dressings or devices
Plantar fasciitis	Gradual onset of heel pain, often worse in the morning	Tenderness on antero medial aspect of calcaneus and proximally Increased pain with passive dorsiflexion	RICE Heel cups Activity modification Stretching and strengthening program
Tarsal Tunnel Syndrome	Intrinsic or extrinsic compression of posterior tibial nerve Burning pain in medial malleolus with radiation to heel and sole	Pain with dorsiflexion and eversion of ankle Weak toe dorsiflexion Positive tinel's sign	Activity modification Anti-inflammatories Physical therapy Surgical release in recalcitrant cases
Deep Peroneal Nerve Entrapment	Dorsal and medial foot pain worse with activity	Tenderness on dorsum of foot Pain with dorsiflexion and plantarflexion Hypoesthesia of 1st and 2nd webspace Limited toe extension	RICE Anti-inflammatories Activity modification
Morton's Neuroma	Burning pain on plantar aspect of foot which radiates to the toes	Pain with palpation of interspace, usually 3rd, or with squeezing forefoot Possible discrete mass (neuroma) Positive Mulder's sign and Morton's test	Shoes with widened toe box Possible trial of corticosteroid injection
Bursitis (Forefoot and Retrocalcaneal)	Pain and swelling to the area usually due to repetitive use or trauma	Tenderness Swelling Possible mild erythema	RICE Anti-inflammatories Activity modification Equipment modification (ie overly tight-fitting shoes), if necessary

Table 8.2 (cont.)

Diagnosis	History	Physical Exam Findings	Treatment
Sever's disease	Aching pain in the heel Overuse	Tenderness of posterior heel Tight heel cord Decreased dorsiflexion	Activity modification Heel cups RICE Stretching of heel cord

*MVA-Motor vehicle accident
*NWB– Non-weight bearing
*RICE– Rest, ice, compression, elevation
*WBAT– Weight-bearing as tolerated

Table 8.3 Indications for Orthopedic Surgery Consultation in the Emergency Department

Fractures	Comments
Any Open Fracture	
Any injury with evidence of neurovascular compromise	
Calcaneus	If fracture is intra-articular
Talus	Major involvement of head, neck, or central portion of the body
Navicular	If fracture is displaced
Lisfranc fracture-dislocation	If there is >2 mm displacement or any evidence of instability
Any significant fracture displacement or angulation that cannot be reduced, any significant intra-articular involvement, any severe fracture comminution	
Dislocations	
Any dislocation that cannot be adequately reduced by ED personnel	
Any open dislocation	
Any dislocation with evidence of neurovascular compromise	
Subtalar	
Soft Tissue Injuries	
Acute compartment syndrome	

Recommended Reading

R.R. Simon, S.C. Sherman. *Emergency Orthopedics*, 6th edition. McGraw Hill; 2011.

D.P. Hanlon. Leg, foot, and ankle injuries. *Emergency Medicine Clinics of North America*. 2010;28(**4**): 885–905.

P.R. Burns, N. Lowery. Etiology, pathophysiology, and most common injuries of the lower extremity in the athlete. *Clinics in Podiatric Medicine and Surgery*. 2011;28(**1**):1–18.

S.M. Oser, T.K. Oser, M.L. Silvis. Evaluation and treatment of biking and running injuries. *Primary Care: Clinics in Office Practice*. 2013; 40(**4**):969–986.

P.H. Seidenburg, A.I. Beutler, eds. *The Sports Medicine Resource Manual*; Philadelphia: Saunders Elsevier; 2008.

References

1. R.R. Simon, S.C. Sherman. *Emergency Orthopedics,* 6th edition. McGraw Hill; 2011.
2. K.A. Egol, K.J. Koval, J.D. Zuckerman. *Orthopedic Handbook of Fractures.* Philadelphia: Lippincott Williams; 2010; 143–162.
3. S.A. Gaines, D.A. Handel, P.N. Ramsey. Foot injuries. In: J.E. Tintinalli et al., eds. *Tintinalli's Emergency Medicine: A Comprehensive Study Guide,* 7th edition. New York: McGraw Hill; 2011; 1875–1880.
4. The Musculoskeletal Exam. The Core Curriculum Lecture Series. 2010. www.acep.org/uploadedFiles/ACEP/Practice_Resources/issues_by_category/sports_medicine/SPORTS MEDICINE MUSCULOSKELETAL EXAM.pdf
5. C.A. Germann, A.D. Perron, M.D. Miller, S.M. Powell, W.J. Brady. Orthopedic pitfalls in the ED: Calcaneal fractures. *American Journal of Emergency Medicine.* 2004; 22(7): 607–611.
6. D.P. Hanlon. Leg, foot, and ankle injuries. *Emergency Medicine Clinics of North America.* 2010; 28(**4**): 885–905.
7. A.D. Perron, W.J. Brady, T.E. Keats. Orthopedic pitfalls in the ED: Lisfranc fracture-dislocation. *American Journal of Emergency Medicine.* 2001; 19(**1**): 71–75.
8. P.R. Burns, N. Lowery. Etiology, pathophysiology, and most common injuries of the lower extremity in the athlete. *Clinics in Podiatric Medicine and Surgery.* 2011; 28(**1**): 1–18
9. S.M. Oser, T.K. Oser, M.L. Silvis. Evaluation and treatment of biking and running injuries. *Primary Care: Clinics in Office Practice.* 2013; 40(**4**): 969–986.
10. F.R. Melio. Soft tissue problems of the foot. In: J.E. Tintinalli et al., eds. *Tintinalli's Emergency Medicine: A Comprehensive Study Guide,* 7th edition. New York: McGraw Hill; 2011; 1933–1937.

Chapter 9

Cervical Spine

Matthew B. Baird

Background/Epidemiology

- Cervical spine (c-spine) injuries are common injuries associated with a wide variety of athletic endeavors.
- The severity of these injuries range drastically from those that resolve spontaneously to those associated with severe morbidity and mortality.
- Although rare, the fear of permanent spinal cord injuries has led to significant attention from athletes, coaches, parents, physicians, governing bodies, media, and the general public. For this reason, the diagnosis and management of c-spine injuries are highly scrutinized.
- As emergency physicians, it is our role to identify unstable injuries and initiate appropriate treatment in a timely manner.
- This chapter focuses on the emergency department (ED) assessment of the athlete with a neck injury and/or radicular upper extremity symptoms.
  - Diagnosis, management in the ED, indications for orthopedic and/or neurosurgical consultation, disposition, and return to sport considerations will be discussed.
- Fortunately, the majority of neck injuries associated with sports are minor, and most athletes return to full function.
- Anatomically, however, the c-spine is unique with respect to sports-related injuries due to the potential for damage to the central nervous system in addition to adjacent musculoskeletal structures.
- Thus, spinal cord injury (SCI) resulting in permanent disability and death is of utmost concern.
  - Head and neck injuries combined account for 70 percent of traumatic deaths and 20 percent of permanent disability associated with sports.[1]
- There are approximately 10,000 cases of SCI annually in the United States,[2] with an estimated incidence of 150–500 cases per 100,000 in the general population.[3]
- Almost 10 percent are associated with athletics, making sports the fourth most common cause of SCI, behind motor vehicle accidents, violence, and falls.[4]
- The National Center for Catastrophic Sports Injury Research (NCCSIR) has defined a catastrophic sports injury as "any severe spinal, spinal cord, or cerebral injury incurred during participation in a school/college sponsored sport."[5]
  - The incidence of catastrophic injuries for all sports is about 1 in every 100,000 high school and 4 in every 100,000 college athletes.
  - Fatality rates are 0.40 of every 100,000 high school and 1.42 of every 100,000 college athletes.
- Cervical trauma accounts for most of these catastrophic injuries, with thoracic and lumbar insults being much less common.[6]
- SCI tends to be associated with youth, with a mean age of 24 years at the time of injury.
  - Sports are the third-leading cause in patients younger than 30 years.[7]
- In athletes, the risk of serious spine injury increases with the age of the athlete.
  - For example, the incidence of quadriplegia in youth American football (ages 5–16 years) is almost zero, but steadily increases from the junior high to high school to college to professional levels.[8]
- The increase in impact force as the athlete matures certainly accounts for the increased

injury rate, which declines when the average player retires from collision sports in the early to mid-twenties.

- Anatomic and biomechanical differences between the adult spine and immature spine predispose athletes of different ages to different patterns of injury.
- Several studies have suggested that children involved in athletics are more likely to suffer neck injuries.
  - Davis et al. performed an ED-based study investigating a large group of pediatric trauma patients in 1993. They found a fourfold increase in neck injuries associated with sport compared to nonsport injuries.[9]
- Gender differences in c-spine injuries have not been thoroughly studied, but trends have been identified.
  - Women seem to have a higher incidence of cervical strains.
  - The incidence of disc herniations appears to be identical.
  - Males seem to suffer more structural spine and spinal cord injuries.[10]
- C-spine injuries seem to be more common in nonorganized sports such as surfing, diving, and skydiving than in organized sports.
- This may account for the assumed underreporting of sport-related spine injuries, as these sports have a much lower public profile.
- Regarding organized sports, American football, ice hockey, rugby, skiing, snowboarding, and equestrian sports have been associated with higher risk for SCI.[11,12,13,14]
- American football accounts for the highest overall number of c-spine injuries, but has a comparable per-participant rate to ice hockey, wrestling, and gymnastics.
  - High school participants account for 80 percent of football injuries due to higher levels of participation and large discrepancies in the size and skill level of the athletes.[15]
  - Up to 15 percent of football players experience a c-spine injury at some point during the playing career.[16]
  - In previously injured players, the risk of subsequent neck injury increases significantly.[17]
  - Up to 50 percent of football players with a history of neck trauma have radiographic changes (i.e., compression fractures, disk disease, abnormal motion segments),[18] suggesting the utility of radiographs in the management of these patients.
  - Almost all c-spine injuries occur when a player is tackled by or tackles an opponent at high velocity, making defensive backs and special teams players most susceptible to these injuries.
- Rule changes have been implemented to try to prevent injuries, especially in collision sports, with varying amounts of success.
  - In 1976 "spear tackling" (using the top of the helmet as the initial point of contact) in American football was prohibited, leading to a 70 percent decrease in c-spine injuries, from 7.72 per 100,000 to 2.31 per 100,000 at the high school level.[19]
  - The incidence of traumatic quadriplegia decreased by 81 percent over this period.[20]
- This successful change indicates that governing bodies may affect safety in sports and play a role in injury prevention.
- Besides American football, many other sports carry a high risk of c-spine injury. These include ice hockey, wrestling, gymnastics, soccer, rugby, skiing/snowboarding, horseback riding, and an array of recreational activities. For the sake of time, these activities will not be discussed in detail here, but share many similar themes with American football.
  - Most injuries are impact related.
  - Risk of injury is position dependent.
  - Rule changes have resulted in decreased incidence of injuries in several sports.
  - Changes in equipment worn during competition have not been shown to change injury incidence.[21]

Anatomy

- Bones (Figure 9.1) and static stabilizers:
  - The bony c-spine is composed of seven cervical vertebrae (C1–C7) with a concave posterior (lordotic) curve.

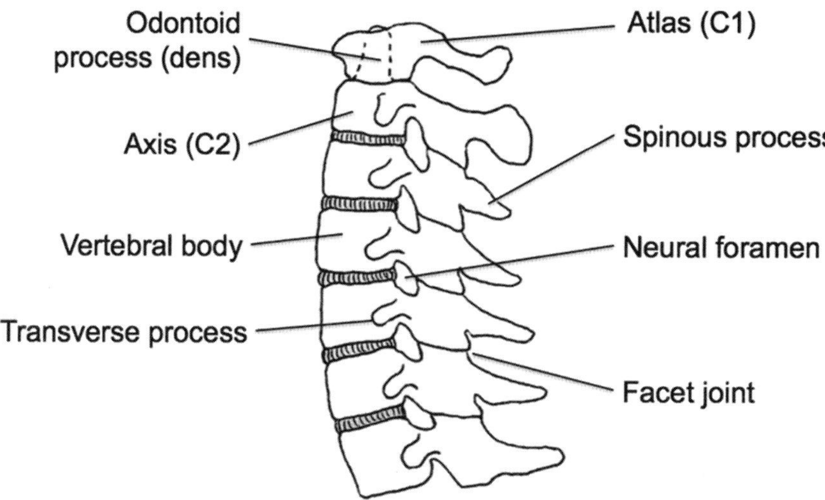

Figure 9.1. Bony anatomy of the cervical spine.

- C1 (the atlas) and C2 (the axis) make up the upper segment of the c-spine, with important anatomic differences from the lower c-spine (C3–C7).
- The C1 vertebra is made up of anterior and posterior arcs with transverse processes projecting laterally.
- The transverse foramen lies lateral to the large vertebral foramen and superior and inferior articular surfaces, which articulate with the skull base and C2 respectively.
- C2 also includes anterior and posterior arcs, transverse processes, and neural foramina. However, it does have a true vertebral body anteriorly and spinous process posteriorly, similar to the lower cervical vertebrae.
- The dens is a fingerlike projection extending superiorly from the vertebral body.
  - It articulates with the atlas, accounting for 60 percent of neck rotation.
- The primary static stabilizer of the upper c-spine is the transverse atlantal ligament, which lies posterior to the dens, supporting the articulation of the dens with the anterior arc of C1.
  - It is disruption of this ligament that causes the vast majority of atlantoaxial instability.
- C1 and C2 are secured to the occiput by the alar ligament, tectorial membrane (superior extension of the posterior longitudinal ligament), and the capsule of the atlantooccipital joint.
  - The atlantooccipital joint accounts for 40 percent of neck flexion.
- The lower cervical vertebrae are each composed of a box-shaped vertebral body, which connect to the transverse processes via the pedicles.
- The neural foramina are adjacent to the pedicle, just lateral to the vertebral body.
- The spinous process protrudes posteriorly and is separated from the transverse processes by the lamina.
- The vertebral arch, which houses the vertebral foramen, is defined by the vertebral body, the pedicles, and lamina.
- The superior and inferior articular processes arise from the junction between the pedicle and lamina and form the facet joints with the vertebrae above and below.
- Primary stability of the lower c-spine is provided by the anterior and posterior longitudinal ligaments, which are located just in front and behind the vertebral bodies respectively.
- Posterior stability is provided by three ligaments:
  - The ligamentum flavum runs on the posterior aspect of the vertebral foramen.

- The intraspinous ligaments run in between the spinous processes.
- The supraspinous ligament runs posterior to the spinous processes.

- The lower c-spine accounts for about 60 percent of flexion/extension (~50–60°), 40 percent of rotation (~60°), and nearly 90 percent of lateral bending (~60°).
  - The majority of this motion occurs between C5 and C7.

Muscles

- The trapezius, rhomboids, and levator scapulae muscles reside posteriorly.
  - The trapezius runs from the spinous processes of the c- and t-spine to the angle of the scapula and is innervated by the spinal accessory nerve and the C3 and C4 nerve roots.
  - It assists in lateral flexion, rotation away from the side of contraction, and extension.
  - The rhomboid major and minor originate at the spinous processes of C7–T5 and insert on the medial border of the scapula.
  - They are innervated by the dorsal scapular nerve, C4, and C5.
  - They assist in adduction and elevation of the scapula.
  - The levator scapula muscle runs from the spinous processes of C1–C4 to the superomedial portion of the scapula.
  - It assists in lateral flexion and rotation.
- The scalene muscles are located laterally.
  - They run from the transverse processes of the cervical vertebrae to the first rib and are innervated by branches of C3–C8.
  - They support lateral flexion, rotation, and forward flexion.
- The sternocleidomastoid (SCM) muscle runs anterolaterally.
  - It runs from the manubrium and medial clavicle to the mastoid process.
  - Nerve supply is C2, C3, and the spinal accessory nerve.
  - It aids in flexion, rotation away from side of contraction, and lateral flexion.
- There are two deep muscles in the neck: the splenius capitis and longus capitis.
  - The splenius capitis arises from the spinous processes of C7–T3 and inserts on the mastoid process.
  - It is innervated by the C4–C8 nerve roots.
  - It helps extend, laterally flex, and rotate the neck.
  - The longus capitis originates from the spinous processes of C3–C6 and inserts on the base of the occiput.
  - It is innervated by C1–C4.
  - It acts as a flexor, lateral flexor, and rotator.

Neurovascular Structures

- There are eight cervical nerves (C1–C8), which exit above the vertebral body for which they are named.
- The spinal canal is funnel shaped, so the cord occupies relatively little space in the upper c-spine and up to 75 percent in the lower c-spine.
- Space available for the spinal cord is normally between 14–23 mm.
  - Stenosis is defined as a canal of less than 13 mm.
  - Cord compression typically occurs at diameters of less than 10 mm.
- The brachial plexus arises from the C5–T1 nerve roots and exits the neck between the anterior and medial scalene muscles.
  - It terminates as the median, radius, ulnar, axillary, and musculocutaneous nerves.
  - Proximal to these branches, it gives rise to several important nerves, including the dorsal scapular nerve and suprascapular nerve.
- The internal carotid and vertebral arteries are the two most important arterial structures that traverse the neck.
  - Both arise from the subclavian artery.
  - The internal carotid accompanies the internal jugular vein and gives off the external carotid artery at about the C4 level, before passing into the skull via the carotid foramen.
  - The vertebral artery runs posteriorly, through the transverse foramina of the cervical vertebrae through the foramen magnum.

Embryologic Considerations

- A basic understanding of cervical embryology may help explain injuries patterns in children and radiographic findings.
- The neural arches of C1 form during the seventh fetal week, but do not fuse until age 3 (posterior arch) and age 7 (anterior arch) on average.
  - This lack of fusion during early childhood may easily be mistaken for a fracture radiographically.
- C2 has two additional ossification centers for the odontoid process.
  - One is present at birth, and the second develops at the tip of the dens between 3 and 6 years of age, fusing at 12 years.
  - The rest of the odontoid process fuses to the body between 3 and 6 years.
  - Remnants of these fusion lines also resemble fractures radiographically.
- The subaxial cervical vertebrae have neural arches that fuse between 2 and 3 years of age.
  - These fuse with the body by age 6.
  - Secondary ossification centers develop for the transverse and spinous processes.
  - These centers may remain unfused until the third decade of life and are often mistaken for fractures.

Initial Stabilization

- As with any trauma patient, a primary survey and initial stabilization of the c-spine is critical in the prehospital setting for any athlete with a suspected head or neck injury. This management precedes a full history and physical exam.
- Universal spine precautions should be observed, with immediate transport to an appropriate ED via emergency medical services (EMS).
- A detailed discussion of prehospital management is beyond the scope of this text, with one exception: the helmeted athlete.
  - Modern American football helmets and pads are designed to provide appropriate alignment of the c-spine. In general, these should be left in place in the athlete with a head, neck, or undifferentiated injury.
    - This practice is starting to change if there are enough prehospital providers who are trained and able to provide in-line cervical immobilization while removing pads and helmets.
  - In other sports, and with football players with ill-fitting equipment, helmet and shoulder pads should be removed while simultaneously observing universal spine precautions.
  - In the unconscious athlete, or when airway compromise is of concern, the facemask alone should be removed.
  - It is generally accepted that all football players requiring transfer to the ED for a potential head/neck injury have the facemask removed.
  - When helmet removal is required, careful attention to head and spine alignment is paramount, to avoid worsening of a potentially unstable injury.
  - There are commercially available devices to assist with removal, but manual removal remains the most common method.
    - Comparison studies have been performed to assess which method minimizes head/neck movement and movement velocity, with pros and cons for both methods. There is not yet clear consensus on the best technique.[22]
  - Hands-on training for helmet and pad removal techniques are highly recommended.

History

- After initial stabilization and appropriate transfer, a more detailed history and physical exam may be obtained (secondary survey).
- As with most medical conditions, a careful, focused history will provide the majority of the information needed to form and narrow the differential diagnosis.

- Understanding the mechanism of injury is an important first step.
  - The most common sport-related mechanism of cervical spinal trauma involves an axial load or a large compressive force applied to the top of the head.
  - More severe injuries tend to occur when the neck is in a slightly flexed position, which negates the lordotic curve. This transfers the force of the impact from the soft tissues to the cervical column.
- The location and nature of the complaint should then be discussed.
  - Location of pain, such as radicular vs. axial, should be noted.
  - Associated upper extremity symptoms such as pain, numbness, paresthesias, or weakness should also be noted.
- The evolution of the pain since the time of injury should be discussed.
  - Note if symptoms are improving, worsening, or staying the same.
- As part of the secondary survey, screening for additional or distracting injuries is also an important aspect of the history.
  - Head injuries, especially concussions, frequently accompany neck injuries, even minor ones.
  - It is important to ask if the athlete has a headache, vision changes, vomiting, or mental status changes.
  - As with all trauma patients, NEXUS criteria and the Canadian c-spine rules pertain, and may help determine which patients require radiographic evaluation. (Table 9.1, Table 9.2)

Table 9.1 NEXUS Criteria

Midline c-spine tenderness
Focal neurologic deficit
Altered level of consciousness
Intoxication
Distracting injury
If none of the above findings are present, the patient's c-spine may be cleared clinically without radiographs.

Physical Exam

- The physical exam of the neck should follow the same general guidelines as all other parts of the musculoskeletal system: inspection, palpation, range of motion, special tests, and neurovascular exam.

Table 9.2 Canadian C-Spine Rules

1. Any high-risk factor that mandates radiographs? If yes, obtain radiographs. If no, proceed to #2.	a) Age greater than or equal to 65 b) Dangerous mechanism i. Fall from > 3 ft or 5 stairs ii. Axial load to head (e.g., driving) iii. MVC high speed (>100km/h), rollover, ejection iv. Motorized recreational vehicle v. Bicycle crash c) Paresthesias in extremities
2. Any low-risk factor that allows safe assessment of range of motion? If yes, proceed to #3. If no, obtain radiographs.	a) Simple rear-end MVC with the following exclusions: i. pushed into oncoming traffic ii. hit by large truck or bus iii. rollover iv. hit by high-speed vehicle b) Sitting position in ED c) Ambulatory at any time d) Delay in onset of neck pain e) Absence of midline cervical spine tenderness
3. Able to actively rotate neck? If yes, no radiographs are necessary. If no, obtain radiographs.	45° to each side

These rules are intended for alert (GCS = 15) and stable trauma patients when cervical spine injury is a concern.

  - Given the presence of the spinal cord and brachial plexus, however, the neurovascular exam is perhaps more important than this list suggests.

Inspection

- In the immobilized patient, the exam will start in a supine position.
- In all other patients, exam is best performed seated.
- Assess the neck for angular or rotational deformities, visual step-offs, and soft tissue injuries.
- Don't forget to inspect the anterior aspect of the neck as well, which may require c-collar removal with an assistant providing manual stabilization.
- Assess the thoracic area and upper extremities for scapular winging and atrophy (in more chronic injuries).

Palpation

- The spinous processes of C2–T1 should be palpated for tenderness.
  - C2 is felt in the midline directly under the occiput.
  - C7 and T1 are quite prominent and easily palpable, but often confused.
    - With active extension C7 will move anteriorly, while T1 remains relatively stable.
  - In thin patients, the transverse processes may often be palpated, especially at C4, which has the shortest spinous process.
- The paraspinal muscles should then be palpated posteriorly, then the scalenes laterally, and sternocleidomastoid muscle anteriorly.
  - Also palpate the trachea, clavicles, and sternal notch.
- Palpation of the brachial plexus laterally is also recommended for pain or to see if it elicits radicular symptoms.

Range of Motion

- If the c-spine has been cleared clinically or radiographically, it is safe to assess range of motion. If not, this step should be postponed until appropriate clearance is obtained.
- Flexion and extension from neutral.
  - Normal flexion is 80 to 90° or two finger widths between the chin and chest.
  - The SCM is the dominant flexor.
  - Normal extension is approximately 70°.
  - The trapezius is the dominant extensor.
- Rotation
  - Normal rotation is 60 to 80°. Young healthy patients may usually rotate enough that the chin is nearly in line with the shoulder.
  - The SCM muscles are the primary rotators.
- Lateral flexion
  - Be sure to tell the patient not to elevate the shoulder.
  - Normal lateral flexion is between 20 and 45°.
  - The scalene muscles are the primary lateral flexors.
- As with any joint, note symmetry of movement, and which movements bring on or exacerbate symptoms.

Neurovascular Exam

- See Table 9.3 for review of spinal nerve function in the c-spine.
- Strength should be assessed for all major upper extremity muscle groups (shoulder shrug, shoulder abduction, elbow flexion and extension, wrist flexion and extension, grip strength).
- *Kumar's sign* (Figure 9.2), is a quick way to assess radial, median, and ulnar nerve function.
  - This test involves extension of the wrist (radial nerve), finger opposition (ulnar), and the "OK sign" with the thumb and index finger (median nerve).
  - If a deficit is identified, further strength and sensation assessment for that particular nerve is indicated.
- Trying to quantify with the standard 0 to 5 scale is appropriate, but it is most important to document comparison to the opposite upper extremity.
- Sensation to light touch should be assessed to both upper extremities, the trunk, and the lower extremities, assessing for deficits that follow a dermatomal distribution.

Table 9.3 Function of Spinal Nerves C5–T1

Nerve	Motor Function	Sensory Function	Reflex
C5	Deltoid, supraspinatous, infraspinatous	Lateral arm	Biceps
C6	Biceps, wrist extensors	Radial forearm, thumb, index finger	Biceps, brachioradialis
C7	Triceps, wrist flexors, finger extensors	Middle finger	Triceps
C8	Finger flexors	Fourth and fifth fingers	None
T1	Finger abductors	Ulnar forearm	None

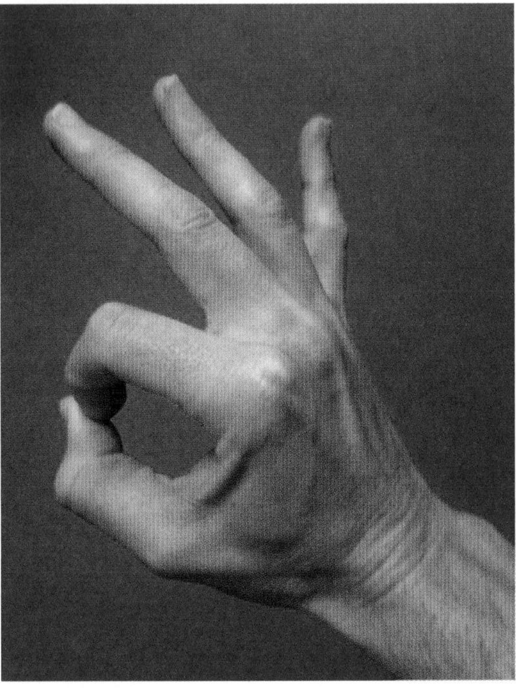

Figure 9.2. Kumar's sign.

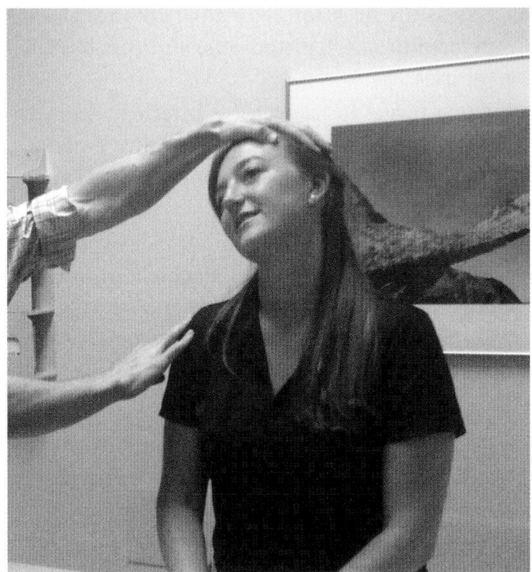

Figure 9.3. Spurling's test.

- If deficits are seen in a specific area, cold-hot and sharp-dull differentiation are appropriate follow-up tests to document.
- Biceps, triceps, and brachioradialis reflexes should be obtained and compared to the contralateral extremity. The standard 0 to 4+ scale is often used to help quantify reflex strength, with 3+ being brisk, 4+ being clonus, and 0 nonexistent.
- Vascular exam may be completed by checking radial and ulnar pulses and capillary refill.

Special Tests

- *Spurling's test*
  - *Spurling's test* (Figure 9.3) is perhaps the most useful special test in assessment for a nerve root impingement syndrome.
  - The examiner passively rotates and extends the neck, then provides a firm, controlled axial load to the patient's head.
  - Pain referred to the ipsilateral upper extremity, beyond the shoulder, is considered a positive test, and should increase index of suspicion for nerve root impingement.
  - The sensitivity of *Spurling's test* is 30–50 percent, with a specificity of 74–93 percent.[23,24]
- *Hoffman's sign*
  - *Hoffman's sign* is a test for an upper motor neuron injury.
  - The examiner flicks the tip of the long finger of a relaxed hand. If this elicits flexion of the thumb and index finger in a pincer motion, the test is considered positive.

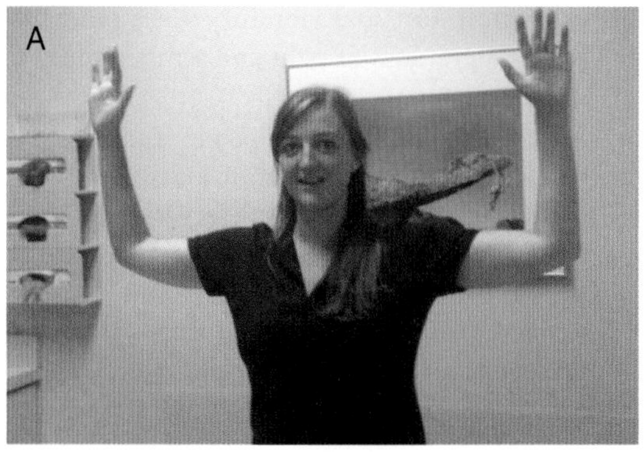

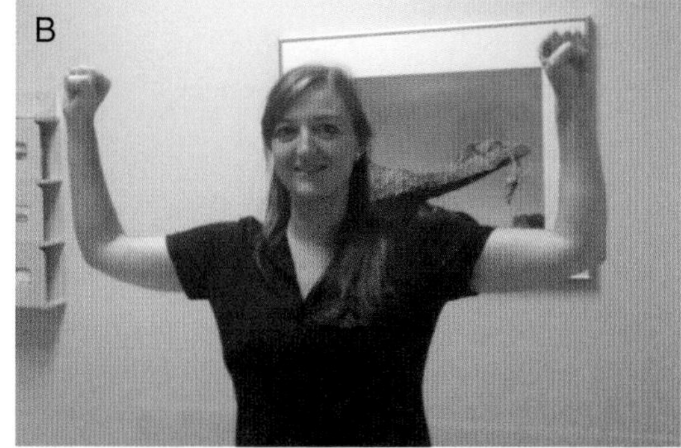

Figures 9.4 A and B. Elevated arm stress test.

  - Trials suggest a sensitivity between 33 and 58 percent, with specificity between 59 and 78 percent, although its reliability as a single test is questionable.[25]
  - When used in combination with other tests, however, its utility increases.
- *Elevated arm stress test (EAST or Roos test)* and *Adson's maneuver.*
  - These tests are assessment tools for thoracic outlet syndrome (TOS) which may present with radicular-type upper extremity symptoms.
  - *Elevated arm stress test* (Figures 9.4 A and B) is performed with the patient sitting with shoulders abducted to 90° and elbows flexed to 90°. The patient then opens and closes the hands for 3 minutes. If reproduction of symptoms occurs during this time, it is considered a positive test.
  - *Elevated arm stress test* (Figures 9.4 A and B) has a sensitivity of 84 percent and sensitivity of 30 percent, based on minimal evidence.[26]
  - *Adson's maneuver* (Figure 9.5) is performed with the examiner palpating the radial pulse on the affected side. The arm is then passively externally rotated, extended, and abducted slightly. The patient rotates the head toward the affected side. If the pulse disappears, this is considered a positive test and concern for vascular TOS is increased.
  - One study suggests that *Adson's maneuver* has a sensitivity of 79 percent and specificity of 76 percent.[27]
- As with all areas of the body, special tests are best used as adjuncts to help increase or decrease the clinical suspicion for a specific injury. They are not meant to be used in isolation.

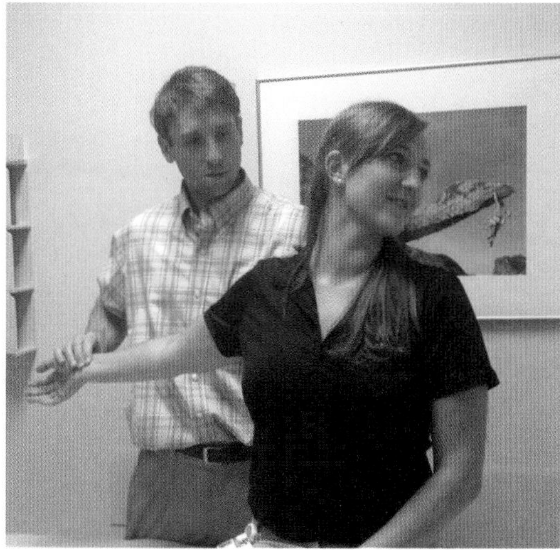

Figure 9.5. Adson's maneuver.

Differential Diagnosis – Emergent and Common Diagnoses

- A reasonable differential diagnosis for neck pain and radicular-type arm pain in the athlete is listed in Table 9.4.
- As with all medical conditions, the differential changes based on history, physical exam, and imaging studies.
- Older patients with nontraumatic or minimally traumatic neck pain may have a broader differential, including cardiac, pulmonary, and even intra-abdominal pathology. These conditions are not included in this text.

Table 9.4 Emergent and Common Diagnoses in the Emergency Department

Emergent	Common
Catastrophic cervical spine injury	Brachial plexus neuropraxia
Cervical spine fracture/ dislocation	Cervical disc herniation
Cervical cord neuropraxia with persistent neurological deficits	Cervical sprains/ strains/contusions
Acute, traumatic cervical disc herniation	Neurologic thoracic outlet syndrome
Any cervical disc herniation with associated neurologic deficits	
Vascular thoracic outlet syndrome	
Any injury with persistent neurological deficits	

Catastrophic C-Spine Injury

Description

- Sport-related c-spine injuries are typically divided into three groups.
- Type 1 injuries are catastrophic spinal cord injuries resulting in permanent neurologic deficits. A catastrophic c-spine injury is defined as "a structural distortion of the cervical spinal column associated with actual or potential damage to the spinal cord."[21] These injuries are discussed in this section.
- Type 2 injuries (discussed separately) result in transient neurologic symptoms with normal radiographic studies. Neuropraxias and most traumatic disc herniations are examples of type 2 injuries.
- Type 3 injuries (discussed separately) are those with radiographic abnormalities but no neurologic deficit. These include fractures (both stable and some unstable), some fracture-dislocations, and certain disc herniations.
- Catastrophic c-spine injuries are categorized into four separate syndromes.
- Brown–Sequard syndrome results from hemisection of the spinal cord. It results in ipsilateral loss of motor function, proprioception, and vibratory sensation, with contralateral loss of pain and temperature sensation.
- Anterior spinal cord syndrome results in damage to the spinothalamic and corticospinal tracts with preservation of the posterior columns. This is manifested by loss of motor function, pain, and temperature below the lesion with preservation of vibration, proprioception, and crude touch.
- Central cord syndrome is caused by damage to the centrally located fibers of the corticospinal and spinothalamic tracts. This results in decreased strength, pain, and sensation predominantly in the upper extremities.
- Mixed injuries usually are a combination of Brown–Sequard syndrome and central cord syndrome. They result in crossed motor and sensory deficits predominantly to the upper extremities.
- Unstable fractures with or without dislocation are the most common cause of catastrophic c-spine injury.

Mechanism

- The most common mechanism of injury in catastrophic c-spine injuries is an axial load to a slightly flexed neck.
- In a neutral position, normal cervical lordosis helps dissipate forces to paraspinal muscles and other soft tissues, avoiding injury to the spinal column itself.

Presentation

- Descriptions of the four categories of catastrophic c-spine injury are discussed earlier. As mentioned, the majority of patients present with mixed injuries and varying degrees of sensory and motor deficits below the level of injury, predominantly in the upper extremities.
- Many patients are comatose or otherwise unable to provide an appropriate history due to head injury or other associated injuries.
- The vast majority of athletes are transported to the ED by EMS on a backboard. If appropriate guidelines are followed, football players have pads and helmet on, with facemask removed. If not, the facemask

should be removed immediately for necessary airway management.

- It should be noted that plain films and CT scans can and should be performed with helmet and pads on, unless there are associated injuries that require removal. Again, helmet and pads should be removed together.
- In other athletes with helmet and pads (i.e., hockey, lacrosse), equipment should be removed.

Physical Exam

- Athletes with c-spine injuries are, and should be treated as typical trauma patients. Thus, physical exam should always begin with a primary survey, with interruptions for cardiopulmonary interventions when indicated.
  - The primary survey should include a brief neurologic evaluation, assessing gross motor and sensory function to the trunk and extremities.
- A secondary survey should follow, including a more detailed neurologic exam in the awake patient who is able to speak and protect their airway.
  - This exam should include sensation to light touch, sharp-dull discrimination, two-point touch discrimination, and basic assessment of extremity proprioception (toe/thumb up, toe/thumb down test).
- It is critical to document as much of a neurologic exam as possible prior to sedation, paralysis, and intubation.
- Full spine precautions should be observed throughout the examination.
- Range of motion testing and the special tests described earlier, with the exception of *Hoffman's sign*, should not be performed in this population.

Essential diagnostics

- Plain c-spine radiographs and/or CT scan should be obtained immediately in patients with suspected catastrophic c-spine injury.
- In those with neurologic deficits on exam, emergent MRI should be performed even if the CT scan is unremarkable.

ED Treatment

- The primary goal of ED management of patients with potentially catastrophic c-spine injury is to prevent secondary neurologic injury due to improper handling of the injured athlete in the ED.
  - Unstable injuries without neurologic compromise may be converted to those with permanent deficits if appropriate precautions are not observed.
  - A proper fitting cervical collar in the non-helmeted athlete or manual c-spine stabilization in the helmeted athlete is essential.
  - Log rolling with at least four people is recommended during the secondary survey.
  - Full thoracic and lumbar spine precautions should continue until an unstable cervical injury is excluded.
- The second goal is a prompt and accurate diagnosis using history, physical exam, and diagnostic imaging.
- The third priority is timely stabilization of unstable injuries. Spine consultants (neurosurgery and/or orthopedics) should be contacted early.
  - Consultation is indicated in any athlete with neurologic symptoms with or without radiographic findings, or those with radiographic findings (fracture, cord edema, ligamentous instability) without neurologic symptoms.
- Supportive care, pain control, management of associated injuries, and communication with family are also important tasks that often fall to the emergency physician.
- The use of high-dose steroids in SCI is controversial, and has been a hotly debated topic for the past several decades.
  - The initial adoption of the practice occurred after the NASCIS (National Acute Spinal Cord Injury Study) II and III trials in 1990 and 1997 respectively.[28,29] These trials concluded that administration of high-dose methylprednisolone within eight hours of injury was beneficial to the patient's neurologic outcome.
  - Subsequent studies brought into question the validity of NASCIS II and III, with more recent studies suggesting

ineffectiveness and potential harm from high-dose methylprednisolone.[30]
  - Thus, high-dose steroids are currently not recommended in patients with SCI.
- The use of hypothermia is also controversial.
  - Currently, there is not sufficient evidence to recommend the use of local or systemic hypothermia for these patients.[31]
  - However, several clinical studies have demonstrated encouraging evidence over the last several years, without large, multi-center trials.[32]
  - Thus, recommendations may change in the near future.
- Consultation with a spine specialist regarding the use of steroids and hypothermia is recommended.

Disposition

- Patients who present with neurologic compromise or unstable injuries should be admitted to an intensive care unit due to the risk of respiratory failure and hemodynamic instability (spinal shock).
- Athletes with stable injuries without neurologic symptoms may often be discharged after consultation with a spine specialist. Follow-up with neurosurgery/orthopedics should be arranged prior to discharge.
- Those with no radiographic abnormalities and no neurologic symptoms may be discharged with follow-up with sports medicine, orthopedics or the PCP in five to seven days.
- Return to play is only considered in athletes with no radiographic abnormalities, no evidence of neurologic compromise, and improving pain.
  - These athletes may gradually return after: (1) resolution of pain, (2) they obtain full range of motion of extremities, and (3) they obtain full strength of extremities.
  - The physician should encourage a stepwise return to sport supervised by an athletic trainer or coach.
- Athletes with permanent neurologic deficits or injuries requiring surgical stabilization are disqualified from contact sports.
  - Those with stable injuries without neurologic compromise may eventually return to sport.
  - The emergency physician should not play a role in clearing these athletes.

Complications

- Improper handling of a patient with an unstable spine injury may lead to, or worsen, permanent neurologic deficits.
- In high cervical lesions, usual above C5, respiratory compromise is likely. This occurs due to damage to the roots of the phrenic nerve, which innervates the diaphragm.
  - It is recommended that these patients be intubated immediately after diagnosis.
- Patients with severe c-spine injury are also at risk for hemodynamic instability, or "spinal shock."
  - If left untreated, this may lead to cardiovascular collapse and death.
  - Thus, close monitoring and supportive care is of utmost importance.

Pediatric Considerations

- Spinal cord injury without radiographic abnormality (SCIWORA).
  - SCIWORA is a well-described phenomenon occurring predominantly in children.
    - It involves clinical evidence of SCI without findings on plain radiographs or CT scan.
    - In the vast majority of cases, abnormalities are found on MRI, however these findings may be subtle.
    - Thus, in any pediatric patient with neurologic complaints or findings, an MRI should be obtained when plain x-ray and CT scans are negative.
  - The mechanism is not well understood, but it is thought to be due to transient deformity of the c-spine due to ligamentous laxity.
  - Spinal cord ischemia may also play a role.
  - Deficits may include partial or complete paralysis.
    - There are reports of SCIWORA that manifests as Brown–Sequard syndrome, central cord syndrome, and anterior cord syndrome.
    - Onset of deficits may be immediate, but may be delayed for hours, and in rare cases up to a few days.

  - Thus, appropriate education for the athlete and their family regarding the possibility of delayed neurologic sequelae is appropriate.
- There is a wide range of symptoms, and the prognosis depends on the severity of deficits.
- Management is the same as for all catastrophic spinal cord injuries.

Pearls and Pitfalls

- It is recommended to assume that any athlete with sport-related neck pain or any neurologic complaints be considered to have a catastrophic or unstable c-spine injury until proven otherwise.
  - Observe full spine precautions until unstable injuries are ruled out.
- Consult with a spine specialist early for any athlete with neurologic compromise and/or radiographic abnormalities.
- Do not administer steroids or begin a hypothermia protocol before discussion with a spine specialist.

Fractures and Dislocations

Description

- Fractures and dislocations of the c-spine are categorized based on the location (upper c-spine vs. lower c-spine), and whether they are stable or unstable.
- Upper c-spine: Upper c-spine injuries involve C1 and C2 and associated ligaments. They are rare in athletes, but several specific injuries deserve discussion. Luckily, most injuries to the upper c-spine do not result in neurologic injury due to the large amount of space available for the cord at these levels.
  - Atlantoaxial instability: Rupture of the transverse atlantal ligament and alar ligaments may lead to anterior translation of C1 on C2.
    - These are considered to be unstable injuries.
  - C1 fracture (Jefferson fracture): C1 fractures were characterized by Jefferson in 1920.[33] This fracture refers to a burst fracture of C1 involving disruption of the anterior and posterior arches.
    - Stability depends on involvement of the transverse ligament.
  - C2 fractures
    - Odontoid fractures are classified into three types.
      - Type 1: Avulsion fracture to the tip of the dens.
        - Type 1 fractures are rare but stable injuries.
      - Type 2: Fracture through the base of the dens.
        - The most common type of c-spine fracture.
        - Unstable.
      - Type 3: Fracture through the body of the axis.
        - Unstable.
    - Hangman's fracture: A traumatic spondylolisthesis of the axis due to fracture through both pedicles. This results in anterior displacement of C2 on C3.
    - An inherently unstable injury.
  - Lower c-spine
    - The majority of fractures/dislocations of C3–C7 in athletes are vertebral body fractures.
    - Vertebral body fractures are divided into five types.
      - Type 1: Anterior wedge compression fractures.
        - These fractures do not involve any posterior structures, making them stable injuries.
      - Type 2: An anterior-inferior "teardrop" fracture.
        - These injuries are stable and do not involve posterior elements.
      - Type 3: A comminuted burst fracture which may or may not involve posterior elements.
        - For the purposes of the emergency physician, these are considered unstable injuries.
      - Type 4: These injuries are described as a "three-part–two-plane" fracture of the vertebral body.
        - They involve (1) a teardrop fracture of the anteroinferior aspect of the vertebral body, (2)

a sagittal fracture through the body, and (3) a fracture through the posterior arch.
        - These are inherently unstable fractures.
    - Type 5: Type 4 fractures with fracture to the posterior element of an adjacent vertebra.
        - Very unstable
- Facet dislocations: Unilateral and bilateral facet dislocations are rare in athletes, but may occur in collision sports and motor sports.
    - Unilateral dislocations without fractures are typically stable injuries without neurologic compromise.
    - Bilateral dislocations are quite unstable and often associated with quadriplegia.
- Clay-shoveler's fracture: This term describes an avulsion fracture of the spinous process of a lower cervical vertebra, typically C7.
    - Isolated clay-shoveler's fractures are stable injuries.

Mechanism

- Upper c-spine injuries
    - Atlantoaxial instability: Transverse and alar ligament rupture is typically the result of a forceful flexion injury causing anterior translation of C1 on C2.
    - Jefferson fractures: Axial load injuries are the predominant mechanism for C1 fractures.
    - Odontoid fractures: There is not a single accepted mechanism, but high-energy axial load with forced flexion (most common) or extension (rare) is suspected.
- Lower c-spine injuries
    - Vertebral body fractures: Axial load
    - Facet dislocations: These high-energy injuries usually involve axial loading, flexion, and rotation.
    - Clay shoveler's fracture: Intense flexion against contracted erector spinae muscles.

Presentation

- Patients with fractures and/or dislocations present with neck pain and pain with range of motion. In unstable injuries, variable amounts of motor or sensory loss is expected.
- Since fractures and dislocations are often associated with catastrophic c-spine injuries, please refer to the discussion in the preceding section.

Physical Exam

- Tenderness to palpation at the injured level is the predominant finding on physical exam.
- Pain with range of motion is seen in most patients who present without a c-collar in place.
- Appropriate neurologic and vascular exams are indicated, as discussed in previous sections.
- *Hoffman's sign* should be performed, but additional special tests should be delayed in athletes with a history/mechanism concerning for an unstable injury.

Essential Diagnostics

- Upper c-spine injuries
    - Atlantoaxial instability: Lateral plain films will demonstrate increase in the atlantodens interval. The normal interval is 3 mm in an adult, but may be widened up to 12 mm if the transverse and alar ligaments are ruptured.
    - Jefferson fractures: Plain films and CT scan will demonstrate bilateral symmetrical overhang of the lateral masses of the atlas in relation to the axis, with an increase in the paraodontoid space on the open mouth view.
        - Overhang of greater than 7 mm suggests a transverse ligament rupture, making this an unstable injury.
    - Odontoid fractures: These fractures are often seen on the open mouth view. With nondisplaced fractures, however, CT scan is often required to make the diagnosis and should be obtained in high-risk individuals.
    - Hangman's fractures: The spondylolisthesis is seen on lateral plain radiograph, with the fractures themselves visible on CT scan.
- Lower c-spine injuries
    - Vertebral body fractures: Most vertebral body fractures are seen on lateral plain film,

although true classification may be difficult. Thus, CT scanning is recommended. MRI may help assess for cervical cord injury in unstable injuries, and help assess acuity of compression fractures.
- Facet dislocations: On plain lateral radiographs, anterior translation of the superior vertebral body on the inferior vertebral body (spondylolisthesis) is seen.
  - Unilateral facet dislocations involve less than 50 percent of anterolisthesis.
  - Translation of over 50 percent is considered a bilateral dislocation.
  - CT and MRI are indicated in the setting of facet dislocation to assess for concomitant fracture and cord injury.
- Clay-shoveler's fracture: Lateral plain films demonstrate these injuries. Additional radiographs are not indicated unless additional injuries are suspected, as this injury is not associated with neurologic compromise.

ED Treatment

- As discussed in the catastrophic c-spine injury section, the initial treatment of patients with c-spine fractures and dislocations involves:
  - Appropriate precautions to avoid exacerbation of an unstable injury
  - Prompt diagnosis
  - Pain control
  - Prompt consultation with a spine surgeon
  - Diagnosis and management of associated injuries
  - Communication with family
- Please refer to the discussion in the previous section for additional details.

Disposition

- For an emergency physician, any fracture or dislocation of the c-spine necessitates consultation with a spine surgeon.
- Admission should be the assumed disposition. In the case of a stable fracture, discharge in an appropriate cervical collar may be reasonable following discussion with the spine consultant.
- The athlete should not be returned to sport by the emergency physician at any time. This decision is the responsibility of the spine specialist after full evaluation, treatment, and rehabilitation goals have been achieved.
- For the sake of completion and patient education, notes on more definitive treatment for select injuries are included here.
  - Atlantoaxial instability: The recommended treatment for this unstable injury is atlantoaxial fusion.
  - Jefferson fractures: Unstable injuries are typically treated with axial traction until muscle spasm resolves, followed by bracing. This treatment should be provided by a spine surgeon.
  - Odontoid fractures
    - Type 1 are treated with a cervical collar for six to eight weeks.
    - Type 2 fractures are difficult conditions to treat definitively, and are a bit of a surgical dilemma. Current practice is predominantly surgical stabilization, although some authors suggest that three months in a halo brace is quite effective.[34]
    - Type 3 fractures are often treated with three months in a halo brace vs. screw fixation, depending on surgeon preference and success of nonoperative care.
  - Hangman's fractures: Typically treated non-surgically with halo immobilization
  - Vertebral body fractures
    - Athletes with types 1 and 2 injuries may safely be discharged home with a collar for comfort after discussion with a spine consultant to assure follow-up in seven to ten days.
    - Admission and surgical stabilization is recommended for types 3, 4, and 5 injuries.
  - Clay-shoveler's fracture
    - Discharge in a cervical collar for comfort in the setting of isolated clay-shoveler's fracture is appropriate. Consultation with a spine specialist, however, is encouraged to establish follow-up in seven to ten days.

Complications

- Many fractures and dislocations are unstable and may result in permanent neurologic deficits, as discussed in the previous section.
- Aside from catastrophic neurologic injuries, inappropriate management of fractures and dislocations may lead to early degenerative changes and chronic pain.

Pediatric Considerations

- Down's syndrome: Patients with Down's syndrome are at risk for atlantooccipital and atlantoaxial instability. For this reason, they are typically restricted from collision sports until instability is ruled out.
  - A higher index of suspicion for ligamentous instability in athletes with Down's syndrome presenting with neck and/or arm complaints is warranted.
  - That being said, natural history studies suggest that one-third of patients with Down's syndrome demonstrate radiographic evidence of instability, but only 3 percent of these individuals suffer neurologic injuries.[35]
  - Clearing athletes with Down's syndrome for sports is a delicate task, aimed at limiting risk but not limiting participation unnecessarily.
  - It is advisable to refer these athletes to a spine specialist and/or sports medicine provider to assist with this decision.
- Atlantoaxial instability
  - In children, the normal atlantodens interval is less than 5 mm (instead of 3 mm as in adults).
- Odontoid fractures
  - As mentioned previously, development of the odontoid process may lead to difficulty interpreting plain radiographs. Thus, MRI should be considered early in children under the age of 7 for further clarification.

Pearls and Pitfalls

- Scrutinizing initial radiographic studies and applying this to information obtained from the history and physical exam is paramount in making an appropriate diagnosis. In the setting of discrepancies, more advanced imaging (CT, MRI) and/or consultation should be obtained immediately.
- In the setting of compression fractures or teardrop fractures, spending the time to obtain old radiographs may help determine acuity.
- Do not clear a patient to return to sport directly from the ED with a fracture or dislocation regardless of when the injury occurs.
  - These decisions are complex and require collaboration between spine surgeons, sports medicine physicians, patients, and families.

Cervical Strains, Sprains, and Contusions

Description

- A strain is a stretch injury to muscle fibers or the musculotendinous junction (most common).
- Similar injury to a ligament is termed a sprain.
- A contusion is a blunt force injury from a direct blow to the soft tissues.
- These three injuries, which often occur in combination, account for the majority of neck injuries in the athlete.

Mechanism

- Strains and sprains are usually a result of a traction-type injury or forceful contraction against resistance. Contusions are due to direct blunt trauma.

Presentation

- The athlete will complain of neck pain, usually unilateral, and pain with range of motion.
- Radicular symptoms are not present

Physical Exam

- Tenderness to the involved muscle(s) is common.
- Pain with range of motion testing
- Normal neurovascular exam

Essential Diagnostics

- If bony tenderness is present, plain radiographs should be obtained.
- In isolated strains, sprains, and contusions, x-rays will be normal.

ED Treatment

- Pain control is the mainstay of treatment.
  - NSAIDs and acetaminophen are first-line agents.
  - Muscle relaxants and opiates may be necessary depending on injury severity and if muscle spasm is present.
  - Ice is encouraged for the first several days for pain relief and edema control.
  - A cervical collar may be provided for the first seven to ten days, until severe pain and spasm have improved.
    - Use of a collar for longer than ten days has been associated with deconditioning and weakness of cervical muscles.[36]
  - Gentle stretching and massage are encouraged when tolerated.

Disposition

- If more serious injury is not suspected, or ruled out, discharge home with primary care or sports medicine follow-up in one to two weeks.
- Orthopedics consult is not indicated.
- The athlete may return to play when pain has resolved and there is full cervical range of motion and normal strength.
- Use of a neck roll or "horse collar" may be considered for football players, although clinical effect is unclear.

Complications

- Sprains, strains, and contusions are self-limiting injuries.
- Under-rehabilitation or return to play prior to symptom resolution may lead to prolonged symptoms or predispose the athlete to other c-spine injuries.

Pediatric Considerations

- Given the ossification pattern of the cervical vertebrae and often normal appearing x-rays in the setting of more significant injury, diagnosing a child with a cervical strain or sprain is fraught with peril unless the clinician is certain of the diagnosis.
- Usually prompt follow-up with the pediatrician or sports medicine provider in three to four days for further evaluation is appropriate management.
- The child should be held from physical activity until follow-up unless pain has resolved at the time of ED assessment (rare).

Pearls and Pitfalls

- Misdiagnosing a more serious injury as a sprain, strain, or contusion is the most concerning pitfall.
- A thorough physical exam and appropriate evaluation for fractures and neurologic injury will help avoid such mistakes and the associated consequences.

Brachial Plexus Neuropraxia (BPN)

Description

- BPN, also called "stingers,", "burners," and transient brachial plexopathies, refer to injuries to the cervical nerve roots or brachial plexus resulting in transient unilateral upper extremity pain and/or paresthesias.
- BPN is quite common and may occur in as many as 50 percent of collision sport athletes.[37]
- The C5 and C6 nerve roots are most commonly affected.
- In most cases, symptoms resolve within seconds to minutes, but may last weeks.

Mechanism

- The most common mechanism is a longitudinal traction injury to the brachial plexus.
- This typically occurs when the ipsilateral shoulder is forcefully depressed with the neck laterally flexed to the contralateral side.
  - Defensive American football players are at highest risk when making a tackle.
- Less commonly, an axial load to the head with the neck rotated in the ipsilateral direction may cause neuroforaminal narrowing and a compression injury to the exiting nerve root.
- Rarely, contusion to the brachial plexus from a direct blow may cause identical symptoms.

Presentation

- The athlete complains of unilateral upper extremity pain, burning, stinging, and/or numbness beginning abruptly after a collision or tackle.

Physical Exam

- The athlete often flexes the neck slightly and holds the affected arm with the other hand to decrease pressure and tension on the affected nerve root.
- Many athletes shake the affected arm to try and relieve symptoms.
- Tenderness to palpation of the neck or brachial plexus may be present shortly after the injury.
- Range of motion is often limited due to pain.
- Sensory and/or strength deficits to the affected limb are common, often in a dermatomal pattern.
- *Spurling's test* may increase or reproduce symptoms.
- Upper motor neuron deficits are not seen.

Essential Diagnostics

- The diagnosis is made clinically, but if midline cervical, shoulder, or clavicular tenderness is present plain x-rays should be obtained.
- If symptoms and deficits are progressing, or if the neurologic exam is significantly abnormal, MRI of the c-spine is the study of choice to assess for SCI, nerve root avulsion, or traumatic disc herniation.

ED Treatment

- By definition, BPN is a transient condition and does not require specific treatment other than avoidance of further injury.
- Once the diagnosis is made, the mainstay of treatment is pain control.
  - For ambulatory patients, first-line agents include NSAIDs and acetaminophen, with the addition of muscle relaxants and opioids if needed.
  - Ice may be soothing to painful areas.
  - A sling may often be useful to support the affected arm and avoid tension on the cervical nerve roots, reducing pain.

Disposition

- Once the clinician is confident with the diagnosis of BPN (i.e., after symptom resolution), discharge with close outpatient management is appropriate.
- Emergent neurosurgical or orthopedic consultation is not indicated.
- Follow-up should be in three to four days with the primary care provider, sports medicine physician, or orthopedist for re-evaluation and to discuss return to sport.
- The athlete should be instructed to return to the ED or call the provider for any worsening of symptoms.
- Athletes should be held from sports until symptoms have resolved completely and they have regained full motion and strength.
- Return to play is a complex decision with multiple factors involved. Often, it is not the place of the emergency physician to make this decision. It is quite reasonable to refer the patient to a sports medicine physician, primary physician, orthopedist, or team physician for final clearance.
- For the sake of completion, for BPN, the following algorithm is recommended:
  - If it is a first occurrence and symptoms resolve within 15 minutes, it is considered safe to return them to play the same day.
  - If symptoms last forty-eight to seventy-two hours, a seven-day delay prior to return to play is recommended.
  - Recurrent neuropraxias (greater than one episode of neuropraxia) have been associated with permanent deficits. In this situation, further outpatient workup is indicated, and the patient should be held from sports until follow-up.

Complications

- Isolated neuropraxias (unless recurrent) do not usually result in long-term complications, although a protracted recovery is possible and should be discussed with the patient.

Pediatric Considerations

- Pediatric patients are treated similarly to adults, with a lower threshold for c-spine imaging.
- Early follow-up in one to two days is also reasonable to assure symptom improvement/resolution.

Pearls and Pitfalls

- Misdiagnosis is certainly the greatest pitfall with cervical neuropraxias.
- Symptoms should always be unilateral and should show steady signs of improvement.
- Bilateral symptoms should be considered an SCI until proven otherwise.

Cervical Cord Neuropraxia (Transient Quadriplegia)

Description

- Cervical cord neuropraxia (CCN) is a transient SCI resulting in bilateral sensory and motor deficits.
- Severity of symptoms may range from mild weakness to complete paralysis.
- Symptoms are usually short-lived, less than 15 minutes, but may last up to 36 hours.

Mechanism

- Hyperflexion, hyperextension, and axial compression injuries all may lead to CCN.
- On a cellular level, segmental demyelination of the axon leading to increased intracellular calcium is the proposed mechanism.

Presentation

- The athlete complains of paresthesias and weakness to bilateral upper and lower extremities, beginning after a collision.

Physical exam

- Decreased sensation and strength below a certain cervical level is seen acutely, often with c-spine tenderness.
  - These symptoms should gradually improve over minutes to hours.
- Other symptoms of catastrophic c-spine injury are often seen acutely, but resolve over a short period of time.

Esential Diagnostics

- In the symptomatic athlete, plain X-rays or CT scan AND MRI are indicated to assess the integrity of the bony and neurologic structures, respectively.
- By definition, imaging will be unremarkable in true CCN, but are essential to rule out fracture, SCI, or unstable injuries.
- Flexion-extension plain films are not indicated in the acute setting, as the presence of pain and spasm do not allow for accurate assessment of stability.
- Historically, the Torg ratio (ratio of the AP diameter of the spinal canal to the AP diameter of the vertebral body on lateral plain x-ray) was proposed as a potential screen for congenital spinal stenosis, which may lead to increased risk of CCN.
  - More recent studies demonstrate that a Torg ratio of less than 0.8 has a high sensitivity (over 90 percent), but very low specificity and positive predictive value for the diagnosis of congenital spinal stenosis.[38]
  - Thus, the Torg ratio is not a useful tool in the emergent setting.

ED Treatment

- Full spinal precautions should be observed until symptoms have resolved and structural damage has been ruled out.
- Pain control should be provided.

Disposition

- Even in the setting of normal radiographic studies, the symptomatic patient with CCN should be managed very conservatively.
- Admission for symptomatic patients is recommended.
- Those with transient symptoms that have completely resolved may be discharged with follow-up with a sports medicine provider in one week.
- The athlete should not be allowed to return to play by the emergency physician.
  - Return to play after a single episode of CCN is controversial and requires an individualized collaborative approach.

Complications

- Like BPN, CCN is transient and usually resolves completely without permanent sequelae.

Pediatric Considerations

- Again, great care with any pediatric patient with neurologic symptoms must be observed.
- Admission is best for those children that remain symptomatic, as it is very difficult to differentiate CCN from SCIWORA in the acute setting.

Pearls and Pitfalls

- As with BPN, making the correct diagnosis is paramount.
- Structural SCI should be suspected in any symptomatic patient.
- The diagnosis of CCN should not truly be made until after symptoms have completely resolved.

- Any patient with c-spine tenderness should be considered to have an unstable fracture until proven otherwise.

Cervical Disc Herniation

Description

- Acute cervical disc herniations are rare in the athlete; significantly less common than lumbar disc herniations. That said, high-level collision sports athletes do seem to be at higher risk than their peers.
- Athletes involved in noncontact sports demonstrate a lower incidence of lumbar and cervical disc herniations. This is thought to be due to improved strength to dynamic stabilizers of the c-spine.
- Disc herniations may lead to transient quadriparesis due to mass effect and contusion to the anterior and lateral portions of the cervical cord. More permanent cord injuries are possible, but much less common.
- American football players, and presumably collision sports athletes in general, are more likely to acquire degenerative changes to the c-spine at an earlier age. Studies of American football college recruits demonstrate radiographically evident changes.[39] Thus, symptoms due to chronic disc herniations are indeed seen in the athletic population.

Mechanism

- Acute disc herniations usually occur from a forceful axial load to the head and c-spine, usually with some aspect of neck flexion.
- An acute tear in the dorsal aspect of the annulus pulposus occurs, allowing the soft nucleus pulposus to extrude posteriorly. This may lead to compression and contusion to the cervical cord and exiting spinal nerve roots.
- Chronic disc herniations occur from repetitive axial load injuries. This leads to disc space narrowing, osteophyte formation, and degenerative tears to the annulus.

Presentation

- Athletes with acute traumatic disc herniations present with neck pain and radicular symptoms to varying degrees.
- Paraspinal muscle spasm is often present, and radiation to the periscapular area is commonly seen.
- Extrusion of disc material into the central spinal canal may rarely lead to catastrophic SCI or CCN.
- Chronic injuries also present with neck pain and radicular symptoms, but with a much more protracted course. Patients typically cannot identify a single inciting event, and symptoms tend to be progressive. Some athletes may report multiple episodes of brachial plexus or CCN due to nerve root/cord injury from acute inflammation of a chronic disc herniation.

Physical exam

- In both acute and chronic injuries, the spectrum of symptoms and physical exam findings is broad, depending on the severity of cord/nerve root injury.
- In acute injuries, limited neck range of motion is a common finding due to spasm and pain.
- Midline and paraspinal tenderness is often present with palpable spasm.
- Radicular symptoms are usually isolated to a single upper extremity and characterized by decreased strength and/or sensation, asymmetric reflexes, and sometimes decreased hand coordination.
- *Spurling's test* may be positive with the head turned toward the side of nerve root impingement.
- In the most severe injuries, complete paralysis to all four extremities with loss of pain and temperature sensation (anterior cord syndrome) may be seen.
- In more chronic injuries, the spectrum of disease begins with neck pain, tenderness, and stiffness, with associated paraspinal muscle spasm.
- As degeneration progresses, pain and paresthesias to the affected arm are common and *Spurling's test* may become positive.
- Weakness tends to develop after the sensory changes, and is a more ominous sign of irreversible injury.
- With time, dysmetria and atrophy may develop.
- *Hoffman's sign* may become positive as myelopathy progresses.
- In advanced disease, lower extremity symptoms may occur, as may ataxia and loss of bowel/bladder control.

Essential Diagnostics

- Definitive diagnosis is made with MRI.
- Plain films are often normal in the acute injury, but should be obtained when bony tenderness is present to assess for fracture.
- In chronic injuries, degenerative changes are commonly seen on plain c-spine x-ray.
  - These include disc space narrowing, mild spondylolisthesis (translation of adjacent vertebrae due to chronic instability), loss of cervical lordosis, and osteophyte changes.

ED Treatment

- ED Treatment greatly depends on the severity of symptoms.
- In mild acute injuries with neck pain, unilateral arm pain, and a normal neurologic exam, symptom control is the most important intervention for the emergency physician.
- If midline tenderness or weakness and/or numbness to the arm is present, a c-collar should be placed and full spinal precautions observed until fracture and significant cord injury have been ruled out with appropriate imaging.
- When this has been achieved and the patient is being discharged, anti-inflammatory drugs and muscle relaxants are first-line agents for symptom relief.
- Often narcotics are needed for several days.
- Gentle stretching and range of motion exercises are encouraged.
- A soft collar may be provided for ambulatory patients for the first seven to ten days for comfort.

Disposition

- Athletes with mild acute injuries (neck and arm pain +/− paresthesias, +/− mild numbness, without additional symptoms) whose c-spines have been appropriately cleared may be discharged home.
- Follow-up with the primary care provider or sports medicine physician should be encouraged in seven to ten days.
- The athlete may return to sport when pain is controlled and there is full neck motion and normal upper extremity strength.
- Mild chronic injuries should be referred to the primary care provider or sports medicine physician in one to two weeks to reassess and discuss referral to physical therapy, potential injection therapy, and additional medications.
- In patients with myelopathy (weakness, dysmetria, evidence of upper motor neuron involvement) or paralysis, consultation with a spine surgeon should be obtained immediately in the ED to assist with appropriate treatment and disposition.
- Athletes with radicular symptoms associated with a disc herniation tend to have a protracted recovery, and should not be cleared for sports by an emergency provider.
  - In these athletes, an average of five months is required before return to sport.[40]
  - However, the majority of patients without SCI improve with a nonoperative treatment plan.

Complications

- Permanent SCI is the most feared outcome in patients with acute disc herniations and associated SCI.
- Proper immobilization to avoid exacerbation of an existing injury and focus on timely decompression when indicated is the job of emergency providers.
- Less severe disc herniations may lead to earlier degenerative changes resulting in chronic pain, and occasionally progressive radicular symptoms, requiring surgical intervention at a later time.
- Educating patients and encouraging follow-up is the most appropriate intervention for ambulatory patients with minor injuries.

Pediatric Considerations

- Cervical disc herniations in preadolescent children are incredibly rare. Several reports suggest that 0.5–4 percent of surgically managed disc herniations occur in children younger than 18 years of age.[41]
- Fractures and SCIWORA are considered more likely.
- True radicular symptoms in a child are ominous and require full radiographic workup and consultation with a pediatric spine specialist if symptoms persist to aid with disposition.

Pearls and Pitfalls

- As mentioned several times earlier, accurate diagnosis of a SCI in the ED is critical to avoiding permanent sequelae.
- A thorough history and exam usually provide the information necessary to decide if imaging is indicated to confirm the suspected diagnosis or narrow the differential.
- In acute injuries, if significant deficits are noted or the patient is showing signs of myelopathy, a consult should be obtained even if imaging is unremarkable.

Thoracic Outlet Syndrome (TOS)

Description

- TOS refers to a constellation of upper extremity symptoms and signs that occur due to compression of the brachial plexus and/or subclavian vessels as they pass between the first rib and clavicle.
  - TOS is categorized as neurologic, venous, or arterial.
  - Neurologic TOS is by far the most common form, accounting for over 95 percent of cases.[42]
  - Vascular TOS may lead to subclavian artery and/or vein stenosis. Over time, a thrombus may develop, which may lead to thromboembolic events.

Mechanism

- Mechanical compression may occur from trauma resulting in swelling, muscle hypertrophy from overtraining neck and chest muscles, masses/tumors, or any condition resulting in mass effect at the thoracic outlet.
  - Cervical ribs and fibrous bands in the area of the scalene muscles are predisposing factors for TOS.

Presentation

- Neurologic TOS: Patients present with extremity pain, paresthesias, numbness, and weakness. This is often accompanied by neck pain and occipital headache.
- Venous TOS: These symptoms are accompanied by arm swelling, dark discoloration, and potentially venous dilation.
- Arterial TOS: The "five p's" are often seen: pain, pallor, pulselessness, poikilothermia (color and temperature change), and paralysis (or weakness).

Physical Exam

- Arm swelling and color changes are often present in vascular TOS.
- Observing for mass or muscle hypertrophy in the area of the thoracic outlet is important.
- Tenderness to the area of the thoracic outlet is occasionally seen.
- Exacerbation of symptoms with full abduction or forward flexion is common.
- *Elevated arm stress test* and *Adson's maneuver* (as described in the physical exam section) may be positive.

Essential Diagnostics

- TOS is a clinical diagnosis, but diagnostic studies may be helpful in establishing a cause for the condition.
- Plain radiographs of the neck and chest may help identify the presence of a cervical rib.
- In the ED, the most important decision is whether or not vascular TOS is a concern. If so, vascular studies are warranted to assess for thrombus, usually in the subclavian vessels.
  - The most appropriate initial step is venous and arterial duplex studies with provocative maneuvers.

ED Treatment

- In the vast majority of cases, treatment for neurologic TOS is not necessary in the ED.
  - Physical therapy is the treatment of choice.
- Patients with vascular TOS are a very different story, however, and require consultation with a vascular surgeon and anticoagulation.
- Pain control is appropriate for these patients.

Disposition

- Athletes with mild neurologic TOS thought to be due to muscle hypertrophy, postural problems, fibrous bands, and even cervical ribs may be safely discharged home.
  - They should follow-up with the primary care or sports medicine physician in the next week for a referral to physical therapy.
  - Those with a cervical rib may require outpatient referral to a vascular surgeon by the primary care or sports medicine provider.
  - Athletes with mild symptoms may return to play when pain is controlled and they

have full range of motion and strength to the upper extremities.

- Admission and prompt consultation with a vascular surgeon is indicated in patients with venous or arterial TOS.

Complications

- Venous TOS may lead to deep vein thrombosis and life-threatening thromboembolic events.
- Arterial TOS may lead to arterial stenosis and limb ischemia if not diagnosed early.
- Chronic vascular TOS may also lead to vascular scarring which may not respond well to surgical intervention.

Pediatric Considerations

- TOS is very rare in young children.
- Suspicion should lead to evaluation for mass, tumor, or lymphadenopathy at the thoracic outlet. This may be done as an outpatient with a pediatrician in the vast majority of cases.

Pearls and Pitfalls

- Diagnosing all TOS as neurologic due to postural or muscular changes may lead to misdiagnosis.
- Look closely for upper extremity swelling, temperature/color changes, and pulse discrepancies, which suggest a vascular etiology.

Table 9.5 Key Diagnoses, Clinical and Radiographic Findings, and Treatment

Diagnosis	Clinical Findings	Radiographic Findings	Treatment
Catastrophic cervical spine injury	Neurologic compromise of various degrees depending on severity: -Anterior cord syndrome -Central cord syndrome -Brown–Sequard syndrome -Mixed syndromes -SCIWORA	Unstable fracture(s), Facet dislocations, Large disc herniations, Cord edema	Full spine precautions, Airway management, Immediate surgical consult, Pain control, Management of other injuries, Athlete should not be returned to play
C-spine fracture and/or dislocation	Neck pain and tenderness, Pain with range of motion, Sensory and motor deficits to trunk and extremities depending upon stability and cord/nerve root involvement.	Plain films: spondylolisthesis, compression fractures, burst fractures, clay-shoveler's fractures CT: C1 and C2 fractures, posterior element fractures MRI: fracture acuity, cord/nerve root involvement	Full spine precautions, Airway management, Immediate surgical referral for all fractures, Admission for unstable fractures, Pain control, Management of other injuries, Athlete should not be returned to play by the ED physician
Cervical cord neuropraxia	Neck pain and tenderness, Pain with range of motion, Bilateral sensory and motor deficits predominantly to arms, Spurling's test often positive, Hoffman's sign positive when upper motor neurons are injured	Usually normal, disc herniations may be seen	Full spine precautions until symptoms resolve, Surgical consult for persistent neurologic deficits for admission, Pain control, Management of other injuries, Athlete should not be returned to play by the ED physician
Brachial plexus neuropraxia	Neck pain and unilateral tenderness common, Tenderness to scalene area common, Motor and/or sensory deficits to unilateral upper extremity, Spurling's test may be positive	Normal findings	Full spine precautions until symptoms resolve, Surgical consult for persistent neurologic deficits, Pain control, Management of other injuries, Athlete may return to play after single episode once completely asymptomatic

Table 9.5 *(cont.)*

Diagnosis	Clinical Findings	Radiographic Findings	Treatment
Cervical disc herniation	Neck pain and tenderness common, Reproductions of symptoms with ROM testing, Neurologic deficits to varying degrees depending on cord/nerve root involvement, Spurling's test often positive	MRI demonstrates disc herniation and assesses cord/nerve root involvement	Full spine precautions in patients with acute injuries and acute neurologic deficits/complaints, Surgical consultation for patients with acute neurologic deficits, Pain control, Athlete should not be returned to play by ED physician
Cervical sprains, strains, and contusions	Neck and paraspinal muscle pain and tenderness, often with palpable spasm, Pain with ROM when affected muscle groups are activated	Normal findings	Full spine precautions until unstable injury has been assessed for and spine cleared using standardized criteria (NEXUS criteria or Canadian C-spine rule), Pain control, and soft collar if needed for comfort, Athlete may return to play once asymptomatic
Thoracic outlet syndrome	Neurologic TOS: tenderness to TO possible, positional numbness/tingling/pain to unilateral arm, scalene hypertrophy possible, supraclavicular mass rare, elevated arm stress test and Adson's maneuver may be positive Venous TOS: upper extremity pain and swelling, venous engorgement possible, elevated arm stress test and Adson's maneuver may be positive Arterial TOS: upper extremity pain, edema possible, pallor, temperature and color changes, weakness, diminished pulses possible, elevated arm stress test and Adson's maneuver may be positive	Radiographs may demonstrate a cervical rib, rarely a mass to lung apex, Venous duplex may demonstrate DVT to subclavian vein, Arterial duplex demonstrates arterial insufficiency	Immediate vascular consult for arterial and venous TOS, Neurologic TOS is treated conservatively with referral to PCP or sports medicine physician for physical therapy, Pain control

Table 9.6 Indications for Surgical Consultation in the Emergency Department

Any fracture or dislocation (stable and unstable)
Any injury with persistent neurologic deficits/complaints
Acute traumatic disc herniations with myelopathy or weakness
Vascular thoracic outlet syndrome (vascular surgery)

Recommended Reading

Miele V, Maroon J: Spinal injuries in sports. In: *Benzel EC, Spine Surgery*, 3rd edition. Saunders, 2012. Chapter 71, 689–700.

Drez D: Spinal injuries. In: Delee JC, Drez D, Miller M (eds). *DeLee and Drez's Orthopedic Sports Medicine*. Saunders, 2010. Chapter 16, 665–768.

Winn HR: Transient quadriparesis and athletic injuries of the cervical spine. In: Winn HR (ed). *Youman's Neurologic Survey*, 6th edition. Saunders, 2011. Chapter 317, 3211–15.

Bailes J.E., Hadley M.N., Quigley M.R., et al.: Management of athletic injuries of the cervical spine and spinal cord. *Neurosurgery* 1991; 29: 491–497.

Snyder RL: Neck injuries. In: Madden CC (ed). *Netter's Sports Medicine*, 1st edition. Saunders, 2010. Chapter 40, 326–331.

References

1. Mueller FO, Cantu RC, Van Camp SP, et al.: Football. In: Mueller FO, Cantu RC, Van Camp SP (eds). *Catastrophic Injuries in High School and College Sports*. Champaign, IL: Human Kinetics, 1996. 41–56
2. Bailes J.E., Hadley M.N., Quigley M.R., et al.: Management of athletic injuries of the cervical spine and spinal cord. *Neurosurgery* 1991; 29: 491–497
3. Kraus J: Epidemiologic features of injuries to the central nervous system. In: Anderson D (ed). *Neuroepidemiology. Florida: CRC*, 1991. 333–357
4. Wilson J.B., Zarzour R., Moorman C.T., et al. Spinal injuries in contact sports. *Curr Sports Med Rep* 2006; 5: 50–55
5. Center NSCIS: Spinal Cord Information Network: Facts and Figures at a Glance. University of Alabama at Birmingham. Available at: www.ncddr.org/rpp/hf/hfdw/mscis/nscisc.html2003
6. Banerjee R., Palumbo M.A., Fadale P.D., et al.: Catastrophic cervical spine injuries in the collision sport athlete, part 1. *Am J Sports Med* 2004; 32: 1077–1087
7. Jackson A.B., Dijkers M., DeVivo M.J., et al.: A demographic profile of new traumatic spinal cord injuries: change and stability over 30 years. *Arch Phys Med Rehabil* 2004; 85: 1740–1748
8. Adickes MS, Stuart MJ.: Youth football injuries. *Sports Med* 2004; 34: 201–207
9. Davis JM, Kuppermann N, Fleisher G, et al.: Serious sports injuries requiring hospitalization seen in a pediatric emergency department. *Am J Dis Child* 1993; 147: 1001–1004
10. Kelley LA: In neck to neck competition are women more fragile?. *Clin Orthop Relat Res* 2000; 372: 123–130
11. Levy A.S., Smith R.H.: Neurologic injuries in skiers and snowboarders. *Semin Neurol* 2000; 20: 233–245
12. Quarrie K.L., Cantu R.C., Chalmers D.J., et al.: Rugby union injuries to the cervical spine and spinal cord. *Sports Med* 2002; 32: 633–653
13. Tator C.H., Carson J.D., Cushman R., et al.: *Hockey injuries of the spine in Canada, 1966–1996. CMAJ* 2000;162(6): 787–788.
14. Schmitt H., Gerner H.J.: Paralysis from sport and diving accidents. *Clin J Sport Med* 2001; 11: 17–22
15. Cantu R.C., Mueller F.O.: Catastrophic spine injuries in American football, 1977–2001. *Neurosurgery* 2003; 53: 358–363
16. Gill SS, Boden BP: The epidemiology of catastrophic spine injuries in high school and college football. *Sports Med Arthrosc* 2008; 16: 2–6
17. Albright JP, McAuley E, Martin RK, et al.: Head and neck injuries in college football: an eight-year analysis. *Am J Sports Med* 1985; 13: 147–152
18. Albright JP, Moses JM, Feldick HG, et al.: Nonfatal cervical spine injuries in interscholastic football. *JAMA* 1976; 236: 1243–1245
19. Torg J.S., Truex R., Quedenfeld T.C., et al.: The National football head and neck injury registry: Report and conclusions 1978. *JAMA* 1979; 241: 1477–1479
20. Torg J.S., Quedenfeld T.C., Burstein A., et al.: National football head and neck injury registry: Report on cervical quadriplegia, 1971 to 1975. *Am J Sports Med* 1979; 7: 127–132
21. Miele V, Maroon J.: Spinal injuries in sports. In: *Benzel EC, Spine Surgery*, 3rd edition. Saunders, 2012. Chapter 71, 689–700.
22. Swartz EE, Mihalik JP, Decoster LC, Hernandez AE.: A study of emergency American football helmet removal techniques. *AJEM* 2012; 30: 1163–1168.
23. Tong H, Haig A, Yamakawa K.: The Spurling's test and cervical radiculopathy. *Spine* 2002; 27:156–159.
24. Wainner R, Fritz J, Irrgang J, et al.: Reliability and diagnostic accuracy of the clinical examination and patient self-report measures for cervical radiculopathy. *Spine* 2003; 28: 52–62.
25. Glaser JA, Cure' JK, Bailey KL, Morrow DL.: Cervical spinal cord compression and the Hoffman's sign. *Iowa Orthop J* 2001; 21: 49–52.

26. Lee J, Laker S, Fredericson M.: Thoracic outlet syndrome. *PM R*. 2010 Jan;2(1):64–70
27. Gillard J, Perez-Cousin M, Hachulla E, et al.: Diagnosing thoracic outlet syndrome: Contribution of provocative tests, ultrasonography, electrophysiology, and helical computed tomography in 48 patients. *Joint Bone Spine* 2001;68:416–424
28. Bracken M.B., Shepard M.J., Collins W.F., et al.: A randomized, controlled trial of methylprednisolone or naloxone in the treatment of acute spinal-cord injury: Results of the Second National Acute Spinal Cord Injury Study. *N Engl J Med* 1990; 322: 1405–1411
29. Bracken M.B., Shepard M.J., Holford T.R., et al.: Administration of methylprednisolone for 24 or 48 hours or tirilazad mesylate for 48 hours in the treatment of acute spinal cord injury: results of the Third National Acute Spinal Cord Injury Randomized Controlled Trial, National Acute Spinal Cord Injury Study. *JAMA* 1997; 277: 1597–1604
30. Bydon M, Lin J, Macki M, Gokaslan Z, Bidon A.: The current role of steroids in acute spinal cord injury. *World Neurosurgery*, in press.
31. Kwon B.W., Mann C., Sohn H.M., et al.: Hypothermia for spinal cord injury. *Spine J* 2008; 8: 859–874
32. Dietrich WD, Levi AD, Wang M, Green BA. Hypothermic treatment for acute spinal cord injury. *Neurotherapeutics*, 2011;8(2):229–39.
33. Jefferson G.: Fracture of the atlas vertebra. *Br J Surg* 1920; 7: 407
34. Cloward R.B.: Acute cervical spine injuries. *Clin Symp* 1980; 32: 2–32
35. Drez D. Spinal Injuries. In: Delee JC, Drez D, Miller M (eds). *DeLee and Drez's orthopedic sports medicine*. Saunders, 2010. Chapter 16, 665–768.
36. Zmurko M.G., Tannoury T.Y., Tannoury C.A., et al.: Cervical sprains, disc herniations, minor fractures, and other cervical injuries in the athlete. *Clin Sports Med* 2003; 22: 513–521
37. Cantu R.C.: Stingers: Transient quadriplegia, and cervical spinal stenosis, return to play criteria. *Med Sci Sports Exerc* 1997; 29: S233–S235
38. Torg J.S., Corcoran T.A., Thibault L.E., et al.: Cervical cord neurapraxia: Classification, pathomechanics, morbidity, and management guidelines. *J Neurosurg* 1997; 87: 843–850
39. Albright JP, Moses JM, Feldick HG, Dolan KD, Burmeister LF.: Nonfatal cervical spine injuries in interscholastic football. *JAMA*. Sep 13 1976;236(11):1243–5
40. Kumano K, Umeyama T: Cervical disk injuries in athletes. *Arch Orthop Traumatic Surg* 1986; 105: 223–226
41. Durham SR, Sun PP, Sutton LN, et al.: Surgically treated lumbar disc disease in the pediatric population: An outcome study. *J Neurosurg* 2000; 92: 1–6
42. Lum YW, Freischlag JA.: Thoracic outlet syndrome. In: Cronenwett JL, Johnson KW (eds). *Rutherford's vascular surgery*, 8th edition. Saunders, 2014. Chapter 125, 1936–1950.

Chapter 10

Lumbar Spine

Jeffrey P. Feden

Background/Epidemiology

- Back pain is the most common musculoskeletal complaint presenting to the emergency department.[1]
- A benign clinical course is expected in the large majority of patients, but a thorough history and physical exam should be conducted on each patient to uncover serious causes of back pain with potentially devastating consequences.
- The term "mechanical low back pain" encompasses all musculoskeletal causes of low back pain in the absence of a specific, identifiable anatomic source.
- Spine injuries account for 9–15 percent of athletic injuries.[2]
- Most athletic spine injuries are benign, but athletes are also affected by more serious spine conditions that are observed in the general population, so a broad range of conditions is reviewed here.

Anatomical Considerations / Pathophysiology

- The lumbar spine (Figure 10.1) consists of five vertebrae, each of which contains a vertebral body, vertebral arch, and several bony processes.
- The vertebral arch protects the neural elements and is composed of the pedicles, laminae, transverse processes, articular processes, and spinous process.
- Beneath each lumbar vertebra lies a pair of intervertebral, or neural, foramina through which the spinal nerve roots, recurrent meningeal nerves and radicular blood vessels pass.
- Vertebrae are connected by intervertebral discs which support axial loading and allow movement.
- Each disc is composed of a central nucleus pulposus, which is surrounded by the annulus fibrosus.

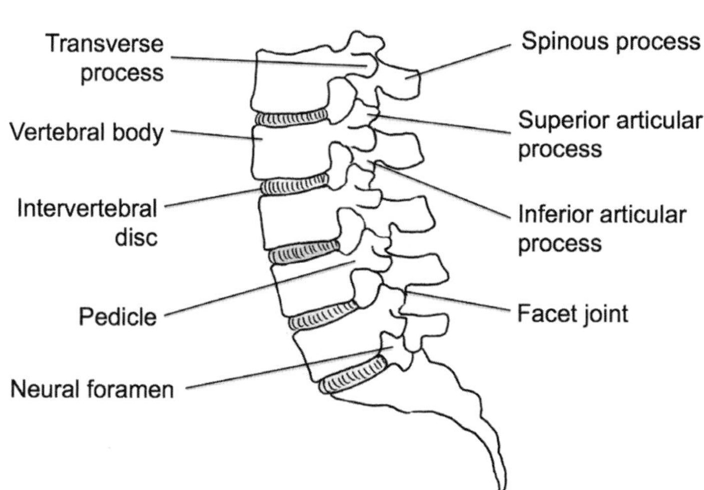

Figure 10.1. Bony anatomy of the lumbar spine, lateral view. Illustration by Yvonne Chow.

- In addition to the lumbar vertebral joints and intervertebral discs, the lumbar spine is supported by several ligaments.
  - The anterior longitudinal ligament covers the anterior surface of the lumbar spine and limits extension.
  - The posterior longitudinal ligament covers the posterior surface of the vertebral bodies within the vertebral canal, and it limits flexion.
  - The ligamentum flavum forms the posterior wall of the vertebral canal and helps to provide constant disc tension.
  - The supraspinous and interspinous ligaments provide attachments to the spinous processes.
- There are four functional groups of muscles that support lumbar spine motion: extensors, flexors, lateral flexors, and rotators.
  - The erector spinae is the primary lumbar spine extensor.
  - The abdominal wall muscles and iliopsoas provide trunk flexion.
  - Lateral flexion and rotation are performed by varying degrees of unilateral contraction of several muscle groups.
- The spinal cord terminates as the conus medullaris, most commonly at the L1 or L2 level.
- The cauda equina is the collection of nerve roots that continue in a caudad direction from the conus medullaris until each exits as a spinal nerve root at its respective intervertebral foramen (i.e., L4 nerve root exits below the L4 vertebra).

Focused History and Physical Exam

General Considerations

- Historical "red flags" should alert the clinician to serious causes of low back pain, such as infection, malignancy, and fracture. (Table 10.1); however, many of these red flags are poorly studied and may offer little diagnostic or predictive value.
- Extraspinal causes of low back pain should always be considered in the differential diagnosis of low back pain, including abdominal aortic aneurysm (AAA), retroperitoneal hemorrhage or mass, nephrolithiasis, and urinary tract infection.
- Patients at the extremes of age warrant special consideration as children and elderly individuals are more likely to have serious causes of back pain.
- Four predictors of serious pathology in adults presenting to the ED with nontraumatic low back pain (91 percent sensitivity, 55 percent specificity)[3] have been identified:
  - Pain that persists despite appropriate treatment.
  - Use of anticoagulant medications.
  - Decreased sensation on physical examination.
  - Pain that is worse at night.
- Axial pain suggests disc disease, while paraspinal pain suggests sacroiliac or facet disease.

Table 10.1 Red Flags

Historical Red Flags[1]	Risk factors for Spinal Epidural Abscess[10]
Persistent pain lasting >6 weeks	Intravenous drug use
Fever/chills	Diabetes
Unexplained weight loss	Chronic liver or kidney disease
History of cancer	Recent spine procedure or indwelling hardware
Intravenous drug use	Concomitant infection
Chronic steroid use	Indwelling vascular catheter
Night pain	Recent spine fracture
Unremitting pain despite analgesics	Immunocompromise
Immunocompromise	
Major trauma	
Minor trauma in the elderly	
Bowel/bladder dysfunction	
Recent bacterial infection	

Physical Exam

- Gait assessment
  - Heel-walking and toe-walking may be used in the assessment of L4 and S1 motor function, respectively.
- Inspection
  - Assess for swelling, deformities, skin changes, scoliosis, asymmetry.
  - Evaluate for rash suggestive of herpes zoster.
- Palpation
  - Distinguish axial vs. paraspinal tenderness, as well as focal vs. diffuse tenderness.
- Range of motion
  - Flexion, extension, lateral rotation, and side-to-side bending should be assessed.
  - Increased pain with flexion suggests disc herniation.
  - Increased pain with extension suggests spinal stenosis, spondylolisthesis, or facet disease.
- Neurologic examination
  - Focuses on assessment of spinal nerve root function and includes testing of muscle strength, sensation and deep tendon reflexes (Table 10.2 and Table 10.3).
  - Bowel or bladder complaints should prompt testing of perianal sensation and rectal tone.
  - Bladder function (e.g., urinary retention, overflow incontinence) may be assessed. with evaluation of post-void residual volume or bedside ultrasound.

Table 10.2 ASIA Muscle Grading Scale

0	Total paralysis
1	Visible or palpable muscle contraction
2	Active movement, full range of motion, with gravity eliminated
3	Active movement, full range of motion, against gravity
4	Active movement, full range of motion, against gravity, provides some resistance
5	Active movement, full range of motion, against gravity, provides normal resistance
NT	Unable to test

- Vascular examination
  - Palpate dorsalis pedis pulses
  - Assess capillary refill
- Special tests
  - *Straight leg raise* (*SLR*) (Figure 10.2) is performed with the patient in a supine position, and the hip is passively flexed with the knee in extension.
    - Reproduction of radicular pain *below the knee* during hip flexion from 30–70° indicates a positive test and suggests nerve root compression from a herniated disc (sensitivity 91 percent, specificity 29 percent).[4]

Table 10.3 Neurologic Examination of the Lower Extremities

Nerve Root	Motor	Sensory	Reflex
L2	Hip flexion	Anterior and medial thigh	None
L3	Knee extension	Medial knee	None
L4	Ankle dorsiflexion	Anterior knee and medial lower leg	Patella
L5	Great toe extension (EHL)	Dorsal foot	None
S1	Ankle plantarflexion	Posterior thigh and calf	Achilles

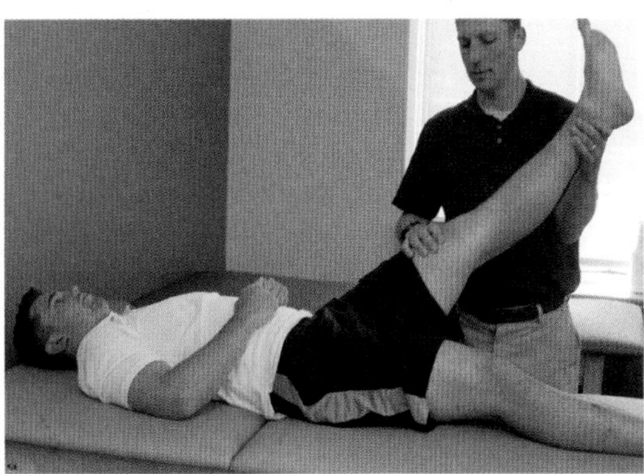

Figure 10.2. Straight leg raise.

- *Braggard's test* is performed after SLR by lowering the leg and then dorsiflexing the ankle to evaluate for reproduction of radicular symptoms.
- *Crossed SLR* is positive when radicular symptoms are reproduced on the affected side by raising the contralateral leg (sensitivity 29 percent, specificity 88 percent).[4]
- The *slump test* (aka slump sit test) is a variant of the SLR and is sensitive for disc herniation. With the patient seated at the edge of the bed and leaning forward, cervical flexion is initiated followed by knee extension and ankle dorsiflexion (Figure 10.3). The patient is then asked to bring their neck back into the neutral position (Figure 10.4). The test is positive if radicular symptoms are reproduced in the slump position and relieved as the patient brings the neck back into the neutral position.
- The *stork test* is a classic test for spondylolysis but has poor sensitivity and specificity. A positive test results from ipsilateral pain with the patient standing on one leg and extending the lumbar spine (Figure 10.5).
- *Waddell signs* are a group of physical exam findings that attempt to differentiate pathologic back pain from nonorganic back pain; positive findings may be associated with worse outcomes and psychosocial factors but not necessarily secondary gain.
  - May indicate symptom magnification but *do not exclude* organic disease.
  - Superficial, diffuse, or nonanatomic tenderness.

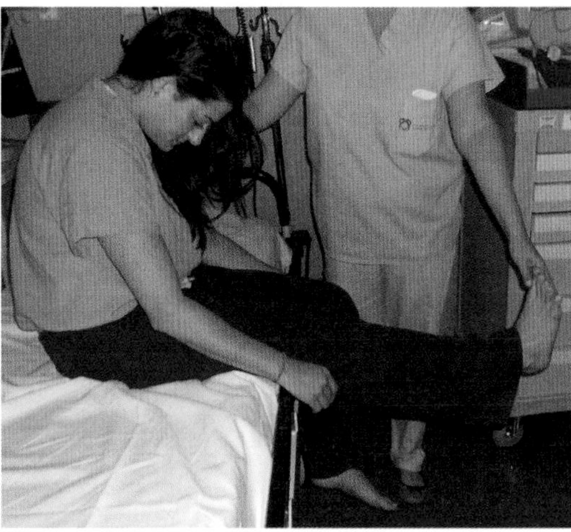

Figure 10.3. Slump test with neck flexion, knee extension and ankle dorsiflexion.

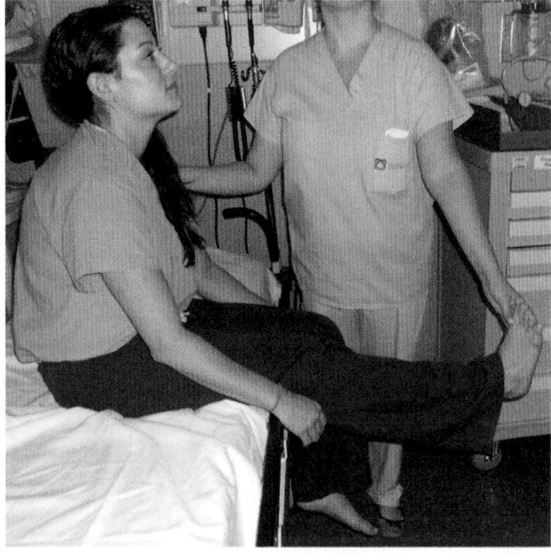

Figure 10.4. Slump test with neck in neutral position.

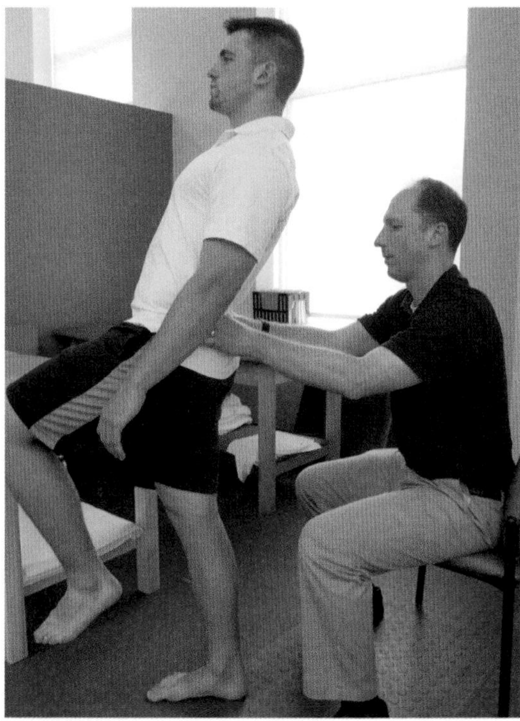

Figure 10.5. Single-leg hyperextension, or stork test.

- Pain provoked by simulated movements, such as axial loading of the head or rotation of the shoulders.
- Positive tests are performed again while distracting the patient.
- Sensorimotor findings that are nondermatomal.
- Gross overreaction to testing.

Diagnostic Testing in the ED

- Routine imaging is generally not indicated in patients presenting to the ED with acute, atraumatic low back pain in the absence of risk factors or exam findings suggestive of serious pathology.
  - Consider imaging for acute low back pain after trauma.
  - Minor trauma may cause fractures in elderly, immunocompromised, or cancer patients.
  - Identification of any spine fracture warrants imaging of the entire spine.
- Laboratory studies provide little diagnostic value unless malignancy or infection is suspected.
  - Consider PT/INR if patient is on anticoagulation.
- Advanced imaging (i.e., MRI) in the ED is reserved for patients with severe or rapidly progressive neurologic deficits, or with signs and symptoms of serious underlying pathology (infection, malignancy, cord compression).
- Advanced diagnostic imaging in the outpatient setting may be considered for failure of conservative management (NSAIDs, physical therapy) after six to eight weeks.

Differential Diagnosis – Emergent and Common Diagnoses

Thoracolumbar (TL) Spine Trauma

- TL spine fractures occur most commonly between T12 and L2 and spinal cord injury (SCI) occurs in 10–25 percent.[5]
- TL fractures usually result from motor vehicle trauma and falls from height (65 percent); the remainder are caused by athletic participation and assault.[6]

Table 10.4 Common and Emergent Diagnoses in the Emergency Department

Emergent Diagnoses	Common Diagnoses
Lumbar spine fracture: Burst fracture Flexion-distraction injury (Chance fracture) Fracture-dislocation	Mechanical low back pain
Infection: Spinal epidural abscess Vertebral osteomyelitis and diskitis	Lumbar disc disease
Neoplasm	Lumbar radiculopathy
Cauda equina syndrome	Myofascial lumbar strain
Any common condition with severe or progressive neurologic impairment (i.e., compression, fracture, spinal stenosis, spondylolisthesis)	Lumbar spinal stenosis
Extraspinal causes: Abdominal aortic aneurysm Retroperitoneal hemorrhage or mass	Spondylosis (degenerative osteoarthritis)
	Spondylolisthesis
	Spondylolysis
	Sacroiliac joint dysfunction
	Lumbar compression fracture

- Treatment is directed toward spine stabilization and preservation of neurologic function.
- Most TL spine fractures are stable and may be managed nonoperatively.
- High-dose steroids are no longer recommended in the acute management of traumatic SCI due to lack of evidence and potential for significant adverse effects.
- There is no existing clinical decision tool that allows for "clearance" of the TL spine or guides the need for imaging following blunt trauma.[7,8]

- Current practice for clinical and radiographic evaluation of the TL spine, though not evidence based, often mirrors evaluation of the cervical spine for which validated guidelines exist (e.g., NEXUS criteria).
- CT often replaces screening radiographs in the patient with high suspicion for fracture.
- Classification systems
  - Denis classification system
    - Widely used in clinical practice but may lack predictive value.
    - Based on radiographic findings and uses a three-column theory to identify instability.
    - Compromise of two or more columns suggests unstable injury.
      - Anterior column = anterior longitudinal ligament and anterior half of vertebral body.
      - Middle column = posterior longitudinal ligament and posterior half of vertebral body.
      - Posterior column = pedicles, facet joints, and supraspinous ligaments.
  - Thoracolumbar injury classification and severity score (TLICS).
    - Newer classification system that is both comprehensive and reliable in determining injury severity and guiding treatment.[9]
    - TLICS is based on three parameters.
      - Fracture morphology
      - Neurologic status of the patient
      - Integrity of the posterior ligament complex

Vertebral Compression Fracture

General Description

- Considered a fragility fracture
- Usually stable fractures affecting only the anterior column.
- May be unstable if more than 50 percent loss of vertebral body height or more than 20–30° of kyphosis, multiple adjacent fractures, or involvement of posterior elements.
- Increased frequency in elderly related to osteoporosis.

Mechanism

- Trauma with anterior or lateral flexion causes injury to the anterior column.
- May result from minor trauma in osteoporotic patients; some may not recall trauma.

Presentation

- Pain is often localized to the area of fracture but may radiate around the torso in some cases.

Physical Exam

- Tenderness is localized to the fracture site and local kyphosis may also be evident
  - Pain is often midline, but may also be paraspinal.
- Neurologic deficits are uncommon.

Essential Diagnostics

- Plain radiographs will demonstrate loss of vertebral height.
- CT is generally unnecessary but may be used to better characterize fracture and may better assess injury to the posterior column.
- MRI is often unnecessary but may be useful to distinguish acute vs. chronic fracture and should be considered for any signs of spinal cord compression.

ED Treatment

- Most patients are treated with observation and pain management.
- Some patients may benefit from bracing with thoracolumbar orthosis (TLSO).
  - Usually not needed if minimal compression.
- Early ambulation is encouraged.
- Surgical decompression is rarely indicated except in cases of progressive neurologic deficits or spine instability.

Disposition

- Most patients may be discharged home with adequate pain control and orthopedic or neurosurgery follow-up.
  - Some may require hospitalization for pain management.
- Patients with simple compression fractures may return to sports or nonstrenuous

occupations once pain is minimal, they have regained near normal range of motion, and there is no evidence of progressive deformity, usually eight to twelve weeks.

  - Isometric back extension and strengthening exercises may be started at this time.

- Consult orthopedics or neurosurgery for unstable fractures, associated neurologic impairment, more than 50 percent vertebral height loss or more than 20 percent angulation.

Complications

- Associated spinal cord compression is rare.
- Kyphoplasty is reserved for failed medical management and persistent, severe pain for greater than six weeks.

Pearls and Pitfalls

- Pathologic fracture should be considered in younger patients without trauma or osteoporosis.
- Consider Chance fracture in patients with high-energy trauma; posterior column injury is an important distinguishing feature and may require advanced imaging.

Spinous Process and Transverse Process Fractures

General Description

- These fractures usually do not affect the stability of the spine and are benign.
- Often times may involve more than one vertebrae.

Mechanism

- Transverse process fractures usually result from a lateral bending force which causes an avulsion fracture.
  - These most commonly occur at L2, L3, and/or L4.
- Spinous process fractures usually result from direct trauma or hyperflexion injuries.

Presentation

- Pain at site of injury.
- Neurological complaints are rare.

Physical Exam

- Tenderness at fracture site and also possibly surrounding paraspinal muscles due to spasm.
- Neurological compromise is rare.
- These injuries may be accompanied by an ileus, so it is important to perform an abdominal exam and ensure patient is able to tolerate oral intake.

Essential Diagnostics

- A minimum of a two-view thoracic and/or lumbar spine x-ray is required.
  - Closely examine the AP view for transverse process fractures.
  - Closely examine the lateral view for spinous process fractures.
- Advanced imaging with CT or MRI is not indicated in the ED unless there is concern for other associated injuries.
- Consider a urinalysis to look for hematuria as renal contusions may be associated with these injuries.

ED Treatment

- Pain control
- Encourage early ambulation and activity as tolerated.
- Bracing is not usually needed for isolated injuries.
  - Except for significant or severe pain, may consider bracing for comfort.

Disposition

- Nearly all of these patients may be safely discharged from the ED unless there is concern for other associated injuries.
- Orthopedic or neurosurgical consultation is not usually necessary for isolated injuries.
- Patient may follow-up with orthopedics, neurosurgery, or sports medicine within one week from discharge.
- Patients may resume normal activity as tolerated over four to six weeks.
- Patients may return to sports after they are pain free and demonstrate near normal range of motion.

Complications

- Neurovascular compromise is unlikely.

- These fractures may result in nonunion but are usually not of any clinical significance.
  - If patients have continued pain, they may be referred for surgical removal of non-united fragment.

Pearls and Pitfalls

- Isolated spinous and transverse fractures of the TL spine are usually benign and self-limited.
- Always evaluate for associated injuries, including ileus and/or renal contusion.

Burst Fracture

General Description

- Spine fracture related to compressive load and associated with significant mechanism of injury.
- Most occur at the TL junction.
- Fracture may be stable despite failure of the anterior and middle columns; adequate assessment of the posterior column is critical in determining the extent of injury.

Mechanism

- Results from axial and/or flexion loading and failure of the anterior and middle columns.

Presentation

- Canal compromise and neurologic deficits may result from retropulsion of bone.

Physical Exam

- Often tenderness at fracture site
- Comprehensive neurologic exam is mandatory.
- Evaluate for concomitant spine and/or pelvic fractures.

Essential Diagnostics

- Plain radiographs demonstrate kyphotic deformity and retropulsed bone fragments.
- Increased space between spinous processes may indicate ligamentous injury and associated instability of the fracture.
- CT is indicated to better characterize fractures identified on plain films or in those with neurologic deficits, and it is useful for showing facet joint diastasis indicative of posterior column injury.
- MRI may be used to evaluate for spinal cord compression or edema, and to assess the integrity of the posterior ligament complex.
- Imaging of the entire spine should be considered as concomitant spine fractures are common.

ED Treatment

- Nonoperative management is reserved for stable injuries without neurologic deficits.
- Operative management is indicated for unstable fractures, as indicated by neurologic compromise, amount of compression, degree of kyphosis, or injury to the posterior ligament complex.

Disposition

- Orthopedic or neurosurgery consultation is recommended for all burst fractures to assist with management and disposition.

Complications

- Retropulsion of bone may result in spinal canal compromise and neurologic. injury

Pearls and Pitfalls

- Most burst fractures are unstable and require emergent consultation in the ED.
  - Evaluation of the posterior column is critical in determining stability

Flexion-Distraction Injury (Chance fractures, seatbelt fractures)

General Description

- A flexion-distraction injury occurs when the anterior/middle and posterior columns fail under compression and tension, respectively.
- Involves bony and/or soft tissue injury.
- By virtue of the significant force required to injure the entire spinal column, these injuries are associated with abdominal solid organ and hollow viscous injuries which may be life threatening.

Mechanism

- Hyperflexion injury involving failure of the anterior column (compression) and posterior column (distraction).

Presentation

- Commonly associated with "seatbelt" injury.
- Patients are often neurologically intact.

Physical Exam

- Often tenderness at fracture site
- Comprehensive neurologic exam is mandatory.
- Evaluate for concomitant abdominal injuries

Essential Diagnostics

- AP and lateral radiographs should be scrutinized for evidence of posterior column injury (increased interspinous process distance on AP view).
- CT may reveal facet fracture or dislocation or may provide additional diagnostic value if plain radiographs are equivocal.
- MRI may detect disruption of the posterior elements.

ED Treatment

- Nonoperative management with immobilization (cast or TLSO brace) may be considered in neurologically intact patients with intact posterior elements (bony injury only).
- Operative management is pursued in patients with neurologic injury and/or disruption of the posterior ligaments.

Disposition

- Orthopedic or neurosurgical consultation is recommended for all Chance fractures to assist with management and disposition.

Complications

- Progressive kyphosis

Pearls and Pitfalls

- Maintain suspicion for abdominal and bowel injuries
- Flexion-distraction injury may be isolated soft tissue injury without fracture.
- Avoid misdiagnosis as compression fracture.

TL Fracture-Dislocation

General Description

- Failure of all three columns renders these injuries highly unstable.
- Frequently associated with SCI and other skeletal injuries.

Mechanism

- Result from a combination of flexion, rotation, distraction, and shearing forces.
- Fractures with posterior facet dislocation are inherently unstable.

Presentation

- Results from high-energy trauma
- High likelihood of neurologic injury

Physical Exam

- Often tenderness at fracture site
- Comprehensive trauma evaluation, including thorough neurologic exam, is mandatory

Essential Diagnostics

- Plain radiographs should demonstrate significant injury.
- CT is frequently utilized in the setting of high-energy or multisystem trauma to better characterize and evaluate injury.

ED Treatment

- Neurologically intact and compromised patients must be equally protected and immobilized.
- Early operative management for decompression and instrumentation improves outcomes.

Disposition

- Immediate orthopedic or neurosurgical consultation is essential.

Complications

- SCI, chronic pain, and spinal deformity.

Pearls and Pitfalls

- Fracture-dislocations require early surgical stabilization.

Spinal Epidural Abscess

General Description

- Spinal epidural abscess (SEA) describes inflammation or a collection of pus located between the dura mater and surrounding adipose tissue.

- Requires early detection to avoid potentially devastating neurologic consequences related to spinal cord compression.

Mechanism

- Etiology[1]
  - Hematogenous spread (25–50 percent)
  - Local contiguous spread (15–30 percent), i.e. diskitis
  - Direct inoculation, i.e. spine surgery or instrumentation
- *Staphylococcus aureus* (including MRSA) accounts for up to two-thirds of cases
- Other causative organisms include gram-negative bacteria (E. coli), streptococci, coagulase-negative staphylococci.

Presentation

- Risk assessment and high index of suspicion are critical to making the diagnosis of SEA because of widely variable presentations (Table 10.1).
- Less than 15 percent of patients demonstrate classic triad of fever, back pain, and neurologic deficit.[1]
- May be associated with insidious onset of severe pain with or without radicular symptoms.

Physical Exam

- Often have tenderness of the affected area of the spine.
- May have neurologic deficit, radiculopathy, or myelopathy.

Essential Diagnostics

- Serum WBC is an unreliable diagnostic indicator.
- Elevated ESR and CRP should prompt further workup for infectious source of back pain.
- In at-risk patients (Table 10.1), ESR (100 percent sensitivity, 67 percent specificity) may guide the need for emergent MRI.[10]
- Blood cultures should be obtained prior to the initiation of antibiotics.
- Plain radiographs are typically normal.
- MRI with gadolinium is the diagnostic imaging modality of choice and may help to guide treatment based on the size and extent of the abscess and degree of cord compression.
- CT has poor diagnostic sensitivity, but CT myelogram is an acceptable alternative to MRI in patients for whom MRI is contraindicated.

ED Treatment

- Treatment is focused on broad-spectrum intravenous antibiotics (anti-staphylococcal/MRSA) and early surgical consultation, as decompression is often indicated, especially in cases with associated neurologic deficits.
- Nonsurgical management may be chosen in patients with small abscesses without cord compression or neurologic deficits.

Disposition

- Hospitalization is required for intravenous antibiotics and consideration of surgical intervention.
- Infectious disease consultation is recommended.
- Orthopedic or neurosurgical consultation is recommended, including nonsurgical cases.

Complications

- Sepsis, permanent neurologic impairment

Pearls and Pitfalls

- Presentations are widely variable; risk assessment is essential.
- Laboratory studies have several limitations.
- Preoperative neurologic impairment is the best predictor of clinical outcome.

Vertebral Osteomyelitis (Spondylodiskitis)

General Description

- Risk factors, pathophysiology, and diagnostic approach are similar to spinal epidural abscess.

Mechanism

- Hematogenous spread, local contiguous spread, or direct inoculation.
- Causative organisms include staphylococci, streptococci, and gram–negative organisms.

Presentation

- Characterized by insidious onset and gradually progressive back pain over weeks to months.

Physical Exam

- Fever is an unreliable diagnostic indicator.
- Neurologic impairment is a late finding associated with vertebral body destruction and/or development of spinal epidural abscess.

Essential Diagnostics

- Serum WBC, ESR, and CRP should be ordered; ESR and CRP may be used to monitor treatment.
- Blood cultures are often negative, but positive cultures are important for directing antibiotic therapy.
- CT-guided biopsy to identify causative organism is considered in nonsurgical cases with negative blood cultures.
- Plain radiographs may demonstrate endplate or other destructive changes to the disc space and vertebral body (Figure 10.6), or may be normal early in the disease process.

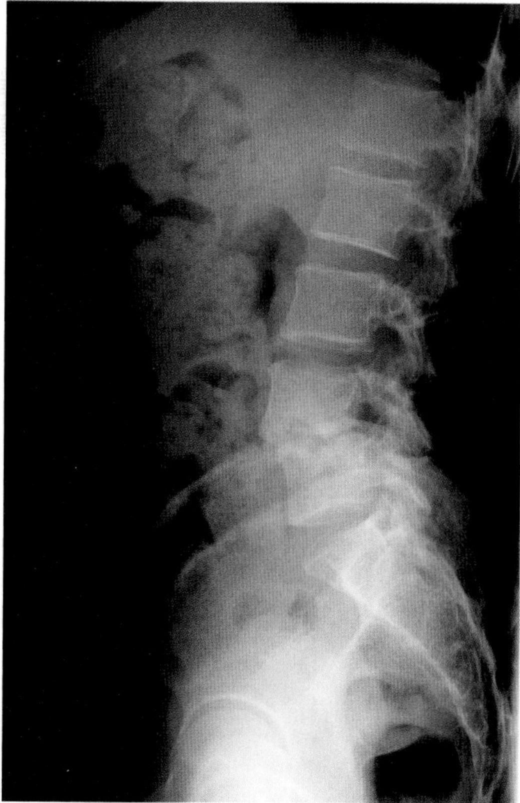

Figure 10.6. Vertebral osteomyelitis. Forty-three-year-old male with several ED visits over two months for intractable back pain, eventually determined to be using IV drugs and found to have a destructive process at L4-5 consistent with vertebral osteomyelitis and diskitis.

- CT may identify bony abnormalities earlier than plain radiographs.
- MRI with gadolinium is the diagnostic imaging modality of choice and allows differentiation from spinal tumors.
- Bone scan is highly sensitive and is an alternative imaging choice for those in whom MRI is contraindicated.

ED Treatment

- Treatment is often nonoperative with bracing and long-term (six to twelve weeks) antibiotics, except in cases with neurologic impairment, spine instability, or failure of conservative measures.

Disposition

- Hospitalization is required initially for both diagnostic and treatment purposes.
- Infectious disease consultation is recommended.
- Orthopedic or neurosurgical consultation is recommended for surgical indications.

Complications

- Sepsis, neurologic impairment, spine instability, or deformity

Pearls and Pitfalls

- Identification of causative organism is essential for treatment.

Cauda Equina Syndrome

General Description

- A true orthopedic and neurological emergency in which terminal lumbosacral spinal nerve root compression results from a space-occupying lesion.

Mechanism

- Large central lumbar disc herniation is the most common cause of cauda equina syndrome (CES), generally occurring in men in the fourth and fifth decades of life.
- Other causes of CES include tumor, trauma, spinal stenosis, epidural hematoma, or abscess.

Presentation

- Acute or insidious bilateral leg pain and sensorimotor deficits, saddle anesthesia,

bladder dysfunction (urinary retention with overflow incontinence), diminished deep. tendon reflexes, decreased rectal tone
- Back pain is usually not a prominent feature.
- Bilateral sciatica, more than 500 mL of urinary retention, and subjective urinary retention or rectal incontinence have high predictive value for CES.[5]

Physical Exam

- Comprehensive neurologic exam must be performed, including assessment of perineal sensation and sphincter tone.
- Urinary retention is a late finding but is highly sensitive and specific.

Essential Diagnostics

- MRI is the preferred imaging modality and is important in identifying compression.
- CT myelogram may be used as an alternative imaging modality in those unable to undergo MRI.

ED Treatment

- Urgent surgical decompression (within forty-eight hours) is critical, and outcome is related to the degree of impairment at the time of clinical presentation.

Disposition

- CES represents a surgical emergency; immediate orthopedic or neurosurgical consultation is essential.
- Hospitalization for urgent surgical intervention is required.

Complications

- Permanent neurologic impairment, including sexual and urinary dysfunction.

Pearls and Pitfalls

- Development of urinary retention indicates a poor prognosis.

Neoplasm

General Description

- Benign and malignant lesions may cause spinal cord compression syndromes, radiculopathy, and pathologic vertebral fractures.

Mechanism

- Metastatic lesions to the epidural space are most common
- Thoracic spine involvement is more common (60 percent) than lumbosacral spine (30 percent).[11]
- Breast, lung, and prostate cancer most commonly metastasize to bone

Presentation

- Night pain and rest pain are characteristic.
- Evaluate for constitutional and neurologic symptoms.

Physical Exam

- Spinal tenderness is common.
- May demonstrate findings of radiculopathy or myelopathy.

Essential Diagnostics

- Plain radiographs may show destructive bone lesions or pathologic fractures.
- CT may demonstrate cortical bone destruction.
- MRI is the diagnostic imaging modality of choice, and imaging of the entire spine should be considered for suspected malignancy as multilevel involvement and distant, asymptomatic metastases are common findings.

ED Treatment

- High-dose corticosteroids, radiation therapy, and early surgical decompression should be considered for neurologic impairment.

Disposition

- Consult orthopedics or neurosurgery for neurologic compromise.
- Outpatient vs. inpatient management is based upon the burden of disease, extent of spinal involvement, and presence of neurologic impairment.

Complications

- Permanent neurologic disability

Pearls and Pitfalls

- Advanced imaging of the entire spine should be obtained if malignancy is diagnosed or suspected, as spinal malignancy often results from metastatic disease.

Lumbar Disc Disease and Radiculopathy

General Description

- Disc disruption (often without herniation) has been described as the most common cause of low back pain between 18 and 50 years of age[4] and is usually not radicular.
- Radiculopathy refers to the constellation of signs and symptoms related to nerve root compression in the distribution of the affected nerve root.
  - Numbness
  - Paresthesias
  - Weakness

Mechanism

- The large majority of lumbar disc herniations occur at L4–L5 and L5–S1, potentially resulting in L5 and S1 radiculopathy, respectively.
- Disc herniations are most commonly posterolateral and affect the traversing (lower) nerve root; they are often asymptomatic.
- Aside from disc herniation, radiculopathy may be caused by degenerative spine changes (spondylosis, spondylolisthesis), foraminal stenosis, cord compression, spinal stenosis, malignancy, or infection.

Presentation

- Symptomatic disc herniations may present with axial low back pain and/or radicular pain (radiating into the leg).
- Radicular pain is worse with sitting and Valsalva maneuvers, improved with standing.

Physical Exam

- Physical exam should include gait assessment, sensory and motor exam, and provocative testing including *SLR* (Figure 10.2), *Braggard's test, crossed SLR* and *slump test* (Figures 10.3 and 10.4).

Essential Diagnostics

- MRI is the diagnostic study of choice but is rarely indicated in the emergency department, except in the following cases:
  - Red flags suggestive of infection or malignancy
  - Signs of cauda equina syndrome, such as bilateral leg pain or weakness, saddle anesthesia, or bowel/bladder dysfunction
  - Rapidly progressive or severe lower extremity weakness
- MRI findings warrant careful interpretation, as abnormal findings are common and must be correlated clinically.

ED Treatment

- Acute pain management and counseling are the goals of treatment in the emergency department.

Disposition

- Physical therapy and NSAIDs are the mainstay of treatment.
- 90 percent of patients improve within six to twelve weeks with conservative measures.
- Bedrest should be avoided in favor of activity modification.
- Epidural corticosteroid injections are considered second-line therapy.
- Follow-up in one week with primary care or sports medicine physician is recommended.
- Orthopedic or neurosurgical consultation and surgical management are reserved for patients with cauda equina syndrome, progressive or significant weakness, or persistent disabling pain despite conservative management.

Complications

- Large central disc herniation is uncommon but may result in cauda equina syndrome.

Pearls and Pitfalls

- While the majority of patients improve with conservative measures, progressive or profound motor weakness warrants advanced imaging in the ED and urgent orthopedic or neurosurgical referral.
- Cauda equina syndrome must be considered and ruled out in all patients presenting with low back pain and/or radiculopathy.

Lumbar Spinal Stenosis

General Description

- Congenital or acquired narrowing of the vertebral canal.

Mechanism

- Usually results from degenerative spine changes (spondylosis), herniated or bulging discs, or hypertrophy of the ligamentum flavum.

Presentation

- Classic symptoms include those of neurogenic claudication and are worsened by extension, standing, and walking.
  - Back pain radiating into buttocks and posterior legs
  - Bilateral sensory changes

Physical Exam

- May cause radiculopathy and focal sensorimotor findings or polyradiculopathy with findings related to multiple nerve roots.
- Distinguish from vascular claudication
  - Neurogenic claudication is related to postural changes (worsened by extension, relieved by flexion).
  - Neurogenic claudication may be provoked by prolonged standing, while vascular claudication is classically relieved with rest.

Essential Diagnostics

- Plain radiographs show degenerative spine changes, such as osteophytes and spondylolisthesis.
- MRI is the preferred diagnostic imaging modality but is rarely necessary in the emergency department.
- Findings of spinal stenosis on advanced imaging are common in asymptomatic individuals, especially those over age 60.

ED Treatment

- Treatment is generally conservative and focuses on pain management

Disposition

- Appropriately managed in the outpatient setting, often with physical therapy and corticosteroid injections
- Follow-up with primary care or sports medicine physician within one week is appropriate for most patients discharged from the ED
- Orthopedic or neurosurgery consultation or referral is indicated for neurologic impairment.
- Surgery is indicated for failure to improve after three to six months of conservative management or for progressive neurologic disability.

Complications

- Cauda equina syndrome is uncommon.

Pearls and Pitfalls

- It is important to distinguish neurogenic claudication from vascular claudication.

Lumbar Myofascial Strain

General Description

- Very common cause of low back pain (up to 70 percent of acute low back pain),[4] especially in athletes and active individuals.

Mechanism

- Results from trauma, overuse, repetitive loading.

Presentation

- Characterized by midline and paraspinal muscle tenderness without radicular or neurologic symptoms.
- Radicular pain suggests disc disease rather than simple muscle injury.

Physical Exam

- Physical exam should include gait assessment, sensory and motor exam, and provocative testing (see special tests in Physical Exam section earlier).
- Neurologic exam is normal with isolated muscle injury.

Essential Diagnostics

- Imaging is generally unnecessary for acute injury without significant mechanism but may be considered for failure to improve after four to six weeks of conservative management.

ED Treatment

- Acute pain management (e.g., NSAIDs) and counseling should be provided.

Disposition

- Primary care or sports medicine follow-up is appropriate.
- Pain and stiffness worsen shortly after acute injury and improvement generally occurs in about one to two weeks.
- Activity modification, analgesics, and physical therapy are the mainstays of treatment.
- Work and athletic activities may resume as tolerated by symptoms.

Complications

- Chronic pain

Pearls and Pitfalls

- Patients with chronic pain (i.e., greater than four to six weeks) warrant plain radiographs and risk assessment for infectious process or other underlying serious etiology of pain.

Spondylolisthesis

General Description

- Described by the position of the vertebral body in relation to the next caudal segment.
  - Anterior translation = anterolisthesis (Figure 10.7)
  - Posterior translation = retrolisthesis
- Grading and treatment is based on percentage of translation (Meyerding Grading System).
  - Grade 1: less than 25 percent translation
  - Grade 2: 25–50 percent translation
  - Grade 3: 50–75 percent translation
  - Grade 4: 75–100 percent translation
  - Grade 5: more than 100 percent translation (aka spondyloptosis)

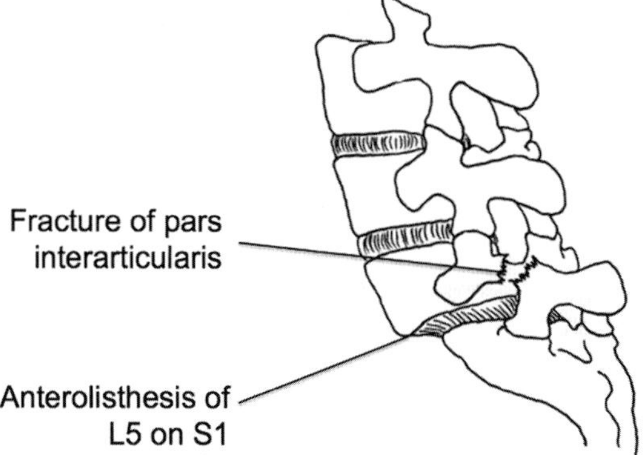

Figure 10.7. Anterolisthesis and fracture of the pars interarticularis. Illustration by Yvonne Chow.

Mechanism

- Vertebral body displacement resulting from acquired bilateral defects in the pars interarticularis (spondylolysis, aka isthmic spondylolisthesis) (Figure 10.7) or from degenerative spine changes (facet and disc degeneration).
- Degenerative spondylolisthesis is most common at L4–L5, while isthmic spondylolisthesis is most common at L5–S1.

Presentation

- Presents with back pain and neurogenic. claudication, similar to lumbar spinal stenosis.
- May also have radicular symptoms.
- Pain worse with extension and range of motion.

Physical Exam

- Tenderness of affected area
- May be able to palpate a step-off with high-grade slip.
- Neurological exam is usually normal.

Essential Diagnostics

- Plain radiographs (lateral view) reveal presence and degree of vertebral body displacement.
  - Flexion-extension views may show dynamic segmental instability.
- MRI is useful for identification of foraminal stenosis and neural impingement.

ED Treatment

- Most patients are managed nonoperatively.
- Pain management and orthopedic or sports medicine referral are usually sufficient.

Disposition

- Outpatient orthopedic or sports medicine follow-up is appropriate unless there is acute, significant neurologic impairment.
- Rehabilitation, and sometimes bracing, complements pain management.
- Epidural corticosteroid injections are second-line therapy.

- Operative management is reserved for failure of conservative measures for several months, progressive neurologic impairment, or high-grade disease (grade 3 with symptoms or grades 4–5).

Complications

- Radiculopathy, neurologic impairment

Pearls and Pitfalls

- It is important to distinguish from vascular claudication.
- Degenerative spondylolisthesis often causes foraminal stenosis and radiculopathy.

Back Pain in Children and Adolescents

General Considerations

- Back pain in the pediatric population is likely more common than originally thought, but vigilance for serious causes of back pain in very young children (<10 years old) should be maintained.
- Incidence of low back pain by late adolescence may be as high as 24–36 percent.[12]
- Sports injuries account for 21 percent of TL spine fractures in adolescents.[12]
- Spondyloarthropathy (i.e., ankylosing spondylitis) should be considered in the adolescent and young adult with low back pain and is characterized by morning stiffness and improvement with activity.

Spondylolysis

General Description

- Spondylolysis describes a stress fracture to the posterior elements, specifically the pars interarticularis (Figure 10.7), and is often referred to as a pars defect.
- Unique to children and may account for source of back pain in up to 47 percent of adolescent athletes.[13]
- May be unilateral or bilateral; bilateral pars defects may progress to spondylolisthesis (Figure 10.7).
- Most common at the L5 level

Mechanism

- Associated with participation in sports that involve repetitive flexion and hyperextension (gymnastics, football, volleyball, dance), thus placing the posterior elements of the developing spine under increased stress.

Presentation

- Pain is typically worse with activity and improves with rest.
- May occasionally have radicular pain.
- Neurologic symptoms are rare.

Physical Exam

- Physical exam often demonstrates pain with hyperextension.
- The *stork test* (performed while standing on one leg and hyperextending) is often provocative for pain but has poor specificity (Figure 10.5).

Essential Diagnostics

- Plain radiographs (AP, lateral, and oblique views) are poorly sensitive but may reveal the characteristic "Scotty dog sign" (Figure 10.8), which is a lucency through the pars. interarticularis (creating a collar at the neck of the Scotty dog) on the oblique views.

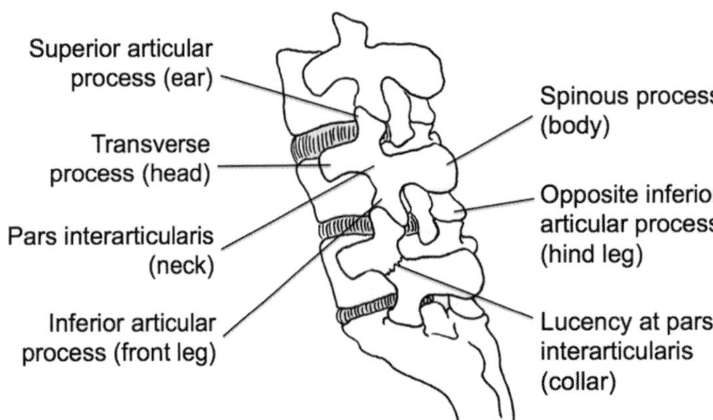

Figure 10.8. Scotty dog sign.

- Advanced imaging is often necessary for diagnosis, but controversy exists over the best method.
- Single positron emission computerized tomography (SPECT) is a reliable diagnostic imaging tool and may help to differentiate symptomatic (active) vs. asymptomatic (inactive) lesions.
- CT shows good bony detail and may be useful to monitor healing, but radiation concerns limit its frequent application.
- MRI has shown marginal sensitivity but good negative predictive value and is often applied using specialized imaging protocols.
- MRI has the advantage of avoiding ionizing radiation and identifying other possible sources of back pain (i.e., disc herniation).

ED Treatment

- Conservative measures (i.e., cessation of activity and physical therapy) are the mainstay of treatment.
- Counseling about activity restriction is important.

Disposition

- Orthopedic or sports medicine follow-up is recommended if spondylolysis is considered.
- Advanced imaging is more appropriate for the outpatient setting than the ED.
- Bracing with a thoracolumbosacral orthosis (TLSO) is controversial and supportive evidence is limited.
- Compliance with both activity restriction and brace wear is challenging.
- Return to athletics is often allowed upon resolution of symptoms (which occurs over weeks to months) and completion of a rehabilitation program.
- Surgical management is rarely necessary but may be considered for symptoms lasting more than nine to twelve months.
- Outcomes are similar for healed fractures and fibrous nonunions.[13]

Complications

- May progress to spondylolisthesis.

Pearls and Pitfalls

- Back pain is children is more common than previously thought, and spondylolysis is considered to be a frequent cause.
- Workup of back pain in children and adolescents is different than in adults.
  - Need to maintain a higher degree of suspicion for concerning underlying etiologies such as spondylolysis, spondylolisthesis, malignancy.
  - Consider early imaging with plain films.

Table 10.5 Key Diagnoses, History, Physical Exam Findings, and Treatment

Diagnosis	History	Physical Exam Findings	Treatment
Vertebral compression fracture	Back pain after trauma	Midline tenderness over fracture site May have paraspinal muscle tenderness Normal neurological exam	Pain management TLSO brace Weight-bearing as tolerated
Spinous process and transverse process fractures	Pain at site of injury after lateral bending force, direct trauma or hyperflexion injury	Tenderness at fracture site and/or surrounding paraspinal muscles Normal neurological exam	Pain management Early ambulation Bracing rarely required
Burst fracture	Pain after axial or flexion loading of spine	Tenderness at fracture site Evaluate for other spine and/or pelvic injuries May have neurologic compromise	Orthopedic and/or neurosurgical consultation

Table 10.5 *(cont.)*

Diagnosis	History	Physical Exam Findings	Treatment
Flexion-distraction injury	Hyperflexion injury	Tenderness at fracture site May be associated with other intra-abdominal injuries Usually normal neurological exam	Orthopedic and/or neurosurgical consultation TLSO brace for stable fractures Operative management for unstable fractures
Thoracolumbar fracture-dislocation	Results from a combination of flexion, rotation, distraction, and shearing forces Usually high-energy trauma	Tenderness at fracture site Frequent neurovascular injury	Early orthopedic or neurosurgical consultation Immobilization Early operative management
Spinal epidural abscess	Classic is back pain, fever, and neurologic complaint but may not be present in all May have pain out of proportion to exam	Back tenderness Fever Neurologic deficit	Early IV antibiotics Often surgical intervention for decompression Infectious disease, orthopedics, and/or neurosurgical consultation
Vertebral osteomyelitis	Insidious onset back pain over weeks to months	Fever may or may not be present Neurologic deficits are late finding	Infectious disease consult Possible orthopedic or neurosurgical consult if operative intervention indicated Admit for IV antibiotics
Cauda equina syndrome	Bilateral leg pain and sensorimotor complaints Saddle anesthesia Bladder dysfunction (urinary retention with overflow incontinence) Back pain is not usually prominent feature	Motor weakness Diminished deep tendon reflexes Decreased rectal tone Urinary retention (> 500 mL)	Emergent orthopedic or neurosurgical consultation for decompression
Neoplasm	Back pain Night and rest pain Constitutional symptoms Radiculopathy and/or neurological complaints	Spinal tenderness May have findings of radiculopathy, myelopathy May have neurological compromise	High-dose corticosteroids Radiation Outpatient vs. inpatient management decision should be made in conjunction with oncologist and orthopedic or neurosurgery if neurological compromise present
Lumbar spine disc disease and radiculopathy	Low back pain with radiculopathy Radiculopathy symptoms worse with sitting, better with standing	May have limited range of motion and antalgic gait Positive straight leg raise and/or slump test Evaluate for neurologic deficit	Anti-inflammatories Activity as tolerated Physical therapy Epidural steroid injection is second-line therapy

Table 10.5 *(cont.)*

Diagnosis	History	Physical Exam Findings	Treatment
Lumbar spinal stenosis	Back pain radiating into buttocks or legs Usually worse with extension, standing, and walking	May have findings of radiculopathy or sensorimotor deficits	Anti-inflammatories (if no contraindications) Physical therapy Corticosteroid injections Surgery usually reserved for recalcitrant cases or neurological compromise
Lumbar myofascial strain	Back pain usually due to minor trauma, overuse, or repetitive loading	Midline and/or paraspinal tenderness No radicular or neurological symptoms	Pain management Physical therapy Activity modification
Spondylolisthesis	Back pain and neurogenic claudication Worse with extension and range of motion	Tenderness of affected area May be able to palpate a step-off	Pain management Physical therapy Occasional bracing Surgery for high-grade slips, progressive neurological impairment or failure of conservative therapy
Spondylolysis	Back pain Often history of participation in repetitive flexion and hyperextension sports	Pain with activity and better with rest Occasional radicular pain Neurological impairment is rare	Activity modification/ restriction Physical therapy Bracing is controversial

Table 10.6 Indications for Surgical Consultation in the Emergency Department

Unstable lumbar spine fractures or ligamentous injuries
Cauda equina or other cord compression syndromes
Spinal epidural abscess or vertebral osteomyelitis
Neoplasm with associated neurologic impairment
Any lumbar spine condition with significant or rapidly progressive neurologic deficits

Recommended Reading

B.N. Corwell. The emergency department evaluation, management, and treatment of back pain. *Emerg Med Clin N Am* 2010;28:811-39.

K.B. Wood, W. Li, D.S. Lebl, et al.. Management of thoracolumbar spine fractures. *Spine J* 2014;14:145-64.

K.H. O'Phelan, E.B. Bunney, S.D. Weingart, et al.. Emergency neurological life support: spinal cord compression. *Neurocrit Care* 2012:17:S96-S101.

K.R. Mautner and M.J. Huggins. The young adult spine in sports. *Clin Sports Med* 2012;31:253-72.

References

1. B.N. Corwell. The emergency department evaluation, management, and treatment of back pain. *Emerg Med Clin N Am* 2010;28:811-39.
2. N. Khan, S. Husain, M. Haak. Thoracolumbar injuries in the athlete. *Sports Med Arthrosc Rev* 2008;16:16-25.
3. V. Thiruganasambandamoorthy, E. Turko, D. Ansell, et al.. Risk factors for serious underlying pathology in adult emergency department nontraumatic low back pain patients. *J Emerg Med* 2014;47:1-11.
4. K.R. Mautner and M.J. Huggins. The young adult spine in sports. *Clin Sports Med* 2012;31:253-72.
5. K.E. Radcliff, C.K. Kepler, L.A. Delasotta, et al.. Current management review of thoracolumbar cord syndromes. *Spine J* 2011;11:884-92.

6. K.J. Koval and J.D. Zuckerman. *Thoracolumbar spine. Handbook of Fractures*, 3rd edition. Philadelphia. Lippincott Williams & Wilkins. 2006;103-18.
7. K. Inaba, J.J. DuBose, G. Barmparas, et al.. Clinical examination is insufficient to rule out thoracolumbar spine injuries. *J Trauma* 2011;70:174-9.
8. B. Mitra, H.A. Thani, P. A. Cameron. Clearance of the thoracolumbar spine: A clinical decision rule is needed. *Injury* 2013;44:881-2.
9. A.A. Patel, A. Dailey, D.S. Brodke, et al.. Thoracolumbar spine trauma classification: the Thoracolumbar Injury Classification and Severity Score system and case examples. *J Neurosurg Spine* 2009;10:201-6.
10. D.P. Davis, A. Salazar, T.C. Chan, et al.. Prospective evaluation of a clinical decision guideline to diagnose spinal epidural abscess in patients who present to the emergency department with spine pain. *J Neurosurg Spine* 2011;14:765-70.
11. K.H. O'Phelan, E.B. Bunney, S.D. Weingart, et al.. Emergency neurological life support: Spinal cord compression. *Neurocrit Care* 2012:17:S96-S101.
12. B.M. Haus and L.J. Micheli. Back pain in the pediatric and adolescent athlete. *Clin Sports Med* 2012;31:423-40.
13. H.J. Kim and D.W. Green. Spondylolysis in the adolescent athlete. *Curr Opin Pediatr* 2011;23:68-72.

Chapter 11

Concussion

Melissa D. Leber

Background/Epidemiology

- A concussion is any injury to the head or neck that alters the way the brain functions. It can also be caused by an injury to any part of the body that causes an impulsive force transmitted to the head.[1] The mechanical insult leads to a metabolic disturbance that causes the symptoms of concussion.[1] It can be from direct trauma to the head, trauma to the neck, or a shaking or sudden severe movement of the head. There does not have to be a loss of consciousness to diagnose concussion.[1]
- Symptoms of a concussion can be transient or prolonged. Symptom onset can be minutes to hours to days after the injury.[1,2]
- Diagnostic criteria: An appropriate mechanism of injury followed by any one, or combination of, possible symptoms (see Table 11.1 for complete list): headache, nausea, dizziness, blurred vision, difficulty concentrating, difficulty sleeping, sleeping more than usual, difficulty remembering, or feeling mentally foggy.[1–3]
    - Symptoms are caused by neuronal functional abnormalities, rather than structural abnormalities.[4]
    - There are no gross anatomic lesions, and therefore there are no pathologic findings on brain imaging.[4]
- Age: There is no minimum or maximum age at which a patient can sustain a concussion. The younger one is, the more susceptible one is to prolonged damage.[4]
- Prognosis: Typically, patients fully recover (symptom free) within seven to ten days of the initial injury.[1–3,5]
    - Risk factors for a longer recovery time include:
        - Progressively longer recovery times after previous concussions.[3,4]
        - History of depression, anxiety, or other psychiatric illness. [4]
        - History of attention deficit hyperactivity disorder (ADHD) or learning disability.[4]
        - Personal or family history of headaches or migraines.
- The more concussions a patient has sustained, the easier it is to sustain a second concussion.[1,3] The brain may be more sensitive to an even more mild impact or trauma because concussed neurons and mitochondria are more vulnerable to further injury.[6,7]
- Post-concussive syndrome: This occurs when symptoms of concussion last for weeks to months to years, or even indefinitely. There is no clear consensus on how long symptoms of concussion must be present prior to making this diagnosis.

Anatomical Considerations / Pathophysiology

- A mechanical insult causes a complex cascade of neurochemical and neurometabolic changes in the brain.[6,8] This results in the following changes:
    - Ion flux of various neurotransmitters and amino acids.
    - Glucose hypometabolism
    - Decreased cerebral blood flow.
    - Influx of calcium ions into mitochondria causes oxidative dysfunction.
    - These changes are usually transient after one concussion but there can be more persistent changes in ion flux after repetitive head injury.[6]
- These changes cause swelling of brain cells which takes time to recover. During this

recovery time, the cells are more vulnerable to further damage, and may be permanently affected, causing cerebral edema, if the brain is impacted again[6,7]. This recovery period typically lasts one to two weeks, and it is during this period, when the cells are more vulnerable to impact, that the patient is susceptible to second impact syndrome (discussed further in the Complications section later).[6,7]

Focused History and Physical Exam

- Initial evaluation of any patient sustaining a head injury should be aimed at ruling out any head injury red flags, which include:
  - Unequal pupils
  - Any focal neurological deficit
  - Extreme drowsiness or unarousable.
  - Worsening headache.
  - Weakness, incoordination
  - Multiple episodes of vomiting.
  - Slurred speech
  - Seizures
  - Confusion or agitation
  - Unusual behavior or observer concern.
- Once a severe head injury, For example, intracranial hemorrhage, has been ruled out, the patient should be further evaluated for other injuries such as concussion.
- ***Concussion specific questions to include in a comprehensive patient history:***
  - For emergency physicians present at the event:
    - Sideline Concussion Assessment Tool (SCAT) and Maddocks questions[9,10]. *To be used at time of injury only*:
      - At what venue are we (name of field/stadium/rink)?
      - Who scored last (which team)?
      - What half/period/quarter/ is it currently?
      - What team did we play last?
      - Did we win the last game?
  - Injury-related questions
    - How did the head injury occur (mechanism of injury)?
    - Did you have any physical symptoms associated with the injury? (e.g., unsteady gait, blurry vision)

Table 11.1 Possible Concussion Symptoms

Headache	Nausea	Vomiting
Balance Problems	Dizziness	Fatigue
Trouble Falling Asleep	Sleeping More than Usual	Sleeping Less than Usual
Drowsiness	Sensitivity to Light	Sensitivity to Noise
Irritability	Sadness	Nervousness
Feeling More Emotional	Numbness or Tingling	Feeling Slowed Down
Feeling Mentally "Foggy"	Difficulty Concentrating	Difficulty Remembering
Visual Problems (blurred vision, double vision, etc.)		

    - How did you react to the injury? (e.g., stand up immediately, hold head in lap, lie down, collapse)
    - Did you lose consciousness?
    - Do you have amnesia to the event?
    - Did you continue participating in the event/activity?
  - Signs and symptoms (see Table 11.1 for complete list)
    - Which signs/symptoms did you have immediately after the injury?
    - Did any of symptoms develop later on?
      - How long after the injury did they begin?
  - Concussion-related history
    - Have you ever had a concussion in the past?
      - If so, when did it occur?
      - How long did it take you to completely recover?
  - Past medical history (pertinent to concussions)
    - Do you have any history of depression, anxiety, or other psychiatric illness?
    - Do you have any history of ADHD or learning disability?
    - Do you have a personal history or family history of headaches or migraines?

- ***Concussion-specific physical exam***
  - Head and face exam
    - Is there evidence of a forceful blow to the head?
    - Is there presence of a hematoma?
      - Is it expanding?
    - Is there a scalp laceration or any other head/face trauma?
  - Musculoskeletal exam
    - Evaluate for neck and back ROM
    - Check for midline spinal tenderness.
  - Neurologic exam
    - Orientation – alert and oriented to person, place, time.
    - Cranial nerve exam (II-XII):
      - II – Optic
      - III – Oculomotor
      - IV – Trochlear
      - V – Trigeminal
      - VI – Abducens
      - VII – Facial
      - VIII – Acoustic
      - IX – Glossopharyngeal
      - X – Vagus
      - XI – Spinal Accessory
      - XII – Hypoglossal
    - Cerebellar testing – Finger to nose.
    - Assess for gait abnormality.
    - Balance test – *Balance Error Scoring System (BESS)*.[11,12]
      - Have the patient close eyes and put hands on hips. With each maneuver below, count the number of errors (see definitions below) made in 20 seconds. Patient is allowed a maximum of 10 errors per stance below:
        - Double leg stance – feet are together, flat on the floor (Figure 11.1).
        - Tandem stance – stand heel-to-toe with nondominant leg in back (Figure 11.2).

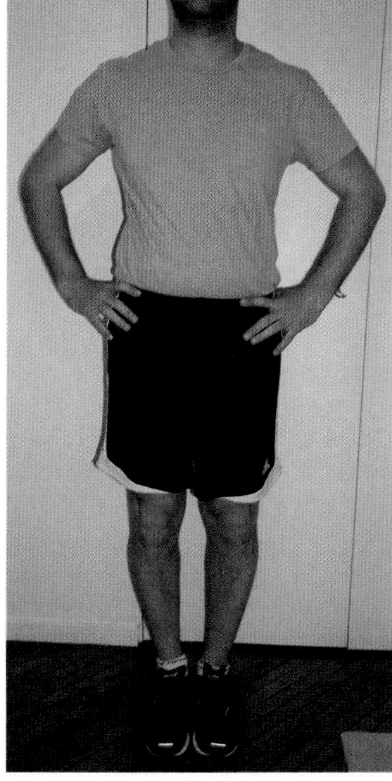

Figure 11.1. Proper positioning for BESS Balance Testing – Double Leg Stance: Feet together, side by side.

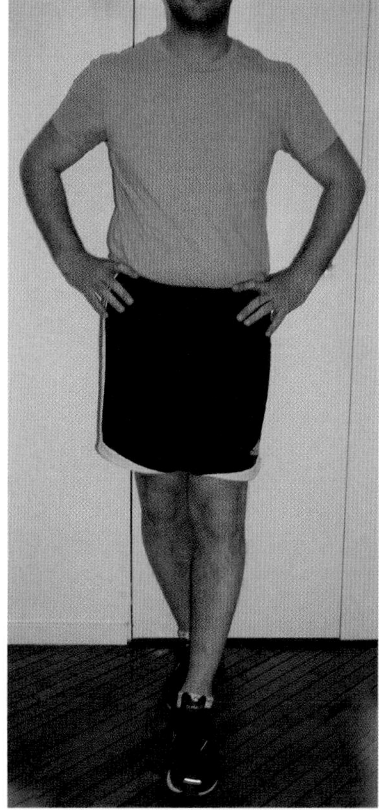

Figure 11.2. Proper positioning for BESS Balance Testing – Tandem Stance: Heel-to-toe with the patient's nondominant leg in the back.

        - Single leg stance – balance on nondominant leg (Figure 11.3).
      - An error is defined as the patient moving the hands off the hips, opening the eyes, taking a step, stumble, or fall, or abduction or flexion of the hips more than 30°.
- Ophthalmic exam
  - Visual acuity
  - Extraocular motions – test smooth pursuits, horizontal saccades, vertical saccades, and convergence.
- Cognitive assessment
  - Concentration tests.
    - Spell the word *world* in reverse (D-L-R-O-W).
    - State the months of the year in reverse order.
      - December, November, October, September, August, July, June, May, April, March, February, January.
    - Repeat numbers in reverse order.
      - 5–7–4
      - 9–6–2–4
      - 3–4–8–8–3
  - Immediate and delayed memory – Give the patient five words to remember. Ask them to repeat the five words immediately and then after a few minutes (three to five) ask them to repeat the same five words. Assess for accuracy.
    - For example, key, carpet, school, banana, ribbon.

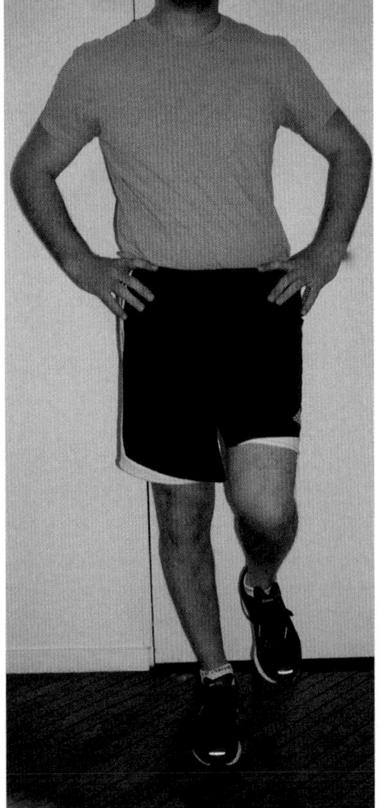

Figure 11.3. Proper positioning for BESS Balance Testing – Single Leg Stance: Balance on the nondominant leg.

Differential Diagnosis – Emergent and Common Diagnoses

- Keep the initial differential diagnosis quite broad.
- Quickly narrow down the differential using history and physical exam, and make sure to rule out the emergent diagnoses.

Management and Clinical Pathway

- If the patient meets the diagnostic criteria for concussion, the majority of the emergency management should involve patient education and counseling.

Table 11.2 Emergent and Common Diagnoses in the Emergency Department

Emergent Diagnoses	Common Diagnoses
Intracranial/subarachnoid hemorrhage	Simple hematoma
Subdural/epidural hematoma	Simple contusion
Second impact syndrome	Cervical muscle strains
Chronic traumatic encephalopathy	Concussion
Skull fracture	Minor head injury
Cervical spine fracture	
Spinal cord injury without radiographic abnormality (SCIWORA)	

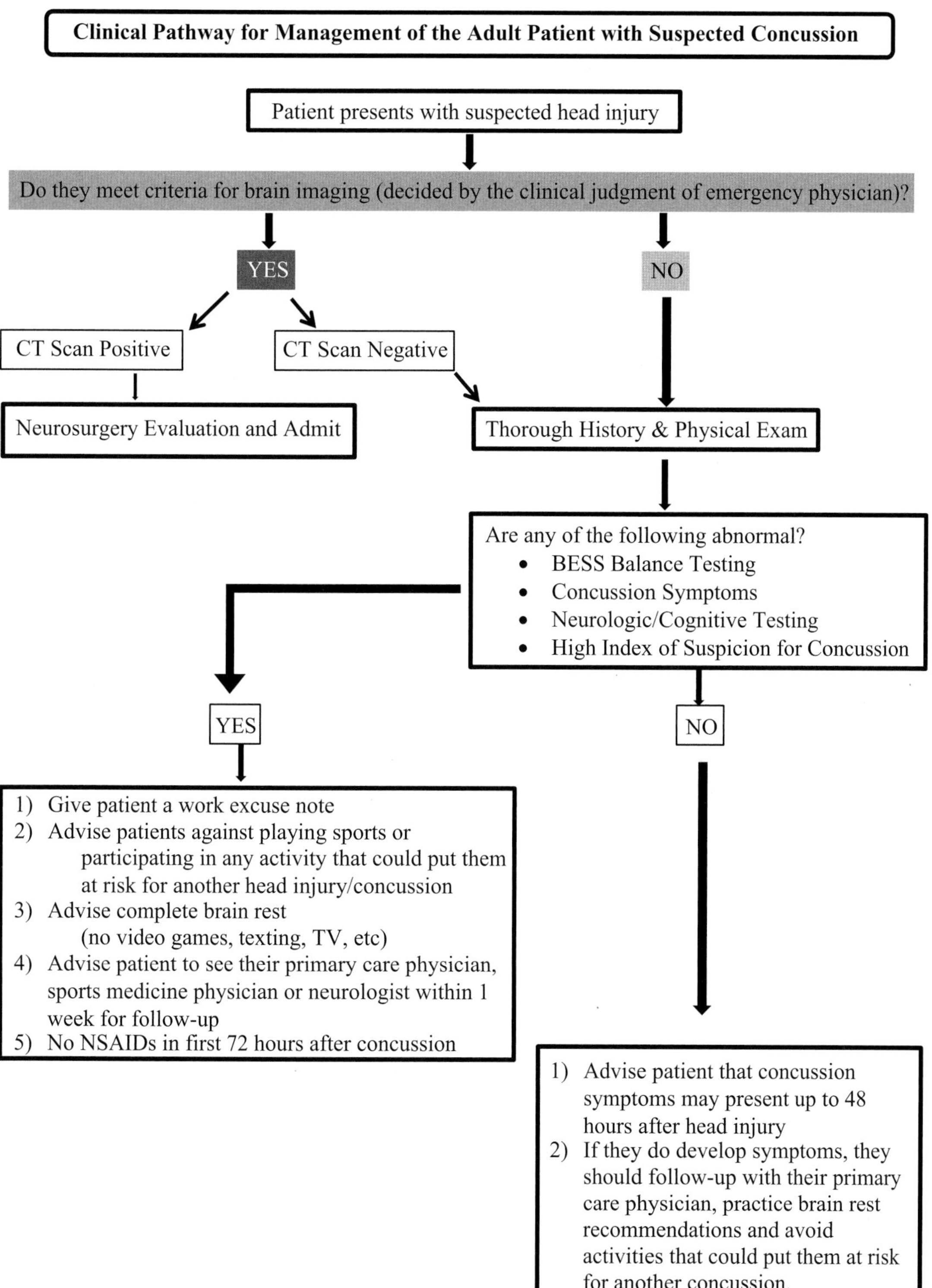

Figure 11.4. Clinical pathway for the adult patient with suspected concussion.

- It is important to always maintain a high degree of suspicion for concussion and err on the side of caution when making this diagnosis.
  - If the diagnosis is uncertain, do not let athletes return to sports until they have followed up with their primary care or sports medicine physician.
  - Follow the mantra, "When in doubt, sit them out."
- Imaging is not indicated in the emergency department for diagnosis of concussion. However, if the patient has focal neurologic deficits or there is concern for underlying severe head injury, brain imaging should be obtained. If the patient has signs of a traumatic blow to the head or face, consider imaging to rule out underlying pathology.
- Medication management: Nonsteroidal anti-informatory drugs (NSAIDs) should **NOT** be taken in the first seventy-two hours after a concussion. This is recommended by the current position statements on concussion in sport because of the theoretical risk of bleeding.[4] If the patient has a headache or neck or back pain, acetaminophen should be taken.
- Brain rest recommendations:
  - The patient should be advised that the more the brain rests, the quicker the recovery. Brain rest entails resting as much as possible, avoiding physical activity, avoiding computer/cellular use, and, when possible, taking one to two days off from work. In general, patients should avoid any activities that make their symptoms worse. While no further damage will ensue from working, texting, or using the brain, it may take slightly longer for symptoms to resolve.[1,4,13]

Disposition

- Follow-up: Every patient should follow-up with their primary care doctor (PCP), sports medicine specialist, or neurologist approximately one to three days after a concussion is sustained.[1,4,5]
- Work/athletics recommendations: The more the patient rests the brain, the quicker the recovery will be.[1,4,5] In addition, stressing the brain with work, studying, reading, and athletics (from increasing the heart rate and blood pressure) may worsen symptoms during and after the activity. If the patient chooses to go to work, it will not cause any further damage to the brain. The patient should not engage in any activity which could potentially risk sustaining a second concussion before fully healing from the current concussion. See the Pediatrics section for school recommendations.
- Brain rest recommendations: The patient should be advised to avoid cellular phone use (including texting), computer use, television, reading, and any activity which raises the heart rate above 100 beats per minute or increases their blood pressure.
- Return to work and return to play recommendations: Patients should be advised to obtain clearance to return to sports from their PCP and/or sports medicine physician. It is important that the emergency physician does not clear patients to return to physical activity or sports from the emergency department. General anticipatory guidance may include advising the patient to slowly begin returning to work as tolerated by symptoms. Athletes should not return to play until after they have been completely symptom free for at least forty-eight hours.[1,3–5,13] The return to play should be a graded progression of activity so that the patient may gradually ease back into the gym and gradually increase the heart rate over many days without triggering any concussion symptoms. The patient may not return to contact sports until completing return to play progression symptom free and being cleared by either the PCP, sports medicine physician, or neurologist.
- Return to play progression:
  - Step 1: Light general conditioning (15- to 20-minute light workout).
  - Step 2: General conditioning and sport-specific skill work (individual 30-minute light workout).
  - Step 3: General conditioning and skill work with team (no contact, workout up to 60 minutes).
  - Step 4: General conditioning, skill work, and team drills (no contact, workout up to 75 minutes).

- Step 5: Full team practice with body contact.

Complications

- Second impact syndrome: This is a rare life-threatening condition that may occur when an individual sustains a second concussion before the brain has completely healed from the first concussion.[6,7].This typically affects young healthy athletes and results in cerebral edema, potential brain herniation, and death.[6,7] It is very important for the emergency physician to educate the patient regarding when to return to play and to warn them of the risk of second impact syndrome, especially with contact sports, while symptoms persist.
- Chronic traumatic encephalopathy (CTE): This is a rare progressive neuropathological disease that results from repetitive brain trauma.[1,5,14] It has been described in athletes such as boxers and football players.[1,5,14] Symptoms of CTE include memory disturbances, behavior and personality changes, and speech and gait abnormalities.[1,5,14]

Pediatric Considerations

Management and Clinical Pathway

- Pediatric Emergency Care Applied Research Network (PECARN)[15] – Use this validated decision rule to determine need for brain imaging in a pediatric patient with head injury.
- History and physical – Complete same H&P as described earlier in the adult section.
    - Determine whether the patient has symptoms of a concussion, more than ten errors on *BESS balance testing*, or if there is a high index of suspicion.[11,12]
        - If any of the above are positive, then follow the six recommendations provided in Figure 11.5.
        - If none of the above are positive, then advise the patient and parents that concussion symptoms may develop up to forty-eight hours after the head injury. If symptoms develop, the patient should stay out of physical education (PE) and any sports and should follow-up with their PCP or sports medicine physician.
- Patient and parent education (see detailed outline later).
- Recommendations for pediatric disposition and management.[1,4]
    - School excuse note – Initially it is best to keep the patient out of school for the first twenty-four to forty-eight hours following a concussion to allow for brain rest. After this period, the child may return to school as able based upon symptoms.
        - Patient and parents should be counseled that certain school accommodations may need to be made if symptoms prevent the patient from doing schoolwork. Accommodations may include:
            - No tests/quizzes/exams; if the patient must take an exam, request open-note and open-book exams, and allow for extra exam time.
            - Allow the child to go to the nurse's office for acetaminophen administration for headaches as needed.
            - Allow the child to go to nurse's office for rest and naps as needed throughout the day.
            - Allow the child frequent breaks from the classroom if experiencing concussion symptoms.
            - Restrict PE and recess until cleared by PCP or sports medicine physician.[13]
            - Allow for use of an elevator (if available) instead of climbing stairs.
            - Allow the child to wear sunglasses in the classroom as needed for light sensitivity.
    - PE/recess/sports excuse note until cleared by PCP or sports medicine physician.
    - Advise parents/patients against doing any activity that puts the patient at risk for another concussion.
    - Complete brain rest – Patients should avoid watching television, playing video games, texting, emailing, using the computer, reading, and so forth. The

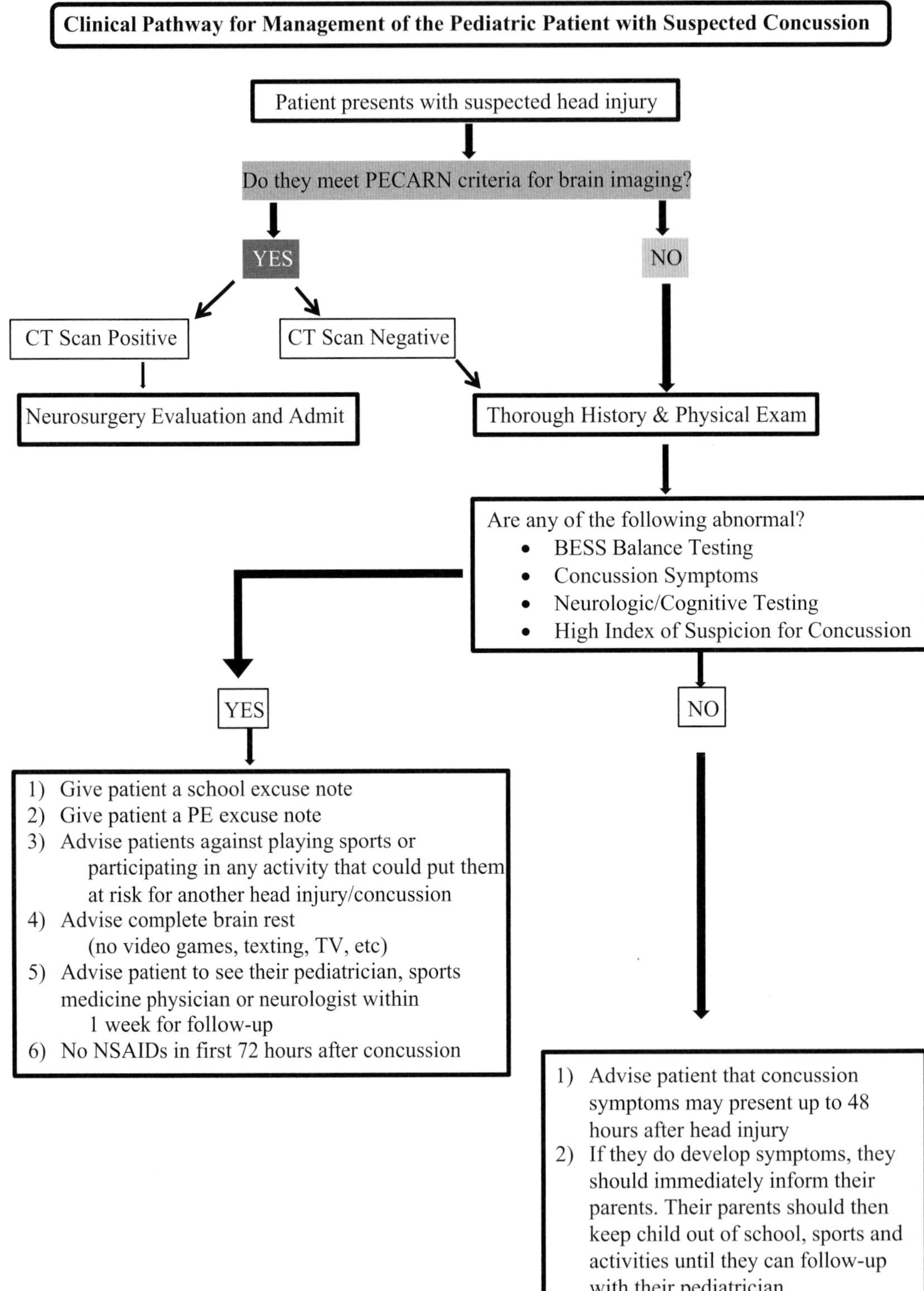

Figure 11.5. Clinical pathway for the pediatric patient with suspected concussion.

  - more the patient rests and relaxes, the better.[1,4]
  - See PCP or sports medicine physician within one to three days for follow-up and potential clearance for return to play and return to school.
  - Advise against taking NSAIDs for symptoms of headache in the first seventy-two hours after a concussion because of the theoretical risk of bleeding.[4]
- Return to play – While the emergency physician will not be guiding the child's return to play, it is important to know what this will involve.
  - Return to play is a guided stepwise progression of activities so as to minimize return of concussive symptoms.
  - Return to play should not begin until the child has been symptom free for at least seventy-two hours.[4,5,13,16]
  - Neurocognitive testing (such as the Impact Test®) is usually completed prior to clearance for return to play. This includes testing of verbal memory, visual memory, and reaction time via a computer-based exam.
    - Baseline testing is completed by most high school and college athletes prior to the start of the athletic season. This has become standard of care.
    - If a concussion is sustained during the season, neurocognitive testing is repeated prior to clearance for return to play. The new composite score is compared to the baseline score.
    - An athlete should not be cleared for return to play until performance is at or near baseline cognitive levels.
    - It is known that physical symptoms resolve prior to complete return of reaction time, memory, and cognition. Therefore, neurocognitive computer-based testing is used as a tool to detect subclinical concussions in athletes.

Pearls and Pitfalls

- The diagnosis of concussion is a clinical diagnosis.
- A patient with a concussion does not have to have had loss of consciousness.
- Proper education of patients and their families is vital in the emergency setting, as this may be the only information they receive post injury.
- Prevention of a subsequent head injury is vital to preventing complications.
- No athlete should return to the game on the same day he or she is suspected of having a concussion[1,4].
  - "When in doubt, sit them out."
- No patient should return to play until symptom free for forty-eight to seventy-two hours and until completing stepwise return to play protocol.[1,4,13]
- Standardizing discharge instructions in the emergency department will ensure that each patient receives the necessary education and counseling.[17]
- Even though an adult may not play on an organized team, advice must still be given regarding recreational sports, exercise, and any activity that may risk a repeat head injury.
- Other mechanisms of injury may cause concussions besides team sports. Make sure to consider this as a possible diagnosis in patients who present after mechanical falls and car accidents.

Recommended Reading

McCrory P, Meeuwisse W, Aubry M, Cantu B, Dvorak J, Echemendia RJ, et al.. Consensus statement on concussion in sport: The 4th International Conference on Concussion in Sport held in Zurich, November 2012. *Clin J Sport Med* 2013 Mar;23(2):89–117.

Harmon KG, Drezner J, Gammons M, Guskiewicz K, Halstead M, Herring S, et al.. American Medical Society for Sports Medicine position statement: concussion in sport. *Clin J Sport Med* 2013 Jan;23(1):1–18.

Guskiewicz KM, McCrea M, Marshall SW, Cantu RC, Randolph C, Barr W, et al.. Cumulative effects associated with recurrent concussion in collegiate football players: The NCAA Concussion Study. *JAMA* 2003 Nov 19;290(19):2549–2555.

References

1. McCrory P, Meeuwisse W, Aubry M, Cantu B, Dvorak J, Echemendia RJ, et al.. Consensus statement on concussion in sport: the 4th International Conference on Concussion in Sport held in Zurich, November 2012. *Clin J Sport Med* 2013 Mar;23(2):89–117.
2. McCrea M, Guskiewicz KM, Marshall SW, Barr W, Randolph C, Cantu RC, et al.. Acute effects and recovery time following concussion in collegiate football players: The NCAA Concussion Study. *JAMA* 2003 Nov 19;290(19):2556–2563.
3. Guskiewicz KM, McCrea M, Marshall SW, Cantu RC, Randolph C, Barr W, et al.. Cumulative effects associated with recurrent concussion in collegiate football players: The NCAA Concussion Study. *JAMA* 2003 Nov 19;290(19): 2549–2555.
4. Harmon KG, Drezner J, Gammons M, Guskiewicz K, Halstead M, Herring S, et al.. American Medical Society for Sports Medicine position statement: Concussion in sport. *Clin J Sport Med* 2013 Jan;23(1):1–18.
5. Makdissi M, Darby D, Maruff P, Ugoni A, Brukner P, McCrory PR. Natural history of concussion in sport: Markers of severity and implications for management. *Am J Sports Med* 2010 Mar;38(3):464–471.
6. Barkhoudarian G, Hovda DA, Giza CC. The molecular pathophysiology of concussive brain injury. *Clin Sports Med* 2011 Jan;30(1):33–48, vii-viii.
7. Cantu RC. Second-impact syndrome. *Clin Sports Med* 1998 Jan;17(1):37–44.
8. Farkas O, Lifshitz J, Povlishock JT. Mechanoporation induced by diffuse traumatic brain injury: An irreversible or reversible response to injury? *J Neurosci* 2006 Mar 22;26(12):3130–3140.
9. Guskiewicz KM, Register-Mihalik J, McCrory P, McCrea M, Johnston K, Makdissi M, et al.. Evidence-based approach to revising the SCAT2: introducing the SCAT3. *Br J Sports Med* 2013 Apr;47(5):289–293.
10. Maddocks DL, Dicker GD, Saling MM. The assessment of orientation following concussion in athletes. *Clin J Sport Med* 1995;5(1):32–35.
11. Bell DR, Guskiewicz KM, Clark MA, Padua DA. Systematic review of the balance error scoring system. *Sports Health* 2011 May;3(3):287–295.
12. Riemann BL, Guskiewicz KM. Effects of mild head injury on postural stability as measured through clinical balance testing. *J Athl Train* 2000 Jan;35(1):19–25.
13. Cantu RC. Return to play guidelines after a head injury. *Clin Sports Med* 1998 Jan;17(1):45–60.
14. McCrory P, Meeuwisse WH, Kutcher JS, Jordan BD, Gardner A. What is the evidence for chronic concussion-related changes in retired athletes: Behavioural, pathological, and clinical outcomes? *Br J Sports Med* 2013 Apr;47(5):327–330.
15. Kuppermann N, Holmes JF, Dayan PS, Hoyle JD,Jr, Atabaki SM, Holubkov R, et al.. Identification of children at very low risk of clinically-important brain injuries after head trauma: A prospective cohort study. *Lancet* 2009 Oct 3;374(9696):1160–1170.
16. West TA, Marion DW. Current recommendations for the diagnosis and treatment of concussion in sport: A comparison of three new guidelines. *J Neurotrauma* 2014 Jan 15;31(2):159–168.
17. De Maio VJ, Joseph DO, Tibbo-Valeriote H, Cabanas JG, Lanier B, Mann CH, et al.. Variability in discharge instructions and activity restrictions for patients in a children's ED postconcussion. *Pediatr Emerg Care* 2014 Jan;30(1):20–25.

Chapter 12

Arrhythmias and Sudden Cardiac Arrest in Athletes

Moira Davenport

Background/Epidemiology

- Participation in athletics and recreational exercise is increasing across all age groups and genders, with the largest increase in activity seen in the elderly age group.
- These active individuals are presenting to the emergency department (ED) with cardiac concerns related to exercise and with cardiac conditions that occur during athletic activity.
- Unfortunately, often the initial presentation of an underlying cardiac problem is sudden cardiac death (SCD).
- However, in some cases there may be prodromal symptoms for which the athlete seeks care in the ED such as chest pain, dyspnea, dizziness, palpitations, near syncope or syncope, or a history of heart disease in young family members.
- For these reasons, the emergency physician should be familiar with basic concepts of sports cardiology as well as both the urgent and emergent management of these conditions.
- Cardiac screening of athletes for potentially catastrophic cardiac conditions has generated much debate. To date, several protocols have been proposed but no universally accepted consensus has been reached.
  - Most of these protocols differ on recommendations for cardiac testing. They have several key features in common and all recommend:
    - Attention should be given to personal and family history, with particular focus on cardiac and pulmonary conditions.
    - This also features a focused review of symptoms, with particular attention given to symptoms that develop during activity.
    - A complete physical exam should be performed, again focusing on cardiac and pulmonary exams.
    - It is advised to assess the cardiac and pulmonary portions of the exam in multiple positions (supine and standing) to try to elicit murmurs and arrhythmias.
- The most widely known position statements follow, with key recommendations regarding cardiac screening:
  - American Heart Association[1]
    - Individualized testing should be performed based on concerning findings.
    - EKG, echocardiography and stress testing are optional in asymptomatic athletes less than 40 years of age.
    - A minimum of an EKG should be performed in the asymptomatic athlete more than 40 years of age, particularly when the individual is starting a new exercise program.
  - European Society of Cardiology
    - EKGs are recommended for all athletes regardless of age and symptomatology.
    - Further testing (echocardiogram, stress testing, MRI, catheterization) is recommended for all athletes with any abnormal finding on physical exam or EKG. The type of testing is based on the initial abnormality detected.
  - National Collegiate Athletic Association (NCAA)[2]
    - There is no recommendation regarding which physician should perform the athletic screening evaluation.

University-affiliated physicians perform 85 percent of these evaluations; 15 percent of exams are performed by a physician of the athlete's choice.
- Repeat cardiovascular screening and examination is required every two years regardless of whether the athlete has been asymptomatic during this time period.
- Despite the NCAA Sports Medicine Handbook guidelines, a recent study found that only 21 of 257 NCAA schools met American Heart Association cardiovascular screening recommendations.[3]

- International Olympic Committee[4]
  - EKGs are required on all athletes.
  - Further testing (echocardiogram, stress testing, MRI, catheterization) is recommended for all athletes with any abnormal finding on physical exam or EKG. The type of testing is based on the initial abnormality detected.

- Research is currently being conducted to determine if a greater focus on family history of SCD at less than 35 years of age (compared to the currently recommended screening for family death at less than 50 years of age) may increase sensitivity of screening[5] in all of the earlier-mentioned protocols.

Anatomical Considerations/ Pathophysiology

- Given that the heart is composed of striated muscle, it stands to reason that a series of morphologic and physiologic changes may result from regular athletic activity, just as is seen in skeletal muscle.
- Several morphologic changes in the heart, particularly in the ventricles, have been linked to regular athletic activity.
  - Increased left ventricle cavity dimension (i.e., increased volume).
  - Increased left ventricle wall thickness.
  - The combination of these two changes typically results in increased cardiac mass.
- The changes seen in the heart are a result of the type of athletic activity preferred by the individual.
  - Isometric activities (such as long distance running and swimming) will increase the fiber length without changing the amount of tension across fibers, thus increasing the ventricular dimension → increased preload.
  - Isotonic activities (such as weight lifting and other power exercises) usually increase the tension across the muscle fibers without changing fiber length, thus increasing the ventricular wall thickness→ increased afterload.
  - Pure examples of isolated isometric or isotonic activities are rare; most athletic activities result in a combination of these changes.
- Genetics also play a role in the extent of changes seen in an individual.
- Male athletes typically have greater amounts of cardiac remodeling than female athletes in the same sport, but female athletes also experience these exercise-related cardiac changes.
  - Female athletes of African/Caribbean ethnicity tend to have greater amounts of cardiac changes than their Caucasian counterparts in the same sports.[6]
- The morphological adaptations seen from regular activity typically result in a slight increase in VO_2 max, which may improve performance slightly, particular in more endurance-based events.
- Structural changes that result from regular athletic activity tend to resolve during periods of decreased training or deconditioning.
- The key clinical challenge is to determine pathologic vs. physiologic adaptations in athletes presenting to the ED.
- EKG guidelines are available to help the clinician distinguish exercise-related cardiac conditions from potentially pathologic cardiac conditions.
- ***EXERCISE-ASSOCIATED EKG CHANGES***[7]
  - The previously discussed morphologic changes in the heart may result in EKG

changes; the emergency physician should be aware of the resultant changes and consider the possibility of athlete's heart when evaluating active patients.

- The extent of EKG changes seen is dependent on gender, genetics, and specific sport; an athlete's underlying medical conditions may also contribute to the EKG changes seen.
- A total of 90 percent of athletes have some degree of bradycardia; the degree of bradycardia seen is sport specific.
  - A heart rate less than 60 is considered bradycardic.
  - A portion of the bradycardia is likely due to increased vagal tone.
  - Athletes with heart rates of 45–60 are typically asymptomatic.
  - If the athlete is asymptomatic and has no other EKG findings, no further workup is required.
  - A heart rate of less than 30 should not be attributed solely to athletic training and warrants further evaluation for pathologic etiology.
- Conduction delays
  - As many as one-third of athletes have a conduction delay on EKG.
  - First-degree AV block is most common and is seen in 35 percent of athletes.
    - This finding is seen in athletes participating in both endurance and power sports.
    - A first-degree AV block is considered a benign finding; athletes with this finding do not require further evaluation.
  - Second-degree heart block is characterized by a conduction delay resulting in the heart skipping (dropping) a beat.
    - The Mobitz type 1 conduction delay is characterized by a gradual increase in the PR interval until a beat is dropped.
    - The Mobitz type 1 block is a common sequela of regular athletic activity; the exact mechanism for the development of this condition remains unclear.
    - Up to 10 percent of athletes have a Mobitz type 1 block on routine EKG testing.
    - Athletes with a Mobitz type 1 block are usually asymptomatic; the change in conduction is typically found on routine EKG testing.
    - If the athlete is asymptomatic, no further evaluation is required. If the athlete is symptomatic, admission is necessary for further testing, including standard cardiac biomarkers and electrophysiologic evaluation.
- Early repolarization (J-point elevation)
  - J-point elevation is defined as a positive notching of the ST segment as it comes off the QRS complex or an upward sloping of the terminal portion of the QRS complex.
  - There are three components:[8]
    - J wave
    - ST elevation (often originating from the J wave).
    - QRS blurring.
  - The location of the J-point elevation is indicative of the risks associated with the condition.
  - J-point elevation in the lateral precordial leads is typically seen in the athletic patient.
  - J-point elevation in these leads is considered benign.
  - J-point elevation may be seen in up to 58 percent of athletes; higher rates are typically seen in endurance athletes.[9]
  - Further evaluation is not currently recommended in asymptomatic athletes with J-point elevation isolated to the lateral precordial leads.[9]
- Increased p-wave amplitude and notched p waves are associated with regular athletic training.
- Incomplete right bundle branch block (iRBBB) is characterized by a wide QRS and is associated with athletic activity.

    - These findings are believed to result from the increased atrial dimensions that result from the increased preload associated with regular athletic activity, particularly endurance exercise.
    - Up to 50 percent of athletes may have an incomplete RBBB.
    - Endurance athletes are more likely to be affected than power athletes.
    - Incomplete RBBB is significantly more common in males than in females.
    - Incomplete and complete RBBB may be seen in patients with atrial septal defects (ASD); attention should be paid to the cardiac exam to rule out murmurs associated with ASD.
    - Asymptomatic athletes with incomplete RBBB may be discharged with cardiology follow-up.
    - Any athlete that is symptomatic with an incomplete RBBB should be admitted for continuous cardiac monitoring, routine lab testing, and electrocardiology testing.
  - Premature atrial complexes (PACs) and premature ventricular contractions (PVCs) are common in athletes, particularly endurance athletes.
    - Athletes with frequent PACs or PVCs may be asymptomatic, or may present with palpitations, lightheadedness, or near syncope.
    - Asymptomatic athletes with PACs require no further evaluation.
    - Symptomatic athletes should have continuous cardiac monitoring, routine blood testing (including cardiac biomarkers), and an echocardiogram. Electrophysiology evaluation should also be considered.
- *CONCERNING EKG CHANGES*[10]
  - Abnormal EKG changes as shown in Table 12.1 should not be attributed to regular athletic activity.
    - When present they should prompt further investigation.

Table 12.1 Comparison of Normal and Abnormal ECG Findings in Athletes

Normal ECG Findings	Abnormal ECG Findings
Sinus bradycardia > 30 bpm	Profound sinus bradycardia < 30 bpm or with sinus pauses > 3 seconds
Sinus arrhythmia	Atrial tachyarrhythmias
Ectopic atrial rhythms	Premature ventricle contractions > 2 per 10-s tracing
Junctional escape rhythms	Ventricular arrhythmias
First-degree AV block	Ventricular pre-excitation with PR < 120 ms with delta wave and wide QRS > 120 ms
Mobitz type I second-degree AV block (Wenckebach)	Mobitz type II and complete heart block
Incomplete right bundle branch block	Right ventricular hypertrophy
Early repolarization (J-point elevation)	T-wave inversions (excludes III, aVR, V1)
Convex ST-segment elevation with T-wave inversions in V1-V4 in black/African males	Brugada EKG pattern
Isolated QRS voltage for left ventricular hypertrophy	Left axis deviation
	Left atrial enlargement
	Complete left bundle branch block
	Pathologic Q waves
	ST-segment depression
	Long QTc (> 470 ms in males; > 480 ms in females)
	Short QTc (< 320 ms)
	Intraventricular conduction delay (QRS > 140 ms)

Table adapted from Drezner, JA, *Br J Sports Med* , 2013. (Seattle criteria)[11]
bpm = beats per minute
AV = atrioventricular
ms = milliseconds

Focused History and Physical Exam

- The emergency physician should rely on structured historical questions, directed family history questions, and a focused physical exam to better evaluate athletes presenting with cardiac-related concerns.
- Regardless of cardiac screening recommendations, most agree that a history and physical exam screening for cardiac abnormalities in athletes should include:
  - Special attention given to personal and family history, with particular focus on cardiac and pulmonary conditions.
    - A focused review of symptoms, with particular attention given to symptoms that develop during activity.
  - A complete physical exam should be performed, again focusing on cardiac and pulmonary exams.
    - It is advised to assess the cardiac and pulmonary portions of the exam in multiple positions (e.g., supine and standing, Valsalva) to try to elicit murmurs and palpitations.
    - It is also important to assess symmetry of radial and femoral pulses on both the right and left sides of the body.
- It is also important to discuss and consider use of (PES) in athletes presenting to the ED with athletic-associated cardiac concerns that seem age inappropriate, particularly those presenting with tachycardia, elevated blood pressure, and/or elevated temperature.
  - PES use is not limited to elite athletes. Multiple studies have documented the use of PES across all demographics.
  - Anabolic steroid use increases total cholesterol, LDL, HDL, VLDL, and triglycerides; use of these substances may lead to premature coronary artery disease in athletes.
  - Stimulants (caffeine, ephedrine, pseudoephedrine) are also considered PES, although caffeine in low to moderate doses is no longer banned by sports governing bodies.
    - Stimulant use may increase heart rate and blood pressure more than expected from regular exercise.
    - Stimulant use may increase an athlete's risk for heat injury, further stressing cardiac function.
    - Caffeine (200 mg, or the amount in two 8-oz cups of coffee) has been shown to decrease myocardial blood flow,[12] with further decreases in myocardial blood flow seen in altitude-simulated conditions.
- ***ED EVALUATION BASICS***
  - All athletes who present to the ED with chest pain should have an EKG and CXR performed.
  - It is very important to differentiate between EKG changes related to sports and exercise vs. pathologic changes.
    - Please see Table 12.1 and discussion in previous section.
  - Depending on clinical circumstances and initial diagnostic evaluation, further evaluation with cardiac biomarkers may be considered.
    - CK, CK MB, and troponin may all increase following prolonged athletic activity.
    - The patient's creatinine level should be considered when evaluating cardiac biomarkers, as dehydration/mild rhabdomyolysis may negatively impact kidney function, thus limiting the kidney's ability to clear cardiac biomarkers.
    - Cardiac biomarkers may rise to a level considered positive in a nonactive patient.[13,14,15] The clinical challenge is to determine reactive versus pathologic elevation in these biomarkers.
    - Biomarker levels typically return to baseline forty-eight to seventy-two hours post event.
    - The amount of biomarker elevation may be related to training intensity, with those running less than 35 miles/week more likely to have significantly increased levels relative to the athlete running more than 45 miles/week.[15]

  - Female athletes are also likely to have elevated biomarkers after athletic activity,[16] however the increase is typically not as significant as in active males in the same sport.
  - Teenagers have also been found to spill markers after a 90-minute run.[17] Age of less than 20 alone is not enough to rule out true cardiac etiology in athletes presenting with exercise-associated cardiac concerns.
  - Research is currently underway to determine if gender-specific cardiac biomarkers may also help better evaluate active patients with cardiac concerns.
- Basic ACLS protocols and guidelines should be followed for all patients whose initial presentation is SCD.[18]
- Symptomatic athletes should be admitted for continuous cardiac monitoring and additional evaluation.
- Asymptomatic athletes with incidental, benign EKG changes may safely be discharged from the ED with close follow-up, either with a PCP, a sports medicine specialist, or a cardiologist.
  - Depending on clinical scenario and risk factors, consider holding athlete from further sports participation until further evaluated as an outpatient by cardiology.

Differential Diagnosis – Structural and Inherited Arrhythmia Disorders

Sudden Cardiac Death

General Description

- The incidence of SCD is increasing in both the general and athletic population.
- The shocking nature of sports-related SCD is drawing increasing attention to these events by the popular press.
- Approximately 300,000 SCDs/year occur in the general population.
- A total of 3/1000 high school athletes per year suffer a SCD.[1]
- Four cardiac related deaths/year occur among NCAA athletes.[19]
- One in 184,000 marathoners experiences sudden cardiac arrest during a race.[20]
- These numbers are likely an underestimation of the true incidence of sudden cardiac arrest among runners. Given the nature and layout of most road races, it is difficult to record the actual number of runners presenting to surrounding EDs, as runners may present to a variety of hospitals in the vicinity of a race.
- A recent study has shown that individuals of African or Caribbean descent are much more likely to suffer an exercise-related sudden cardiac event than those of other ethnic backgrounds.[21]
- Males are much more frequently affected by SCD during exercise than are females; the ratio is 9:1.[1]
- Although both the general population and the active population suffer SCD, the risk factors for a cardiac event differ between the two groups (Table 12.2).

Mechanism

- The mechanism of SCD during exercise is unknown.
  - Several theories about the etiology of sudden cardiac arrest have been proposed.
  - Various arrhythmias, including atrial fibrillation, ventricular fibrillation, and atrial fibrillation triggering ventricular fibrillation, have been linked to SCD in athletes. The trigger for these arrhythmias also remains the focus of current research.

Table 12.2 Risk of Sudden Cardiac Death in the General vs. the Athletic Population

Risk Factor	General Population	Athletic Population
Coronary artery disease	80%	2.5%
Hypertrophic cardiomyopathy	5%	80%
Coronary artery anomalies		14%
Mitral valve prolapse	5%	
Acquired valve disease	5%	2.5%

- Inadequate cardiac output has also been considered a trigger of SCD in athletes; it is not clear if this reduced output is a result of structural changes, genetic characteristics, or increased heart rate associated with exercise.
- Current leading theory is that the true etiology of SCD during athletic activity is likely a combination of inadequate cardiac output and an arrhythmia.

Presentation

- Patient may be in fulminant cardiac arrest on presentation to the ED or may have been resuscitated in the field by bystanders and/or emergency medical system (EMS) providers.
- The most common presenting arrhythmia is ventricular fibrillation.
  - Patients may present with tachyarrhythmias, bradyarrhythmias or asystole.

Physical Exam

- An exam appropriate to the clinical presentation should be performed. However, patients in cardiac arrest will not have pulses and will not be breathing spontaneously.

Essential Diagnostics

- As appropriate to the urgency of the clinical situation.
  - If patient is stable, essential workup includes:
    - IV, O2, monitor
    - EKG, CXR
    - Laboratory evaluation, including CBC, CMP, and cardiac biomarkers.

ED Treatment

- Treat arrhythmias per current ACLS guidelines.[18]

Disposition

- Admit all to the intensive care unit.
- Emergent cardiology consult.
- Return to sports will be determined by the etiology of the cardiac arrest, in consultation with a cardiologist.

Pearls and Pitfalls

- Treat all cardiac arrest patients per current ACLS guidelines.
- Current 2010 guidelines emphasize high-quality CPR and rapid defibrillation.[18]

Inherited Arrhythmia Disorders

Sport-Related Syncope

General Description

- Sudden collapse that occurs either during or immediately after a period of exercise.
- Exercise does not have to be particularly intense.
- Collapse during activity is more likely to have underlying cardiac etiology than collapse immediately after exercise; this is often referred to as exercise-associated collapse (EAC) or heat syncope.
  - EAC is commonly the result of fatigue, mild dehydration, or orthostasis; however sport-related syncope should also be considered to rule out any underlying cardiac abnormalities.

Mechanism

- Several possible mechanisms for sport-related syncope have been considered, but no definitive causative theory has been proven.
  - Orthostatic hypotension
  - Electrolyte abnormality
  - Structural cardiac abnormality.
  - Cardiac dysrhythmia

Presentation

- Athletes experiencing a sport-related syncopal episode often present to the ED after prehospital care has been provided. Event physicians caring for these patients may arrive on scene when the patient is still in an altered state of consciousness.
- If the collapse occurred after the athletic event it may be beneficial to keep the athlete supine and elevate the legs by flexing the hips and holding the feet in the air.

Physical Examination

- The initial physical exam should ensure that no concurrent trauma was sustained during the sport-associated syncopal event. If there is

any concern for a cervical spine injury or head injury, basic immobilization should be instituted.
- Initial physical exam should include vital signs, blood glucose, and EKG/cardiac monitoring.
- A thorough cardiopulmonary examination should be performed, with attention focused on cardiac murmurs and arrhythmias.

Essential Diagnostics
- A formal EKG should be performed.
- A chest x-ray may help be beneficial to evaluate for cardiomegaly or pulmonary edema.
- Continuous cardiac monitoring should be performed.
- Standard laboratory testing should include cardiac markers, electrolytes, and CBC. Additional tests to consider include D-dimer and thyroid studies.
- If associated trauma is suspected appropriate imaging studies should be performed.

ED Treatment
- Patients with exercise-associated syncope or collapse should remain on continuous cardiac monitoring while initial diagnostic studies are completed.
- If an underlying cause of the syncope is identified (e.g., dehydration, electrolyte abnormality) this abnormality should be treated appropriately.
- Cardiology consultation should be considered in all patients with exercise-associated syncope in whom no identifiable cause is identified.

Disposition
- If no identifiable cause of the exercise-associated syncopal event is identified the patient should be admitted to cardiology to continue the evaluation.
- If a noncardiac cause of the syncopal event is identified and corrected in the ED the patient may be discharged home with PCP or sports medicine follow-up. The patient should not return to athletic activity until cleared by the PCP or sports medicine physician.
- If a cardiac cause of the syncopal event is identified the patient should be admitted to cardiology to continue the evaluation.
- If no cause of the syncopal event is identified the patient should be admitted to cardiology to continue the evaluation.

Pediatric Considerations
- Pediatric patients suffering a syncopal event during a sporting event should be admitted for further evaluation.

Pearls and Pitfalls
- It is important to differentiate between whether syncope occurred during or after exercise.
  - Syncope that occurs during exercise is always concerning and needs further evaluation.
- Causes of sports-related syncope vary from benign to life threatening, thus a high degree of suspicion should be maintained at all times.

Wolff Parkinson White syndrome (WPW)

General Description
- WPW is a pre-excitation condition triggered by the presence of an accessory conduction pathway between the atria and ventricles.
- The rate of WPW among athletes is similar to that of the general population, with 1 in 1000 people afflicted with this condition.[11]

Mechanism
- The trigger(s) that leads to the development of the accessory pathway remains to be determined in both the active and in the general population.
- The presence of the accessory pathway may lead to tachyarrhythmias such as supraventricular tachycardia and atrial fibrillation.
  - However, atrial fibrillation triggered by WPW often leads to ventricular fibrillation during exercise likely due to the further decrease in blood flow.

Presentation
- Patients with WPW typically present to the ED with a tachydysrhythmia, near syncope, syncope, palpitations, or sudden cardiac arrest (particularly during exercise).

Physical Examination

- Vital signs should be performed as soon as the patient arrives in the ED.
- A thorough cardiovascular examination should be performed.

Essential Diagnostics

- An EKG should be performed as soon as the patient arrives at the ED.
  - Several EKG findings are characteristic of WPW including:
    - Short PR interval
    - Widening of the QRS complex.
    - Presence of a delta wave
- Routine lab testing, including cardiac markers, should be performed.
  - Thyroid studies should be considered.
- Chest x-ray (PA and lateral) should be performed.

ED Management

- If an athlete sustains a tachydysrhythmia or sudden cardiac arrest due to presumed WPW, standard ACLS resuscitation protocols should be followed.[18]
- If circulation returns, the affected athlete should be admitted for further cardiac monitoring and evaluation, specifically electrophysiologic evaluation.
- If an athlete presents to the ED with sport-related syncope, ED management is as previously described.

Disposition

- All patients diagnosed with WPW in the ED should be admitted for further evaluation and testing, particularly electrophysiologic evaluation.
- Cardiology should be consulted while the patient is in the ED.
- Athletes found to have WPW (without associated tachydysrhythmia) on routine screening may be referred for outpatient electrophysiologic evaluation as long as the athlete remains asymptomatic.

Pediatric Considerations

- WPW has been diagnosed in teenage athletes and should be considered in this patient population.

Pearls and Pitfalls

- All EKGs performed in the ED should be evaluated for presence of an accessory pathway.
  - If an accessory pathway is suspected, the athlete needs evaluation by cardiology prior to return to sport even if asymptomatic.
- All symptomatic athletes should not be allowed back to sports and need further evaluation by cardiology.

Catecholaminergic Polymorphic Ventricular Tachycardia

General Description

- Catecholaminergic polymorphic ventricular tachycardia (CPVT) is a ventricular arrhythmia due to abnormalities in cardiac metabolism of calcium.
- This genetically transmitted condition typically results in ventricular tachycardia (and occasionally ventricular fibrillation) and is typically triggered by exercise.

Mechanism

- Significant research is being conducted to isolate the specific abnormality in calcium metabolism.
- Several genetic mutations have been identified that likely contribute to this condition.

Presentation

- Individuals suffering from CPVT often present to the ED after an sport-related syncopal event.
- These patients may be in polymorphic ventricular tachycardia or may be in ventricular fibrillation.
- Like the other channelopathies, the initial presenting symptom of CPVT may be SCD.

Physical Examination

- A focused cardiopulmonary examination should be performed.

Essential Diagnostics

- The patient with suspected CPVT should be immediately placed on a continuous cardiac monitor with pulse oximetry and blood pressure monitoring capacity.

- A formal EKG should be performed.
  - The baseline EKG of patients with CPVT is typically normal (with the exception of mild bradycardia).
  - Patients with CPVT presenting in PVT will have the typical findings of polymorphic ventricular tachycardia.
  - There are no specific EKG findings unique to CPVT.
- Bedside echocardiography should be considered to evaluate for other potential causes of the presenting dysrhythmia.
- Routine laboratory testing should include cardiac markers, electrolytes, CBC, and thyroid studies. Additional testing may include a D-dimer.
- Chest x-ray (PA and lateral) should also be performed to rule out other potential causes of the dysrhythmia.

ED Treatment

- Any patient with suspected CPVT that presents with sudden cardiac arrest should have basic resuscitative measures continued until such efforts are deemed futile by the treating physician.
- CPVT patients presenting with stable ventricular tachycardia should have the essential diagnostic procedures performed to attempt to elucidate the cause of the episode.
  - Once the essential diagnostic studies are complete, these patients should receive IV hydration during the initial evaluation process.
- Possible CPVT patients with unstable ventricular tachycardia or ventricular fibrillation should be cardioverted as per ACLS protocols.

Disposition

- All patients with suspected CPVT should be admitted to continue the evaluation.
- Cardiology should be consulted for all suspected cases of CPVT.
  - Exercise testing is typically performed to try to trigger an episode of CPVT.
  - Cardiology will determine when (and if) a patient is able to return to sports.
  - If cardiology determines that CPVT is the diagnosis, patients may be started on calcium channel blockers or beta blockers. Some patients ultimately require pacemaker/defibrillator placement.

Pediatric Considerations

- The diagnosis of CPVT should be considered in children with a family history of presenting with sport-related syncope or SCD.

Pearls and Pitfalls

- A high degree of suspicion should be maintained for any symptomatic athletes.
  - Athletes should always be counseled against further sports participation when there is concern for CPVT or another cardiac abnormality.
- Symptomatic athletes and/or athletes with abnormalities on their EKGs need either admission for further workup or close outpatient follow-up with cardiology.

Brugada Syndrome

General Description

- This syndrome is a sodium channelopathy known for its characteristic EKG changes and often leads to ventricular dysrhythmias and SCD.
- The condition is inherited via an autosomal-dominant transmission.
- Males are much more commonly affected than females.
- Young patients are much more commonly affected than those over 50.

Mechanism

- Many theories exist regarding the mechanism of Brugada syndrome, with the leading theory that the condition is an autosomal-dominant inherited sodium channelopathy.
- Arrhythmias may also occur due to an imbalance in sympathetic and parasympathetic tone.

Presentation

- Patients with Brugada syndrome typically present with SCD.
  - Patients may also present after a syncopal episode.
  - Up to 20 percent of patients with Brugada syndrome may be asymptomatic.

Physical Examination

- A focused cardiopulmonary examination should be performed.
  - The physical examination, however, is usually unremarkable.

Essential Diagnostics

- The patient with suspected Brugada syndrome should be placed on continuous cardiac monitoring, including blood pressure and pulse oximetry.
- An EKG should be performed immediately.
  - Characteristic EKG changes are often but not always present and include:
    - Pseudo–RBBB
    - ST/T-wave changes in V1-V3.
- Basic laboratory studies include cardiac markers, basic electrolytes, point of care glucose testing, and a D-dimer (based on clinical suspicion for pulmonary embolism).
- Chest x-ray (PA and lateral) should be performed to detect other possible causes of the presentation.
- An echocardiogram should be performed to evaluate for other potential causes of the presentation.

ED Treatment

- Patients presenting in sudden cardiac arrest should have ACLS resuscitative protocols[18] followed until the treating physician determines the effort to be futile.
- Patients with syncopal episodes associated with Brugada syndrome or those successfully resuscitated should have cardiac pacing (preferably transvenous) until a permanent pacemaker/defibrillator can be placed.

Disposition

- All patients with suspected Brugada syndrome (previously undiagnosed) should have emergent cardiology consultation and be admitted to cardiology (preferably the cardiac care unit) to facilitate further evaluation and management.
- Decisions regarding return to activities is to be made by cardiology.
  - These patients are not typically allowed to return to sports.

Pediatric Considerations

- The diagnosis of Brugada syndrome should be considered in children, particularly males, with a family history of presenting with sport-related syncope or SCD.

Pearls and Pitfalls

- Most often patients are not diagnosed with this condition until they are symptomatic and present with syncope or sudden cardiac arrest.
- All family members of patients suspected of having this condition should be notified and screened.
- Treatment is placement of an implantable defibrillator to prevent sudden cardiac arrest from ventricular arrhythmia.

Commotio Cordis

General Description

- Sudden cardiac arrest triggered by direct, blunt chest wall trauma.
- Multiple sports have had deaths related to commotio cordis, including baseball, lacrosse, and the martial arts.
- Protective gear (i.e., chest protectors for baseball) has not been shown to reduce the incidence of commotio cordis.

Mechanism

- Forces are transmitted directly from the chest wall to the precordium, altering the normal electrical conduction of the heart.
- EKG studies have demonstrated that the transmission of forces generates an R wave prior to completion of the previously initiated T wave (R on T phenomenon) resulting in ventricular fibrillation.
- Chest wall impact 30–15 milliseconds before T-wave peak is most likely to generate ventricular tachycardia.[22]
- Chest wall impact at 40 mph is most likely to generate ventricular tachycardia.[23]

Presentation

- If a patient is successfully resuscitated in the field, presentation to the ED will be as a standard post-arrest patient.
- There may be obvious signs of chest wall trauma resulting from the blunt force that triggered commotio cordis.

Physical Examination

- The treating physician should carefully examine the chest wall for signs of trauma (rib fracture, sternal fracture, contusion) in addition to the commotio cordis.
- A thorough cardiopulmonary examination should be performed.

Essential Diagnostics

- The post–commotio cordis patient should be placed on a cardiac monitor.
- An EKG should be performed.
- Routine lab testing, including cardiac markers, should be performed.
- Chest x-ray (PA and lateral) should be performed to assess for pulmonary contusions, rib fractures, and sternal fractures.

ED Management

- If a patient is successfully resuscitated in the field, the mainstay of ED therapy is supportive care.

Disposition

- Post–commotio cordis patients should be admitted for continued cardiac monitoring and evaluation.
- Cardiology should be consulted while the patient is in the ED.
- The decision regarding return to school/sports should be made by cardiology.

Pediatric Considerations

- Commotio cordis is primarily a pediatric diagnosis based on the increased chest wall compliance in younger patients.

Pearls and Pitfalls

- Time to defibrillator application is key to survival.
- This highlights the need for AED presence and appropriate placement at youth sporting events.

Atrial Fibrillation

General Description

- Atrial fibrillation is the asymmetric and irregular contraction of the atria, resulting in significantly decreased blood flow to the ventricles.
- The incidence of atrial fibrillation among middle-aged athletes is five times higher than in the general population.[24]
- Atrial fibrillation is more common in endurance athletes with years of training than in power athletes and athletes with shorter training histories.

Mechanism

- Multiple etiologies of atrial fibrillation have been identified, including accessory pathways, thyroid dysfunction, valvular dysfunction, structural cardiac changes, and genetic mutations.
- Atrial fibrillation is not attributed to regular athletic training and warrants further evaluation.

Presentation

- Patients with atrial fibrillation may present with palpitations, decreased exercise tolerance, sport-related syncope or SCD.
- Athletes with atrial fibrillation may experience a decrease in exercise capacity (due to decreased purposeful blood flow and subsequent decreased ability to meet oxygen demands of exercise).

Physical Examination

- Vital signs should be performed upon the patient's arrival.
  - Patients with atrial fibrillation may be tachycardic or may have a normal heart rate.
- A thorough cardiopulmonary examination should be performed.
  - These patients will often have a classic irregularly irregular rhythm.

Essential Diagnostics

- An EKG should be performed immediately.
- Standard lab studies should be sent, including CBC, CMP, cardiac biomarkers, thyroid studies, and coagulation studies.

ED Management

- Athletes with atrial fibrillation should have basic resuscitation principles followed based upon severity of presentation.

- Athletes with atrial fibrillation without sudden cardiac arrest should be placed on a monitor and have IV access established.
- If the athlete is in atrial fibrillation with rapid ventricular response and is hemodynamically stable, medications should be considered to lower the heart rate to less than 100 beats per minute.
- Anticoagulation should be initiated if the patient has had atrial fibrillation for an unknown length of time.
- If the athlete can ensure that the symptoms have been present for less than forty-eight hours, anticoagulation may not be immediately needed.
- If the athlete is in atrial fibrillation with rapid ventricular response and is hemodynamically unstable, consider cardioversion.

Disposition

- Athletes presenting to the ED with exercise-associated symptoms should be admitted to the hospital to continue the cardiac evaluation and initiate medications as needed.
- Cardiology consultation may be considered in the ED.
- Athletes who are rate controlled and do not have underlying structural heart disease may be able to participate in sports.
    - Beta blockers, which are commonly used in the management of atrial fibrillation, are prohibited in some competitive sports. These medications can also limit the athlete's ability to compete in some sports due to the physiologic effect on heart rate.
- Consideration should also be given to ablative therapy, as this may allow return to sport without restrictions.

Complications

- Long-term anticoagulation may be required for athletes with atrial fibrillation.
    - This may limit an athlete’s ability to compete, particularly in contact sports.

Pediatric Considerations

- Atrial fibrillation has been diagnosed in adolescent athletes and should be part of the differential diagnosis for sport-related syncope.

Pearls and Pitfalls

- Etiology of atrial fibrillation should be sought in all athletes presenting with this arrhythmia.
- Treatment of athletes with atrial fibrillation is similar to that of the general population.
- Depending on the severity of symptoms and treatment, athletes may still be able to participate in sports.

Long QT Syndrome

General Description

- This syndrome is characterized by an increased QTc interval on EKG.
- The incidence of long QT syndrome is approximately 1 in 10,000.[11]

Mechanism

- This is a genetically transmitted potassium channelopathy.

Presentation

- Individuals with long QT syndrome are often asymptomatic until presentation with syncope or cardiac arrest (often due to ventricular fibrillation).

Physical Examination

- Vital signs should be performed as soon as the patient arrives in the ED.
- A thorough cardiopulmonary exam should be performed.

Essential Diagnostics

- An EKG is essential to making the diagnosis of long QT syndrome; this should be performed as soon as the patient arrives in the ED.
- EKG criteria are used to make the diagnosis of long QT syndrome and are the basis of referral for further evaluation.
    - Heart rate should be more than 60 beats per minute when calculating the QTc; the standard formula is not reliable when a patient is bradycardic.
    - Age- and gender-specific norms have been established.
    - See Table 12.1 for general guidelines.

ED Management

- Athletes presenting with sport-related syncope or with exercise-associated SCD should be resuscitated using standard ACLS protocols.
- If the athlete has return of spontaneous circulation, continuous cardiac monitoring should be performed.
- An EKG should be completed as soon as possible. Attention should be paid to the standard EKG parameters, with particular focus on the QT and the QTc.
- Standard blood testing should be performed, including CBC, CMP, cardiac biomarkers, and coagulation studies.
- Treatment with pharmacotherapy or an implantable defibrillator may be considered, but does not necessarily need to be initiated from the ED, depending on the clinical scenario.

Disposition

- Any athlete that presents to the ED for sport-related syncope should be admitted for further evaluation and possible electrophysiologic testing.
- Cardiology consultation may be considered in the ED but is not required for hemodynamically stable patients.
- Asymptomatic athletes with EKG findings concerning for long QT syndrome should be sent for emergent outpatient evaluation.
- These athletes should be counseled to avoid exercise and training until this evaluation has been completed.
- Most athletes with this condition are restricted from participating in competitive sports.[25, 26]

Complications

- Athletes with long QT syndrome frequently require pacemaker/defibrillator placement.

Pediatric Considerations

- Pediatric athletes with a family history of long QT syndrome should be evaluated by cardiology prior to starting regular athletic activity, even if asymptomatic.

Pearls and Pitfalls

- The clinician should maintain a high index of suspicion for long QT syndrome when evaluating athletes with exercise-related sport-related syncope.

Short QT Syndrome

General Description

- Short QT syndrome is an inherited channelopathy.

Mechanism

- The short QT interval leads to abnormally short repolarization periods, predisposing the affected individual to cardiac dysrhythmias, especially ventricular fibrillation.

Presentation

- Individuals with short QT syndrome typically present with SCD, syncope, or palpitations.

Physical Examination

- Vital signs should be performed as soon as the patient arrives in the ED.
- A thorough cardiopulmonary exam should be performed.

Essential Diagnostics

- An EKG is essential to making the diagnosis of short QT syndrome; this should be performed as soon as the patient arrives in the ED.
- EKG criteria are used to make the diagnosis of short QT syndrome and are the basis of referral for further evaluation.
- The same heart rate criteria apply for calculating QTc as discussed in the long QT section.
- QTc of less than 320 milliseconds is diagnostic.

ED Management

- ACLS resuscitation protocols should be followed in patients presenting in cardiac arrest.[18]
- Patients presenting with syncope or palpitations should have the standard ED evaluation performed to further evaluate these conditions.

Disposition

- All patients found to have a short QT/QTc should be admitted for further evaluation.

- Symptomatic patients should be seen by cardiology prior to admission.
- Athletes may be managed with pharmacotherapy or an implantable defibrillator.
- Athletes are usually restricted to low-level sports.[25, 26]

Complications

- Patients with short QT syndrome often require pacemaker/defibrillator placement for long-term management.

Pediatric Considerations

- Short QT syndrome has been diagnosed in children as young as one year of age.
- The ED physician should consider this diagnosis in children presenting with acute life-threatening events.

Pearls and Pitfalls

- Don't forget to evaluate EKGs not just for prolonged QTc, but also short QTc.
- Short QT syndrome has a much more varied presentation among affected family members than does long QT syndrome.
  - Family history is important but may not be as revealing as the family history in a patient with long QT syndrome.

Structural Disorders

Myocarditis

General Description

- Myocarditis is the inflammation of the cardiac muscle.

Mechanism

- Myocarditis is typically caused by a viral infection; several viruses have been implicated, including:
  - Coxsackie virus
  - Parvovirus
  - Enterovirus
  - Hepatitis C
  - HIV
  - CMV
- Myocarditis has both an acute phase and a chronic phase.
- The causative viral agent is rarely detected in the acute phase.
- Autoimmune causes of myocarditis have also been identified, but this is significantly less common in the athletic population.

Presentation

- The most common presenting symptoms of myocarditis include fever, chills, and sweats.
- A history of a viral illness in the last two to three weeks is common.
- Chest pain is rare in isolated myocarditis.
- Patients with myocarditis may present with a variety of cardiac complications, including bradycardia or tachycardia, heart block, heart failure, or SCD.
- Myocarditis is responsible for a small percentage of SCD in athletes.

Physical Examination

- The physical examination should focus on the cardiopulmonary examination, with particular attention paid to the sequelae of heart failure, including:
  - Murmur
  - Gallop
  - Rales and/or rhonchi
  - Peripheral edema

Essential Diagnostics

- The key to diagnosing myocarditis is to maintain a high suspicion for the condition.
- The patient with suspected myocarditis should be immediately be placed on continuous cardiac monitoring (including blood pressure and pulse oximetry).
- An EKG should be performed immediately.
  - Global ST segment elevations are the hallmark of myocarditis.
- Standard laboratory testing includes cardiac markers, CBC with differential, ESR, CRP, blood cultures times two, and basic electrolytes.
- Chest x-ray (PA and lateral)
- Echocardiography

ED Management

- Patients with suspected myocarditis should remain on continuous cardiac monitoring

while the essential diagnostic studies are performed.
- Patients should be treated based on their initial presenting symptoms. Blood pressure support, diuresis, and temporary pacing may be required.
- Cardiology consultation should be obtained when the diagnosis of myocarditis is considered.
- Infectious disease consultation may also be considered, based on patient presentation.
- Cardiothoracic surgery consultation may also be considered in severely decompensated myocarditis patients.

Disposition

- All patients with suspected myocarditis should be admitted to cardiology; several of these patients may require admission to the cardiac care unit.
- The definitive diagnosis of myocarditis is made via biopsy; this is not usually performed in the ED.
- Athletes with myocarditis should never be allowed to return to play.
    - Return to sports may be considered once there is no evidence of structural heart disease or significant EKG abnormalities.

Complications

- In some cases, athletes with myocarditis may develop dilated cardiomyopathy or other segmental wall motion abnormalities which increase their risk for SCD.

Pearls and Pitfalls

- A high index of suspicion is required to make the diagnosis of myocarditis. Consider this condition in any athlete presenting with general concerns following a viral illness.

Marfan Syndrome

General Description

- Marfan syndrome is a congenital defect (autosomal dominant) in the fibrillin gene, leading to a variety of connective tissue abnormalities.
- Marfan syndrome is characterized by several physical characteristics:
    - Lens dislocation
    - Unusually long, thin fingers
    - Limbs longer than expected relative to trunk length.
    - Thoracic wall deformities
    - Scoliosis
    - Aortic root dilation
    - Aortic aneurysms

Presentation

- Individuals with Marfan syndrome are typically identified based on the previously described physical characteristics.
- Patients are usually identified prior to presenting with catastrophic cardiac complications (i.e., ruptured aortic aneurysm or aortic root dissection).

Physical Examination

- The emergency physician should perform a thorough family history, focusing on identifying family members with Marfan syndrome.
- The emergency physician should focus on identifying the previously described characteristic physical findings of Marfan syndrome.

Essential Diagnostics

- Specific diagnostic criteria exist to formally make the diagnosis of Marfan syndrome (Table 12.3).
- The presence of major criteria in two organ systems and one minor criteria in a different organ system confirms the clinical diagnosis of Marfan syndrome in an individual with no family history of the condition.
- If a patient has a family history of Marfan syndrome, one major and one minor criteria in different organ systems will confirm the diagnosis.
- Genetic testing is available to identify Marfan syndrome (FBN1 mutation).
- Echocardiography should be performed to evaluate aortic root parameters and aortic contours.
- Any patient with suspected Marfan's related musculoskeletal abnormalities should have x-rays of these anatomic areas performed.
- Either CT scan or MRI may identify dural ectasia.

Table 12.3 Diagnostic Criteria for Marfan's syndrome[27]

	Major Criteria	Minor Criteria
Musculoskeletal	Severe pectus excavatum Upper to lower extremity ratio <0.85 Wing span: height ration > 1.05 Thumb-index finger overlap around wrist Scoliosis >20^0 Hind foot collapse	Hypermobile joints High palate Marfan facies Minor to moderate pectus excavatum
Ocular	Lens dislocation	Flat cornea Myopia
Cardiovascular	Ascending aorta dilation Ascending aorta dissection	Descending aortic dissection or dilation Mitral valve calcification MVP Pulmonary artery dilation
Pulmonary	None	Blebs (typically apical) Spontaneous pneumothorax
Skin	Dural ectasia (lumbosacral)	Recurrent hernia Striae

Abstracted from Sonh GH et al.[27]

- A slit lamp exam should be performed to evaluate for lens dislocation or retinal detachment.

Treatment

- ED treatment should be tailored to the patient's presentation.
- The emergency physician should focus on blood pressure control in patients with aortic root dilation or aortic dissection.

Disposition

- Previously undiagnosed but asymptomatic Marfan's patients should be urgently evaluated as an outpatient. If this rapid outpatient evaluation cannot be arranged the patient should be admitted. Symptomatic patients should be admitted for evaluation.
- Patients with aortic root or aortic pathology should be emergently evaluated by both cardiology and cardiovascular surgery.
- Athletes need close monitoring but may perform low-level activities depending on amount of aortic root dilation or mitral regurgitation and family history.[25]
- The decision regarding return to sports should be made by cardiology.

Complications

- Aortic root and descending aorta dilatation may lead to aortic dissection and rupture.
  - May also cause left ventricular dysfunction and mitral valve prolapse.

Pediatric Considerations

- Pediatric patients may display several of the characteristic findings of Marfan syndrome. Presence of these sequelae should prompt the emergency physician to inquire about family history and to initiate the evaluation regardless of whether the patient is symptomatic.

Pearls and Pitfalls

- Patients without a known family history of Marfan syndrome may not be aware of the diagnosis. Physicians should initiate the evaluation for the syndrome if the physical features are present.

Mitral Valve Prolapse

General Description and Mechanism

- Mitral valve prolapse (MVP) is the incomplete closure of the mitral valve typically due to

structural abnormalities (congenital or acquired).
    - This incomplete closure of the valve may result in the valve intruding into the atrium during cardiac contraction.
- Despite this abnormal valvular motion, the majority of patients with MVP are asymptomatic.
- There is a low rate of adverse cardiac events with MVP.
- Approximately 5 percent of the population has MVP.
- Women are more likely than men to have MVP.

Presentation

- The majority of patients with MVP are asymptomatic.
- Patients may become symptomatic due to autonomic difficulties or natural progression of the abnormal anatomy.
- Patients with autonomic-associated symptoms may present with:
    - Palpitations
    - Anxiety
    - Excess fatigue
    - Syncope/near syncope
- Patients with natural progression of underlying abnormal anatomy may present with typical symptoms of heart failure.

Physical Examination

- Particular focus should be given to the cardiac examination.
- The hallmark finding of MVP is a late systolic click; a late apical murmur may or may not be associated with the click.
- The emergency physician should also pay attention to the sequelae of heart failure.

Essential Diagnostics

- The patient with suspected MVP should immediately be placed on continuous cardiac monitoring, including pulse oximetry and blood pressure monitoring.
- An EKG should be performed immediately.
- Echocardiography should be performed in the ED.
    - Specific criteria have been described to aid in the diagnosis of pathologic MVP.[28]
- Basic laboratory testing should include cardiac markers, basic electrolytes, thyroid studies, and possibly a D-dimer (based on presentation and clinical suspicion).
- Chest x-ray (PA and lateral) should be performed in patients with suspected progression of known disease to evaluate for heart failure.

ED Treatment

- No treatment is needed for asymptomatic patients.
- Patients with autonomic-associated MVP that have returned to baseline typically do not require emergent treatment.
- Patients with progression of underlying anatomic abnormalities should have treatment based on the extent of heart failure present.
- Most athletes with MVP may continue to participate in sports as long as they are asymptomatic and there is no personal or family history of significant cardiac events.[29]

Disposition

- Asymptomatic patients may be safely discharged from the ED to follow-up with a PCP.
- Patients with autonomic-associated symptoms of MVP that have returned to baseline may also be discharged from the ED.
- These patients should avoid caffeine and other stimulants until seen by a PCP or by cardiology (as an outpatient).
    - These patients should also avoid exercise until seen for follow-up.
- These patients may be discharged with twenty-four-hour cardiac monitoring.
- Emergency physicians are not advised to start this patient group on long-term management medications (e.g., beta blockers).
- Patients with progression of underlying anatomic abnormalities should be admitted to cardiology for further management of heart failure.
- These patients may benefit from emergent consultation with cardiovascular surgery to evaluate the need for emergent valve replacement.

Pediatric Considerations

- The characteristic click and murmur of MVP are commonly seen in the pediatric population. If these are incidental findings the patient may be advised to refrain from exercise until seen by a pediatrician or pediatric cardiologist.

Pearls and Pitfalls

- MVP has a low risk of adverse cardiac events.
- Most athletes may continue sports participation as long as they are asymptomatic and have no personal or family history of significant cardiac events.

Hypertrophic Cardiomyopathy (HCM)

General Description

- This is the most common cause of SCD in young athletes in the United States.
- It is characterized by an increase in left ventricular size.
- It may affect any portion of the left ventricle, but most commonly the intraventricular septum.
- A family history of SCD before the age of 35 should raise suspicion of a familial component to the presentation.
- Multiple alleles causing HCM have been identified.
  - Genotype testing is increasingly used to identify at-risk athletes, particularly those with a concerning family history.

Mechanism

- The left ventricular wall increases in thickness due to genetics, pathologic conditions, exercise, or a combination of factors.
- Left ventricular cavity diameter may also change due to the previously mentioned factors.
  - Normal left ventricular wall thickness is less than 11 mm.
  - Measurements between 12–15 mm are considered indeterminate.
  - Left ventricular wall thickness of greater than 15 mm is considered frank hypertrophy.
- This increase in wall thickness may not be symmetric around the ventricle, further limiting cardiac output.
- Many athletes have changes in both left ventricular wall thickness and cavity diameter.
- A small percentage of athletes also have changes to the right ventricle.

Presentation

- Patients with hypertrophic cardiomyopathy may present to the ED with a variety of symptoms ranging from chest pain, dyspnea (at rest or with exertion), decreased exercise tolerance, near syncope/syncope, to sudden cardiac arrest.

Physical Examinations

- Always check vital signs first.
- A thorough cardiopulmonary examination is mandatory.
  - Cardiac auscultation listening for murmurs.
    - An outflow murmur present with Valsalva but not at rest is pathognomonic for HCM.
  - Also assess for signs of heart failure.
    - Listen to lung sounds.
    - Assess for jugular venous distention (JVD) and for peripheral edema.

Essential Diagnostics

- An EKG should be performed immediately.
  - Among individuals with hypertrophic cardiomyopathy, 90–95 percent have EKG changes.[30]
  - Left ventricular hypertrophy is the most common (using standard criteria).
- Routine lab testing (CBC, CMP, cardiac biomarkers, coagulation studies) should be sent to monitor patient status and to evaluate for possible triggering etiologies.
- Chest x-ray (PA and lateral) should be performed to evaluate cardiac size.
- An echocardiogram should be performed to more clearly delineate cardiac parameters.
  - Echocardiogram measurement is considered the current gold standard for determining wall thickness.

ED Management

- Patients experiencing SCD should have the basic principles of ACLS followed.[18]

- In stable patients, further management should be based upon symptoms and acuity of presentation.

Disposition

- Patients who are otherwise stable may be considered for discharge with close outpatient follow-up with cardiology.
  - Decision to discharge vs. admit will be determined by the acuity of the presentation and should be done in consultation with a cardiologist.
- Patients should be instructed to not engage in any physical activity until they have followed up with cardiology.

Pediatric Considerations

- Pediatric patients, particularly any teenage athletes or a teenager with a family history of hypertrophic cardiomyopathy, are at risk for the condition and should be evaluated for HCM, even if they are asymptomatic.

Pearls and Pitfalls

- Hypertrophic cardiomyopathy should be considered in any athletic patient presenting with cardiac complaints.
- It is critical to obtain a thorough family history as well as a thorough athletic history.
- It is also critical to auscultate for cardiac murmurs both at rest and with Valsalva.

Arrhythmogenic Right Ventricular Cardiomyopathy (ARVC)

General Description

- ARVC is characterized by fatty infiltration of the right ventricular muscle cells, not an increase in the muscle cells as is typically seen in left ventricular hypertrophy.
- The true incidence of this condition is still under investigation, but is as high as 1 in 1000 in the general population.
- Individuals from the Veneto region of Italy have a significantly higher rate of ARVC.

Mechanism

- This condition is due to a genetic mutation.
- Inheritance is believed to be an autosomal dominant.

Presentation

- The initial presentation of ARVC is often SCD.

Physical Examination

- The emergency physician should complete a thorough cardiopulmonary examination, focusing on vital signs, presence of a cardiac murmur, presence of a cardiac dysrhythmia, abnormal breath sounds, and signs of right heart failure.

Essential Diagnostics

- An EKG should be performed immediately.
  - No characteristic EKG abnormality is associated with ARVC.
- Routine lab testing (CBC, CMP, cardiac biomarkers, coagulation studies) should be sent to monitor patient status and to evaluate for possible triggering etiologies.
- Chest x-ray (PA and lateral) should be performed to evaluate cardiac size.
- An echocardiogram should be performed to more clearly delineate cardiac parameters.

ED Management

- Patients that arrive to the ED with pulses should be placed on a monitor immediately.
- An EKG should be performed as soon as possible after the patient arrives in the ED.
- Further management is based upon presenting symptoms and acuity of presentation.

Disposition

- Patients arriving in the ED with suspected ARVC should be evaluated by cardiology.
- Patients should be admitted to facilitate completion of the evaluation, initiation of medications (as needed) and for further counseling.
- The time to return to sports should be determined by cardiology.

Pediatric Considerations

- Pediatric patients, particularly any teenage athletes or a teenager with a family history of ARVC, are at risk for the condition and should be evaluated for the genetic mutation.

Pearls and Pitfalls

- ARVC should be considered in any athletic patient presenting with cardiac concerns. It is critical to obtain a thorough family history as well as a thorough athletic history.
- Patients experiencing SCD in the field should have the basic principles of resuscitation followed and ACLS protocols followed.[18]
- Patients should be transported to the nearest ED as soon as possible.

Coronary Artery Anomalies

General Description

- Atypical anatomy of the coronary arteries.
- These are fairly common in athletes; variants are seen in up to one-third of athletes.[31]

Mechanism

- The anomalous artery often leads to decreased myocardial blood flow and potential catastrophic consequences, particularly during exercise.

Presentation

- Presenting symptom is typically sport-related syncope or cardiac arrest.
- The artery affected and the athlete's dominance (right vs. left coronary artery) may affect the athlete's presentation.

Physical Examination

- A thorough cardiopulmonary examination should be performed with particular attention paid to any murmurs heard, or any signs of heart failure.

Essential Diagnostics

- The patient should be placed on a cardiac monitor.
- An EKG should be performed.
- Routine lab testing, including cardiac markers, should be performed.
- Chest x-ray (PA and lateral) should be performed.

ED Management

- Standard principles of ACLS resuscitation should be followed when an athlete has a sudden cardiac arrest during sports.[18]

Disposition

- If circulation returns, patients should be admitted for cardiac monitoring and further testing, including:
  - Echocardiogram
  - Stress exercise testing
  - Cardiac MRI
  - Cardiac catheterization
    - Anomalous coronary arteries are difficult to detect on routine testing; cardiac catheterization is often required to detect the anatomic variants.
- The decision regarding return to sports should be made by cardiology.

Pediatric Considerations

- Teenage patients presenting with sudden cardiac arrest during sports may have anomalous coronary arteries.
- The condition is rarely diagnosed in preteen patients.

Pearls and Pitfalls

- A high index of suspicion is required to make the diagnosis of anomalous coronary arteries.

Recommended Reading

Pellaccia A and Crawford MH, eds. The athlete's heart: On the border between physiology and pathology. *Cardiology Clinics.* 2007 August;25(3).

Maron BJ and Zipes DP. 36th Bethesda Conference: Eligibility recommendations for athletes with cardiovascular abnormalities. *J Am Coll Cardiol.* 2005:45(8):1313–75.

Lawless CE, Olshansky B et al.. Sports and exercise cardiology in the United States: Cardiovascular specialists as members of the athlete healthcare team. *J Am Coll Cardiol.* 2014;63(15):1461–1472.

References

1. Maron BJ, Thompson PD et al.. Recommendations and considerations related to preparticipation screening for cardiovascular abnormalities in competitive athletes: 2007 update, a scientific statement from the American Heart Association Council on Nutrition, Physical Activity and Metabolism. *Circulation* 2007;115:1643–55.
2. 2013-2014 NCAA Sports Medicine Handbook, 11. Accessed 14 May 2014. www.princeton.edu/uhs/pdfs/2013-14-NCAA-Sport Medicine-Handbook.pdf
3. Charboneau ML, Mencias T and Hoch AZ. *Cardiovascular Screening Practices in Collegiate Student-Athletes.* PMR. In press.
4. The International Olympic Committee (IOC) Consensus Statement on Periodic Health Evaluation of Elite Athletes. March 2009. 3-36-10-36. Accessed 14 May 2014. www.olympic.org/Documents/Reports/EN/en_report_1448.pdf
5. Asif IM and Drezner JA. Detecting occult cardiac disease in athletes: History that makes a difference. *Br J Sports Med.* 2013;47:669–70.
6. Rawlins J, Carre F et al.. Ethnic differences in physiological cardiac adaptation to Intense physical exercise in highly trained female a thletes. *Circulation.* 2010;121:1078–1085.
7. Corrado D, Pelliccia A et al.. Recommendations for interpretation of 12-lead electrocardiogram in the athlete. *Eur Heart J* (2010) 31, 243–259.
8. Muramoto D, Yong CM et al.. Patterns and prognosis of all components of the J-wave pattern in multiethnic athletes and ambulatory patients. *Am Heart J.* 2014;167;259–66.
9. Noseworthy PA and Baggish AL. The prevalence and clinical significance of J wave patterns in athletes. *J Electrocard.* 46 (2013) 424–6.
10. Schmied C and Borjesson M. Sudden cardiac death in athletes. *J Intern Med.* 2014; 275:93–103.
11. Drezner JA, Ackerman MK, Cannon BC et al.. Abnormal electrocardiographic findings in athletes: Recognizing changes suggestive of primary electrical disease. *Br J Sports Med* 2013;47:153–67.
12. Namdar M et al.. Caffeine decreases exercise-induced myocardial flow reserve. *J Am Col Card.* 2006;47(2): 405–10.
13. Leers MPG et al.. Effects of a long-distance run on cardiac markers in healthy athletes. *Clin Chem & Lab Med.* 2006;44(8):999–1003.
14. Saenz AJ et al.. Measurement of a plasma stroke biomarker panel and cardiac troponin T in marathon runners before and after the 2005 Boston Marathon. *Am J Clin Path.* 2006 August;126(2):185–9.
15. Neilan TG et al.. Myocardial injury and ventricular dysfunction related to training levels among nonelite participants in the boston marathon. *Circulation.* 2006;114:2325–2333.
16. Frassl W, Kowoll R et al.. Cardiac markers (BNP, NT-pro-BNP, troponin I, troponin T) in female amateur runners before and up until three days after a marathon. *Clin Lab.* 2008;54(3-4):81–7.
17. Fu F, Nie J and Tong TK. Serum cardiac troponin T in adolescent runners: effects of exercise intensity and duration. *Int J Sports Med.* March 2009;30(3):168–72.
18. circ.ahajournals.org/content/122/18_suppl_3/S639
19. Maron BJ, Haas TS et al.. Incidence and causes of sudden death in U.S. college athletes. *J Am Coll Cardiol* 2014;63:1636–43.
20. Kim JH, Malhotra R et al.. Cardiac arrest during long distance races. *N Engl J Med* 2012; 366:130–140.
21. Papakakis M, Carre F et al.. The prevalence, distribution, and clinical outcomes of electrocardiographic repolarization patterns in male athletes of African/Afro-Caribbean origin. *Eur Heart J.* 2011 Sep;32(18):2304–13.
22. Link MS et al.. An experimental model of sudden death due to low energy chest wall impact (commotio cordis). *NEJM.* 1998;338:1805–11.
23. Link MS et al.. Upper and lower limits of vulnerability to sudden arrhythmic death with chest wall impact (commotio cordis). *J Am Coll Cardiol.* 2003 Jan;41(1):99–104.
24. Abdulla J, Nielsen JR. Is the risk of atrial fibrillation higher in athletes than in the general population? A systematic review and meta-analysis. *Europace* 2009;11:1156–9.
25. Mitchell JH, Haskell W, Snell P, Van Camp SP. Task Force 8: Classification of sports. *J Am Coll Cardiol.* 2005;45(8):1364.
26. Zipes DP, Ackerman MJ, Estes NA III, Grant AO, Myerburg RJ, Van Hare G. Task Force 7: Arrhythmias. *J Am Coll Cardiol.* 2005;45(8):1354.
27. Sohn GH, Jang SI, Moon JR et al.. The usefulness of multidetector computed tomographic angiography for the diagnosis of Marfan Syndrome by Ghent criteria. *Int J Cardiovasc Imaging* (2011):679–688.

28. Perloff JK et al.. New guidelines for the clinical diagnosis of mitral valve prolapse. *Am J Cardiol.* 1986;57(13):1124–9.

29. Maron BJ, Ackerman MJ, Nishimura RA, Pyeritz RE, Towbin JA, Udelson JE. Task Force 4: HCM and other cardiomyopathies, mitral valve prolapse, myocarditis, and Marfan syndrome. *J Am Coll Cardiol.* 2005; 45(8):1340.

30. Ryan MP et al.. The standard electrocardiogram as a screening test for hypertrophic cardiomyopathy. *Am J Cardiol* 1995; 76: 689–94.

31. Chandra N Bastiaenen R, Papadakis M, Sharma S. Sudden cardiac death in young athletes: Practical challenges and diagnostic dilemnas. *J AM Coll Cardiol.* 2013; 61(10):1027–40.

Chapter 13

Exertional Heat Illness

Brian Springer

Background/Epidemiology

- Much like sudden cardiac death, exertional heat illness receives a great deal of public attention. High profile cases of heat-associated death have occurred at the high school, collegiate, and professional level. It also remains a major concern of U.S. military forces in basic training and during training and operations, domestically and overseas.[1,2]
- Exertional heat stroke (EHS) is currently the third leading cause of death in athletes, behind sudden cardiac death and head/cervical spine trauma.[2,3]
- For reasons not yet understood, under identical environmental conditions some athletes go on to develop exertional heat illness while others do not.
- Many cases of exertional heat illness occur without the presence of a medical professional.
  - Lack of knowledge on heat illness prevention, recognition, and treatment by athletes and coaches puts athletes at unnecessary risk.
  - Efforts should focus on prevention in order to reduce the morbidity and mortality associated with exertional heat illness. Athletes and coaches should be educated on proper acclimatization, equipment, and fluid replacement strategies. When practicing/playing in challenging environmental conditions, athletes, coaches, and medical staff must monitor closely for early signs of heat illness.
- True incidence of exertional heat illness remains unknown.
  - There is no large, systematic database that tracks prevalence of exertional heat illness during athletic activities. Smaller studies tend to focus on specific groups and settings (high school athletes, military recruits, popular road races, etc.). While deaths are often reported to the press, nonfatal exertional heat illness is usually not reported to the press unless it is a high profile athlete.
  - Cases are often misdiagnosed, and terminology such as EHS and exertional heat exhaustion are often used without a uniform case definition.
  - Exertional heat exhaustion is the most common heat-related disorder in active populations.[3]
  - Prevalence of EHS in sport, military, and industrial populations seems to be on the increase, with a greater number of reported deaths being reported in the past several years.[4]
  - While reports vary, between 400 and 800 deaths may be attributed to all types of heat-related illness in the U.S. annually.[1,5]
  - Highest rates of death are among elderly adults and those with comorbid disease. Among teenage athletes, heat illness is the third leading cause of death, behind trauma and cardiac causes of death.[6]
  - Over 9,000 high school athletes are treated for exertional heat illness annually, occurring at a rate of 1.2 per 100,000 athlete exposures:[7]
    - Among American high school students, exertional heat illness rates in football (4.42 per 100,000 athlete exposures) is over ten times greater than all other sports combined.
    - Over one-half (60.3 percent) of high school cases occur in August. Of those cases reported during practice,

one-third occur over two hours into practice.

- Heat illness occurs worldwide with prolonged activity in almost any intensely physical sport.
- EHS and exertional heat exhaustion occur most frequently in hot and humid conditions, but may occur in cool conditions with prolonged activity:[3,7]
  - Fatal EHS occurs in American football most frequently during the first days of preseason conditioning (1 in 350,000), when high temperatures and high humidity are present.
  - High overall incidence of EHS is seen during road races and other activities involving continuous exercise.
  - Studies of exertional heat exhaustion among religious pilgrims in desert conditions and soldiers in summer maneuvers show individuals affected at a rate of 4–13 per 10,000 individuals per day.
  - Fit competitors in a 14-K road race in mild temperatures, that is 52–68°F (11–20°C), are affected at 14 per 100,000 individuals per day, presumably demonstrating the effect of high-intensity exercise in lower heat.
  - Competitors in a multi-day youth soccer tournament in hot weather are affected by heat exhaustion at 85 per 10,000 individuals per day, with a sharp increase on the second day, presumably due to cumulative effects of heat exposure.

Pathophysiology

- The human body eliminates excess heat through four basic mechanisms: convection, conduction, radiation, and evaporation.
- Environmental, physiologic, and equipment factors all may play a role in impairing those mechanisms.
  - Convection is minimized in still air and when overlying clothing and equipment prevent moving air from contacting the skin.
  - Air is an insulator and conduction provides only minimal heat loss. An exception is when the individual is submerged in cold water. Conduction then becomes the most effective means of heat loss, an important concept in the treatment of heat illness.
  - Radiation is ineffective when the environmental temperature exceeds skin temperature, and may also be impeded by overlying equipment and clothing.
  - Evaporation of sweat from the skin surface becomes less efficient as humidity increases. In addition, medications and dehydration may impair the body's sweating mechanism, rendering evaporation ineffective as a heat-loss method.
- The common element to exertional heat illness is the effect of heat stress on the exercising individual.
- Heat stress is cumulative. Presence of any heat illness indicates presence of heat stress and should be taken seriously, with the individual closely monitored.
- Heat illness is often looked at as a continuum from mild (heat edema, heat rash, heat cramps, heat syncope) to severe (heat exhaustion, heat stroke). There is no evidence that mild illness will progress to severe disease if untreated. However, heat exhaustion left untreated may lead to development of heat stroke.[1]
- Heat stroke may occur in athletes exercising in hot conditions without any prodromal signs of dehydration or heat exhaustion.
- In general, inability to continue exercise (exhaustion) occurs due to a combination of hyperthermia-induced central and peripheral reduction of muscle activation, diminished hydration, electrolyte imbalance, and energy depletion.[3,4]
  - In hot conditions this is more pronounced due to rapid depletion of energy stores.
  - Variables affecting the individual athlete include duration/intensity of exercise, environmental conditions, acclimatization, VO2 max, conditioning, hydration status, medications, sleep, and recent illness.
  - Combined effects of heat stress and dehydration reduce exercise performance greater than either alone.
  - The removal of body heat is controlled by the central nervous system (CNS) centers in the hypothalamus and spinal cord and by peripheral centers in skin and organs.

Table 13.1 Risk Factors for Development of Exertional Heat Illness (3,4,19)

Weather conditions	High ambient temperatures, relative humidity, and solar load all decrease time to development of heat stress and increase risk of illness
Lack of acclimatization	Individual acclimatization up to 14 days reduces heat illness risk; benefit is lost following 18–28 days inactivity
Exercise duration/ Intensity	Prolonged or intense activity without adequate recovery creates immediate and cumulative heat stress
Dehydration	Reduced volume creates reduced removal of heat from the core and reduced heat loss via evaporation from the skin
Overweight/Obese/ Sedentary	Diminished VO2 max and excess body fat have both been linked to risk of exertional heat stroke. Excess body fat may also exacerbate the heat-retaining effects of athletic clothing/protective equipment
Sleep loss	Linked to risk of exertional heat stroke and death, exact etiology currently unknown
Recent illness	Fever, gastroenteritis, diarrhea, and vomiting all impair heat dissipation and increase heat stress
Medications	Prescription medications, over-the-counter medications, and supplements may increase risk of heat illness by reducing sweating, diminishing blood flow to skin, and increasing heat production

- Exertional hyperthermia with a core temperature above 104°F (40°C) occurs during physical exertion when muscle-generated heat accumulates faster than heat dissipation via sweating and skin blood flow.
- Heat tolerance and risk for exertional heat illness is affected by exercise intensity, environmental conditions, clothing, equipment, and individual host factors.[8] (See Table 13.1)
- Wide variations of heat tolerance exist among individuals. Some athletes tolerate prolonged hyperthermia well above 104°F (40°C) and show no signs of heat illness.
- Dehydration occurs more rapidly in hot environments where sweat loss occurs faster than fluid intake. Fluid deficits as little as 3–5 percent of body weight result in diminished sweat production and declining skin blood flow with resultant impaired heat dissipation.
- Excessive sweating results in salt loss which may result in muscle cramps. Prolonged endurance events in the heat may also lead to hypovolemic hyponatremia.
- Elevated core temperatures and dehydration both diminish compensatory splanchnic and skin vasoconstriction. This results in reduced total vascular resistance, decreased removal of heat from exercising muscle, and increased cardiac insufficiency.

- Acclimatization:[9]
  - Defined by a marked improvement in physiologic response of healthy humans to exercise in heat.
  - Effects of acclimatization demonstrated by reduction in occurrence and severity of heat illness, and increased work output concurrent with reduced cardiovascular, thermal, and metabolic strain.
  - Both passive exposure to hot conditions and intensive exercise in cool conditions aid with acclimatization, but the most effective means of acclimatization is exercise in a hot environment.
  - Physiologic adaptations include:
    - Sweating begins at lower core temperature.
    - Increased skin blood flow facilitates heat dissipation to environment.
    - Increased plasma volume facilitates heat removal from core.
    - Diminished excretion of NaCl in sweat and urine produces expanded extracellular fluid volume.
    - Improved exercise economy and diminished heart rate decrease overall cardiovascular strain.

- Complete acclimatization takes up to fourteen days. Increased fluid and electrolyte intake do not enhance speed of acclimatization, but dehydration may result in delay.
- Host factors may influence acclimatization capacity:
  - When matched for pertinent physical and morphological characteristics, males and females show little difference in acclimatization capacity.
  - Heat intolerance in older individuals is most likely due to diminished training intensity and reduced aerobic output as opposed to the aging process itself.
- Adaptations to exercise in the heat disappear after eighteen to twenty-eight days of inactivity. Cardiovascular adaptations are the first to diminish.

- Pediatric considerations
  - Anatomic and physiologic differences between children and adults affect response to heat.
  - These differences alone do not appear to put children at higher risk for heat illness.
  - Differences include:[7,10]
    - Children produce greater metabolic heat per kilogram than adults due to higher basal metabolic rate.
    - Young children have a greater surface area to mass ratio, allowing greater environmental heat absorption.
    - In older children and adolescents, increased body fat and diminished fitness levels increase risk of heat illness.
    - Children have lower cardiac output and absolute blood volume than adults, impeding transfer of heat from core to body surface during physical activity.
    - Children begin sweating at higher body temperature than adults.
    - Children have lower sweat rates per gland than adults.
    - Children tend to acclimatize to a hot environment more slowly than adults.
    - Children are less likely to replenish fluid losses following exercise.
  - Classic heat stroke (as opposed to EHS) is more common in younger children unable to escape from a hot environment (for example, a locked automobile) or having chronic underlying medical conditions that impair thermoregulation.[11]

Focused History and Physical Exam

- Priority in any individual experiencing exertional heat illness is assessment of circulatory status, airway/breathing, and evidence of neurologic disability.
- Neurologic disability in early EHS may be subtle. Confusion, disorientation, and personality changes may precede more pronounced findings such as delirium, seizure or coma.[3,4]
- Core temperature in suspected exertional heat illness must be accurately measured. This generally means a rectal temperature in the field, and a rectal or esophageal temperature in the emergency department.
- Tympanic and temporal thermometers are not sufficiently accurate at temperature extremes to be used in suspected exertional heat illness. [12]
- Elevation in core temperature in the digestive tract measured by swallowed monitors have correlated with core temperature elevations and risk of exertional heat illness.[13]
- In cases of suspected associated trauma (such as a fall from a height or significant collision with another athlete) initiate cervical spine precautions.

Differential Diagnosis – Emergent and Common Diagnoses

Table 13.2 Emergent and Common Diagnoses in the Emergency Department

Emergent Diagnoses	Common Diagnoses
Heat stroke	Heat Cramps
Heat exhaustion	Heat Syncope
Exertional hyponatremia	

Exertional Heat Stroke

General Description

- Characterized by hyperthermia (core temperature of more than 104°F (40°C), CNS disturbances and (if untreated) multiple organ failure.
- When heat production outpaces heat loss, core temperature rises to levels that ultimately cause end organ damage.
- Most EHS patients present initially with profuse sweating, as opposed to the hot dry skin seen in classic heat stroke.
- In cases of suspected heat illness where the core temperature is less than 104°F (40°C) but mental status is abnormal, consider EHS as some cooling may have occurred prior to assessment.[14]
- Classic vs. exertional heat stroke:[1,15]
  - In classic heat stroke, the environment plays a major role in an individual's ability to dissipate heat. In EHS, intrinsic heat production is the major source.
  - Most cases of classic heat stroke are linked to heat waves. Elderly and other vulnerable individuals, often on medications that may impair thermoregulation, develop thermoregulatory dysfunction over time with resultant hyperthermia and end organ damage. EHS occurs in all types of weather.
  - Anhidrotic skin is a hallmark of classic heat stroke, whereas those with EHS demonstrate profuse sweating. Therefore, presence or absence of sweating has no role in the diagnosis of EHS.
  - Treatment for both conditions is identical: rapidly cool the individual as quickly as possible to minimize organ dysfunction.

Mechanism

- When internal organ tissue temperature reaches critical threshold levels of 104°F (40° C) cell dysfunction occurs.
- Temperatures above threshold levels impair cell volume, metabolism, and membrane permeability. Initial dysfunction may lead to cell death and organ failure.
- Organ systems typically affected include brain, heart, kidneys, GI, muscle, and hematologic.
- Degree of multisystem injury and death correlate directly to time spent subjected to elevated body temperature.[16,17,18]
- Rapid cooling and return to normal range of body temperature within one hour allows full recovery in most cases of EHS.
- Athletes with unrecognized EHS or delay in cooling have increased morbidity and mortality.
  - Athletes who present comatose and with evidence of multiorgan injury but are cooled in less than one hour do well.
  - The primary difference between mild and severe EHS appears to be the duration of time from collapse to cooling.[18]
- Once organ dysfunction begins, without rapid cooling a life-threatening spiral begins.[3]
  - Cardiac hyperthermia reduces cardiac output, impairing oxygen delivery to tissues as well as vascular transport of heat from core to periphery. This accelerates hyperthermia and worsens tissue hypoxia.
  - CNS hyperthermia results in hypothalamic dysfunction, further impairing thermoregulation and circulatory maintenance.
  - Hyperthermia increases muscle membrane permeability, promoting rhabdomyolysis.
  - Both renal tissue hypothermia as well as impaired renal flow due to the earlier mentioned mechanisms may lead to renal failure and increased susceptibility to rhabdomyolysis.
- Predisposing factors to development of EHS include:[4,19]
  - Exercise in hot and humid environment. Greatest risk exists with wet bulb globe temperature (WBGT) exceeding 82°F (28° C), high-intensity exercise, especially when longer than one hour.
  - Lack of acclimatization.
  - Poor physical fitness.
  - EHS may occur in cool to moderate environments, suggesting significant individual variation in susceptibility.[20,21]
- Why people die from EHS:[4]
  - No treatment or delayed treatment: most often this is due to failure to recognize EHS. Having qualified medical personnel (physicians, athletic trainers) on site can mitigate this risk.

- Ineffective cooling: cold water immersion is the gold standard of rapid cooling; however, access to this modality may be limited. Also, now-debunked concerns over creation of shivering or monitoring difficulties may result in use of less effective methods of cooling.
- Immediate or delayed transport: if means exist to rapidly cool on-site, they should be utilized. Rapid transport either prior to cooling or interrupting cooling begun in the field may delay time to reduction of core temperature to safe levels. Delayed transport may lengthen time to treatment if no means of effective cooling are available/begun in the field.
- Rapid return to activity: sufficient time must pass for an individual to fully recover from heat illness; otherwise, the patient may be at risk for recurrence of EHS.

Presentation

- Rapid recognition of EHS is critical so that cooling may be initiated as soon as possible.
- Appearance of signs and symptoms of EHS depends on the degree and duration of hyperthermia. Signs and symptoms may be nonspecific. They include:[16,22]
  - Confusion, disorientation, unusual behaviors or inappropriate comments, changes in personality and increased irritability, headache, fatigue, nausea and vomiting, diarrhea, seizure, or frank coma. The patient may be stumbling, clumsy, or completely collapse.
  - Abnormal vital signs may include tachycardia, tachypnea, and hypotension.
  - Skin is often cool and sweaty.
  - Any change in personality or performance, especially in hot conditions, should prompt consideration of EHS.
- Body core temperature estimate is critical in establishing the diagnosis.
  - Measure a rectal temperature in any athlete with suspected EHS.
  - Tympanic, oral, temporal, and axillary temperature measurements are susceptible to inaccuracy, especially at extremes of temperature, and should not be used.[12]
  - Ingested devices to measure gastrointestinal core temperature are useful, but only if they have been ingested prior to onset of heat illness.[13]

Physical Exam

- Rapid initial assessment of circulatory status, airway and breathing, and neurological status.
- Obtain vital signs, to include heart rate, respiratory rate, and blood pressure.
- Obtain a rectal temperature.
  - Lay the individual on the side and pull down shorts to easily access the rectum.
  - Shielding for privacy is optimal but should not delay measurement.
- Auscultate heart and check peripheral pulses to assess adequate perfusion.
- Check mucous membranes and skin turgor for signs of dehydration.
- Examine extremities for signs of edema, which may be present in overhydration.
- Auscultate lungs for wheezes to ensure athlete has not collapsed secondary to asthma, allergy, or anaphylaxis.
- Perform a focused neurological exam, being especially alert for subtle changes in CNS function. Some individuals may present with a deceptive "lucid interval." In retrospect, subtle CNS changes (such as irritability or personality changes) are usually present.[22]

Essential Diagnostics

- Initial recognition of EHS via careful assessment for subtle CNS dysfunction.
- Rapidly obtaining a rectal or core temperature.

ED Treatment

- Remember that the most critical element of treating EHS is rapid lowering of core temperature.
  - If not begun in the field or during transport, it should commence immediately upon ED arrival.
  - Cooling that has begun in the field should be continued in the ED in conjunction with assessment.
  - Goal is to bring the temperature down to 104°F (40°C) or less in under 30 minutes.

Table 13.3: Rapid Cooling of Patients with Exertional Heat Stroke: Good, Better, Best [1,3,4,23,24,25]

GOOD	BETTER	BEST
Water Mist/Fan	Ice Water-Soaked Towels	Cold/Ice Water Immersion
Pros: Simple, requires minimal equipment (mist-sprayer and fan), can be applied in remote locations	Pros: Simple, effective, does not require lifting/immersion of patient, can be applied in remote locations	Pros: Most rapid means of cooling patient with suspected EHS
Cons: Slower cooling than immersion, most effective when relative humidity is low	Cons: Requires proper equipment on-hand (towels, ice water)	Cons: Requires access to tub and very cold/ice water, requires personnel to lift/place patient in water

  - If cooling is started in the field via an effective modality such as cold water immersion, consideration should be given to delaying transport until the core temperature is between 102°F–104°F (38.9–40°C).
- Assess circulatory status, airway, and breathing.
- Recheck core temperature to guide therapy.
- The patient should have vital signs monitored. However, repeat vital signs, cardiac monitoring, IV access, and so forth, should NOT interfere with cooling. The most important initial monitoring should be placement of a rectal temperature probe.
- The gold standard for treatment is cold water/ice water immersion.[4,23,24,25] If a tub is available in the field or in the ED, it should be utilized. (See Table 13.3)
  - Immerse individual in cold 35–57°F (1.7–13.9°C) or ice water over as much of the body as possible.
  - Apply a wet towel around the head.
  - Water should be continually stirred to maintain contact of cold water on the skin surface.
  - This modality of cooling may bring the patient's core temperature to under 104°F (40°C) in under 20 minutes.
- If cold/ice water is not available, temperate water may be used, although it is a less effective modality.[4]
  - Peripheral vasoconstriction and shivering may be less with temperate water immersion.
  - Cold water immersion, however, cools more rapidly, and minimizes time of exposure to the cooling modality. Thus, heat production via shivering is limited.
- If cold water immersion is not available in the field or ED, an alternative cooling modality is use of towels soaked in ice water.[18]
  - Maintain twice the number of towels needed to cover the patient.
  - Rotate towels used every several minutes to ensure cold towels are on the patient while the others are recooled.
  - Maintain this modality until a tub for immersion is available or core temperature goal has been achieved.
  - Combined with application of icepacks to the neck, axillae, and groin, this method provides a rapid method of cooling.
- The use of warm air mist and fanning has been shown to be effective for rapid cooling of large numbers of individuals. This method relies heavily on evaporative cooling and is effective only when relative humidity is low.
- Cooling should cease when rectal temperature reaches 102°F–104°F (38.9–40°C). Continued cooling may result in hypothermia.[26]
- Even if the patient regains lucidity, continue cooling until rectal temperature is below 104°F (40°C). Observe to ensure maintenance of normal temperatures and mental status once recovered.
- Replace intravascular volume losses with normal saline.
  - Fluid resuscitation improves renal blood flow and protects from rhabdomyolysis.

- Optimized volume status improves tissue perfusion, enhancing heat exchange, oxygenation, and removal of waste products.
- Patients who fail to respond to cooling should be checked for other potential life-threatening causes of collapse.
  - Check bedside glucose and treat for hypo- or hyperglycemia as indicated.
  - Obtain a 12-lead EKG.
  - Check serum electrolytes for hyper- or hyponatremia or hypokalemia. Check renal function for evidence of prerenal azotemia or kidney injury due to rhabdomyolysis.
  - Check serum creatine kinase (CK) levels. Urinalysis positive for blood on dipstick but negative for blood on microscopic may indicate myoglobinuria and subsequent risk of rhabdomyolysis.
  - Check coagulation studies including PT/INR and PTT, as EHS may cause a coagulopathy.
- EHS patients with prolonged core temperature elevations and development of multiple organ failure require more extensive interventions.
  - Clinical markers of disseminated intravascular coagulopathy, multiple organ failure, and prolonged elevations of CK carry a poor prognosis.[27]
  - Do not allow testing to interfere with ongoing cooling efforts.

Disposition

- In patients who have a rapid return of normal mental status and normalized core temperature, consideration may be given for discharge.
  - There are multiple reports of road race competitors with rectal temperatures above 107.6°F (42°C) and profound CNS dysfunction who, following rapid diagnosis and treatment with ice water cooling, are discharged home from the medical tent without hospitalization.[22]
- Return-to-play decision making is a complex and sometimes controversial subject that is based on limited evidence.
- Current guidelines vary widely; suggested return to play varies from seven days to fifteen months.[3]
  - Athletes who receive prompt cooling have an excellent prognosis for full recovery and return to play.
  - In some individuals, thermoregulation, exercise heat tolerance, and acclimatization ability may take months to return to normal following EHS.
  - In those who experience severe hepatic injury, full recovery may take over one year.
- Decision making on RTP (return to play) requires input from physicians, athletic trainers, coaches, as well as the athlete.
- American College of Sports Medicine has five recommendations for RTP following EHS:
  - Refrain from exercise at least seven days following release from medical care.
  - Follow-up in one week for physical exam and repeat testing of affected organs (based on the clinical course of illness).
  - Once cleared for RTP, begin exercise in a cool environment. Gradually increase duration, intensity, and heat exposure for two weeks to allow for acclimatization and demonstrated heat tolerance.
  - If return to activity has not been achieved in one month, consider a laboratory-based exercise heat tolerance test.[28,29,30]
    - No standard of care exists in the performance of HTT (heat tolerance test).
    - Classic walking HTT may not be appropriate for the elite athlete.
    - Tailor HTT protocol to duplicate the demands of the elite athlete.
  - If heat tolerance exists after two to four weeks of full training, the athlete may be cleared for full activity.

Pearls and Pitfalls

- Duration of hyperthermia is linked to outcome: the sooner cooling is commenced, the lower the risk of morbidity and mortality.
- Recognition of EHS is critical. Early signs may be subtle and include behavioral disturbances.

- Core temperature should be measured with a rectal thermometer, or correlated to GI temperature via a swallowed monitor.
- Cold water or ice water immersion is the gold standard of cooling in EHS and should not be delayed nor ceased for transportation until core temperature is below 104°F (40°C).
- Proper acclimatization and education for athletes and coaches are essential.

Heat Exhaustion

General Description

- May be the initial presentation of heat illness.
- Inability to continue exercise; may occur with heavy exertion in all temperatures and may or may not be associated with physical collapse.
- Often presents with complaints of malaise, dizziness, headache, and nausea.
- Core temperature may be normal or elevated, but is below 104°F (40°C).
- Unlike heat stroke, the athlete with heat exhaustion will have normal mentation and neurological exam.

Mechanism

- Evidence suggests heat exhaustion results from central fatigue inducing peripheral vasodilation and subsequent collapse.
- This central failure may be a mechanism of protecting the body against overexertion in hot/stressful environments.[3,9]
- Heat exhaustion related to dehydration is more common in hot and humid conditions.
- Combination of tachycardia, high cardiac output, and lowered peripheral vascular resistance result in hypotension and cardiovascular insufficiency.
- Blood volume pooling in skin impairs heat transport from core to surface. This is compounded by high humidity, where evaporative cooling is impaired, signaling the body to increase cutaneous blood flow to increase non-evaporative heat loss.
- Predisposing factors for development of heat exhaustion include:[1,3,19]
  - Increased body mass index (>27 kg/m^2).
  - Exertion during the hottest months of the year.
  - Inadequate fluid intake.
  - Increased air temperature (>91.4°F, 33°C) and diminished air velocity (<2.0 m/s).

Presentation

- Signs and symptoms of heat exhaustion are nonspecific.[1]
- Athletes may present with generalized weakness, headache, nausea and vomiting, diarrhea, dizziness, and irritability.
- Acutely, athletes are tachycardic, tachypneic, and have low blood pressure.
- Athletes may appear sweaty and pale and have cool and clammy skin.
- Piloerection may be present.
- Muscle cramping may accompany heat exhaustion.
- Rectal temperature may be normal or elevated, but should be less than 40°C.

Physical Exam

- Rapid initial assessment of circulatory status, airway and breathing, and neurological status.
- Obtain vital signs, to include heart rate, respiratory rate, and blood pressure.
- Obtain a rectal temperature.
- Auscultate heart and check peripheral pulses to assess adequate perfusion.
- Check mucous membranes and skin turgor for signs of dehydration.
- Examine extremities for signs of edema, which may be present in overhydration.
- Perform a focused neurological exam, being especially alert for changes in sensorium that may indicate more severe EHS.
- Orthostatic vital signs add little to assessment, especially early in evaluation.

Essential Diagnostics

- Obtaining a rectal temperature in the field may help discriminate between heat exhaustion and heat stroke. (See Table 13.4)
- In heat exhaustion, rectal temperature is <104°F (40°C) whereas in EHS temperature is >104°F (40°C).
- If a rectal temperature cannot be rapidly obtained, consider instituting rapid cooling for empiric treatment of EHS, particularly if there are signs of CNS dysfunction.

Table 13.4 Exertional Heat Exhaustion vs. Exertional Heat Stroke [1,3,16,22]

Heat Exhaustion	Heat Stroke
Core temperature < 104°F (40°C)	Core temperature ≥ 104°F (40°C)
Significant dehydration	May not be significantly dehydrated
Unaltered sensorium and neurologic exam	CNS disturbances (confusion, disorientation, personality changes, irritability, seizure, coma)
Profuse sweating	Profuse sweating early; anhidrosis is a late finding in EHS

- Altered sensorium should prompt pursuit of hyperthermia, hypoglycemia, hyponatremia, or other medical problem.

ED Treatment

- Treatment should begin in the field by moving the athlete out of the heat and into a shaded or air-conditioned area.
- Remove athletic equipment and constrictive clothing.
- Place athlete in supine position with legs elevated to improve central and cerebral blood flow.
- The majority of athletes improve symptomatically with removal from hot environment, rest, and oral rehydration.
  - Continually monitor vital signs and neurologic status.
  - Recheck a rectal temperature following field treatment.
  - Should the athlete not improve with these measures, transport to an emergency facility.
- Once in the emergency department, the same basic measures should be instituted as in the field:
  - Remove any equipment or constrictive clothes.
  - Keep athlete in a cool environment.
  - Monitor heart rate and blood pressure and check rectal temperature.
  - Do frequent neurological checks looking for CNS dysfunction.
- Routine labs are unnecessary unless the physician suspects another cause of collapse or the athlete fails to respond to initial treatment.
- A bedside blood glucose check may be useful to determine if hypoglycemia is present.
- In athletes who are awake, alert, able to swallow well, and not severely nauseated or losing fluids rapidly through diarrhea or emesis, oral rehydration is preferred.[1,3,9]
  - As electrolyte losses may contribute to the patient's symptoms, hypotonic fluids should be avoided for oral resuscitation.
  - Sport drinks, oral rehydration fluids, or Pedialyte are all reasonable options to facilitate rehydration.
- If blood pressure, pulse, and temperature improve with treatment and there are no ongoing fluid losses (such as diarrhea) then IV fluids are not required.
- If the athlete has ongoing abnormal vital signs, cannot tolerate oral rehydration, or has ongoing fluid losses, institute resuscitation with IV fluids.
  - IV fluids have been shown to enhance rapid recovery from heat exhaustion in those who cannot ingest oral fluids or have severe dehydration.
  - Normal saline is the most recommended resuscitation fluid for the dehydrated athlete.
  - Administer 1–4 liters. The end goal is improvement of vital signs and symptoms.
  - If the athlete is hypoglycemic, 5% dextrose in NS may be used.
  - Cooled fluids may be used initially for the moderately hyperthermic athlete, but be careful not to create hypothermia.
  - Routine IV rehydration on the sidelines of games is neither evidence based nor recommended.
  - If the collapsed athlete is not clearly clinically dehydrated or showing signs of overhydration, consider exertional hyponatremia.[1]
- Worsening of mental status or failure to clinically improve should prompt a more detailed medical assessment.
  - Recheck rectal temperature, looking for hyper- or hypothermia.

  - Recheck bedside glucose.
  - Obtain serum electrolytes, looking for hyper- or hyponatremia and hypoglycemia.
  - Obtain 12-lead EKG in cases of suspected electrolyte abnormalities, dysrhythmias, ACS, or in the collapsed athlete with ongoing hemodynamic instability.

Disposition

- As noted, most athletes with heat exhaustion quickly recover with treatment on site or in the emergency department.
- Once clinically stable, they may be discharged home with instructions for continued rest and rehydration.
  - Urine color can be a useful gauge for hydration status.
  - Advise maintenance of pale yellow to clear urine for the next forty-eight hours, prior to resumption of activity.
- If asymptomatic and hydrated after twenty-four to forty-eight hours, the athlete may resume activity with caution.[30]
  - Immediate return to activity is not advised.
  - Even with rest and cooling, athletes should not return to full exercise capacity the same day.
- More severe cases of heat exhaustion (delayed recovery, severe symptoms) should follow-up with a physician or athletic trainer prior to resumption of activity.
- Athletes who remain severely symptomatic in the ED (ongoing nausea, vomiting, diarrhea, or abnormal vital signs) should be brought into the hospital for continued IV therapy and monitoring.

Pearls and Pitfalls

- In athletes with changes in mental status or neurologic dysfunction, treat as EHS and cool rapidly.
- Failure to recognize heat exhaustion or to fully recover from heat exhaustion prior to resumption of activity may lead to cumulative heat stress and the possibility of development of EHS.
- Proper acclimatization and modification of activity in extreme heat may reduce risk of heat exhaustion.
- Rehydrate with a sports drink or another electrolyte containing fluid, or use NS for IV resuscitation if needed in the ED.

Heat cramps

General Description

- One of the earliest indicators of heat stress in the individual athlete.
- Painful muscle cramps/spasm occurring in active muscle groups following exercise challenge.
- Cramps most likely to occur after prolonged exercise (more than two hours) but may occur anytime.
- High incidence among football players, tennis players, and military.[1,3]

Mechanism

- Poorly understood, multifactorial etiology.
- Most likely results from some combination of dehydration, salt loss, and neuromuscular fatigue.[3,9,31]
- Sodium (as opposed to potassium) appears to be the predominant electrolyte deficiency linked to heat cramp development.
- Individuals with more concentrated (saltier) sweat develop heat cramps more commonly.

Presentation

- Painful contractions usually inhibit athlete's ability to continue participation/play.
- Occurs most often in gastrocnemius, hamstrings, quadriceps, or abdominal muscles.
- May occur alone or in conjunction with heat exhaustion.
- Heat cramps alone do not indicate increased risk of development of heat stroke.

Physical Exam

- If the athlete has collapsed to the ground, quickly assess circulatory status, airway/breathing, and neurologic function.
- Assess for any acute injury that may have caused the athlete to collapse or may have occurred if the athlete collapsed to the ground due to cramping.
- Physical exam may reveal tight, actively contracting muscle.

Essential Diagnostics

- Beyond a focused history and physical exam, further diagnostic testing is not indicated.
- Should cramps occur in conjunction with other symptoms (altered sensorium, nausea and vomiting, etc.), obtain a core temperature and consider assessing serum electrolytes to look for significant hyponatremia.

ED Treatment

- Massage and stretching of affected muscles is often effective.
- Muscles may be cooled via application of ice.
- Encourage intake of sodium-containing fluids such as a sports drink.
- In cases of severe, recalcitrant cramping, administer IV normal saline to restore euvolemia and sodium stores.[1,9,31]

Disposition

- Athletes may be safely discharged home following resolution of symptoms.
- Advise against vigorous physical activity until fully rested, rehydrated, and asymptomatic. Athlete should not return to vigorous activity on the same day.
- Further acclimatization and conditioning may be beneficial prior to resumption of vigorous activity.
- Encourage the athlete to consume adequate hydration to restore body weight and to consume sodium-containing meal.

Peals and Pitfalls

- Acclimatized, hydrated, and conditioned athletes are less likely to develop heat cramps.
- Treat cramps with massage, stretching, ice, and consumption of sodium-containing fluids.
- Sodium is the key electrolyte deficiency in heat cramps, not potassium. Emphasis on potassium supplementation (such as bananas, potassium salt, etc.) in severe cramps is misguided.
- Do not miss an acute musculotendinous injury such as a gastrocnemius or hamstring tear.
- Do not miss concurrent heat exhaustion or stroke.

Heat Syncope

General Description/Mechanism

- Syncope or near syncope occurring secondary to orthostatic hypotension. This may also be referred to as exercise- associated collapse (EAC).
- Orthostasis results from peripheral vasodilation, venous pooling, and relative hypovolemia.
- Prolonged standing in the heat, prolonged standing after significant exertion, and rapid changes of body position following exertion all may precipitate heat syncope.[1,9]
- Prolonged standing or a change in position tend to create venous pooling in the lower extremities. This pooling is exaggerated when peripheral vasodilation occurs in response to heat production.
- Cessation of intense activity such as running also results in venous pooling, along with the loss of muscle action contributing to venous return.

Presentation

- Athletes most commonly present with heat syncope after they have stopped exercising.[1,16,22]
- Medical providers should be particularly vigilant for this condition at the end of an event (such as at the chute of a cross-country event) and keep athletes moving until they have cooled down.
- Athletes with heat syncope tend to recover rapidly once supine, as cerebral blood flow is restored.
- Extra concern is required for the athlete who collapses *before* reaching the finish line. In these cases consider EHS or cardiac syncope as likely mechanisms for loss of consciousness.[16,22]

Physical Exam

- Initial exam should focus on circulation, airway and breathing, and neurologic function.
- Obtain vital signs, to include heart rate and blood pressure. Orthostatic readings, especially early, are likely to be abnormal and contribute little to evaluation.
- If concern exists for more significant illness, obtain an accurate temperature.

- Look for evidence of trauma that may have occurred when the athlete collapsed. Immobilize the cervical spine if there is clinical suspicion of neck injury or significant head injury.
- Athletes with heat syncope should improve rapidly once supine. If an athlete with suspected heat syncope remains altered in the field or arrives altered in the emergency department, consider an alternate diagnosis.
- Assess mucous membranes and skin turgor for evidence of dehydration.
- Perform a cardiac and pulmonary exam, listening for abnormal murmurs, dysrhythmias, or wheezes. Check strength of peripheral pulses.
- Perform a focused neurologic exam, checking for level of consciousness, orientation, and any focal deficits.

Essential Diagnostics

- If suspicion exists for EHS, an accurate temperature (rectal, esophageal) must be obtained.
- If suspicion exists for a cardiac cause of syncope, obtain a 12-lead EKG.
- Imaging is only indicated in cases of suspected trauma.

ED Treatment

- Many cases of heat syncope will not ever be brought in for ED evaluation.[3]
- Allow the athlete to remain supine/recumbent and in a cool environment.
- It may help to elevate the legs to enhance venous return.
- In most cases, oral rehydration will be appropriate to compensate for heat-related fluid losses. If the athlete is significantly dehydrated (persistent abnormal vital signs) or is having difficulty taking adequate oral fluids due to nausea, weight-appropriate boluses of IV fluid may be used.

Disposition

- Athletes with heat syncope may be safely discharged once they are sufficiently asymptomatic and are able to ambulate and tolerate oral fluids.
- Advise rest and rehydration prior to resumption of any athletic activity.
- If the diagnosis is unclear and there is any concern for cardiac syncope, consultation with cardiology should be obtained. If the athlete is subsequently discharged, any exertion should be avoided pending further evaluation.

Pearls and Pitfalls

- Exertional heat syncope may be avoided by supervising athletes in the field and ensuring they remain moving and cool down gradually at the cessation of intense activity.
- Always consider alternate diagnoses such as EHS or cardiac syncope in the athlete with a syncopal episode.
- In the athlete with heat syncope and persistent altered level of consciousness, obtain a rectal temperature, looking for EHS.

Exertional Hyponatremia

General Description/Mechanism

- Clinically defined by a serum sodium of less than 130–135 mmol/L.
- Occurs from excessive intake of free water before, during, and after endurance events.
  - Most commonly occurs during sustained, high-intensity endurance activities such as marathons or triathlons.[32]
  - "Blanket" hydration advice in which one recommendation fits all has led to overdrinking by well-meaning athletes.[33]
  - They will typically consume more fluid than they lose in sweat, and may actually gain weight over the course of an event.
  - As the event proceeds, the athlete may develop lethargy and nausea secondary to low sodium. These symptoms may inadvertently be taken as signs of dehydration, prompting even greater fluid intake.[1]
- Risk factors for exertional hyponatremia differ from those for heat stroke.[1,34,35] They include:
  - Female gender
  - Younger age
  - Slower race times
  - Lower body weight
  - Increased availability of fluids.
  - Use of NSAIDs.

- May occur in as many as 2–7 percent of participants.[36]
- Most cases lead to few or no complications and may be treated with close monitoring and fluid restriction.

Presentation

- Appears clinically similar to exertional heatstroke, with altered mental status, nausea and vomiting, and diminished level of consciousness.
- Exertional hyponatremia is distinguished from heat illness by presence of a normal core temperature.[1]
- Severe hyponatremia (serum sodium <120 mmol/L) can precipitate seizures, coma, and death.
- Typically occurs during or up to twenty-four hours after prolonged physical activity.[37]

Physical Exam

- Initial exam should focus on circulation, airway and breathing, and neurologic function.
- Obtain vital signs, to include heart rate, respiratory rate, and blood pressure.
- Check mucous membranes and skin turgor for signs of dehydration.
- Examine extremities for signs of edema, which may be present in overhydration.
- Promptly obtain a rectal temperature.

Essential Diagnostics

- If suspicion exists for EHS, an accurate temperature (rectal, esophageal) must be obtained.
- Point of care testing of serum sodium should be made available in the medical tent of any large endurance event. Otherwise, obtain it as quickly as possible in the emergency department.
- Serum sodium should be rapidly assessed in any endurance athlete presenting with a history of altered mental status, diminished level of consciousness, excess water consumption, and a normal core temperature.

ED Treatment

- Initial support of the hyponatremic patient in the emergency department should focus on circulation, airway, and breathing.
- Minimally symptomatic patients who are able to drink may be treated with concentrated oral hypertonic solution.
- Minimally symptomatic patients should be fluid restricted until they have urinated adequately and approach their normal body weight.
- Patients who are comatose or seizing should be treated with 3% hypertonic saline.
  - Initial treatment is up to three 100-mL boluses of 3% saline spaced at ten-minute intervals.[38]
  - Goal of therapy is resolution of neurologic symptoms.
  - In cases refractory to initial treatment, large volume hypertonic saline therapy (up to 1 L) may be considered.[39]
  - Concern over central pontine myelinolysis from rapid correction of exercise-associated hyponatremia is unsupported, as development of the electrolyte imbalance is an acute (as opposed to chronic) condition.[40]

Disposition

- Athletes with mild exertional hyponatremia (>120 mmol/L) who are asymptomatic may be placed on fluid restriction and observed until they are urinating and approaching their normal body weight.
- Symptomatic patients at any level should be observed to ensure that they urinate and that symptoms do not worsen.
- Patients discharged to home should be warned to return immediately should they develop weakness, nausea, vomiting, or other concerning symptoms.[38]
- Symptomatic patients requiring hypertonic saline treatment should admitted to intensive care where they can be closely monitored and have seizure precautions instituted.
- Athletes should not return to sports without physician clearance.
  - Mild cases may resume activity in a few days.
  - Athlete education on safe hydration practices and prevention of exertional hyponatremia is strongly encouraged.

Pearls and Pitfalls

- Exertional hyponatremia may be mistaken for EHS, syncope, or another entity. The athlete with neurological dysfunction and a normal core temperature should prompt evaluation of serum sodium levels.
- A partially cooled patient with EHS may be difficult to discern from a patient with exertional hyponatremia. When in doubt, continue the cooling process while evaluating serum electrolytes.
- Treatment for exertional hyponatremia with neurological dysfunction (altered mental status, seizures, coma) is hypertonic saline. End goal is resolution of symptoms.
- Educate athletes and coaches that the key preventive intervention is moderate fluid consumption based on perceived need ("ad libitum") rather than on a rigid rule.[34]

Preventive Strategies

- Environmental awareness
  - Athletic activities should be modified or restricted when weather conditions pose risk for heat illness.
  - WBGT is a combined measure of ambient temperature, humidity, sun angle/cloud cover (solar load), and wind speed.[41]
  - Heat index is a combined measure of ambient temperature and humidity only. It is usually easier to obtain than WBGT.
  - For given levels of WBGT or heat index, specific activity restrictions are recommended. These range from increased hydration breaks and more frequent player substitutions to rescheduling or canceling games.[42]
- Hydration
  - Dehydrated athletes are more likely to suffer heat illness.[1,3,4]
  - Different sports organizations have different recommendations for fluid management.
  - As a general rule, athletes should drink ad libitum to maintain output of clear to light yellow urine.
  - Water is an adequate replacement for activity lasting one hour or less. In prolonged activity, a sports drink may aid in maintenance of electrolyte balance.
  - Since children are less likely to adequately replenish fluid losses, they should have scheduled hydration breaks and be encouraged to drink.
  - Measurement of pre- and post-exercise body weight may guide fluid replacement.
    - Athletes should consume between 8–16 ounces of fluid for every pound lost during activity.
    - Athletes with persistent weight loss of 2 percent or greater should be held from activity.
- Clothing and equipment
  - Clothes should be loose fitting and light colored to allow convective heat loss and reduce absorption of solar radiation.
  - Helmets, protective pads, jerseys, gloves, and other garments impair dissipation of heat.
    - During heat acclimatization, protective equipment should be modified to allow heat loss and prevent hyperthermia.
    - The National Collegiate Athletic Association (NCAA) heat acclimatization regulations for American football gradually introduce protective padding over the course of five days.
    - NCAA regulations should serve as a minimal standard for acclimatization of athletes.[42]
- Acclimatization
  - Heat acclimatization results in increased minimal temperatures at which fatal EHS occurs.[3]
  - Enhanced fitness levels reduce prolonged, near-maximal exertion associated with EHS risk.
  - Heat cramps, heat syncope, and heat exhaustion all involve deficiencies in fluid-electrolyte balance, extracellular volume and tonicity, or cardiovascular adaptation.[9,13]
    - Sport-specific training in the heat reduces incidence of exertional heat illness via improved cardiovascular function and fluid-electrolyte homeostasis.[3]

Table 13.5 Exertional Heat Illness Do's and Don'ts

DO	DON'T
Check a rectal temperature in collapsed/ altered athletes	Rely on an external temperature
Initiate cooling of EHS as soon as possible	Allow transport or other interventions to delay cooling
Use cold or ice water immersion as the primary modality for cooling EHS	Overcool and cause hypothermia
Consider all causes of collapse in athletes, to include cardiac and metabolic causes	Be overly concerned about cardiac monitoring during the cooling phase of exertional heat stroke: priority one is rapid cooling
Encourage oral rehydration in mild to moderate cases of exertional heat illness	Allow athletes to return to play until fully recovered from heat illness, no matter how mild
Educate athletes, coaches, and parents on prevention and treatment of heat illness	Allow pressure from athletes, coaches, or parents to keep you from speaking up when conditions are unsafe or an athlete is at risk

Table 13.6 Key Diagnosis, History, Physical Exam Findings, and Treatment

Diagnosis	History	Physical Exam Findings	Treatment
Exertional heat stroke	Altered mental status, confusion, irritability or personality changes, nausea and vomiting, dizziness, fatigue, seizure, or coma	Core temperature ≥ 104°F (40°C)	Rapid cooling with ice water bath immersion May need laboratory evaluation and cool IV fluids Consider hospital admission (depending on severity of illness)
Heat exhaustion	Generalized weakness, headache, nausea and vomiting, diarrhea, dizziness, and irritability during or after exercise Normal mental status Usually recover quickly after period of rest	Tachycardia, tachypnea, hypotension Elevated core temperature, but < 104°F (40°C) Sweaty, clammy, and pale	Place in cool, shaded environment Remove athletic equipment and restrictive clothing Place in supine position with legs elevated Encourage oral rehydration Frequent monitoring
Heat cramps	Painful muscle contractions during or after exercise	Tight, contracting muscles	Massage and stretching of affected muscles Ice Oral salt solution Intravenous hydration only in recalcitrant cases
Heat syncope	Syncope after exercise Rapid recovery	Normal core temperature	Place patient in supine position with legs elevated Encourage oral rehydration
Exertional hyponatremia	Altered mental status, nausea and vomiting	Normal core temperature Low serum sodium (<130–135 mmol/L)	PO hypertonic solution, if able Fluid restriction Intravenous hypertonic solution, if needed

Recommended Readings

Armstrong LE, et al.. American College of Sports Medicine position stand: Exertional heat illness during training and competition. *Medicine and Science in Sports and Exercise* 2007 Mar; 39(3): 556–72.

Casa DJ, et al.. Exertional heat stroke: New concepts regarding cause and care. *Current Sports Medicine Reports* 2012 May–Jun; 11(3):115–23.

Howe AS, Boden BP. Heat-related illness in athletes. *American Journal of Sports Medicine* 2007 Aug; 35(8):1384–95.

References

1. Howe AS, Boden BP. Heat-related illness in athletes. *American Journal of Sports Medicine* 2007 Aug; 35(8):1384–95.
2. Carter R, et al.. Epidemiology of hospitalizations and deaths from heat illness in soldiers. *Medicine and Science in Sports and Exercise* 2005 Aug; 37 (8):1338–44.
3. Armstrong LE, et al.. American College of Sports Medicine position stand: Exertional heat illness during training and competition. *Medicine and Science in Sports and Exercise* 2007 Mar; 39(3): 556–72.
4. Casa DJ, et al.. Exertional heat stroke: New concepts regarding cause and care. *Current Sports Medicine Reports* 2012 May-Jun; 11(3):115–23.
5. Maron BJ, et al.. Sudden deaths in young, competitive athletes: Analysis of 1866 deaths in the United States, 1980–2006. *Circulation* 2009 March; 119 (8):1085–92.
6. Centers for Disease Control and Prevention. Heat-related deaths: United States, 1999–2003. *MMWR Morbidity and Mortality Weekly Report* 2006; 55(29):796–98.
7. Kerr ZY, et al.. Epidemiology of exertional heat illness among US high school athletes. *American Journal of Preventive Medicine* 2013 Jan; 44(1):8–14.
8. Cheung SS, McClellan TM. Heat acclimation, aerobic fitness, and hydration effects on tolerance during uncompensable heat stress. *Journal of Applied Physiology* 1998 May; 84: 1731–39.
9. Armstrong LE. Heat acclimatization. In Fahey TD (ed.), Encyclopedia of Sports Medicine and Science 1998 Internet Society for Sports Science. http://sportsci.org
10. Council on Sports Medicine and Fitness and Council on School Health. Climatic heat stress and exercising children and adolescents. *Pediatrics* 2011 August; 128(3):e741–47.
11. McLaren C, Null J, Quinn J. Heat stress from enclosed vehicles: Moderate ambient temperatures cause significant temperature rise in enclosed vehicles. *Pediatrics* 2005; 116: e109–112.
12. Pryor RR, et al.. Estimating core temperature with external devices after exertional heat stress in thermal protective clothing. *Prehospital Emergency Care* 2012; 16(1):136–41.
13. Coris EE, et al.. Gastrointestinal temperature trends in football linemen during physical exertion under heat stress. *Southern Medical Journal* 2009 Jun; 102(6):569–74.
14. Marom T, et al.. Acute care for exercise-induced hyperthermia to avoid adverse outcome from exertional heat stroke. *Journal of Sport Rehabilitation* 2011 May; 20(2):219–27.
15. Glazer JL. Management of heatstroke and heat exhaustion. *American Family Physician* 2005 June; 71(11):2133–40.
16. Druyan A, Janovich R, Heled Y. Misdiagnosis of exertional heat stroke and improper medical treatment. *Military Medicine* 2011 November; 176(11): 1278–80.
17. Sithinamsuwan P, et al.. Exertional heatstroke: Early recognition and outcome with aggressive combined cooling: a 12-year experience. *Military Medicine* 2009 May; 174(5):496–502.
18. Smith JE. Cooling methods used in the treatment of exertional heat illness. *British Journal of Sports Medicine* 2005 August; 39(8):503–7.
19. Wallace RF, et al.. Risk factors for recruit exertional heat illness by gender and training period. *Aviation, Space, and Environmental Medicine* 2006 April; 77(4):415–21.
20. Roberts WO. Exertional heat stroke during a cool weather marathon: A case study. *Medicine and Science in Sports and Exercise* 2006 July; 38 (7):1197–203.
21. Robertson B, Walter E. Cool runnings': Heat stroke in cool conditions. *Emergency Medicine Journal* 2010 May; 27(5):387–8.
22. Hostler D, et al.. Recognition and treatment of exertional heat illness at a marathon race. *Prehospital Emergency Care* 2014 Jan; 24: epub ahead of print.
23. Newport M, Grayson A. Towards evidence-based emergency medicine: Best BETs from the Manchester Royal Infirmary; BET 3: In patients with heatstroke is whole-body ice-water immersion the best cooling method? *Emergency Medical Journal* 2012 October; 29(10):855–6.
24. McDermott BP, et al.. Acute whole-body-cooling for exercise induced hyperthermia: A systematic review. *Journal of Athletic Training* 2009 January-February; 44(1):84–93.
25. Casa DJ, et al.. Cold water immersion: The gold standard for exertional heatstroke treatment.

Exercise and Sports Science Reviews 2007; 35(3):141–9.

26. Makranz C, Heled Y, Moran DS. Hypothermia following exertional heat stroke treatment. *European Journal of Applied Physiology* 2011 September; 111(9):2359–62.
27. Leon LR, Helwig BG. Heat stroke: Role of the systemic inflammatory response. *Journal of Applied Physiology* 2010 December; 109(6): 1980–1988.
28. Kazman JB, et al.. Exertional heat illness: The role of heat tolerance testing. *Current Sports Medicine Reports* 2013 March–April; 12(2):101–110.
29. Johnson EC, et al.. Specific exercise heat stress protocol for a triathlete's return from exertional heat stroke. *Current Sports Medicine Reports* 2013 March–April; 12 (2):106–109.
30. O'Connor FG, et al.. Guidelines for return to duty (play) after heat illness: A military perspective. *Journal of Sports Rehabilitation* 2007 August; 16(3):227-237.
31. Miller KC, et al.. Exercise-associated muscle cramps: Causes, treatment and prevention. *Sports Health* 2010 July; 2(4):279–283.
32. O'Connor RE. Exercise-induced hyponatremia: Causes, risks, prevention, and management. *Cleveland Clinic Journal of Medicine* 2006 September; 73 (Supplement 3):S13–18.
33. Beltrami FG, Hew-Butler T, Noakes TD. Drinking policies and exercise-associated hyponatremia: Is anyone still promoting overdrinking? *British Journal of Sports Medicine* 2008 October; 42 (10):796–501.
34. Rogers IR, Hew-Butler T. Exercise-associated hyponatremia: Overzealous fluid consumption. *Wilderness & Environmental Medicine* 2009 Summer; 20(2):139–143.
35. Wharam PC, et al.. NSAID use increases the risk of developing hyponatremia during an Ironman triathlon. *Medicine and Science in Sports and Exercise* 2006 April; 38(4):618–22.
36. Rosner MH. Exercise-associated hyponatremia. *Seminars in Nephrology* 2009 May; 29 (3):271–281.
37. Bennett BL, et al.. Wilderness Medical Society practice guidelines for treatment of exercise-associated hyponatremia. *Wilderness & Environmental Medicine* 2013 September; 24(3):228–40.
38. Hew-Butler T, et al.. Consensus statement of the Second International Exercise-Associated Hyponatremia Consensus Development Conference, New Zealand 2007. *Clinical Journal of Sports Medicine* 2008 April; 18(2):111–121.
39. Elsaesser TF, et al.. Large-volume hypertonic saline therapy in endurance athlete with exercise-associated hyponatremic encephalopathy. *Journal of Emergency Medicine* 2013 June; 44 (6):1132–1135.
40. Hoffman MD, et al.. Exercise-associated hyponatremia with exertional rhabdomyolysis: Importance of proper treatment. *Clinical Nephrology* 2014 June; 16: epub ahead of print.
41. National Weather Service Weather Forecast Office. WetBulb Globe Temperature. www.srh.noaa.gov/tsa/?n=wbgt
42. Exertional Heat Stroke. Korey Stringer Institute. http://ksi.uconn.edu

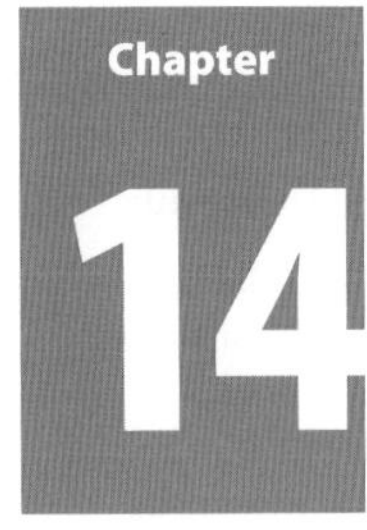

Basic Principles of Splinting in the Emergency Department

Anna L. Waterbrook
Illustrations by Yvonne Chow

Introduction

- Splints are generally used as a temporary method of immobilization.
- Indications for splinting include fractures, dislocations, sprains, tendon and ligament partial or complete disruptions, joint infections, tenosynovitis, and lacerations.
- Equipment needed includes:
  - Padding
  - Plaster or fiberglass
  - Bucket + water
  - ACE wrap
  - Scissors or trauma sheers
  - Gloves

Splint Application

- Tips for application of the splint include:
  - Make sure to always use two to three layers of padding prior to placement of the splint.
    - Be sure to add extra layers of padding over bony prominences such as elbows and ankles, between digits and at each end of the splint border.
    - Avoid wrinkles.
    - Do not tighten as it can cause ischemia.
  - May use plaster or fiberglass material to make a splint.
    - Plaster should be used anytime that it is essential to help maintain stability of the bone or joint, that is, after any reduction is performed or for any potentially unstable fracture.
      - Generally, eight to ten layers of plaster are needed for upper extremity splints, and twelve to fifteen layers of plaster are needed for lower extremity splints.
        - As plaster dries it creates an exothermic reaction.
        - The more layers used increases the risk of burns.
      - Plaster may take up to twenty-four hours to fully cure.
    - Fiberglass is easier to use and more breathable, but is less moldable and therefore does not offer as much stability as a plaster splint.
      - Cures in approximately 20 minutes.
      - Increased risk of burns due to faster setting time.
      - Lighter weight
      - More radiolucent.
      - Fiberglass often comes readymade with one layer of padding, however it is still essential to use extra padding prior to placement of the splint.
    - If possible, include joints above and below the fracture or dislocation in the splint.
    - In general, splint in the position of function.
    - Always assess and document neurovascular status before and after application of a splint.

Complications

- Complications include:
  - Burns
    - Increased risk with increasing layers of plaster.
  - Ischemia
    - Less likely than with a cast.
    - When in doubt, take off the splint if there is ANY concern for ischemia.

Table 14.1. Common Immobilization Techniques and Associated Common Clinical Indications

Common Immobilization Techniques	Common Clinical Indications
Upper Extremity	
Sling	• Shoulder dislocation • Clavicle fracture • Acromioclavicular separation • Shoulder sprains, strains and other causes of shoulder discomfort, or for mechanical support if splinting the upper extremity
Sling and Swath	• Rarely used but may be used for same indications as a sling if extra immobilization is needed
Cuff and Collar	• Proximal humerus fracture
Burkhalter (Figure 14.1)	• Metacarpal fracture and proximal phalanx fracture
Radial Gutter (Figure 14.2)	• Second and third metacarpals, proximal and middle phalanx fracture
Ulnar Gutter (Figure 14.3)	• Fourth and fifth metacarpals, proximal and middle phalanx fracture, hamate or pisiform fracture
Volar Wrist (Figure 14.4)	• Soft-tissue injuries, sprains/strains and stable fractures of the wrist • Carpal tunnel syndrome
Thumb Spica (Figure 14.5)	• Scaphoid fracture • Thumb metacarpal or proximal phalanx fracture or dislocation
Posterior Long Arm (Figure 14.6)	• Stable elbow and forearm injuries
Proximal Sugar-Tong	• Humeral fractures
Forearm Sugar-Tong (Figure 14.7)	• Wrist and distal forearm fractures
Double Sugar-tong (Figure 14.8)	• Elbow and forearm fractures
Lower Extremity	
Knee Immobilizer	• Patella fracture • Patella dislocation or subluxation • Knee dislocation after reduction • Unstable ligament injury • Tibial plateau fracture
Posterior Long Leg (Figure 14.9)	• Used in place of knee immobilizer if unavailable or if extremity is too large to fit in an immobilizer • Temporary immobilization of femur, knee, or tibia and fibula shaft fractures requiring immediate orthopedic evaluation or surgery
Posterior Short Leg (Figures 14.10A and B)	• Distal leg, ankle, tarsal, and metatarsal fractures • Reduced dislocations • Severe sprains
Ankle Stirrup (Figure 14.11)	• Used in combination with the posterior short leg splint (Figures 14.12A and B) for added stability to prevent inversion and eversion of the ankle • Ankle sprains, fractures and dislocations
Short-Leg Walking Boot	• May be used in place of short-leg splint anytime weight-bearing is allowed. • Stable ankle or foot fractures • Severe sprains • Achilles tendon rupture with a heel lift
Hard-Sole Shoe	• Sprains, strains, or contusions • Stable toe fractures • Stable metatarsal fractures

- Advise the patient to ice and elevate the extremity to decrease swelling and risk of ischemia.

- Pressure sores
  - Avoid wrinkles.
  - Make sure there is plenty of padding, especially over bony prominences.

- Infection
  - Ensure there is no open fracture prior to placement of any splint.
  - Clean and dress all wounds prior to placement of the splint.
  - If a high-risk wound is present, consider cutting out a window in splinting material to perform dressing changes and monitor wound.
  - Prophylactic antibiotics are controversial.

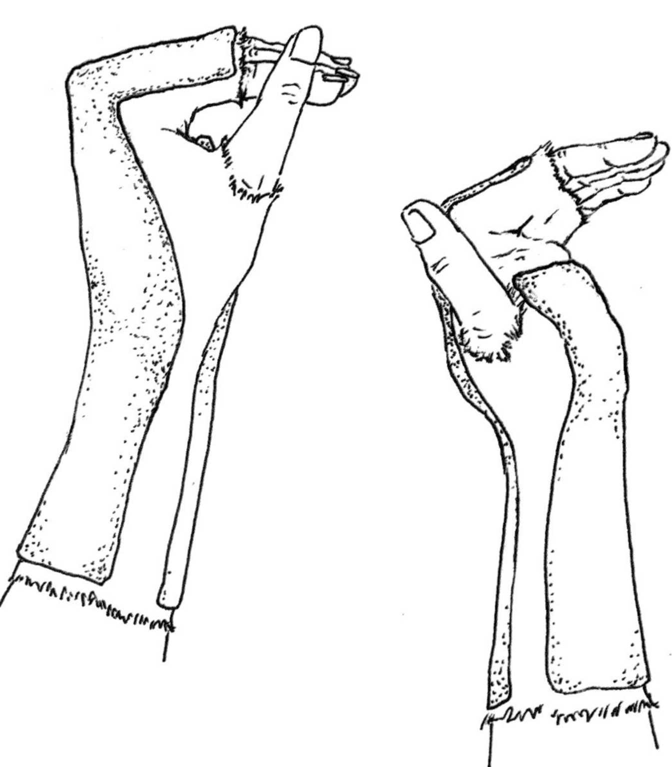

Figure 14.1. Burkhalter splint.

Upper Extremity Splints

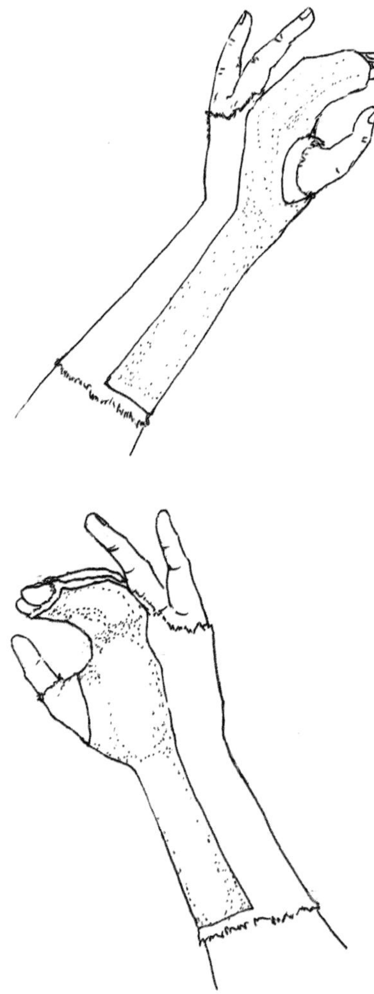

Figure 14.2. Radial gutter splint.

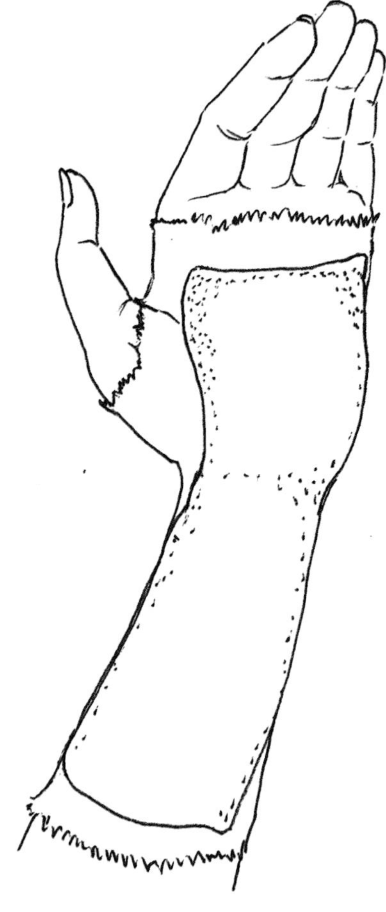

Figure 14.4. Volar wrist splint.

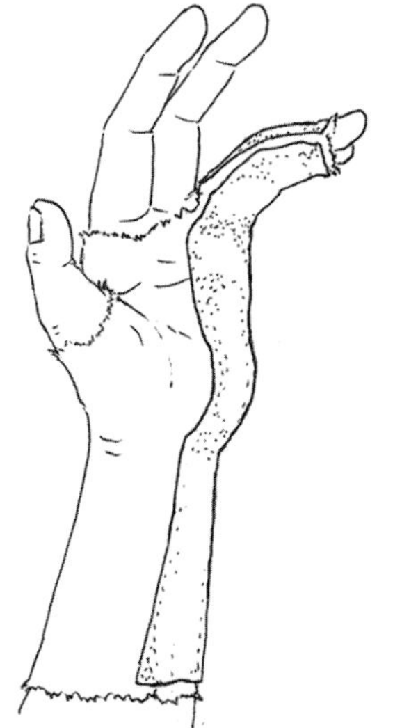

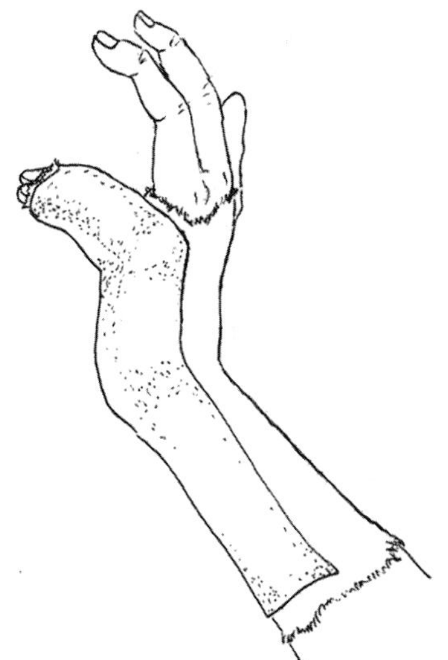

Figure 14.3. Ulnar gutter splint.

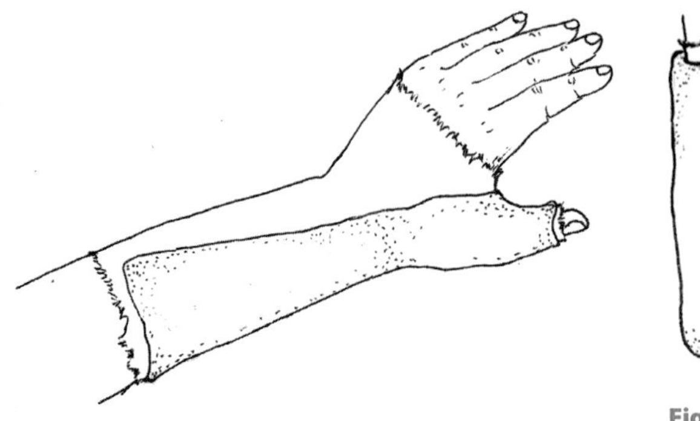

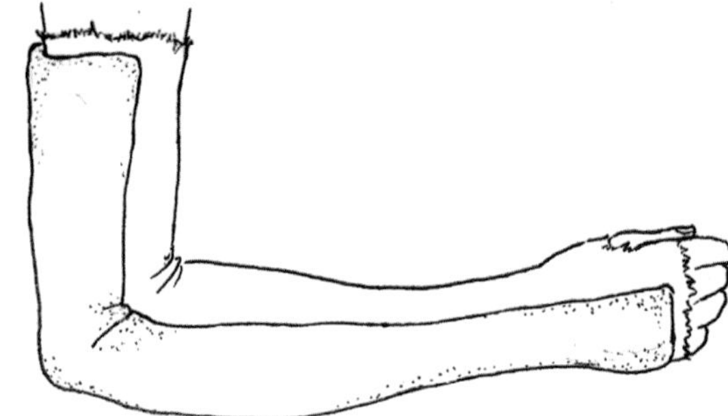

Figure 14.6. Posterior long arm splint.

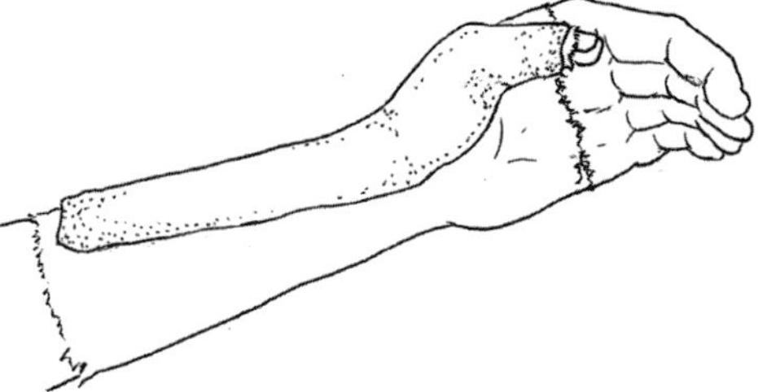

Figure 14.5. Thumb spica splint.

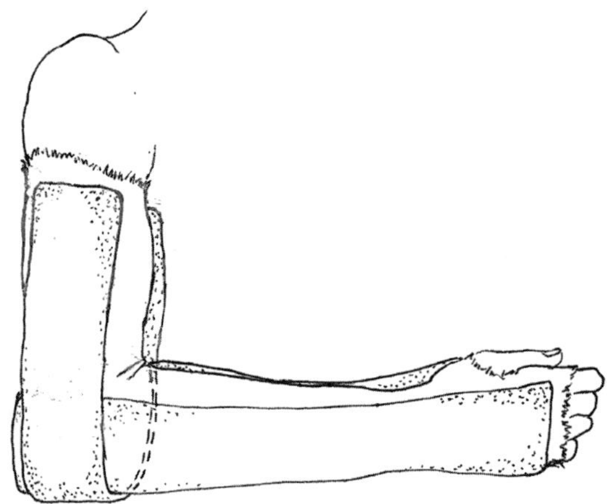

Figure 14.8. Double sugar-tong splint.

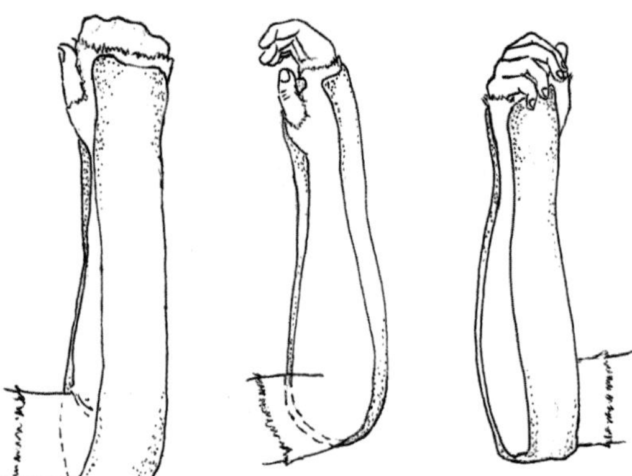

Figure 14.7. Forearm sugar-tong splint.

Lower Extremity Splints

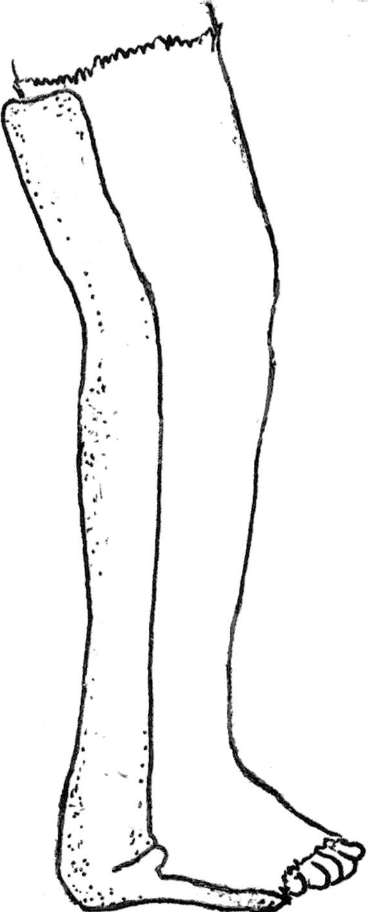

Figure 14.9. Posterior long leg splint.

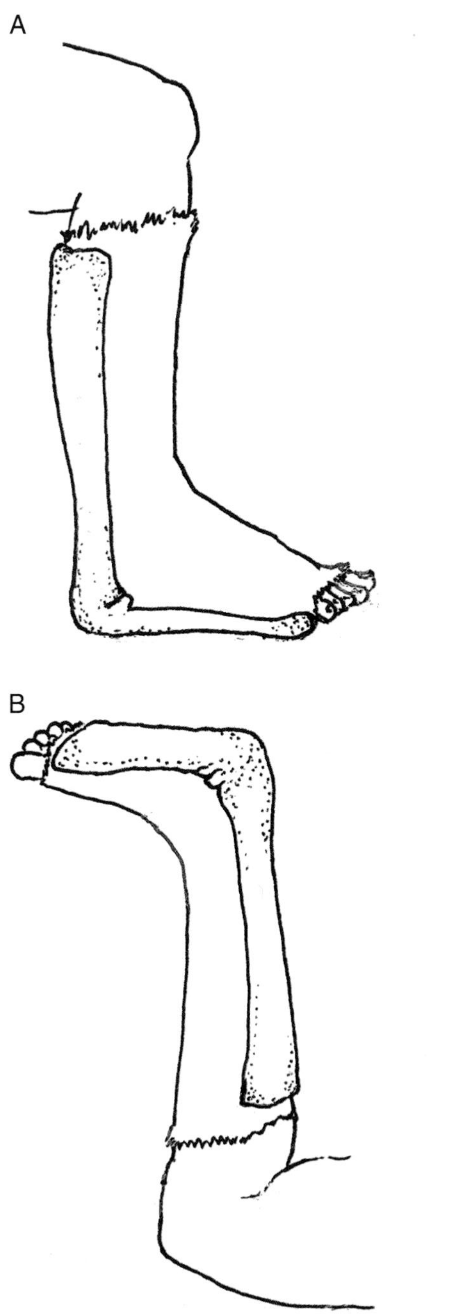

Figures 14.10A and B. A) Posterior short leg splint and B) Posterior short leg splint (prone).

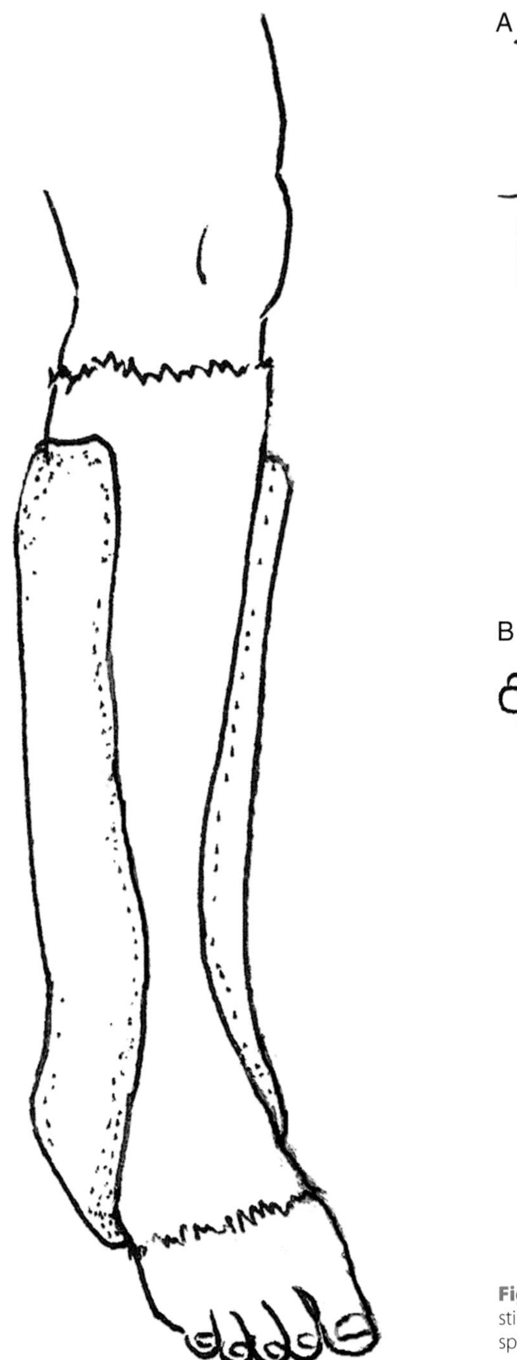

Figure 14.11. Ankle stirrup splint.

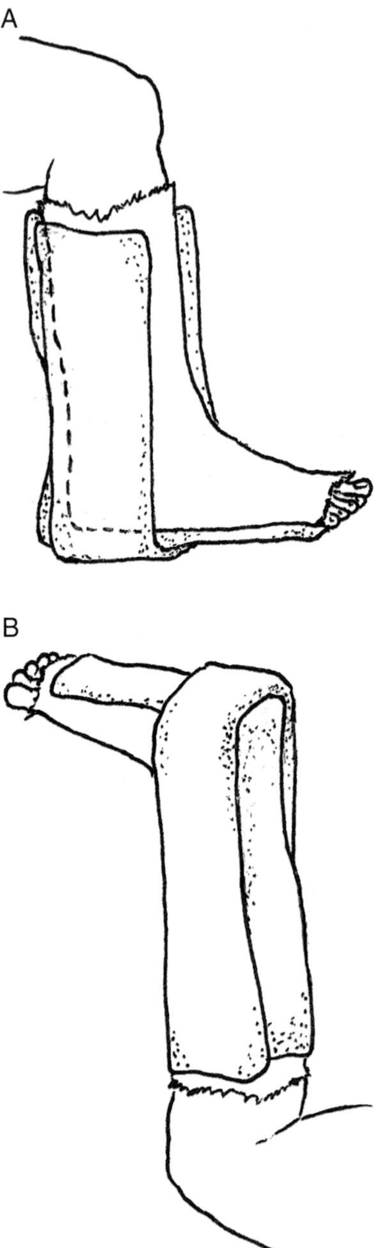

Figures 14.12A and B. A) Posterior short leg with ankle stirrup splint and B) Posterior short leg with ankle stirrup splint (prone).

Recommended reading

Roberts JR, Custalow CB, Thomsen TW, et al. , eds. *Roberts and Hedges' Clinical Procedures in Emergency Medicine, 6th edition*; Elsevier Saunders; Philadelphia; 2014.

Seidenberg PH, Beutler AI, eds. *The Sports Medicine Resource Manual*; Saunders Elsevier; Philadelphia; 2008.

Tintinalli J, Stapczynski J, Ma OJ, et al., eds. *Tintinalli's Emergency Medicine: A Comprehensive Study Guide, 7th edition*; McGraw Hill Medical; New York; 2011.

Index